A————
Consumer's
Dictionary
of
Food
Additives

D0172282

ALSO BY RUTH WINTER

A Consumer's Dictionary of Cosmetic Ingredients

Vitamin E

The Anti-Aging Hormones

Super Soy

A Consumer's Dictionary to Medicines in Food

A Consumer's Dictionary of Medicines: Prescription, Over-the-Counter, Homeopathic, and Herbal

A Consumer's Dictionary of Household, Yard, and Office Chemicals

Poisons in Your Food

Ageless Aging

Cancer-Causing Agents

Beware of the Food You Eat

A
Consumer's
Dictionary
of
Food
Additives

FIFTH EDITION

Ruth Winter, M.S.

Three Rivers Press
New York

To my husband, Arthur Winter, M.D., my daughter, Robin Winter-Sperry, M.D., my sons, Craig and Grant, and my grandchildren, Samantha, Hunter, and Katelynd.

Published by Three Rivers Press, 201 East 50th Street, New York, New York 10022. Member of the Crown Publishing Group.

Random House, Inc. New York, Toronto, London, Sydney, Auckland
www.randomhouse.com

THREE RIVERS PRESS is a trademark of Random House, Inc.

Printed in the United States of America

Library of Congress Cataloging-in-Publication Data

Winter, Ruth, 1930– .
    A consumer's dictionary of food additives / Ruth Winter.—
5th ed.
        p.   cm.
    Includes bibliographical references (p. 481).
    1. Food additives—Dictionaries.   I. Title.
TX553.A3W55   1999
664′.06′03—dc21   98-31668
                                                              CIP

ISBN 0-609-80366-2

10 9 8 7 6 5 4 3 2 1

Fifth Edition

CONTENTS

A
Consumer's
Dictionary
of
Food
Additives

WHY YOU NEED THIS BOOK

What additives—direct and indirect—are in your foods? Who's not only watching the store but the ports of entry? Although we do have an alphabet soup of agencies—the FDA (Food and Drug Administration), USDA (U.S. Department of Agriculture), EPA (Environmental Protection Agency), and CDC (Centers for Disease Control)—with dedicated agents trying their best to do a good job, they are understaffed, underfinanced, and without the sophisticated technology to completely check the additives and undesirable contaminants that may be hidden in raw and processed products.

Michael Friedman, M.D., deputy commissioner for operations at the FDA, admitted before a congressional committee: "Given the current constraints on government resources, it is unlikely the FDA will ever have sufficient resources to inspect, sample, and analyze more than a small percentage of all food products, domestic, as well as imported."[1]

The FDA budget has been cut so that inspections of domestic food supplies have fallen from 21,000 in 1981 to just 5,000 last year. The FDA inspects an FDA-regulated plant on average only once every ten years.[2] At the same time, foreign food imports have doubled to 2.2 million shipments a year while FDA border inspections have been cut in half and only 2 percent of imported foods are sampled for contamination at the docks.[3]

The FDA's Dr. Friedman has said: "The current system of regulatory controls is reactive, not preventive. That is, the system generally relies on detecting and correcting problems after they occur rather than preventing them in the first place."[4]

He went on to say that it is the FDA's goal to use the agency's resources in the most effective way to minimize consumer exposure to unsafe products. This includes steps the agency has taken to "reduce the number of regulations and environmental assessments." What has been the result of such efforts?

- Lax enforcement of the Delaney Amendment that mandated no cancer-causing additive could be added to food.

- The determination that a food additive is "generally recognized as safe" (GRAS) left up to the manufacturer.

- The presence of some unidentified additives listed as "natural" flavorings or colorings—a potentially dangerous situation for a number of allergic citizens.

- The inability to control the residues of more than ninety antibiotics in meat, poultry, and vegetable crops that may be contributing to the increasingly alarming antibiotic-resistant bacteria.

---

[1]Michael Friedman, deputy commissioner for operations, FDA, testifying before the Subcommittee on Human Resources and Intergovernmental Relations: Committee on Government Reform and Oversight, May 10, 1996, Washington, D.C.
[2]"Food Safety from Farm to Table: A National Food Safety Initiative," report to the President, May 1997.
[3]President Bill Clinton, speech, October 2, 1997, Washington, D.C.
[4]Friedman, op. cit.

- Eighty percent of U.S. livestock and poultry are treated with animal drugs (*see* Appendix C).

- The continued use of nearly one hundred pesticides, many of which are known cancer-causing agents, on food crops and on animals (*see* Appendix D).

For all the FDA's best intentions, you must be the primary gatekeeper to protect your family's health by being a conscientious and informed consumer.

This fifth edition of *A Consumer's Dictionary of Food Additives* contains many more listings of food additives with more information about them than any other reference. The information has been gathered from multiple sources, including the World Health Organization, government reports, and scientific and trade organizations. This new edition of the book describes what is known so far about some of those new and proposed additives such as CF-3 (Prempt) a blend of twenty-nine beneficial microbes found in the gastrointestinal tract of mature, healthy chickens that can reduce salmonella colonization that causes human illness and bovine somatotropin (BST), a protein produced by the pituitary gland of cattle given to cows to make them produce more milk.

With this book, you will be better able to:

- Evaluate foods
- Read labels
- Identify nutritious foods
- Understand what labels do not reveal
- Avoid salt
- Avoid hidden sugars
- Avoid allergens
- Plan your diet to avoid certain additives
- Find foods abundant in desirable ingredients

When it comes to food additives we must first ask ourselves and our government if these chemicals are added for our benefit or just for the food producer's economic gain. Then we must inform ourselves, take responsibility for urging our legislators to increase funding, personnel, and methodology to protect us, and above all, we must make informed choices about what we purchase for our tables. Some food additives are highly beneficial. Many are absolutely unnecessary and some are known to cause cancer or nerve damage. This dictionary can be used to help you find those additives in the first category—those that are harmless and sometimes beneficial.

Reading Labels

The first place to begin is with the food label. It's more important than ever that you read and understand it so that you have enough knowledge to make informed choices. This book tells you about where additives come from, how they are used, and what is known about how they may affect your health.

LABELING

A food label is a contract between the manufacturer and us. Like most contracts, it may be difficult to understand, and what is not included may be as important as what is. The government estimates that over the next twenty years, labels will reduce national health care costs substantially by making it easier for the public to choose more healthful diets.

Newer regulations give more realistic serving sizes (*see* page 11). Instead of a food manufacturer presenting a low calorie or fat count for half a teaspoonful they give the count for a half a cup—the realistic serving size.

The FDA and USDA previously established a standard of identity for about three hundred foods, such as peanut butter, mayonnaise, and fruit cocktails, fixing the ingredients by law (*see* page 389). Many of these foods were exempted from the need to list ingredients. Labeling now requires full ingredient listing for all foods including those with standards of identity. It also allows manufacturers for the first time to produce healthier versions of some products and still use the recognized name. For instance, a reduced fat ice cream does not have to be called "imitation" or "ice milk" but can be called "low fat ice cream."

Nutrients, such as folic acid and calcium, are the chemical substances found in food that can be used and are necessary for your health. There are more than forty nutrients, including minerals, vitamins, and the amino acids from proteins.

Additives are substances or mixture of substances other than basic foodstuffs present in food as a result of any aspect of production, processing, storage, or packaging. BHT and BHA are examples of preservatives and Red No. 3 is an example of a coloring. Some substances—vitamins E and C, for example—are both nutrients and additives. The two vitamins are sometimes added for their ability to retard rancidity.

Can you decipher the chemicals on the label? How do you know which ones are good, bad, or unnecessary? You can look them up in this dictionary. For example, there is a list of those ingredients Generally Recognized As Safe (GRAS). Are they really safe?

Generally Recognized as Safe (GRAS) List

Congress established the GRAS list in 1958. Those substances that had been added to food over a long time, which under the conditions of their intended use were generally recognized as safe by qualified scientists, would be exempt from premarket clearance. At that point, Congress had acted on a very marginal response—on the basis of returns from those scientists sent questionnaires. Approximately 355 out of 900 responded, and only about 100 of those responses had substantive comments. Three items were removed from the originally published list.

In recent years, developments in the scientific fields and in consumer awareness brought to light the inadequacies in food additive testing. The difficulties in listing some additives as GRAS without adequate testing have also been illuminated. For example, cyclamates, the artificial sweeteners, were shown to be cancer-causing agents in laboratory animals and were removed from the market. They had been on the GRAS list. As a result of these inadequacies in 1969 President Richard M. Nixon directed the FDA to reevaluate all of the items on the GRAS list.

By 1980, 415 substances that had been in use prior to the 1958 Food Additives Amendment to the Food, Drug and Cosmetic Act were reviewed. The committee's evaluations were based on a review of medical and scientific literature and unpublished reports. In some cases the research extended back sixty years. The number of references obtained for a given GRAS substance ranged from twenty-three reports for carnauba wax to two thousand for vitamin A.

Food ingredients whose use is determined GRAS by qualified experts have not been required by law to receive FDA approval before marketing. Until 1997, however, a manufacturer who wanted FDA affirmation that a food additive was GRAS had to submit a formal petition to FDA. In 1997, the FDA wanted to simplify GRAS notification and save personnel time and money. The agency said that manufacturers can make a self-determined GRAS declaration claiming exemption from the premarket approval requirement for food additives. However, instead of petitioning FDA for affirmation, they simply notify FDA of their GRAS determination for a substance and provide some evidence that supports the claim. The manufacturers' notification then serves as a basis for informing FDA without the need for a lot of paperwork. The FDA says that letting the manufacturer determine what is generally recognized as safe and making it simpler to obtain FDA approval will allow the FDA to "gain increased awareness of ingredients in the nation's food supply and the cumulative dietary exposure to GRAS substances."

Then, in the late 1990s, the federal government enfeebled the generally-recognized-as-safe category. GRAS food ingredients were no longer required by law to receive FDA approval before marketing nor required to go through evaluation by FDA appointed experts. Under former procedures, a manufacturer determined that a food substance was GRAS without a formal petition to FDA. But if FDA affirmation was wanted as of its additive's GRAS, the company had to submit a petition and go through a rule-making process. The agency proposed in 1997 that instead of petitioning FDA for affirmation, manufacturers could simply notify the FDA of their additive's GRAS status and provide some evidence to support it. The FDA says that letting the manufacturer determine what is generally recognized as safe and making it simpler to obtain FDA approval will allow the FDA to "gain increased awareness of ingredients in the nation's food supply and the cumulative dietary exposure to GRAS substances."

Despite this backtracking, most of the ingredients that appear on the GRAS list are safe, and some are even desirable. Those entries that have been generally recognized as safe have the designation GRAS at the end of their listing in the dictionary.

Identifying Nutritious Foods

The goal of this dictionary is not only to help you find foods that used safe ingredients but to find nutritious foods that will aid your own family's health. Again the label is a key tool for locating and evaluating the nutritional content of foods. The nutritional chart required on almost every foodstuff since the middle of the 1990s provides valuable information, but it can be somewhat confusing. Following are explanations that will make it clearer and more useful for you.

Daily Reference Values (DRVs)

Daily Values (DV) comprise two sets of references for nutrients:

1. Daily Reference Values (DRVs)
2. Reference Daily Intakes (RDIs).

These designations are for nutrients for which no set of standards previously existed, such as fat, cholesterol, carbohydrates, proteins, and fibers. DRVs for these energy-producing nutrients are based on the number of calories consumed per day. For labeling purposes, two thousand calories has been established for calculations. This level was chosen, in part, because many health experts say it approximates the maintenance calorie requirements of the group most often targeted for weight reduction: postmenopausal women.

DRVs for the energy-producing nutrients are calculated as follows:

- Fat based on 30 percent of calories
- Saturated fat based on 10 percent of calories
- Carbohydrates based on 60 percent of calories
- Protein based on 10 percent of calories
- Fiber based on 11.5 grams of fiber per 1,000 calories

The DRVs for cholesterol, sodium, and potassium, which do not contribute calories, remain the same no matter what the calorie level.

Because of the links between certain nutrients and specific diseases, DRVs for some nutrients represent the uppermost limit considered desirable. Eating too much fat or cholesterol, for example, has been linked to heart disease and too much sodium to the risk of high blood pressure. Therefore, the label shows you a product has less than the *uppermost limits* of DRVs for fats, cholesterol, and sodium which are:

- Total fat: less than 65 g
- Saturated fat: less than 20 g

- Cholesterol: less than 300 mg
- Sodium: less than 2,400 mg

Reference Daily Intakes (RDIs)

RDIs are a set of dietary references based on and replacing the recommended dietary allowances (RDAs, *see* Appendix E) for essential vitamins and minerals and, in selected groups, protein. You will continue to see vitamins and minerals expressed as percentages on the label, but these figures now refer to the daily values.

Here are the RDIs—once familiar to us as RDAs:

Nutrient	Amount
vitamin A	5,000 International Units (IU)
vitamin C	60 milligrams (mg)
thiamin	1.5 mg
riboflavin	1.7 mg
niacin	20 mg
calcium	1.0 gram (g)
iron	18 mg
vitamin D	400 IU
vitamin E	30 IU
vitamin B_6	2.0 mg
folic acid	0.4 mg
vitamin B_{12}	6 micrograms (mcg)
phosphorus	1.0 g
iodine	150 mcg
magnesium	400 mg
zinc	15 mg
copper	2 mg
biotin	0.3 mg
pantothenic acid	10 mg

The mandatory and voluntary dietary components on the label and order in which they must appear are:

- total calories
- calories from fat
- calories from saturated fat
- total saturated fat

- stearic acid (on meat and poultry products only)
- polyunsaturated fat
- monounsaturated fats
- cholesterol
- sodium
- potassium
- total carbohydrates
- dietary fiber
- soluble fiber
- insoluble fiber
- sugars
- sugar alcohol (for example, the sugar substitutes xylitol, mannitol, and sorbitol)
- other carbohydrates (the difference between total carbohydrate and the sum of dietary fiber, sugars, and sugar alcohol, if declared)
- protein
- vitamin A
- percent of vitamin A present as beta-carotene
- vitamin C
- calcium
- iron
- other essential vitamins and minerals

If a food is fortified or enriched with any of the optional components, or a claim is made about any of them, pertinent additional nutrition information becomes mandatory. These mandatory and voluntary components are the only ones allowed on the nutrition panel.

Tip: When a caloric value for a serving of food is less than 5 calories, the FDA allows the label to read "zero" calories. If a fat calorie is less than 0.5 grams, it can be listed as "calories from fat zero."

No Nutrition Information

Some foods are exempt from nutrition labeling. Due to space limitations, small packages, such as a candy bar, do *not* have to provide nutrition information on the label. However, the address or telephone number must be provided for shoppers who wish to obtain this material. It is important for consumers to realize that products produced and sold in the same state or that do not have ingredients that move interstate are not subject to FDA regulations.

Other foods that do not have to provide nutrition labeling include:

- Food produced by small businesses. The FDA defines a small business as one with food sales of less than $50,000 a year or total sales of less than $500,000. The U.S. Department of Agriculture Food Safety and Inspection Service (FSIS) defines a small business as one employing five hundred or fewer employees and producing no more than a certain amount of product per year.

- Food served for immediate consumption, such as that served in restaurants and hospital cafeterias, on airplanes, and by food service vendors (such as mall cookie counters, sidewalk vendors, and vending machines).

- Ready-to-eat foods that are not for immediate consumption, as long as the food is primarily prepared on-site—for example, many bakery, deli, and candy-store items.

- Food shipped in bulk, as long as it is not for sale in that form to consumers.

- Medical foods.

- Plain coffee and tea, flavor extracts, food colors, some spices, and other foods that contain no significant amounts of any nutrients.

- Donated foods.

- Products intended for export.

- Individually wrapped FSIS-regulated products weighing less than half an ounce and making no nutrient content claims.

Although these foods are exempt, they are free to carry nutrition information when appropriate as long as it complies with the new regulations.

A great controversy occurred concerning the labeling of bioengineered foods such as the "Flavr Savr" tomato and milk produced with bovine somatotropin (BST) *(see)*. The FDA has said that there is no need to identify genetically engineered foods on the label, and in fact has warned dairy food producers against saying that *no* BST was used in their products.[5]

Besides the label panel giving specific information about the nutritional value (or lack thereof) of foods, there are other terms that indicate nutritional value:

- *Food grade.* The USDA has established grades for more than three hundred food products. Grading for most products is done voluntarily at the manufacturer's request (and expense) by a USDA inspector, and a USDA grade symbol may then appear on the package; lack of a symbol does not mean substandard product. Unfortunately, these grades lack continuity among product categories (Grade AA is the highest grade for eggs; Grade A is the highest for milk). Meat and poultry, however, whether fresh or processed and packaged, must be inspected and carry an inspection stamp.

---

[5] Keith Schneider, "FDA Warns the Dairy Industry Not to Label Milk Hormone-Free," *New York Times,* February 8, 1994, p. 1.

- *Low calorie* . . . fewer than 40 calories per serving.

- *Low sodium* . . . 140 mg or less preserving.

- *Very low sodium* . . . less than 35 mg per serving.

- *Sodium free* . . . less than 5 mg per serving.

- *Low fat* . . . 3 g or less per serving.

- *Low saturated fat* . . . means 1 g or less per serving.

- *Low cholesterol* . . . signifies 20 mg or less per serving.

- *High* or *source of* . . . denotes the beneficial presence of a nutrient, such as fiber or vitamins.

- *High* or *excellent source of* . . . contains 20 percent or more of the daily value *(see)* for a particular nutrient in a serving.

- *Good source of* . . . supplies 10 to 19 percent of the daily value for a particular nutrient.

- *Reduced* . . . means a product has been nutritionally altered and contains at least 25 percent less of a nutrient (such as fat) or 25 percent fewer calories than the regular product.

- *Less* . . . means a product contains 25 percent less of a nutrient or 25 percent fewer calories than the reference food. For example, pretzels that have 25 percent less fat than potato chips could carry a "less" claim.

- *Light* or *lite* . . . signifies a product contains one-third fewer calories or one-half the fat of the comparison food. "Light in sodium" may be used on food in which the sodium content has been reduced by at least 50 percent.

- *More* . . . means a product contains at least 10 percent more of the daily value for a desirable nutrient, such as fiber, than the regular food.

- *Fresh* . . . signifies a food that has not been heat processed or frozen and contains no preservatives.

- *Lean* and *extra lean* . . . describe the fat content of meats, poultry, seafood, and game meats. *Lean* = fewer than 10 g fat per serving. *Extra lean* = fewer than 5 g fat per serving.

- *Percent fat free* . . . is used only to describe foods that qualify as low fat.

- *High potency* . . . describes a nutrient in a food that is 100 percent or more of the RDI *(see)* established for that product. The term may also be used with multiingredient products if two-thirds of the nutrients are present at 100 percent of the RDI.

- *Antioxidant* . . . may be used in conjunction with currently defined claims for "good source of" and "high" to describe a nutrient scientifically shown to be absorbed in a sufficient quantity such as vitamin E to inactivate free radicals *(see* in dictionary) or prevent free radical-initiated chemical reactions in the food.

Natural or Organic

The demand for *natural* or *organic* products has increased by 20 percent each year since 1990. With the expansion of the market, thirty-five different certifying private organizations tried to offer definitions of this category of food. Food labels appeared on many products claiming that a product is "natural" and contains "no preservatives or MSG," but they had no legal meaning. The very same product might be next to it on the shelf, make no health claims, also contain no preservatives or MSG, and be a fraction of the price.[6] To clear up the confusion, Congress passed the Organic Foods Production Act in 1990 to standardize the terms and practices for organic farming. The guidelines set were:

- Livestock could be fed 20 percent nonorganic feed, yet still be labeled organic.
- Genetically engineered organisms could be allowed.
- Irradiated foods were not prohibited.

These guidelines did not go over well with true believers in organic or natural foods, especially since municipal sludge containing heavy metals and other toxic wastes could be used as organic compost and rules about animal confinement and the use of antibiotics were lax. Furthermore, farmers could only use the word *organic* on the label and could not advertise that their animals were antibiotic-free or that their plants were not genetically engineered.

Who Checks the Nutritional Analysis of a Product?

The author, being on a low-salt diet, has often wondered who checks the analysis of a product for the amount of sodium or any other ingredient. The FDA does not approve, and is not in a position to endorse or recommend, specific laboratories. The FDA tells food processors: "Assistance may be available through the following sources: trade and professional associations, trade publications, colleges and universities, and by looking in local phone books under testing or analytical laboratories. For compliance purposes, FDA uses appropriate methods published by the Association of Analytical Chemists in *Official Methods of Analysis of the AOAC International.*

When researchers at Columbia University in New York City checked the calorie content of packaged foods, they found the actual calories as much as three-and-one-half times higher than the labels indicated. The blatant underestimations occurred with regionally sold foods rather than with national brands.[7]

---

[6]Laura Loro, "Sales Blood for Natural Foods," *Advertising Age,* November 8, 1993. p. 39.
[7]Roger Field, "Calorie Counts on Food Labels Can Be Misleading," *Medical Tribune,* October 21, 1993, p 3.

What Counts as a Serving?

One of the problems that occurs with the amount of ingredients listed on a label is not knowing what consists of a serving. For instance, a low-sodium soy sauce may appear to be lower in sodium than another, but when you check the bottles, the serving size of the first is smaller, accounting for the decrease in sodium. The second may actually contain less salt although the serving size is larger. So you have to check the serving size as well as the ingredients. The following are common serving sizes:

GRAIN PRODUCTS GROUP (BREAD, CEREAL, RICE, AND PASTA)

1 slice of bread

1 ounce of ready-to-eat cereal

½ cup of cooked cereal, rice, or pasta

VEGETABLE GROUP

1 cup of raw leafy vegetables

½ cup of other vegetables, cooked or chopped raw

¾ cup of vegetable juice

FRUIT GROUP

1 medium apple, banana, orange

½ cup of chopped, cooked, or canned fruit

¾ cup of fruit juice

MILK GROUP (MILK, YOGURT, AND CHEESE)

1 cup of milk or yogurt

1–1½ ounces of natural cheese

2 ounces of processed cheese

MEAT AND BEANS GROUP (MEAT, POULTRY, FISH, DRY BEANS, EGGS, AND NUTS)

2–3 ounces of cooked lean meat, poultry, or fish

½ cup of cooked dry beans

1 egg

2 tablespoons of peanut butter

⅓ cup of nuts

Some foods fit into more than one group. Dry beans, peas, and lentils can be counted as servings in either the meat and beans group or vegetable group. These "crossover" foods can be counted as servings from either one or the other group, but not both. Serving sizes indicated here are suggested for adequate nutrient intake.

Understanding What Labels Don't Have to Say

Despite the fact that labels are the first place you as a consumer will turn to to understand what you are eating, do not forget that there is some information manufacturers are not required to list. To help you be a savvier label reader, one who can read between the lines, this book again will help you.

Terms on packages may be misleading. For example, "unsalted," "processed without salt," or "no salt added" may signify that the producer didn't *add* salt in during processing, but the food may still be naturally high in sodium. For example, a low-sodium soy sauce has 390 mg of sodium per teaspoon (and who can use only a teaspoon of soy sauce on a dish?) and a popular tomato-vegetable drink with "no salt added" has 90 mg per 4.5 fluid ounces. Salt can also be listed under dozens of "sodium" designations, such as monosodium glutamate and sodium caseinate, adding additional salt to your diet.

Sugar labeling, like salt, can be deceptive. A food can be labeled "sugar free" or "sugar-less" and still contain calories from sugar alcohols such as xylitol, sorbitol, and mannitol.

Label Health Claims

How realistic are the health claims made on label? The FDA lists the following criteria to determine the "propriety of the health-related claims and information": The health message or claims made on food labels must be truthful and not misleading to consumers, and they "should not imply that a particular food (can) be used as part of a druglike treatment or therapy-oriented approach to health care." Further, the information "must not overemphasize or distort the role of a food" in promoting good health.

Claims linking a nutrient or a food to the risk of a disease or health-related condition are allowed only under certain circumstances on FDA-regulated products. The FDA permits statements only about the relationships between:

- calcium and osteoporosis
- fat and cancer
- saturated fat and cholesterol and coronary heart disease (CHD)
- fiber-containing grain products, fruits, and vegetables and cancer
- fruits, vegetables, and grain products that contain fiber, particularly soluble fiber, and coronary heart disease (CHD)
- sodium and hypertension
- oats and oat flour and cholesterol
- the Food and Drug Association, at this writing, is proposing to authorize the use on food labels of the association between soy protein and the reduced risk of coronary heart disease

The claims must be supported by "valid, reliable, publicly available scientific evidence . . . and should conform to generally recognized medical and nutritional principles" for a sound, total diet.

The claims must clearly indicate that good nutrition is the result of the total diet and not a result of eating a specific food or foods. That requirement conforms to the traditional advice most nutrition experts give that people should eat a varied but balanced diet of nutritious foods. (Nutrition labeling is mandatory on any product making a health claim.)

But should you "swallow" everything a food processor puts on the label about the health benefits of a product? A soup company, for example, created a conflict when it claimed: "You can get as much fiber from a serving of home-style bean soup as you can from a serving of many bran cereals . . . and fiber is important because the National Cancer Institute says that a diet high in fiber and low in fat may help reduce the risk of some kinds of cancer."

The Cancer Institute found the advertisement misleading because the company's bean and pea soups contained 600 to 700 milligrams of sodium, excessively higher than the Department of Health and Human Services maintains is prudent. The Cancer Institute's name was removed from advertising in 1987–88.

In another example of questionable advertising, the Dairy Board highlighted the benefits of calcium in dairy products, but left out that they are also high in fat and sodium.

Even that old home remedy, chicken soup, is not immune. How about a product that is promoted as very low sodium? "The ingredients in descending order of content are: Dextrose, potassium chloride, hydrolyzed cereal solids, autolyzed yeast, chicken fat, onion powder, monoammonium glutamate, gelatin, natural chicken flavor, spices, garlic powder, turmeric, disodium inosinate, disodium guanylate, and carrot powder. Chances are neither your mother nor a chicken would recognize it. Very low sodium is desirable for persons with cardiovascular problems, but chicken fat and the largest ingredient, dextrose (a sugar), are not.

Another "instant" chicken soup aimed at the general public proclaims "no preservatives," but it not only has sugar, cottonseed oil, sodium pyrophosphate, potassium pyrophosphate, sodium carbonate, potassium carbonate, monosodium glutamate (notice all those fancy sodium words?), but a whopping 1,435 milligrams of sodium.

Saving Money in the Store: Unit Pricing

Finding the best buys at the supermarket takes some know-how. You must consider quality, nutrition, convenience, family tastes, storage space, and economy when shopping for food. Unit pricing is the key to knowing which product is most economical.

Unit pricing is a tool for comparing prices at a glance. The package price tells you how much you pay for a food item; the unit price tells you the price of each "unit" in a package.

A unit can be an ounce, a pound, a quart, a square foot, or an individual piece in a package. For example, the *unit price* shows you the cost of each ounce in a can of soup. The *package price* just tells you the price of the whole can.

By using unit pricing, you can easily compare the cost of any brand and any package size. But remember, compare only similar items. For example, comparing the unit prices of a carton of orange juice, bottled apple juice and a can of fruit punch tells you which is least expensive, because all are liquid, ready-to-drink beverages. Comparing unit prices of canned, frozen and powdered drinks is misleading, however, because you add water to frozen concentrates and powdered mixes.

Why You Buy

Did you ever notice that staples that you always need—such as sugar and flour—are at the bottom of store shelves while the "impulse" buying products are at eye level? Just one way to lure you to buy. Some stores even use fresh pizza or strawberry aromas in the frozen food sections and the smell of fresh baked bread in the bakery section to subconsciously lure you to purchase these items.

Putting "New!" on the label is also a lure and now University of Illinois at Urbana-Champaign researchers have found another of our vulnerabilities: quantity numbers. The researchers discovered we will buy more if we see a supermarket display that advertises a specific purchase quantity number, such as:

- Three bags of chips for $3
- Limit twelve cans of soup per person
- Buy six candy bars for Saturday

By varying the displays in eighty-nine supermarkets in Chicago, Philadelphia, and Iowa, it was discovered these larger quantities nearly doubled how much the typical grocery shopper would otherwise buy of that item.[8] For instance, when shoppers in Sioux City, Iowa, saw a grocery display that advertised canned soup as "79 cents—No Limit per Person," they typically bought three or four cans. When the display was changed to read "79 cents—Limit Twelve per Person," they purchased twice as many—seven cans per person. "Three for $3" instead of "One for $1" increased average sales by over 30 percent. Seeing the number is suggestive to shoppers.

If you realize you have been a sucker for such manipulations, don't fret. Studies have shown that numerical displays influence almost everyone—including math professors, physicians, and U.S. senators. Even if you buy more than you intended don't feel too badly. You'll eventually eat the extra products.

---

[8]Brian Wansink, Robert Kent, and Stephen Hoch. *Journal of Marketing,* February 1998.

Tip: If you want to be certain not to overpurchase the next time, just write a number next to the items on your shopping list. Studies show that this technique will help you resist the enticement of "two-fers," etc.

Making Sure Your Food Hasn't Expired

A large percentage of food additives are preservatives to extend shelf life, but even "embalmed" foods can spoil or become less appetizing.

Want a date? You can use the dates that are given on food packaging if the manufacturer is using "open dating." On the other hand, "code dating" is not useful to the consumer. In open dating, dates are stated alphanumerically, such as Oct. 15, or numerically, such as 10-15 or 1015. In code dating, the information is coded letters, numbers, and symbols so that usually only the manufacturer can translate it.

Open dating may be used for:

- *Pull date.* This is the last day that the manufacturer recommends that the product remain for sale. This date takes into consideration additional time for storage and use at home. If the food is bought on the pull date, it still can be eaten at a later date. How long the product should be offered for sale and how much home storage is allowed is determined by the manufacturer, based on knowledge of the product and the product's shelf life.

- *Quality assurance or freshness date.* This date shows how long the manufacturer thinks a food will be of optimum quality. On the label, it often appears as: "Best if used by March 2, 2000." This doesn't mean, however, that the product can't be used after the suggested date.

- *Pack date.* This is the date the food was packaged or processed. It may enable you to determine how old a product really is.

- *Expiration date.* This is the last day on which a product should be *eaten*. State governments regulate these dates for perishable items, such as milk and eggs. FDA regulates only the expiration dates of infant formula.

Of considerably less use to you is the code date. A common type of code dating is the product code. This code enables the manufacturer to convey a relatively large amount of information with a few small letters, numbers, and symbols. It tells when and where a product was packaged. In the case of a recall, this makes it easier for the grocer and manufacturer to quickly identify and track down the product and take it off the market. FDA encourages manufacturers to put product codes on packaging, especially for products with a long shelf life.

Food processors are often masters at making codes inconspicuous. On frozen-food packages, the dates are usually indented on the wrapper or the carton. These colorless indentations are most often found at one end of the package. Another method of dating frozen food involves putting a small letter or number on the food wrapper. It is stamped, but is part of the printing on the wrapper. Cans have the code numbers embossed on one end, usually the bottom. Boxes have either stamped or indented codes on one end of the package.

Most supermarkets keep a thick book of master codes in their offices. If you have no success in breaking the code of a particular product, ask the store manager to see the codebook.

Avoiding Certain Additives

What do you want from your food? You are part of the market force. By using this book to understand the labels and by selecting wisely, you can affect the sales of more wholesome foods and protect the health of your family. There are more than five thousand indirect and direct common food additives in our diet, nearly two-thirds of them flavorings used to replace the natural flavors lost during processing.

Contrary to public belief, food additives are not a modern innovation. Adding chemicals to food began at the dawn of civilization, when man first discovered that by adding salt to meat, the meat would last longer.

The father of modern food additives laws was Dr. Harvey W. Wiley, who in the early 1900s led the fight against chemical preservatives such as boric acid, formaldehyde, and salicylic acid. He dramatized the problem with his famous "Poison Squad," made up of young men willing to be guinea pigs, which meant eating measured amounts of these chemicals to determine toxicity. As a result of Dr. Wiley's pioneering work, the first Federal Food and Drug Act was passed in 1906.

Since this book was first published in 1972, thirty-five widely used additives that had been approved as safe have been removed from the market as unsafe, most because they were found to be capable of causing cancer. In 1978, food additives were a $1.3 billion a year business. Today, it is a $4.73 billion a year enterprise. Consumers like "new" foods. This means that in any given year, U.S. food processors spend $1.4 billion annually to introduce 10,000 new food products, some with new additives and many with new combinations of additives.[9]

My intention is to help you understand these chemicals, how they are used, and what is known about how they may affect your health, so that you can make better choices. Your knowledge is your best protection for understanding how to keep undesirable chemicals away from you and your loved ones.

Today, food processors have in their armamentaria an estimated thousands of chemicals they can add to what we eat. Some are deleterious, some are harmless, and some are beneficial.

Every chemical used in food processing is *supposed to* serve one or more of the following purposes:[10]

- Improve nutritional value.

- Enhance quality or consumer acceptability.

---

[9]Office of the Food Safety Center Director, U.S. Department of Agriculture, 1998.
[10]The Food Protection Committee of the National Academy of Sciences evaluated the safety of additives in a 1998 report.

- Improve the keeping quality.
- Make the food more readily available.
- Facilitate its preparation.

The majority of food additives have nothing to do with nutritional value, as anyone can see from the contents of this dictionary. Most of the chemicals added to enhance consumer acceptability are there to feed our illusions. We want enhanced food because all our lives we have been subjected to the beautiful pictures of foods in our magazines and on television. We have come to expect an advertiser's concept of perfection in color and texture, even though Mother Nature may not turn out all her products that way. As a result, the skin of the oranges we eat are dyed bright orange to match our mental image of an ideal orange. Our poultry is fed a chemical to turn the meat yellower and more appetizing, and our fruits and vegetables are kept unblemished by fungicides, pesticides, herbicides, and other antispoilants.

Other chemicals are added to improve the keeping quality of some products. Processors embalm them. Bread has sixteen chemicals to keep it feeling "fresh." One type of bread, balloon bread, undergoes rigor mortis thanks to its additive plaster of paris. Ironically, when nothing is added to the foods, they cost us considerably more. Unbleached flour is four times as much as bleached; untreated tomatoes, five times as much as regular canned tomatoes, and unsulfured raisins are six times the cost of treated ones.

The purpose of this dictionary is to enable you to look up any additive under its alphabetical listing to determine whether it is something you want to be eating. In this way you can reject cancer-causing agents or toxins.

AVOIDING SALT

The basic sources of cereals, on the other hand, are salt-free—wheat, corn, rice, and oats. Yet instant oatmeal contains about 360 mg per serving, instant corn grits 590 mg, and instant cream of wheat 180 mg. If you're willing to cook the cereals a little bit, you can avoid the high salt. It's providing the "instant" that dishes out the sodium. Some seventy sodium compounds are used in foods, as you will see in this book. The National Academy of Sciences, whose experts establish dietary guidelines, recommends that we ingest no more than 1,100 to 3,000 milligrams of sodium for the entire day. The average American ingests 5,000 to 7,000 milligrams. If the numbers for sodium look very low on a label, look again and be aware of the difference between milligrams and grams. Some companies make you think there is less by saying 2 grams (g) of sodium, for example, which is really 2,000 milligrams (mg).

AVOIDING SUGAR

Sugar, as you may recall, also masquerades under a variety of names and can be difficult to avoid. Common names such as sucrose, fructose, and corn syrup may be familiar to readers, but a food can be labeled "sugar free" or "sugar-less" and still contain calories from sugar alcohols such as xylitol, sorbitol, and mannitol. Saccharin is a nonnutritive sweetener—that is, it has no calories. Aspartame has the same calories as sugar, but is so much sweeter that only small amounts are needed to provide the desired sweetness in a product.

We may even be getting more than we bargained for when we get our sweets from fruit juice. A popular brand of diet fruit juice has a beautiful picture of an open pineapple and a cut orange on its label proclaiming it to be "sugar free" and "low sodium." It is, however, artificially sweetened and flavored with FD and C Yellows No. 5 and No. 6, both recognized allergens, and benzoate of soda—a flavoring agent and also a common allergen—saccharin, and aspartame. Now from what tree was that concoction harvested?

AVOIDING ALLERGENS

An allergic reaction to certain food additives may range from an itchy, runny nose or sore throat to indigestion and even death. Any food may cause an allergic reaction, but the most common offenders are milk, fish, shellfish, mollusks, soybeans, chicken, nuts, berries, eggs, peanuts, and fresh fruits such as peaches and apples. The only specific treatment for food allergy is avoidance, but escaping a food allergen in the form of a hidden additive is not simple.

For example, if you were allergic to corn, you would have to avoid corn sugar, dextrose, and corn syrup. You would have to know that they are used in maple, nut, and root beer flavorings for beverages, ice cream, ices, candy, and baked goods. The syrup is also used in bacon, baking mixes, powders, beers, bourbon, breads, cheese, cereals, chop suey, chow mein, confectioners' sugar, cream puffs, fish products, ginger ale, hams, jellies, processed meats, peanut butter, canned peas, plastic food wrap, sherbets, whiskeys, and American wines. It may also be found in corn chips, fritters, frostings, canned or frozen fruit, graham crackers, gravies, grits, gum, monosodium glutamate, oleomargarine, pablum, tortillas, vinegar, yeasts, bologna, baking powders, bath powders, frying fats, and fruit juices.

Sulfites and peanuts (*see* both in dictionary) which may be in foods as additives, are among the most common cause of the life-threatening allergic reaction, anaphylaxis *(see)*.

As pointed out, it is difficult to avoid certain allergenic food additives, but it can help if you read the listing for the additive you know you are allergic to and note the foods to which it may be added (*see also* Appendix B).

AVOIDING SUSPECTED CANCER-CAUSING ADDITIVES

A major report on the relationship between nutrition and the development of cancer concludes that 3 to 4 million cases of cancer per year could be prevented by appropriate diet.[11]

---

[11]John R. Seffrin, Ph.D., CEO of the American Cancer Society and American Association for Health Educators School, in "Personal Behaviors Are What Really Matters When It Comes to Avoiding Cancer," paper presented to the American Association for Health Educators, St. Louis, March 22, 1997.

The Delaney Amendment

Written by Congressman James Delaney, the amendment was part of the 1958 law requested by the Food and Drug Administration. The law stated that food and chemical manufacturers had to test additives before they were put on the market, and the results had to be submitted to the FDA. Delaney's amendment specifically states that "no additive may be permitted in any amount if the tests show that it produces cancer when fed to man or animals or by other appropriate tests."

Ever since the amendment was enacted, it has been severely attacked by food and chemical manufacturers, the Nutrition Council of the American Medical Association, and several FDA commissioners. The FDA commissioners claim it is unenforceable and point to the problem with saccharin, a proven carcinogen. The artificial sweetener has been in use since 1879, and when it was shown to cause cancer in laboratory animals in 1977, the FDA announced that saccharin in foods and beverages would be banned. There was a public outcry from dieters led by the Calorie Control Council, a trade organization that spent over a million dollars in just six months to stop the ban. The Council in 1997 successfully requested the National Toxicology Program to review new data that could lead to a delisting of the sweetener as a carcinogen.

The problem with identifying exposure to a cancer-causing additive is:

- In most instances exposure to cancer-causing agents (carcinogens) takes place twenty to thirty years before a statistically significant increase in cancer can be detected. Only then can it be adduced that the increase in cancer may have been caused by exposure to specific cancer-causing agents.

- Animal studies may give clues, but laboratory conditions and the bodies of other creatures may not result in valid conclusions for us.

- Each of us is unique in the way our bodies process chemicals based on our age, sex, heredity, medical history, diet, and behavior. Epidemiologists estimate that approximately one-third of all cancer deaths can be attributed to diet.[12]

The Delaney Amendment, as pointed out, is being ignored in a significant number of instances. The listings in this dictionary cite the known or suspected additives that can be carcinogenic. There are well-known ones such as nitrates and nitrites *(see)*. If you can't resist bacon and processed meats that contain them, then you can reduce their effects by eating or drinking something high in vitamin C.

If you want to avoid other additives such as saccharin or vinyl chlorides, you can by not buying the products that contain them.

---

[12]Robert J. Scheuplein, "Perspectives on Toxicological Risk—An Example: Food-borne Carcinogenic Risk," *Critical Reviews in Food Science and Nutrition* 32 (1992): 105–21.

Avoiding Neurotoxins

While the testing of additives in our food for carcinogenicity may be imperfect, little if any testing is being done to determine if food additives may be toxic to the brain and nerves, although a number of scientists believe that neurotoxins are even more of a problem in food than carcinogens.[13] Thomas Sobotka, Ph.D., of the FDA's Inter-Center neurobiology group points out:

In humans, neurotoxins can adversely affect a broad spectrum of behavioral functions, including the ability to learn, to interact appropriately with others, and to perceive and respond to environmental stimuli; basically these represent everyday functions that enable people to live productive lives. The focus placed on neurotoxicity will encourage the development of more relevant information about the potential adverse effects of chemicals on the structural and functional integrity of the nervous system, and should help obtain the information needed for a reasonable assessment of potential neurotoxic hazard."[14]

In the meantime, the dictionary cites those chemicals such as monosodium glutamate and Red No. 3 (*see* both) that have been found to be suspected neurotoxins. Most of the chemicals identified as neurotoxins here are pesticides, since they have long been identified with nerve damage. They are hard to avoid unless you grow your own food, without chemicals. You can reduce your intake by avoiding those few products that are thus far known to contain neurotoxins.

Understanding Additive Uses

This dictionary includes virtually all of the food additives in common use. For the sake of clarity and ease of use, I have grouped their nearly fifty functions under the broad categories that follow.

Preservatives

These "antispoilants" are used to help prevent microbiological spoilage and chemical deterioration. They are of many different types, of which about one hundred are in common use. Preservatives for fatty products are called antioxidants, which prevent the production of off-flavors and off-odors. Some common antioxidants include benzoic acid used in margarine and butylated hydroxyanisole (BHA) used in lard, shortenings, crackers, soup bases, and potato chips.

In bread, preservatives are usually "mold" inhibitors. They include sodium and calcium propionate, sodium diacetate, and such acetic substances as acetic acid

---

[13]Bernard Weiss, Ph.D., University of Rochester School of Medicine, *Nutrition Update* 1 (1983): pp. 21–38; Charles Vorhees and R. E. Butcher, *Developmental Toxicology,* ed. K. Snell (London: Croom Helm, 1982), pp. 247–98.
[14]Thomas J. Sobotka, Ph.D., "Revisions to the FDA's Redbook Guidelines for Toxicity Testing: Neurotoxicity," *Critical Reviews in Food Science and Nutrition* 32 (1992): 165–71.

and lactic acid. Sorbic acid and sodium and potassium salts are preservatives used in cheeses, syrups, and pie fillings. Preservatives used to prevent mold and fungus growth on citrus fruits are called "fungicides." Sequestering agents, still another type of preservative, prevent physical or chemical changes that affect color, flavor, texture, or appearance. Ethylenediaminetetraacetic acid (EDTA) and its salts, for instance, are used to prevent the adverse effects of the presence of metals in such products as soft drinks where metal ions can cause clouding. Sequestrants used in dairy products to keep them "fresh and sweet" include sodium, calcium, and potassium salts of citric, tartaric, and pyrophosphoric acids. Other common multipurpose preservatives are the gas sulfur dioxide, propyl gallate, and, of course, sugar, salt, and vinegar.

Food processors have explored some novel food preservation systems. Consumers evidently prefer a preservative from a natural source, which enables the processors to use the word "natural" on the label. Bacteriocins are not new; however, like nisin—derived from the starter bacteria for yogurt—they are now being used to extend shelf life and enhance the safety of a variety of food products. The use of bacteriocins is likely to be expanded in the future. Inhibitory strains of lactic acid bacteria can be selected for use in dairy cultures or be added to refrigerated foods to extend shelf life and enhance safety.

Modified and controlled atmosphere packaging are also used by the food industry. They have the potential for even wider use, particularly with fresh fruits and vegetables sold at retail. These methods rely on inhibiting microbial growth by excluding oxygen or by inhibitory concentrations of carbon dioxide. Among other sterilizing techniques:

Irradiated Food

When food is irradiated, it is loaded onto a conveyor belt and passed through a radiation cell where it is showered with beams of ionizing radiation produced by high radioactive isotopes. The radiation can inhibit ripening and kill certain bacteria and molds that induce spoilage, so that food looks and tastes fresh for up to several weeks. The process does not make food radioactive, does not change the food's color or texture in most cases. Does it destroy nutrients? Does it create radiolytic products in food after exposure that may cause genetic damage? Is irradiation less dangerous than some of the other chemicals added to foods as preservatives? These questions are being hotly debated.

Radiation of red meat was cleared on December 2, 1997. It had been first used on a food product in 1963 when radiation-treated wheat and wheat flour was allowed to be marketed. Dr. Michael Friedman of the FDA said the agency was satisfied that radiation was safe, that it did not demonstrably alter the nutritional content of food, that it did not change the flavor or aroma of meat, and that it killed nearly all bacteria on meat that can sicken and kill. Irradiation was already approved for poultry, where it reportedly can kill salmonella, and for fruits and vegetables to kill molds and fungi that cause rot.

Food	Approved Use	Dose
Spices and dry vegetable seasoning	Decontaminates and controls insects and microorganisms	30 kGy
Dry or dehydrated enzyme preparations	Controls insects and microorganisms	10 kGy
All foods	Controls insects	1 kGy
Fresh foods	Delays maturation	1 kGy
Poultry	Controls disease-causing microorganisms	3 kGy
Red meat such as beef, lamb, and pork	Controls spoilage and disease-causing microorganisms	4.5 kGy (fresh) 7 kGy (frozen)

APPROVED USES OF IRRADIATION

The FDA sets the maximum radiation dose the product can be exposed to, which is measured in units called kiloGray (kGy). The following is a list of all approved uses of radiation on foods to date, the purpose for irradiating them, and the radiation dose allowed.

Jeremy Rifkin, president of the Pure Food Campaign, says more attention should be placed on raising healthier livestock, which he says would reduce pathogens and make irradiation unnecessary. The Center for Science in the Public Interest calls irradiation expensive and "an end-of-the-line solution to contamination problems that can and should be addressed earlier."

Many organizations in addition to the FDA endorse irradiation of food, including the World Health Organization, the American Medical Association, and the American Dietetic Association.

The FDA requires that foods that have been irradiated must say so on the label and display an international logo, a flower in a circle, so you will be able to decide for yourself.

Ohmic Heating

Ohmic heating involves passing an electric current through the food. Unlike conventional heating when liquids heat faster than solids, the reverse can occur with ohmic. Sterilization is also faster with less loss of quality, according to its advocates. Ohmic reportedly works best with liquids and mixtures containing very small particles.

Pulsed Electric Field Processing

Pulsed electric field processing uses a very strong pulsed electric current to disrupt microbial cells and pasteurize foods with little or no heating.

Bright Light Processing

Bright light processing uses an intense white light to kill bacteria on the surface of foods. This light does not penetrate deeply and can only be used for surface pasteurization.

Aseptic Processing

Aseptic processing dates back to the mid-1940s but has yet to realize its full potential. The most widely used of the new technologies, aseptic processing involves sterilizing a food product in a continuous process through a heat exchanger and then filling that food in an aseptic filler. The aseptic filler is a highly specialized piece of equipment designed to sterilize the packaging material, pour the sterile product into its container in a sterile environment, and then seal the package.

Biotech Foods

Biotechnology is an umbrella term covering a vast variety of processes for using living organisms—such as plants, animals, and microbes—or any part of these organisms to create new or improved products. It is aimed at faster, more precise, and controllable manipulation of genes than traditional breeding and selection techniques.

Although the idea of genetic manipulation frightens a lot of consumers, biotechnology is not really new. For thousands of years humans have used bacteria and yeast to produce foods such as cheese and bread. In the 1860s the scientist Gregor Mendel discovered the genetic principles of selective and cross-breeding. Using Mendelian genetics, the agricultural community bred hybrid forms of many crops, selecting traits that made them more resilient and otherwise desirable. Such breeding methods largely accounted for the phenomenal gains in food productivity during the twentieth century.

The most common goals of biotechnology today are to create a longer shelf life, expand the ability to grow and ship perishable products, and to make produce and animals more productive and disease-resistant.

Biotechnology is often divided into old and new varieties. The older forms include plant and animal breeding and fermentation, which are based on the use of whole living organisms. The newer biotechnologies use parts of living organisms, manipulating the chromosomes or DNA strands—or the genetic sequences that control specific traits. Biotech tomatoes, for example, travel better, look more appealing, and reportedly have more resistance to fungus and insects. Biotech canola oil has more unsaturated fats, and biotech soybeans reportedly have more nutritive value.

Questions have been raised about whether genetic manipulation may introduce toxins and allergens into foods. Naturally occurring toxins are present at low levels in many foods. Although they have seldom posed a safety problem, they could cause illness if concentrated at high levels and consumed in large quantities. The introduction of allergens creates hazards for sensitive individuals, which has prompted the Food and Drug Administration to require special labeling for such products. Indeed, there may be changes in some products but producers claim that in many cases these alterations improve nutritive value

The FDA is fairly relaxed about biotech foods. In May 1992, FDA issued a policy statement on regulating biotechnology food products. It developed a science-based safety assessment based on objective characteristics of the food, such as new substances, increased toxins, changes in important nutrients, and potential allergic reactions. The FDA requires premarket review only for foods into which substances are intentionally introduced, significantly changing the structure or function.

The FDA only requires labeling in two circumstances: if the characteristics significantly differ from what is normally expected and/or if safety issues arise. One reason for this precaution is primarily to warn people of allergens. For example, if a walnut protein were inserted into a tomato, consumers allergic to walnuts must be alerted. Labeling could also be required if the nutritional content of the food has been changed significantly.

The FDA says that it will review genetically altered foods if:

- The concentration of any naturally occurring toxins in the plant has been increased.
- An allergen not commonly found in the plant has been introduced.
- The levels of important nutrients have changed.
- New substances have been introduced into food that raise safety questions.
- There is a problem with an environmental effect.
- Accepted, established scientific practices have not been followed.

The U.S. Department of Agriculture regulates the products of biotechnology but not the process itself. It has responsibility for assessing the ecological effects of new plants developed through biotechnology. Initially, the USDA plans to regulate transgenic animals (those with genetic material from a different species) under existing guidelines covering experimental animals in the Code of Federal Regulations for Meat and Poultry.

On March 31, 1993, the USDA issued a final rule on the notification procedures for genetically engineered organisms and products. This rule establishes a notification system to replace the existing permit process for genetically engineered crops that are field-tested with specific safety criteria.

In addition, the system introduces special requirements that companies would have to satisfy before slaughtering transgenic animals. They would have to describe any drugs or chemicals given to the animals, along with the biological techniques and products used. Before granting approval for slaughter, the USDA plans to scrutinize safety on three levels:

1. Hazards introduced by the transgene; that is, by the genetic material introduced into the animal

2. Safety of the final food product

3. Secondary changes in the animal caused by the insertion of new DNA

Some consumer and environmental groups believe that the FDA's approach fails to protect public health because, in their view, genetic engineering poses unique food and environmental safety risks that warrant premarket testing and review. These groups contend that the FDA's policy allows manufacturers too much discretion in determining the safety of new food products before marketing them. Some believe that genetic engineering is a radical new technology—not an extension of traditional breeding—and will introduce products that have not been a part of the food supply. Some argue that the new techniques allow genetic modifications that were not possible with traditional breeding methods.

The Pure Food Campaign, led by Jeremy Rifkin, president of the Foundation on Economic Trends, Washington, D.C., says that consumers will have no way of knowing which whole and processed foods are genetically engineered. Vegetarians and religious groups with dietary restrictions could unwittingly eat fruits and vegetables that contain unlabeled genetic material from insects, fish, fowl, pigs, and other animals. This consumer group is also concerned that bioengineered plants may have elevated levels of allergens or toxins.

Michael Jacobson of the Center for Science in the Public Interest believes that biotechnology should be monitored in the first few years and that companies that market such products should have to register.

What other countries have been developing biotechnology products? Japan and China have developed many products similar to those under development in the U.S. and are actively working on more. Japan, for example, has developed a low-allergen variety of rice. China currently has many test plots of transgenic plants under cultivation. Europe is actively exploring biotechnology. The nations of Europe, however, have been unable to reach a uniform agreement on the regulations governing biotechnology. As a result, the research remains mostly in the laboratory with few field studies under way.

Fresh Refrigerated Products

Fresh refrigerated products are expected to grow at 14 percent per year. These processed foods are designed to offer the convenience of frozen and canned foods while providing homemade taste and appearance. Typically, they are cooked just enough to ward off spoilage for a short period of time. As a further aid to freshness, they are often sealed in packaging that contains little or no oxygen, which can extend shelf life for several weeks. Scientists, however, are concerned that some dangerous bacteria may not be killed during the minimal precooking and that microorganisms that cause botulism can flourish in an oxygen-free environment. One publicized outbreak of botulism associated with this category could devastate it.

The following are more conventional methods of adding additives directly to food for various purposes:

ACIDS, ALKALIES, BUFFERS, NEUTRALIZERS

The degree of acidity or alkalinity is important in many processed foods. An acid such as potassium acid tartrate, sodium aluminum phosphate, or tartaric acid acts on the leavening agent in baked goods and releases the gas that causes the desired "rising." The flavor of many soft drinks, other than cola types, is modified by the use of an acid such as citric acid from citrus fruits, malic acid from apples, or tartaric acid, a component of grapes. Phosphoric acid is used to give colas the "tangy" taste. The same acids that are used in soft drinks are also used in churning cream to help preserve the flavor and keeping quality of butter. Alkalies such as ammonium hydroxide in cocoa products and ammonium carbonate in candy, cookies, and crackers are employed to make the products more alkaline. Buffers and neutralizing agents are chemicals added to foods to control acidity or alkalinity, just as acids and alkalies are added directly. Some common chemicals in this class are ammonium bicarbonate, calcium carbonate, potassium acid tartrate, sodium aluminum phosphate, and tartaric acid.

MOISTURE CONTENT CONTROLS

Humectants are necessary in the production of some types of confections and candy to prevent drying out. Without a humectant, shredded coconut, for example, would not remain soft and pliable. Substances used for this purpose include glycerin (which retains the soft, moist texture in marshmallows), propylene glycol, and sorbitol. On the other hand, calcium silicate is used to prevent table salt from caking due to moisture absorption from the air.

PHYSIOLOGIC ACTIVITY CONTROLS

The chemicals in this group are added to fresh foods to serve as ripeners or antimetabolic agents. For instance, ethylene gas is used to hasten the ripening of bananas, and maleic hydrazide is used to prevent potatoes from sprouting. Coming into increasing use are enzymes that are of natural origin and generally believed to be nontoxic. Of all food enzyme additives, amylases that act on starch have the most numerous applications. Various amylases from plant, animal, fungal, and bacterial sources have been used to break down the components of starch to make it more digestible. Enzymes are also used in the fermentation of sugar to make candy, in brewing beer, and in the manufacture of artificial honey, bread, and frozen milk concentrates.

BLEACHING AND MATURING AGENTS, BREAD IMPROVERS

Fresh ground flour is pale yellow. Upon storage, it slowly becomes white and undergoes an aging process that improves its baking qualities. For more than fifty years, processors have added an oxidizing agent to the flour to accelerate this process, thus reducing storage costs, spoilage, and insect infestation. Compounds such as benzoyl peroxide bleach the flour without affecting baking qualities. Other compounds, such as oxides of nitrogen, chlorine dioxide, nitrosyl chloride, and chlorine have both a bleaching and maturing, or "improving" ability. Bread improvers used by the baking industry contain oxidizing substances such as potassium bromate, potassium iodate, and calcium peroxide. They also contain inorganic salts such as ammonium or calcium sulfate and ammonium phosphates, which serve as yeast foods and dough conditioners. Quantities used are relatively small, since too much can easily result in an inferior product. Bleaching agents may also be used in other foods, such as cheese, to improve the appearance of the finished product.

PROCESSING AIDS

Many chemicals fall into this category. Sanitizing agents, for instance, used to clean bacteria and debris from products, are considered such aids. So are clarifying agents, which remove extraneous materials. Tannin, for example, is used for clarifying liquids in the wine and brewing industries. Gelatin and albumen remove small particles and minute traces of copper and iron in the production of vinegar and some beverages.

Emulsifiers and emulsion stabilizers help to maintain a mixture and assure a consistency. They affect characteristics such as volume, uniformity, and fineness of grain (bakery products have a softer "crumb" and slower "firming" rate). They influence ease of mixing and smoothness, such as the whipping property of frozen desserts and the smoothness of cake mixes, and they help maintain homogeneity and keeping quality in such products as mayonnaise, candy, and salad dressing. Some common emulsifiers are lecithin, the monoglycerides and diglycerides, and propylene glycol alginate. Sorbitan derivatives are used to retard "bloom," the whitish deposits of high-melting components of cocoa butter that occasionally appear on the surface of chocolate candy. Food chemists sometimes call emulsifiers "surfactants" or "surface-active agents."

Texturizers or stabilizers are added to products to give them "body" and maintain a desired texture. For instance, calcium chloride or some other calcium salt is added to canned tomatoes and canned potatoes to keep them from falling apart. Sodium nitrate and sodium nitrite are used in curing meats to develop and stabilize the pink color. Nitrogen, carbon dioxide, and nitrous oxide are employed in pressure-packed containers of certain foods to act as whipping agents or as propellants. The texture of ice cream and other frozen desserts is dependent on the size of the ice crystals in the product. By addition of agar-agar, gelatin, cellulose gum, or some other gum, the size of the ice crystals is stabilized. Texturizer gums are also used in chocolate milk to increase the viscosity of the product and to prevent the settling of coca particles to the bottom of the container. Gelatin, pectin, and starch are used in confectionery products to give a desired texture. Artificially sweetened beverages also need bodying agents to give a desired texture because they do not contain the "thickness" normally contributed by sugar. The thickeners employed include such natural gums as sodium alginate and pectins. The foaming properties of brewed beer can also be improved by the addition of texturizers.

COLORING AGENTS

Food colors of both natural and synthetic origin are extensively used in processed foods and play a major role in increasing the acceptability and attractiveness of these products. However, the indiscriminate use of color can conceal damage or inferiority, or make the product appear better than it actually is. The World Health Organization in delineating some 140 different kinds of colorants found many to be unsafe. Coal tar colors were subject to a special provision in a 1938 law that required every coal tar color used in food to be listed with the government as "harmless and suitable for use," and every batch of the color intended for use in food had to be certified by a government agency as safe. Some of the colors originally listed as "harmless" were found to produce injury when fed to animals and were removed from the list. In 1960, the federal government required manufacturers to retest all artificial colors to determine safety. At present, nine are permanently listed as safe. Among them FD and C Blue No. 1 and FD and C Citrus Red No. 2 have been shown to cause tumors at the site of injection in animals, but the FDA does not consider this significant because the experiment concerned injection by needle and not ingestion in food or application on the skin. FD and C Red No. 40, one of the most widely used colorings, is also being questioned because it is made from a base known to be carcinogenic and because many scientists feel that it should not have been given permanent listing based solely on the manufacturer's tests.

Among the natural colors used in foods are annatto, carotene, chlorophyll, cochineal, saffron, and turmeric. Foods that are frequently colored include candies, baked goods, soft drinks, and such dairy products as butter, cheese, and cream.

FLAVORINGS

A wide variety of spices, natural extractives, oleoresins, and essential oils are used in processed foods. In fact, of the three thousand food additives known to be added to our food supply, two thousand are flavorings to replace the flavors lost during processing. In addition, the modern flavor chemist has produced many synthetic flavors. Both types of products are used extensively in soft drinks, baked goods, ice cream, and confectionery. Flavoring agents are the most numerous additive, with over two thousand in use. Of these, some five hundred are natural, and the balance are synthetic. These are usually employed in amounts ranging from a few to three hundred parts per million. Amyl acetate, benzaldehyde, carvone, ethyl acetate, ethyl butyrate, and methyl salicylate are typical compounds employed in the preparation of flavoring materials. However, many of the compounds used in synthetic flavorings are also found in natural products or derive from natural acids. Essential oils, such as oil of lemon and oil of orange, are natural flavors made by extraction of the fruit rind. There are also flavor enhancers, the commonest being monosodium glutamate (MSG) and maltol.

NUTRITION SUPPLEMENTS

Enrichment of food means that the natural nutrients have been removed during processing and then replaced. Enrichment of cereal foods, according to the big producers, is supposed to provide 12 to 23 percent of the daily supply of thiamin, niacin, and iron, and 10 percent of the riboflavin recommended for human consumption.

Fortification of food means that additional nutrients are added to the product to make it more nutritious than it was before. For instance, vitamin C is added to orange drinks and vitamin A to margarine. Vitamin D is used to fortify milk to prevent rickets, and potassium iodide is added to iodized salt to prevent goiter, a thyroid tumor caused by iodine deficiency.

Amino acids, the building blocks of protein, may become commonly used as additives. The major use of amino acids in the food industry today is monosodium glutamate, which enhances flavor. Actually, the human body needs certain amino acids not manufactured in the body in sufficient amounts and some processors add certain amino acids to increase the protein component of their product.

A number of additional substances are employed for various purposes. Certain sugar substitutes are used in food for persons who must restrict their intake of ordinary sweets. Saccharin and sorbitol are commonly used for this purpose. Glazes and polishes such as waxes and gum benzoin are used on coated confections to give luster to an otherwise dull surface. Magnesium carbonate and tricalcium phosphate are employed as anticaking agents in table salt, and calcium stearate is used for a similar purpose in garlic salt.

More Information Is Needed on Food Additives

Although officially the FDA claims to know what additives are being used in food, FDA researchers report that it is impossible to check small manufacturers. Efforts have been made through the years to have food manufacturers register and provide the information, but as yet, there is no law requiring them to do so.

There is still much to learn about additives. As you will learn when you read the entries in this book, many additives are beneficial and necessary and others should be removed from our food supply as soon as possible.

One of the greatest advances for the consumer as far as knowing what is in the foods they purchase was the passage of the Nutrition Labeling and Education Act (NLEA) and the Dietary Supplement Act of 1992, the first major change in food labeling regulations since 1974. As of May 8, 1994, food producers have had to comply with most of the FDA's new labeling requirements. (Advertising is not covered by NLEA; the Federal Trade Commission, however, has indicated it may apply the same criteria to advertising that the FDA does to labels.)

HOW TO USE THIS BOOK

While unique in content, this dictionary follows the format of most standard dictionaries. The following are sample entries with any explanatory notes that may be necessary.

MARJORAM, POT • Sweet Marjoram. The natural extract of the flowers and leaves of two varieties of the fragrant marjoram plant. The *oleoresin (see)* is used in sausage and spice flavorings for condiments and meats (3,500 ppm). The *seed* is used in sausage and spice flavorings for meats and condiments. Sweet marjoram is used in sausage and spice flavorings for beverages, baked goods, condiments, meats, and soups. The *sweet oil* is used in vermouth, wine, and spice flavorings for beverages, ice creams, ices, candy, baked goods, and condiments. Also used in hair preparations, perfumes, and soaps. Can irritate the skin. The redness, itching, and warmth experienced when applied to the skin are caused by the local dilation of the blood vessels or by local reflex. May produce allergic reactions. Essential oils such as marjoram are believed to penetrate the skin easily and produce systemic effects. GRAS.

This entry says that pot marjoram is a natural flavoring extract, that there are two kinds of marjoram—pot and sweet. Both are utilized as an oleoresin, a seed, and as a sweet oil. By looking up *oleoresin* we learn that it means a natural plant product consisting of essential oil and resin extracted from a substance, such as ginger, by means of alcohol, ether, or acetone, and that oleoresins are usually more uniform and more potent than the original product. The *ppm* stands for "parts per million," that is, 3,500 parts of marjoram is added to a million parts of meat. However, because ppm amounts (which do not appear on labels) represent maximum rather than actual usage, they are not reliable estimates of consumption and are included here only to show how amounts can be relatively large or small. GRAS means, of course, that the item is on the government's generally recognized as safe list although they may not have undergone laboratory testing. ("GRAS in packaging" means that even though substances from the containers may migrate into the food, they are assumed not harmful.)

WORMWOOD • Absinthium. A European woody herb with a bitter taste, used in bitters and liquor flavoring for beverages and liquors. The *extract* is used in bitters, liquor, and vermouth flavorings for beverages, ice cream, candy, and liquors, and in making absinthe. The *oil* is a dark green to brown and a narcotic substance. Used in bitters, apple, vermouth, and wine flavorings for beverages, ice cream, ices, candy, baked goods, and liquors. In large doses or frequently repeated doses, it is a narcotic poison, causing headache, trembling, and convulsions. Ingestion of the volatile oil or of the liquor, absinthe, may cause gastrointestinal symptoms, nervousness, stupor, coma, and death.

Absinthium is another name for wormwood and is cross-referenced in the dictionary. Source materials for the comments on toxicity is indicated in the Bibliography at the end of the dictionary. A similar example is the entry for lye.

SODIUM SESQUICARBONATE • Lye. White crystals, flakes, or powder produced from sodium carbonate. Soluble in water. Used as a neutralizer for butter, cream, fluid milk, ice cream, in the processing of olives before canning, cacao products, and canned peas. Used as an alkalizer in bath salts, shampoos, tooth powders, and soaps. Irritating to the skin and mucous membranes. May cause allergic reaction in the hypersensitive. The final report to the FDA of the Select Committee on GRAS Substances stated in 1980 that it should continue its GRAS status with no limitations other than good manufacturing practices.

Terminology has generally been kept to a middle road between technician and the citizen of average interest, while at the same time oversimplification of data has been avoided. If in doubt, look up any term, such as *isolate* (used in its chemical context), *extract,* or *anhydride.* Each is in entries to describe chemicals, but each also has its own entry to help you clarify its meaning.

With *A Consumer's Dictionary of Food Additives* you will be able to work with the current labels to determine the purpose and the desirability or toxicity of the additives listed. You will be able to assert your right to wholesome food along with a wholesome environment. By having options in the marketplace, by rejecting those products that are needlessly costly or unsafe or unpalatable in favor of "clean" food, you strike back at greed and ignorance as practiced by too many in the food industry. And you reward those manufacturers who deserve your purchases.

There is little doubt that what we eat affects our health. Our bodies are wonderful machines that can detoxify and render harmless many poisons we ingest; don't want to overburden our bodies by taking unnecessary chances. Certainly, not all food additives are harmful. Some, in fact, are greatly beneficial. It is all a matter of judgment. I hope this book will allow you to make wiser choices.

CONSUMER COMPLAINTS

The widespread distribution of food additives and consequent public safety concerns necessitate timely and reliable evaluation of suspected adverse reactions. However, few criteria exist to evaluate consumer-initiated reports of adverse medical reactions after the products have been marketed.

Currently, consumer complaints related to food additives as well as other food products, are monitored by passive surveillance, carried out primarily by the Food and Drug Administration. Therefore, it is important that if you have had an adverse reaction to a food, you report it. To report an incident or to ask a question about a processed food ingredient, contact:

- The FDA Food and Seafood Information Line at 1-800-FDA-4010 (1-800-332-4010).
- If the problem involves meat or poultry, which are regulated by the U.S. Department of Agriculture, call the USDA hotline at 1-800-535-4555. Operates toll-free weekdays, 10–4 EST.
- The Office of Consumer Affairs, Food and Drug Administration, HFE-88, 5600 Fishers Lane, Rockville, MD 20857.

General Guidelines About Reporting

Report what happened as soon as possible. Give names, addresses, and phone numbers of person(s) affected. Include your name, address, and phone number, as well as that of the doctor or hospital if emergency treatment was provided. State the problem clearly. Describe the product as completely as possible, including any codes or identifying marks on the label or container. Give the name and address of the store where the product was purchased and the date of purchase. You should also report the problem to the manufacturer or distributor shown on the label and to the store where you purchased the product.

What the FDA Doesn't Handle

Reports and complaints about the following should be made to the agencies listed. Phone numbers can be found in your local phone directory:

- Restaurant food and sanitation—Local and state health departments
- Unsolicited products in the mail—U.S. Postal Service
- Accidental poisonings—Poison control centers or hospitals
- Pesticides or air and water pollution—the U.S. Environmental Protection Agency (EPA)

- Hazardous household products, including toys, appliances, and chemicals—Consumer Product Safety Commission, 1-800-638-2772
- Alcoholic beverages—Department of Treasury's Bureau of Alcohol, Tobacco and Firearms
- Drug abuse and controlled substances—Department of Justice's Drug Enforcement Administration
- Hazardous chemicals in the workplace—Department of Labor's Occupational Safety and Health Administration
- Warranties—Federal Trade Commission
- Dispensing and sales practices of pharmacies—State board of pharmacy
- Medical practice—State certification board

If you want regulations strengthened and agencies such as the FDA and USDA well funded so they can more adequately protect our food supply, contact your senators and representatives. The phone number for the House and Senate office buildings is 202-224-3121.

If you want to contact any federal agency, including the White House, the Federal Information Center (FIC) is 800-688-9889.

It can be frustrating trying to report a problem to an agency, especially if it has a "push this number" type of voice-mail. But eventually, with persistence, you will be able not only to make yourself feel better, you will be protecting the rest of us from a similar adverse experience.

A

ABIES ALBA MILL • *See* Pine Needle Oil.

ABIETIC ACID • Sylvic Acid. Chiefly a texturizer in the making of soaps. A widely available natural acid, water insoluble, prepared from pine rosin, usually yellow and composed of either glassy or crystalline particles. Used also in the manufacture of vinyls, lacquers, and plastics. Employed to carry nutrients that are added to enriched rice in amounts up to .0026 percent of the weight of the nutrient mixture. Little is known about abietic acid toxicity; it is harmless when injected into mice but causes paralysis in frogs and is slightly irritating to human skin and mucous membranes. May cause allergic reactions.

ABSINTHIUM • Extract or Oil. *See* Wormwood.

ABSOLUTE • The term refers to a plant-extracted material that has been concentrated, but that remains essentially unchanged in its original taste and odor. For example, *see* Jasmine Absolute. Often called "natural perfume materials" because they are not subjected to heat and water as are distilled products. *See* Distilled.

ACACIA • Acacia vera. Gum Arabic. Egyptian Thorn. Catechu (from the Latin *Acacia catechu,* which is interchangeable with acacia). Acacia is the odorless, colorless, tasteless dried exudate from the stem of the acacia tree grown in Africa, the Near East, India, and the southern United States. Its most distinguishing quality among the natural gums is its ability to dissolve rapidly in water. The use of acacia dates back four thousand years when the Egyptians employed it in paints. Its principal use in the confectionery industry is to retard sugar crystallization and as a thickener for candies, jellies, glazes, and chewing gum. As a stabilizer, it prevents chemical breakdown in food mixtures. Gum acacia is a foam stabilizer in soft drink and brewing industries. Other uses are for mucilage, and the gum gives form and shape to tablets. In 1976 the FDA placed acacia in the GRAS category as an emulsifier, flavoring agent, processing aid, and stabilizer in beverages at 2.0 percent, chewing gum at 5.6 percent; as a formulation aid, stabilizer and humectant in confections and frostings at 12.4 percent; as a humectant stabilizer and formulation aid in hard candy at 46.5 percent; in soft candy at 85 percent; in nut formulations at 1.0 percent; and in all other food categories at 8.3 percent of the product. Medically, it is used as a demulcent to soothe irritations, particularly of the mucous membranes. It slightly reduces cholesterol in the blood. It can cause allergic reactions such as skin rash and asthmatic attacks. Oral toxicity is low. *See also* Vegetable Gums and Catechu Extract. GRAS.

ACCEPTABLE DAILY INTAKE (ADI) • An estimate of the amount of a food additive, expressed on a body-weight basis, that can be ingested daily over a lifetime without appreciable health risk, according to the World Health Organization (1987).

ACE K • *See* Acesulfame.

ACENAPHTENE • White needles derived from coal tar, insoluble in water. Used as a dye intermediate in pharmaceuticals, insecticides, fungicides, and plastics. *See* Coal Tar.

ACEPHATE (0-S-DIMETHYL ACETYLPHOSPHERAMIDOTHIOATE and 0,S-DIMETHYL PHOSPHORAMIDO THIOATE) • A contact and systemic pesticide used on cottonseed meal resulting from application to growing crops. The FDA permits a tolerance of 8 ppm in cottonseed and 4 ppm in soybean meal resulting from application to growing crop.

ACER SPICATUM LAM • *See* Mountain Maple Extract.

ACEROLA • Used as an antioxidant. Derived from the ripe fruit of the West Indian or Barbados cherry grown in Central America and the West Indies. A rich source of ascorbic acid. Used in vitamin C. No known toxicity.

ACESULFAME K • Acesulfame Potassium. Sunette. Ace K. In a petition filed in September 1982, the American Hoechst Corporation asked for approval to make this nonnutritive sweetener two hundred times sweeter than table sugar for use in chewing gum, dry beverage mixes, confections, canned fruit, gelatins, puddings, custards, and as a tabletop sweetener. The petition, including fifteen volumes of research studies, said the sweetener is not metabolized and would not add calories to the diet. The FDA approved acesulfame K on July 27, 1988, for use in dry food products and for sale in powder form or tablets that can be applied directly by the consumer. It has about the same sweetening power as aspartame *(see),* but unlike aspartame, has no calories. Hoechst obtained approval to use acesulfame K as an ingredient in liquids and baked goods and candies. The sweetener had previously been approved for use in twenty countries including France and Britain. Pepsi and Coca-Cola use it in Europe and Canada in their diet drinks.

The Food and Drug Administration said that four long-term animal studies in dogs, mice, and rats had not shown any toxic effects that could be pinned on the sweetener. However, the Center for Science in the Public Interest, a Washington, D.C.–based consumer group, sent a warning to the FDA more than six months before the sweetener's approval saying that animals fed acesulfame K in two different studies suffered more tumors than others that did not receive the compound. In another study cited by CSPI, diabetic rats had a higher blood level of cholesterol when fed the sweetener.

The FDA said in a press release that it had considered the Center's concerns and concluded that "any tumors found were typical of what could routinely be expected and were not due to feeding with acesulfame K."

Hoechst said that acesulfame is not metabolized by the body and is excreted unchanged by humans and animals. When heated to decomposition emits toxic fumes.

ACETAL • A volatile liquid derived from acetaldehyde *(see)* and alcohol and used as a solvent in synthetic perfumes such as jasmine. Also used in fruit flavorings (it has a nutlike aftertaste) and as a hypnotic in medicine. It is a central nervous system depressant, similar in action to paraldehyde but more toxic. Paraldehyde is a hypnotic and sedative whose side effects are respiratory depression, cardiovascular collapse, and possible high blood pressure reactions. No known skin toxicity.

ACETALDEHYDE • Ethanal. An intermediate *(see)* and solvent in the manufacture of perfumes. A flammable, colorless liquid, with a characteristic odor, occurring naturally in apples, broccoli, cheese, coffee, grapefruit, and other vegetables and fruit. Also used in the manufacture of synthetic rubber and in the silvering of mirrors. It is irritating to the mucous membranes, and ingestion of large doses may cause death by respiratory paralysis. Its ability to depress the central nervous system is greater than that of formaldehyde *(see),* and ingestion produces symptoms of "drunkenness." Acetaldehyde is thought to be a factor in the toxic effect caused by drinking alcohol after taking the anti-alcohol drug Antabuse. Inhalation, usually limited by intense irritation of lungs, can also be toxic. Skin toxicity not identified. GRAS.

ACETALDEHYDE ETHYL CIS-3-HEXENYL ACETAL • A synthetic flavoring. The FDA has as of this writing not yet done a thorough toxicology search. *See* Acetaldehyde.

ACETALDEHYDE PHENETHYL PROPYL ACETAL • Petital. A synthetic fruit flavoring agent for beverages, ice cream, ices, candy, and baked goods. *See* Acetaldehyde for toxicity.

p-**ACETAMIDOBENZOIC ACID** • *See* Benzoic Acid.

ACETANISOLE • A synthetic flavoring agent, colorless to pale yellow solid, with an odor of hawthorn or hay, moderately soluble in alcohol and most fixed oils. Acetanisole is used in butter, caramel, chocolate, fruit, nut, and vanilla flavorings, which go into beverages, ice cream, ices, candy, baked goods, and chewing gum.

ACETATE • Salt of acetic acid *(see)* used in liquor, nut, coffee, vanilla, honey, pineapple, and cheese flavorings for beverages, ice cream, sherbets, cakes, cookies, pastries, and candy. Also used in perfumery. May be irritating to the stomach if consumed in large quantities.

ACETIC ACID • Occurs naturally in apples, cheese, cocoa, coffee, grapes, skimmed milk, oranges, peaches, pineapples, strawberries, and a variety of other fruits and plants. Vinegar is about 4 to 6 percent acetic acid and essence of vinegar is about 14 percent. It is used in cheese, baked goods, and animal feeds. Can be used in standardized foods and thus need not be listed on the label. Solvent for gums, resins, and volatile oils. Styptic, it stops bleeding when applied to a cut on the skin. It is used in freckle-bleaching lotions, hand lotions, and hair dyes. Potential adverse skin reactions include irritation or itching, hives, and overgrowth of organisms that do not respond to germ-killers. In its glacial form (without much water) it is highly corrosive and its vapors are capable of producing lung obstruction. Less than 5 percent acetic acid in solution is mildly irritating to the skin. It caused cancer in rats and mice when given orally or by injection. GRAS.

ACETIC ACID, CITRONELLYL ESTER • A flavoring agent found in oils of citronella geranium, and about twenty other oils. Colorless liquid; fruity odor. Used as a flavoring agent in mayonnaise, salad dressings, and sauces. Mildly toxic by ingestion. A human skin irritant.

ACETIC ANHYDRIDE • Acetyl Oxide; Acetic Oxide. Colorless liquid with a strong odor, it is derived from oxidation of acetaldehyde *(see)*. It is used as a dehydrating and acetylating agent (*see* Dehydrated and Acetylated) and in the production of dyes, perfumes, plastics, food starch, and aspirin. It is a strong irritant and may cause burns and eye damage. The FDA says there is no reported use of the chemical and no toxicology information is available.

ACETIC ETHER • A synthetic agent, transparent, colorless liquid with a fragrant, refreshing odor, used in butter, butterscotch, fruit, nut, and spice flavorings for beverages, ice cream, ices, candy, baked goods (1,000 ppm), and chewing gum (4,000 ppm). Also used to coat vegetables.

ACETISOEUGENOL • White crystals with a clove odor, used as a flavoring agent. It is moderately toxic by ingestion. When heated to decomposition, it emits acrid smoke and irritating fumes. The FDA permits it use at a level not to exceed an amount reasonably required to accomplish the intended effect.

ACETOACETIC ESTER • *See* Ethyl Acetoacetate.

ACETOIN • Acetyl Methyl Carbinol. A flavoring agent and aroma carrier used in perfumery, it occurs naturally in broccoli, grapes, pears, cultured dairy products, cooked beef, and cooked chicken. As a product of fermentation and of cream ripened for churning, it is a colorless or pale yellow liquid or a white powder, has a buttery odor, and must be stored in a light-resistant container. It is used in raspberry, strawberry, butter, butterscotch, caramel, coconut, coffee, fruit, liquor, rum, nut, walnut, vanilla, cream soda, and cheese flavorings for beverages, ice cream, ices, candy, baked goods, margarine, gelatin desserts, cottage cheese, and shortenings. Mildly toxic by injection under the skin. A moderate skin irritant. When heated to decomposition it emits acrid smoke and fumes. GRAS.

2-ACETONAPHTHONE • Orange Crystals. 2-Naphthyl Ketone. White crystalline solid with an orange blossom odor. Used as a flavoring agent. Moderately toxic by ingestion. A human skin irritant. When heated to decomposition it emits acrid smoke and fumes.

ACETONE • A colorless ethereal liquid derived by oxidation or fermentation and used as a solvent for spices. Not more than 30 ppm may be a residual in the product. It is also frequently used in nail polish removers and nail finishes and as a solvent for airplane dope, fats, oils, and waxes. It can cause peeling and splitting of the nails, skin rashes on the fingers and elsewhere, and nail brittleness. Inhalation may irritate the lungs, and in large amounts it is narcotic, causing symptoms of drunkenness similar to ethanol *(see)*. In 1992, the FDA proposed a ban on acetone in astringent *(see)* products, because it had not been shown to be safe and effective as claimed.

ACETONE PEROXIDE • Acetone *(see)* to which an oxygen-containing compound has been added. A maturing agent for bleaching flour and dough, it has a sharp, acrid odor similar to hydrogen peroxide. A strong oxidizing agent, it can be damaging to the skin and eyes. The FDA says that although it is allowed as a food additive, there is no current reported use of the chemical, and therefore, although toxicology information may be available, it is not updated.

ACETOPHENONE • Acetyl Benzene. Benzoyl Methide. A synthetic agent derived from coal tar, with an odor of bitter almonds, used in strawberry, floral, fruit, cherry, almond, walnut, tobacco, vanilla, and tonka bean flavorings for beverages, ice creams, ices, candy, baked goods, gelatin desserts, and chewing gum. It occurs naturally in strawberries and tea and may cause allergic reactions. Poisonous by injection. Moderately toxic by ingestion. A skin and severe eye irritant. Narcotic in high concentrations. When heated to decomposition it emits acrid smoke and fumes. The FDA has up-to-date toxicology information available on this additive.

ACETOSTEARIN • Obtained from fats and oils, it is a glyceride *(see)* that the Select Committee on GRAS Substances stated in 1980 should be GRAS with no limitations. It is used as a protective coating for food and as a plasticizer. *See also* Stearic Acid.

ACETYL ACETONE • Acetoacetone. Diacetyl methane. Colorless to slightly yellow liquid with a pleasant odor. Used as a flavoring agent in food. The FDA requires it not be used in excess of the amount reasonably required to accomplish the intended effect. Moderately toxic if ingested, injected, or inhaled.

ACETYL BENZENE • *See* Acetophenone.

ACETYLAMINO-5-NITROTHIAZOLE • Acinitrazole. Trichloral. Tritheom. An animal drug used in turkeys and limited to 0.1 ppm in the bird's flesh by the FDA. When heated to decomposition emits toxic fumes.

ACETYL BENZOYL PEROXIDE • White crystals decomposed by water and organic matter. Used in medicine as a germicide and disinfectant. It is used to bleach flour. Toxic when ingested.

ACETYL BUTYRYL • *See* 2,3-Hexandione.

ACETYL-*o*-CREOSOL • *See* *o*-Tolyl Acetate.

3-ACETYL-2,5-DIMETHYL FURAN • Yellow liquid with a strong roasted-nut odor, it is used as a flavoring agent. When heated to decomposition it emits acrid smoke and irritating fumes. The FDA has toxicology information on this food additive. GRAS.

2-ACETYL;-3,(5 or 6)-DIMETHYLPYRAZINE, MIXTURE OF ISOMERS • Flavoring agent. The FDA has toxicology information on this food additive.

3-ACETYL-2,5-DIMETHYLTHIOPHENE • A flavoring agent.

2-ACETYL-3-ETHYLPYRAZINE • A flavoring agent.

ACETYL EUGENOL • *See* Eugenyl Acetate.

ACETYL FORMALDEHYDE • *See* Pyruvaldehyde.

ACETYL FORMIC ACID • *See* Pyruvaldehyde.

ACETYL HEXAMETHYL TETRALIN • Used in perfumes. It is closely related to acetyl ethyl tetramethyl tetralin, which was voluntarily removed from perfumes when it was reported to cause nerve damage in animals. The "hexa" component was inserted to make the fragrances less volatile and less allergenic.

***n*-ACETYL-L-METHIONINE** • (Free, Hydrated, Anhydrous, or Sodium or Potassium Salts.) Nutrient in foods except infant foods and products containing added nitrites/nitrates *(see both)*. Limited to 3.1 percent by weight of the total protein in the food. When heated to decomposition emits toxic fumes.

ACETYL METHYL CARBINYL ACETATE • *See* Acetoin.

2-ACETYL-5-METHYLFURAN • A synthetic flavoring.

ACETYL NONYRYL • *See* 2,3-Undecadione.

ACETYL PELARGONYL • *See* 2,3-Undecadione.

ACETYL PENTANOYL • *See* 2,3-Heptanedione.

ACETYL PROPIONYL • Yellow liquid. Soluble in water. Used as a butterscotch or chocolate-type flavoring. *See* 2,3-Pentanedione.

2-ACETYL PYRAZINE • Colorless to pale yellow crystals or liquid with a sweet popcornlike odor. Used as a flavoring agent. Skin and eye irritant. When heated to decomposition emits toxic fumes. GRAS.

2-ACETYL PYRROLE • Light beige to yellow crystals with a breadlike odor used as a flavoring agent. When heated to decomposition emits toxic fumes. GRAS when used at a level not in excess of the amount reasonably required.

4-ACETYL-6-TERT-BUTYL-1,1-DIMETHYL-INDANE • A synthetic flavoring.

2-ACETYLTHIAZOLE • Used in the manufacture of fungicides and dyes.

***p*-ACETYL TOLUENE** • *See* 4-Methyl Acetophenone.

ACETYL-*p*-TOLYL ACETATE • *See p*-Tolyl Acetate.

ACETYL TRIBUTYL CITRATE • *See* Citric Acid.

ACETYL TRIETHYL CITRATE • A clear oily, essentially odorless liquid used as a solvent and plasticizer. Moderately toxic by ingestion. When heated to decomposition it emits acrid smoke and fumes. *See* Citric Acid.

ACETYL TRIOCETYL CITRATE PECTIN • Citrus Pectin. A jelly-forming powder obtained from citrus peel and used as a texturizer and thickening agent to form gels with sugars and acids. Light in color. It has no known toxicity.

ACETYL VALERYL • Yellow liquid used as a cheese, butter, and miscellaneous flavors. *See* 2,3-Heptanedione.

ACETYL VANILLIN • *See* Vanillin Acetate.

ACETYLATED • Any organic compound that has been heated with acetic anhydride or acetyl chloride to remove its water. Acetylation is used to coat candy and other foods to hold in moisture. Acetic anhydride produces irritation and necrosis of tissues in vapor state and carries a warning against contact with skin and eyes.

ACETYLATED MONOGLYCERIDES • Acetylated Mono- and Diglycerides. Esters *(see)* of glycerin with acetic acid and edible fat-forming fatty acids. May be white to pale yellow liquids or solids. Bland tasting. Used as coating agents, emulsifiers, lubricants, solvents, and texture-modifying agents in baked goods, cake shortening, desserts, fruits, ice cream, margarine, meat products, nuts, oleomargarine, peanut butter, puddings, shortening, and whipped toppings. Use permitted by the FDA at a level not in excess of the amount reasonably required to accomplish the intended effect. When heated to decomposition it emits acrid smoke and irritating fumes.

ACETYLATED DISTARCH ADIPATE and PHOSPHATE • Starches *(see)* that have been modified to change their solubility and digestibility. The Select Committee on GRAS Substances stated in 1980 that there is no available evidence that demonstrates or suggests a hazard to the public when they are used at levels now current and in the manner now practiced. However, it is not possible to determine, without additional data, whether a significant increase in consumption would constitute a dietary hazard. They can continue GRAS with limitations on amounts that can be added to food.

ACETYLATED DISTARCH PROPANOL • A starch *(see)* that has been modified to change it solubility and digestibility. The final report to the FDA of the Select Committee on GRAS Substances stated in 1980 that although no evidence in the available information on it demonstrates a hazard to the public at current use levels, uncertainties exist requiring that additional studies be conducted. GRAS status is continued while tests are being completed and evaluated, the FDA said in 1980. Since then, no action has been reported.

ACETYLATED HYDROGENATED COTTONSEED GLYCERIDE • *See* Cottonseed Oil.

ACETYLATED HYDROGENATED LARD GLYCERIDE • *See* Lard and Lard Oils.

ACETYLATED HYDROGENATED VEGETABLE GLYCERIDE • *See* Vegetable Oils.

ACETYLATED MONOGLYCERIDES • Emulsifiers used in food, food processing, and food packaging restricted only according to good manufacturing practices to accomplish the intended effect.

ACETYLATED SUCROSE DISTEARATE • The acetyl ester of sucrose distearate (*see* Ester and Sucrose Distearate).

ACETYLISOEUGENOL • Isoeugenol acetate. White crystals with a spicy, clove-like odor, it is used as an aroma and flavor carrier in foods. In perfumery, it is used especially for carnation-type odors.

ACETYLMETHYL CARBINOL • Slightly yellow liquid or crystals used as an aroma and flavor carrier. *See* Acetoin.

2- or 3-ACETYLPYRIDINE • Additives used in making synthetic food additives.

2-ACETYLTHIAZOLE • Used in the manufacture of fungicides and dyes.

ACHILLEIC ACID • *See* Aconitic Acid.

ACID • An acid is a substance capable of turning blue litmus paper red and of forming hydrogen ions when dissolved in water. An acid aqueous solution is one that has a pH *(see)* of less than 7. Citric acid *(see)* is an example of a widely used acid in foods.

ACID HYDROLYZED PROTEINS • Acid Hydrolyzed Milk Protein. Hydrolyzed Plant Protein (HPP). Hydrolyzed Vegetable Protein (HVP) Hydrolyzed (Source) Protein Extract. Composed mainly of amino acids, small peptides, and salts resulting from almost complete hydrolysis *(see)* of peptide bones in edible protein materials treated with heat or food-grade acids. The edible proteins used as raw materials are derived from corn, soy, wheat, yeast, peanuts, rice, or other suitable vegetable or plant sources, or from milk. Produces maybe in liquid, paste, powder, or granular form. Used as a flavoring agent or flavor enhancer in bologna, salami, sauces, and stuffing. Use at level not in excess of the amount reasonably required to accomplish the intended effect. When heated to decomposition it emits acrid smoke and irritating fumes.

ACID-MODIFIED STARCHES • Usually made by mixing an acid—such as hydrochloric or sulfuric—water, and starch at temperatures too low for gelatinization. When the starch has been reduced in viscosity to the degree desired, the acid is neutralized and the starch is filtered, washed, and dried. It is done so that starches can be cooked and used at higher concentrations than unmodified starches. Acid-modified starches are often used for salad dressings and puddings and as inexpensive thickening agents. The final report to the FDA of the Select Committee on GRAS Substances stated in 1980 that acid-modified starches are GRAS with no limitations.

ACID POTASSIUM SULFITE • *See* Sulfites.

ACIDOPHILUS • A type of bacteria that ferments milk and has been used medically to treat intestinal disorders.

ACIDS • *See* Acidulants.

ACIDULANTS • Acids. An acid is a substance capable of turning blue litmus paper red and of forming hydrogen ions when dissolved in water. An acid aqueous solution is one with a pH less than 7 (*see* pH). Acidulants are acids that make a substance more acid and function as flavoring agent to acidify taste, to blend unrelated flavoring characteristics, and to mask any undesirable aftertaste. Acidulants are also used as preservatives to prevent germ and spore growths that spoil foods. Acidulants control the acid-alkali (pH) balance and are used in meat curings to enhance color and flavor and as a preservative. Among the most common acids added to foods are acetic, propionic, and sorbic *(see all)*.

ACIFLUOREN, SODIUM • Herbicide. FDA tolerances are 0.02 ppm residues in cattle and sheep, kidney and liver. Residues in rice, milk, and eggs is tolerated at 0.1 ppm.

ACIMETON • Lobamine. Banthionine. Cynaron. Methilanin. Neston. White crystalline platelets with a characteristic odor. Used as a dietary supplement and nutrient. Moderately toxic by ingestion and other routes. When heated to decomposition it emits toxic fumes. *See* Methionine.

ACONITIC ACID • Citridic Acid. Equisetic Acid. Achilic Acid. A flavoring agent found in beetroot and cane sugar. Most of the commercial aconitic acids, however, are manufactured by sulfuric acid dehydration of citric acid. It is used in fruit, brandy and rum flavorings for beverages, ice cream, ices, candy, baked goods, liquors, and chewing gum. Also used in the manufacture of plastics and buna rubber. As of this writing, the FDA's data bank has not yet done a toxicology search of the literature concerning this additive. GRAS.

ACROLEIN • A yellow, transparent liquid byproduct of petroleum produced by the oxidation of propylene. Sources include combustion of wood, paper, cotton, petroleum products, and polyolefins. Used in modifying food starch. Used in making plastics and metal products. Toxic, causes tearing and intense irritation of the upper respiratory tract. It is also a skin irritant and a fire hazard from heat and flame. The FDA's data bank says there is no reported use of the chemical and there is no toxicology information available.

ACRYLAMIDE • Colorless, odorless crystals soluble in water and derived from acrylonitrile and sulfuric acid. It is used in clarifying beet sugar or cane sugar juice and in cornstarch. It is also used as a thickener and suspending agent in nonmedicated animal feeds. It is toxic by skin absorption.

ACRYLAMIDE-SODIUM ACRYLATE RESIN • Used to dilute pesticides for application.

ACRYLATE-ACRYLAMIDE RESIN • Acrylic Acid. Colorless, odorless crystals soluble in water and derived from acrylonitrile and sulfuric acid. It is used as a clarifying agent in beet sugar and cane sugar juice and liquor or corn starch hydrolysate (5 ppm by weight of juice, 10 ppm by weight of liquor or hydrolysate). It is also used in the manufacture of dyes, adhesives, and in permanent-press fabrics, nail enamels, and face masks. It is toxic by skin absorption.

ACRYLIC ACID • Colorless liquid with an acrid odor, it is derived by condensing ethylene oxide with hydrocyanic acid followed by reaction with sulfuric acid. It is used for making plastics and resins.

ACRYLIC RESINS • Polymers *(see)* of acrylics. Used in waxy oils, base coats, protective coatings, and waterproofing. Acrylates *(see),* if inhaled, can cause allergic reactions in humans.

ACRYLONITRILE COPOLYMERS • Used in packaging materials. When heated to decomposition it emits acrid smoke and irritating fumes.

ACRYLONITRILE POLYMER WITH STYRENE • Used in coatings and films in packaging materials. No restrictions, but cyanide and its compounds are on the Community Right-To-Know List *(see)*. *See also* Styrene.

ACTADECYLSILOXYDIMETHYLSIOLOXYPOLYSILOXANE • A component of defoaming agents *(see)* used in processing beets and yeast. No known toxicity.

ACTIVATED CHARCOAL (CARBON) • Charcoal is obtained by destructive distillation of organic material such as vegetables or animal bones and is activated by heating with steam or carbon dioxide, which results in a porous material. It is used to relieve intestinal discomfort and diarrhea and to counteract poisons. It is the main ingredient in the "universal antidote." Activated charcoal is recognized by the FDA for the treatment of swallowed poisons. It adheres to many drugs and chemicals inhibiting their absorption from the GI tract. Potential adverse reactions include black stools and nausea. Used to remove impurities that cause undesirable color, taste, or odor in liquid. The major sources are lignite, coal, and coke. The Select Committee of the Federation of American Societies for Experimental Biology (FASEB), under contract to the FDA, concluded that it is not a hazard to human health at current or possible future use levels. However, the Committee said because the substance is extensively used in the food industry, it would be prudent to have purity specifications for food-grade activated carbon to assure the absence of any cancer-causing hydrocarbons in food. It can cause a dust irritation, particularly to the eyes and mucous membranes.

ACTIVATED 7-DEHYDROCHOLESTEROL • *See* Vitamin D$_3$.

ADENOSINE • White crystalline powder with mild saline or bitter taste. It is isolated by the hydrolysis of yeast nucleic acid.

ADENOSINE PHOSPHATE • *See* Adenosine Triphosphate.

ADENOSINE TRIPHOSPHATE • Adenylic Acid. An organic compound that is derived from adenosine *(see)*. A fundamental unit of nucleic acid, it serves as a source of energy for biochemical transformation in plants, photosynthesis, and also for many chemical reactions in the body, especially those associated with muscular activity.

ADI • Abbreviation for Acceptable Daily Intake *(see)*.

ADIPATES • The salt of adipic acid *(see)* used in food packaging. Some are suspected cancer-causing agents.

ADIPIC ACID • Hexanedioic Acid. Colorless needlelike formations, fairly insoluble in water; found in beets. A buffering and neutralizing agent impervious to humidity. Used in flavorings for baked goods, baking powder, condiments, dairy products, meat products, oils, oleomargarine, relishes, snack foods, canned vegetables, beverages, and gelatin desserts (5,000 ppm) to impart a smooth-tart taste. Also used as a buffer and neutralizing agent in confections, but limited to 3 percent of contents and in the manufacture of plastics and nylons, and as a substitute for tartaric acid *(see)* in baking powders because it is impervious to humidity. No known toxicity. The final report to the FDA of the Select Committee on GRAS Substances stated in 1980 that it should continue its GRAS status with no limitations other than good manufacturing practices. Poison by injection and moderately toxic by other routes. A severe eye irritant. Combustible when exposed to flame; can react with oxidizing materials.

ADIPIC ANHYDRIDE • A starch-modifying agent, not to exceed .12 percent of the starch compound. There is no reported use of the chemical and there is no toxicology information available, according to the FDA's data bank. *See* Modified Starch.

ADSORBATE • A powdered flavor made by coating liquid flavoring on the surface of a powder such as cornstarch, salt, or maltodextrin *(see* all).

AEROSOL • Small particles of material suspended in gas.

AFLATOXIN • A mold that contaminates corn and peanuts. Poisonous by ingestion and moderately toxic by other routes. Carcinogenic and mutagenic.

AGAR-AGAR • Japanese Isinglass. A stabilizer and thickener, it is transparent, odorless, and tasteless, and obtained from various seaweed found in the Pacific and Indian oceans and the Sea of Japan. Agar was the first seaweed to be extracted, purified, and dried. Discovered by a Japanese innkeeper around 1658 and introduced in Europe and the United States by visitors from China in the 1800s as a substitute for gelatin, it goes into beverages, ice cream, ices, frozen custard, sherbet, meringue, baked goods, jelly, frozen candied sweet potatoes, icings, confections, artificially sweetened jellies and preserves. It can be 1.2 percent of candy and .25 percent of frozen desserts, jelly, and preserves. Agar serves as a substitute for gelatin and is used for thickening milk and cream. It is also a bulk laxative, and aside from causing an occasional allergic reaction is nontoxic. The final report to the FDA of the Select Committee on GRAS Substances stated in 1980 that there is no evidence in the available information that it is a hazard to the public when used as it is now, and it should continue its GRAS status with limitations on amounts that can be added to food. Mildly toxic by ingestion.

AGAVE LECHUGUILLA • American Aloe. Native to the warm part of the United States and known by its heavy, stiff leaf and tall panicle or spike of candelabralike flowers. The leaves are used for a juice employed in cosmetics as an adhesive and in medicines as a diuretic. The fermented juice is popular in Mexico for its distilled spirit (mescal). Some species are cultivated for their fibers, which are used in thread and rope. No known toxicity.

AGRIMONY EXTRACT • An extract of *Agrimonia eupatoria,* an herb found in north temperate regions. It has yellow flowers and bristly fruit.

AI • Abbreviation for Adequate Intake. A value based on observed or experimentally determined approximations of nutrient intake by a group of healthy people. It is used when the RDA *(see)* cannot be determined.

AKLOMIDE • Gray scales from alcohol, it is used as an animal drug to combat fungus infections in chickens. The FDA residue tolerances are: 4.5 ppm in liver and muscle of uncooked edible tissue of chickens and 3 ppm in skin and fat.

ALACHLOR • Lasso. Alanex. A preemergent herbicide. The FDA permits its use. The EPA has determined it is a cancer-causing agent in rats and mice.

ALANEX • *See* Alachlor.

ALANINE (B-, L-, and DL-) • Colorless crystals derived from protein. A nonessential amino acid, it is used in microbiological research and as a dietary supplement in the L and DL forms. It is used as a flavor enhancer at 1 percent for pickling spice. It is now GRAS for addition to food. It caused cancer of the skin in mice and tumors when injected into their abdomens.

ALAR • *See* Daminozide.

ALBENDAZOLE • Zental. Valbazen. A worm medicine given to cattle. The FDA tolerances for residues are: 0.2 ppm in uncooked edible cattle tissue; 0.6 in muscle; 1.2 ppm in liver; 1.8 ppm in kidney; 2.4 ppm in fat.

ALBUMEN • *See* Albumin.

ALBUMIN • (Albumen). A group of simple proteins composed of nitrogen, carbon, hydrogen, oxygen, and sulfur that are soluble in water. Albumin is usually derived from egg white and employed as an emulsifier in foods and cosmetics. May cause a reaction to those allergic to eggs. In large amounts can produce symptoms of lack of biotin, a growth factor in the lining of the cells.

ALBUMIN MACRO AGGREGATES • Used as a binder and firming agent in sausage, soups, stews, and wine. Poisonous by injection.

ALCOHOL • Ethyl Alcohol. Ethanol. Alcohol is widely used as a solvent in the cosmetic and food fields. Alcohol is manufactured by the fermentation of starch, sugar, and other carbohydrates. It is clear, colorless, and flammable, with somewhat pleasant odor and a burning taste. Medicinally used externally as an antiseptic and internally as a stimulant and hypnotic. *Absolute alcohol* is ethyl alcohol to which a substance has been added to make it unfit for drinking. *Rubbing alco-*

hol contains not less than 68.5 percent and not more than 71.5 percent by volume of absolute alcohol and a remainder of denaturants, such as perfume oils. Toxic in large doses. *See also* Anisyl Alcohol.

ALCOHOL, DENATURED • This refers to ethyl alcohol, which is deliberately made unfit for drinking.

ALCOHOL, SDA-3A • *See* alcohol denatured.

ALCOHOLS / PHOSPHATE ESTERS • May be used at a level not to exceed 0.2 percent to assist in the lye peeling of fruit and vegetables.

ALDEHYDE, ALIPHATIC • A class of organic chemical compounds intermediate between acids and alcohols. Aldehyde contains less oxygen than acids and less hydrogen than alcohols. Formaldehyde *(see)*, a preservative, is an example of an aldehyde widely used in cosmetics. Benzaldehyde and cinnamic aldehydes are used to scent perfumes. Most are irritating to the skin and gastrointestinal tract.

ALDICARB • Temik. Crystals from isopropyl ether used as an insecticide, spider killer, and worm killer on citrus pulp in growing crop. FDA tolerance is 0.6 ppm, 0.3 ppm in cottonseed hulls, and 0.5 ppm in sorghum.

ALDRIN • Aldrex. Altox. Drinox. A pesticide. Poison by ingestion, skin contact, intravenous, intraperitoneal and other routes. Causes tumors, cancer, and birth defects. Human systemic effects by ingestion: excitement, tremors, and nausea or vomiting. Continued acute exposure causes liver damage.

ALFALFA • Herb and Seed. Lucerne. Extract of *Medicago sativa*. A natural cola, liquor, and maple flavoring agent for beverages and cordials. Alfalfa is widely cultivated for forage and is a commercial source of chlorophyll. GRAS.

ALGAE, BROWN • Kelp. Ground, dried seaweed used to carry natural spices, seasonings, and flavorings. A source of alginic acid *(see)*. Also used in chewing-gum base. All derivatives of alginic acid are designated "algin." The food industry is one of the major users of alginates *(see)* along with the pharmaceutical, cosmetic, rubber, and paper industries. The United States is the largest producer of alginates. Algae is claimed to prevent wrinkles and to moisturize the skin, but the American Medical Association denies any validity for algae's therapeutic benefits. However, seaweed products are widely used in cosmetics for many purposes. The final report to the FDA of the Select Committee on GRAS Substances stated in 1980 that it should continue its GRAS status with no limitations other than good manufacturing practices. Nontoxic. *See* Alginates.

ALGAE MEAL, DRIED • Permanently listed to be used in chicken feed to enhance color of chicken skin and egg yolks. No known toxicity.

ALGAE, RED • A natural extract of seaweed used to carry natural spices, seasonings, and flavorings. Nontoxic GRAS. *See* Alginates.

ALGANET • Coloring agent used in casings and rendered fats.

ALGIN • The sodium salt of alginic acid *(see)*, it is used in cheeses, frozen desserts, soda water, jellies, and preserves as a stabilizer. GRAS.

ALGINATES • Ammonium, Calcium, Potassium, and Sodium. All derivatives of alginic acid are designated "algin." Gelatinous substances obtained from certain seaweed and used as stabilizers and water retainers in beverages, ice cream, ices, frozen custard, emulsions, desserts, baked goods, and confectionery ingredients. A clarifying agent for wine, chocolate milk, meat, toppings, cheeses, cheese spreads, cheese snacks, salad dressings, and artificially sweetened jelly and jam ingredients. Alginates are used also as stabilizers in gassed cream (pressure-dispensed whipped cream). The alginates assure a creamy texture and prevent formation of ice crystals in ice creams. Alginates have been used in the making of ice pops to impart smoothness of texture by ensuring that the fruit flavors are uniformly distributed throughout the ice crystals during freezing, helping the pops to retain flavor and color, and to stop dripping. The final report to the FDA of the Select Committee on GRAS Substances stated in 1980 that there is no evidence in the available information that calcium, sodium, or potassium alginates are a hazard to the public when used as they are now, and their GRAS status will continue with limitations on the amounts that can be added to food. Alginates are also used as emulsifiers in hand lotions obtained from certain seaweed and used as emulsifiers in hand lotions and creams, as thickening agents in shampoos, wave sets, and lotions. Ammonium alginate is used in boiler water and is not GRAS.

ALGINIC ACID • Obtained as a highly gelatinous precipitate from seaweed. It is odorless and tasteless and is used as a stabilizer in ice cream, frozen custard, ice milk, fruit, sherbet, water ices, beverages, icings, cheeses, cheese spreads, cheese snacks, French dressing, and salad dressing. It is also used as a defoaming agent in processed foods. Capable of absorbing 200 to 300 times its weight of water and salts. Also used in sizing paper and textiles and as a stabilizer in cosmetics. The sodium carbonate *(see)* extracts of brown dried seaweed are treated with acid to achieve the result. Resembles albumin or gelatin *(see both)*. Alginic acid is slowly soluble in water, forming a thick liquid. The World Health Organization Committee on Food Additives observed that in a 90-day study in rats, 15 percent alginate in the diet resulted in an enlarged, distended, heavy lower intestine, bumpy urinary bladder, and calcium deposits in the renal pelvis. A slight decrease in growth was also seen. The Committee noted that alginic acid and its salts have a laxative effect at high level of intake. The Committee did not offer an ADI *(see)* for alginic acid. GRAS.

ALITAME • A candidate for approval as an artificial sweetener, it has two thousand times the sweetness of sugar and has no calories. Its potential use is in all areas requiring sweetening. It is derived from the amino acid alanine *(see)* and is related to aspartame *(see)*. The benefits include a clean, sweet taste, good stability at high temperatures, broad pH *(see)* range, and high water solubility. The drawbacks are the off-flavor from prolonged storage in some acidic solutions.

ALKALI • The term originally covered the caustic and mild forms of potash and soda. Now a substance is regarded as an alkali if it gives hydroxyl ions in solution. An alkaline aqueous solution is one with a pH *(see)* greater than 7. Sodium bicarbonate is an example of an alkali that is used to neutralize excess acidity.

ALKALOID • A compound of vegetable origin. Usually derived from a nitrogen compound such as pyridine, quinoline, isoquinoline, or pyrrole, designated by the ending -ine. Examples are atropine, morphine, nicotine, quinine, codeine, caffeine, cocaine, and strychnine. The alkaloids are potent and include the hallucinogen mescaline and the deadly poison brucine. There are alkaloids that act on the liver, nerves, lungs, and digestive systems.

ALKANE • *See* Alkanet Root.

ALKANET ROOT • Alkane Ferrous Sulfate. A red coloring obtained from extraction of the herblike tree root grown in Asia Minor and the Mediterranean. Used as a copper or blue coloring (when combined with metals) for hair oils and other cosmetics. It was also used as a coloring for wines, inks, and sausage casings. The FDA withdrew the authorization for use in 1988.

ALKANNIN • A red powder and the principal ingredient of alkanet root *(see)*. Used as an astringent in cosmetics and to color cosmetics.

ALKANOMIDE • Produced by condensation of coconut oil, fatty acids, and diethanolamine *(see);* used in delinting cotton seeds. FDA tolerance is less than 0.2 percent of weight by application. *See* diethanolamine for potential cancer hazard.

ALKYL • Meaning "from alcohol," usually derived from alkane. Any one of a series of saturated hydrocarbons such as methane. The introduction of one or more alkyls into a compound is to make the product more soluble. The mixture is usually employed with surfactants *(see),* which have a tendency to float when not alkylated.

ALKYL BETAINES • *See* Alkyl Sulfates.

ALKYL ETHER SULFATES • *See* Alkyl Sulfates.

ALKYL SULFATES • Surfactants *(see)* used in foods, drugs, and cosmetics. The Germans during World War II developed these compounds when vegetable fats and oils were scarce. A large number of alkyl sulfates have been prepared from primary alcohols by treatment with sulfuric acid; the alcohols are usually prepared from fatty acids *(see)*. Alkyl sulfates are low in acute and chronic toxicity but may cause skin irritation.

ALKYLENE OXIDE ADDUCTS OF ALKYL ALCOHOLS • Used to assist in lye peeling of fruits and vegetables. FDA permits less than 0.2 percent in lye.

ALLERGEN • A substance that provokes an allergic reaction in the susceptible but does not normally affect other people. Plant pollens, fungi spores, and animal danders are some of the common allergens.

ALLERGIC CONTACT DERMATITIS • ACD. Skin rash caused by direct contact with a substance to which the skin is sensitive. Symptoms include a red rash, swelling, and intense itching. Blisters may develop and break open, forming a crust. ACD may develop at any age and may be acute or chronic. Symptoms may appear seven to ten days after the first exposure to an allergen. More often, the allergic reaction doesn't develop for many years and may require many repeated low-level exposures. Once the sensitivity does develop, however, contact with the triggering allergen will produce symptoms within 24–48 hours. An attack builds in severity from one to seven days. Even without treatment, healing often occurs in one or two weeks, though it may take a month or longer.

ALLERGIC REACTION • An adverse immune response following repeated contact with otherwise harmless substances such as pollens, molds, foods, cosmetics, and drugs.

ALLERGY • An altered immune response to a specific substance, such as ragweed, pollen, on reexposure to it.

ALLOMALEIC ACID • *See* Fumaric Acid.

ALLSPICE • A natural flavoring from the dried berries of the allspice tree. Allspice is used in liquor, meat, and spice flavorings for beverages, ice cream, ices, candy, baked goods (1,400 ppm), chewing gum, condiments (1,000 ppm), and meats. Allspice oleoresin (a natural mixture of oil and resin) is used in sausage flavoring for baked goods, meat, and condiments. Allspice oil is used in sausage, berry cola, peach, rum, nut, allspice, cinnamon, ginger, nutmeg, and eggnog flavorings for beverages, ice cream, ices, candy, baked goods, chewing gum (1,700 ppm), condiments, pickles, meats, liquors, and soups. A weak sensitizer that may cause skin rash on contact. GRAS.

ALLYIC SULFIDES • Found in garlic and onions, these compounds may protect against cancer-causing agents by stimulating production of a detoxification enzyme, glutathione-S-transferase.

ALLYL- • Prefix meaning, "derived from allyl alcohol" *(see)*.

ALLYL ALCOHOL • A colorless, pungent liquid made chiefly from allyl chloride heated to a thick substance in the presence of oxygen. It is used to make resins and plasticizers and as the basis for many synthetic flavorings.

***p*-ALLYL ANISOLE** • Esdragol. Isoanethole. Tarragon. Isolated from the rind of *Persea gratissima garth,* and from oil of estragon, found in oils of Russian anise, basil, fennel, turpentine, and others. A flavoring agent used in bakery products, both alcoholic and nonalcoholic beverages, chewing gum, confections, fish, ice cream, salads, sauces, and vinegar.

ALLYL ANTHRANILATE • A synthetic citrus fruit and grape flavoring agent for beverages, ice cream, ices, candy, baked goods, and gelatin desserts. No known toxicity.

ALLYL BUTYRATE • A synthetic butter, fruit, and pineapple flavoring agent for beverages, ice cream, ices, candy, baked goods, and gelatin desserts. No known toxicity.

ALLYL CAPROATE • 2-Propenyl-N-Hexanoate. Flavoring agent used in candy, gelatin desserts, puddings. Poison by ingestion and skin contact. An irritant to human skin.

ALLYL CINNAMATE • A light to yellow liquid with a cherry odor, it is used as a synthetic fruit and grape flavoring agent for beverages, ice cream, ices, candy, baked goods. Moderately toxic by ingestion. Human skin irritant. When heated to decomposition emits acrid smoke and irritating fumes.

ALLYL CROTONATE • Used in the manufacture of vitamins and flavorings.

ALLYL CYCLOHEXANE ACETATE • A synthetic pineapple flavoring agent for beverages, ice cream, ices, candy, baked goods.

ALLYL CYCLOHEXANE BUTYRATE • A synthetic pineapple flavoring agent for beverages, ice cream, ices, candy, baked goods.

ALLYL CYCLOHEXANE HEXANOATE • A synthetic fruit flavoring agent for beverages, ice cream, ices, candy, baked goods.

ALLYL CYCLOHEXANE PROPIONATE • A synthetic, liquid and colorless with a pineapplelike odor, used in pineapple flavorings for beverages, ice cream, ices, candy, baked goods, gelatin desserts, puddings, chewing gum, and icings. No known toxicity. Poisonous by ingestion. When heated to decomposition it emits acrid smoke and irritating fumes.

ALLYL DISULFIDE • Found naturally in garlic and leeks but considered a synthetic flavoring. It is used in garlic, onion, and spice flavorings for meats and condiments. No known toxicity.

ALLYL ENANTHATE • *See* Allyl Heptanoate.

ALLYL 2-ETHYLBUTYRATE • A synthetic berry, fruit, and brandy flavoring agent for beverages, ice cream, ices, candy, baked goods, gelatin desserts, and puddings. GRAS.

ALLYL 2-FUROATE • A synthetic coffee and pineapple flavoring agent for beverages, ice cream, ices, candy, baked goods, and gelatin desserts. GRAS.

ALLYL HEPTANOATE • A synthetic berry, fruit, and brandy flavoring agent for beverages, ice cream, ices, candy, baked goods, gelatin desserts, and chewing gum. Moderately toxic by ingestion and skin contact. A human skin irritant. Combustible liquid. When heated to decomposition it emits acrid smoke and irritating fumes. GRAS.

ALLYL HEXANOATE • A synthetic orange, strawberry, apple, apricot, peach, pineapple, and tutti-frutti flavoring agent for beverages, ice cream, ices, candy, baked goods, gelatin desserts, and toppings. GRAS.

ALLYL a-IONONE • Cetone V. A synthetic agent, yellow, with a strong fruity, pineapplelike odor, used in fruit flavorings for beverages, ice cream, ices, candy, baked goods, gelatin desserts, and toppings. A skin irritant. GRAS.

ALLYL ISOTHIOCYANATE • Mustard Oil. A naturally occurring agent in mustard, horseradish, and onion used in meat and spice flavorings for beverages, ice cream, ices, candy, condiments, meat, and pickles. Colorless or pale yellow with a pungent, irritating odor and acrid taste. It is used also in the manufacture of war gas. Can cause blisters and other skin problems. Toxic.

ALLYL ISOVALERATE • Derived from valeric acid *(see)*, it is used as a flavoring.

ALLYL MERCAPTAN • A synthetic spice flavoring agent for beverages, ice cream, ices, candy, baked goods, and meats. Poison by inhalation and ingestion. Strong irritant to the skin and mucous membranes. Dangerous fire hazard.

4-ALLYL-2-METHOXY PHENOL • *See* Eugenol.

ALLYL METHYL DISULFIDE • A synthetic flavoring. *See* Allyl Alcohol and Sulfides.

ALLYL METHYL TRISULFIDE • *See* Allyl Alcohol and Sulfides.

ALLYL NONANOATE • A synthetic fruit and wine flavoring agent for beverages, ice cream, ices, candy, baked goods, and meats.

ALLYL OCTANOATE • A synthetic pineapple flavoring agent for beverages, ice cream, ices, candy, baked goods, and gelatin desserts. Moderately toxic by ingestion. A skin irritant.

ALLYL PELARGONATE • Liquid, fruity odor used in flavors and perfumes.

ALLYL PHENOXYACETATATE • Acetate PA. A synthetic fruit and grape-flavoring agent for beverages, ice cream, ices, candy, baked goods, and gelatin desserts. Moderately toxic by ingestion and skin contact.

ALLYL PHENYLACETATE • A synthetic pineapple and honey flavoring agent for beverages, ice cream, ices, candy, baked goods.

ALLYL PROPIONATE • A synthetic pineapple flavoring agent for beverages, ice cream, ices, candy, baked goods.

ALLYL SORBATE • A synthetic fruit and grape-flavoring agent for beverages, ice cream, ices, candy, baked goods, and gelatin desserts.

ALLYL SULFHYDRATE • *See* Allyl Mercaptan.

ALLYL SULFIDE • A synthetic fruit and grape-flavoring agent for beverages, ice cream, ices, candy, baked goods, condiments, and meats. Occurs naturally in garlic and horseradish. Irritates the eyes and respiratory tract. Readily absorbed through the skin. Acute exposure can cause unconsciousness. Long-term exposure can cause liver and kidney damage.

ALLYL THIOPROPIONATE • A flavoring derived from the onion.

ALLYL TIGLATE • A synthetic fruit and grape-flavoring agent for beverages, ice cream, ices, candy, baked goods.

ALLYL 10-UNDECENOATE • A synthetic fruit flavoring agent for beverages, ice cream, ices, candy, baked goods.

ALLYL UNDECYLENATE • *See* Allyl 10-Undecenoate.

p-**ALLYLANISOLE** • *See* Estragole.

ALLYL THIOL • *See* Allyl Mercaptan.

4-ALLYLVERATROLE • *See* Eugenyl Methyl Ether.

ALMOND OIL • Bitter Almond Oil. A flavoring agent from the ripe seed of a small tree grown in Italy, Spain, and France. Colorless or slightly yellow, strong almond odor, and mild taste. Used in cherry and almond flavorings for beverages, ice cream, ices, candy, baked goods, chewing gums, maraschino cherries, and gelatin desserts. Used also in the manufacture of liqueurs and perfumes. It is distilled to remove hydrocyanic acid (prussic acid), which is toxic. Nontoxic without the hydrocyanic acid. GRAS.

ALOE VERA • A compound expressed from the aloe plant leaf from a South African lilylike plant. Used in bitters, vermouth, and spice flavorings for beverages (2,000 ppm) and alcoholic drinks. It contains 99.5 percent water, with the remaining .5 percent composed of some twenty amino acids *(see)* and carbohydrates. It has been used as a cathartic but was found to cause severe intestinal cramps and sometimes kidney damage. Cross-reacts with benzoin and balsam Peru in those who are allergic to these ingredients. There is reported use of the chemical; it has not yet been assigned for toxicology literature.

ALPHA-AMYLASE • An enzyme used to modify food starch. (*See* modified starch.)

ALPHA-GALACTOSIDASE FROM MORTIERELLA VINACEAE • An enzyme used in the product of sugar from sugar beets to increase sugar yield. No residue is permitted in finished product.

(ALPHA RS, 2R)-FLUVALINATE (RS)-ALPHA-CYANO-3-PHENOXYBEN-ZYL(R)-2[2-CHLORO-4-TRIFLUOROMETHYL)ANILINO]-3-METHYL BUTONATE • An insecticide. FDA residue tolerances are 1.0 ppm as a residue on cottonseed; 1.0 ppm as a residue in cottonseed oil; 0.3 ppm in cottonseed hulls; 0.05 ppm as a residue in meat byproducts and fat of cattle, goats, hogs, poultry, and sheep; 0.01 ppm as residues in milk, eggs, fat, meat of cattle, goats, hogs, poultry, and sheep. Contains cyanide *(see)*.

ALPHA TOCOPHEROL • There is reported use of the chemical; it has not yet been assigned for toxicology literature. *See* Tocopherols and Vitamin E.

ALTHEA FLOWERS or ROOT • Marshmallow Root. A natural flavoring substance from a plant grown in Europe, Asia, and the United States. The dried root is used in strawberry, cherry, and root-beer flavorings for beverages. The boiled root is used as a demulcent in ointments to soothe mucous membranes. The roots, flowers, and leaves are used externally as a poultice. Nontoxic. There is reported use of the chemical, it has not yet been assigned for toxicology literature.

ALUM • Potash Alum. Aluminum Ammonium. Potassium Sulfate. A colorless, odorless, crystalline, water-soluble solid used in astringent lotions, after-shave lotions, and as a styptic (stops bleeding). A double sulfate of aluminum and ammonium potassium, it is also employed to harden gelatin, size paper, or waterproof fabrics. In concentrated solutions alum has produced gum damage and fatal intestinal hemorrhages. It has a low toxicity in experimental animals but ingestion of thirty grams (an ounce) has killed an adult human. It is also known to cause kidney damage. Concentrated doses have damaged gums. Liquid alum has been found by Penn State researchers to be capable of removing over 99 percent of phosphates from waste water. GRAS when used in packaging only.

ALUMINUM • Silvery white, crystalline solid. It is frequently used in food additives and cosmetics. Ingestion or inhalation of aluminum can aggravate kidney and lung disorders. Aluminum deposits have been found in the brains of Alzheimer's victims but its part, if any, in this degenerative brain disorder is not clear.

ALUMINUM AMMONIUM SULFATE • Odorless, colorless crystals with a strong astringent taste. Used in purifying drinking water, in baking powders, as a buffer and neutralizing agent in milling, and in the cereal industries. Used also for fireproofing and in the manufacture of vegetable glue and artificial gems. In medicine, it is an astringent and styptic (stops bleeding). Ingestion of large amounts may cause burning in mouth and pharynx, vomiting, and diarrhea. The final report to the FDA of the Select Committee on GRAS Substances stated in 1980 that it should continue its GRAS status with no limitations other than good manufacturing practices.

ALUMINUM CALCIUM SILICATE • Anticaking agent used so that it is 2 percent of table salt. Used also in vanilla powder to prevent caking. Essentially harmless when given orally. GRAS.

ALUMINUM DISTEARATE • A binder that holds loose powders together when compressed into a solid cake form. *See* Aluminum Stearates.

ALUMINUM HYDROXIDE • An alkali used as a leavening agent in the production of baked goods. Mild astringent and alkali used in antiperspirants, dentifrices, and dusting powders. A white gelatinous mass used as a drying agent, catalyst, adsorbent, and coloring agent in many cosmetic processes. Also used as a gastric antacid in medicine. Practically insoluble in water but not in alkaline solutions. Aluminum hydroxide has a low toxicity but may cause constipation if ingested. The final report to the FDA of the Select Committee on GRAS Substances stated in 1980 that it should continue its GRAS status for packaging only, with no limitations other than good manufacturing practices.

ALUMINUM ISOSTEARATES / LAURATES / STEARATES • The aluminum salt of a mixture of isostearic acid, lauric acid, and stearic acid *(see all)*. Used as a gelling agent. No known toxicity.

ALUMINUM ISOSTEARATES / MYRISTATES • Myristates is the aluminum salt of a mixture of isostearic acid and myristic acid *(see both)*. Used as a gelling agent. No known toxicity.

ALUMINUM ISOSTEARATES / PALMITATES • Palmitate is the aluminum salt of palmitic acid *(see)*, and isostearic acid *(see)*. Used as a gelling agent. No known toxicity.

ALUMINUM LACTATE • The aluminum salts of lactic acid *(see both)*.

ALUMINUM MONOSTEARATE • Anticaking agent, binder, emulsifier, and stabilizer used in packaging materials and various foods. Must conform to FDA specifications for salts, fats, or fatty acids derived from edible oils.

ALUMINUM MYRISTATES / PALMITATES • Myristates is the aluminum salt of a mixture of palmitic acid and isostearic acid *(see both)*. Used as a gelling agent. No known toxicity.

ALUMINUM NICOTINATE • Used as a source of niacin in special diet foods, also as a medication to dilate blood vessels and to combat fat. Tablets of 625 milligrams are a complex of aluminum nicotinate, nicotinic acid, and aluminum hydroxide. Side effects are flushing, rash, and gastrointestinal distress when taken in large doses.

ALUMINUM OLEATE • A yellow, thick, acidic mass practically insoluble in water. Used in packaging, as lacquer for metals, in waterproofing, and for thickening lubricating oils. Low toxicity. The final report of the FDA of the Select Committee on GRAS Substances stated in 1980 that it should continue its GRAS status for packaging only, with no limitations other than good manufacturing practices.

ALUMINUM PALMITATE • White granules, insoluble in water, used as a lubricant and waterproofing and packaging material. Also used to thicken petroleum and as an antiperspirant. The final report to the FDA of the Select Committee on GRAS Substances stated in 1980 that it should continue its GRAS status for packaging only, with no limitations other than good manufacturing practices.

ALUMINUM PHOSPHIDE • Used to fumigate processed foods including corn grits, brewer's malt, and brewer's rice. The FDA requires that processors aerate the finished food for forty-eight hours before it is offered to the consumer. It further warns that under no conditions should the formulation containing aluminum phosphide be used so that it or its unreacted residues will come into contact with any processed food. Reacts with moist air to produce the highly toxic phosphine.

Residues of phosphine in or on processed food may not exceed .01 parts per million, according to the FDA. Phosphine may cause pain in the region of the diaphragm, a feeling of coldness, weakness, vertigo, shortness of breath, bronchitis, edema, lung damage, convulsions, coma, and death.

ALUMINUM POTASSIUM SULFATE • Colorless, odorless, hard, transparent crystals or powder with a sweet antiseptic taste used for clarifying sugar and as a firming agent and carrier for leaching agents. It is used in the production of sweet and dill pickles, cereal, flours, bleached flours, and cheese. Ingestion of large quantities may cause burning in the mouth and throat and stomach distress. The final report to the FDA of the Select Committee on GRAS Substances stated in 1980 that it should continue its GRAS status with no limitations other than good manufacturing practices.

ALUMINUM SALTS OF FATTY ACIDS • Used as binders, emulsifiers, and anticaking agents. Regulated and used according to good manufacturing practices. *See* Aluminum Sodium Sulfate.

ALUMINUM SODIUM SULFATE • Colorless crystals used as a buffer, firming agent, neutralizing agent, and carrier for bleaching agents. For other uses, *see* Aluminum Potassium Sulfate. The final report to the FDA of the Select Committee on GRAS Substances stated in 1980 that it should continue its GRAS status with no limitations other than good manufacturing practices. A weak sensitizer. Local contact may cause skin rash.

ALUMINUM STEARATES • Hard, plasticlike materials used in waterproofing fabrics, thickening lubricating oils, and as a chewing-gum base component and a defoamer component used in processing beet sugar and yeast. *Aluminum tristearate* is a hard plastic material used as a thickener and coloring in cosmetics. No known toxicity.

ALUMINUM SULFATE • Cake Alum. Patent Alum. Colorless crystals, soluble in water. Odorless, with a sweet, mildly astringent taste. Used in producing sweet and dill pickles and as a modifier for starch. It is used in packaging materials, pickle relish, potatoes, and shrimp packages. Also used as an antiseptic, astringent, and detergent in antiperspirants, deodorants, and skin freshener; also purifies water. It may cause pimples under the arm when in antiperspirants and/or allergic reactions in some people. Moderately toxic by ingestion and injection. May affect reproduction. The final report to the FDA of the Select Committee on GRAS Substances stated in 1980 that it should continue its GRAS status with no limitations other than good manufacturing practices.

AMARANTH • Red No. 2, banned by the FDA in 1976. The ban was reaffirmed in 1980.

AMARANTH FLOUR • A grain grown in Central and South America for thousands of years, it is high in protein and fiber. Because it costs more than other grains, it is usually found only in health food stores.

AMBERGRIS • Concretion from the intestinal tract of the sperm whale found in tropical seas. About 80 percent cholesterol, it is a gray to black waxy mass used for fixing delicate odors in perfumery. It is also used in a flavoring for food and beverages. No known toxicity. GRAS.

AMBRETTE • A natural flavoring agent from the seed of the hibiscus plant, clear yellow to amber as a liquid, with a musky odor. Seed used in berry and floral flavorings for beverages, ice cream, ices, candy, baked goods. The tincture is used in a black walnut and vanilla flavorings for the same products and in cordials. The seed oil is used in fruit flavoring for beverages, ice cream, candy, and baked goods. No known toxicity. GRAS.

AMBRETTOLID • Formed in ambrette seed oil. Used as a flavoring, perfume fixative. No known toxicity.

AMBUSH • Ectiban. Exmin. Permethrin. A pesticide, poisonous by inhalation and injection. Moderately toxic by ingestion. May be mutagenic. A skin irritant.

AMERICAN DILLSEED OIL • See Dill.

AMES TEST • Dr. Bruce Ames, a biochemist at the University of California, developed a simple, inexpensive test in the early 1970s using bacteria that reveals whether a chemical is a mutagen. Almost all chemicals that are known carcinogens have also been shown to be mutagenic on the Ames Test. Whether the test can identify carcinogens is still controversial.

AMINE OXIDES • Surfactants derived from ammonia (see both).

AMINO ACIDS • The body's building blocks, from which proteins are constructed. Of the twenty-two known amino acids, eight cannot be manufactured in the body in sufficient quantities to sustain growth health. These eight are called "essential" because they are necessary to maintain good health. A ninth, histidine, is thought to be necessary for growth only in childhood. Widely used in moisturizers and emollients because they are thought to help penetrate the skin. Certain amino acid deficiencies appear to have tumor-suppressing action. The amino acids of protein foods are separated by digestion and go into a general pool from which the body takes the ones it needs to synthesize its own personal proteins.

4-AMINO-6-tert-BUTYL-3-(METHYL THIO)-1,2,4-TRIAZIN-5-ONE • Sencoral. Secorex. An herbicide used on barley, potato chips, processed potatoes, sugar cane, molasses, and wheat, except flour. Under the EPA Genetic Toxicology Program. Poison by ingestion. A selective residue herbicide.

4-AMINO-6-(1,1-DIMETHYL-ETHYL)-3-(METHYL THIO)-1,2,4-TRIAZINE-5 (4H)-ONE • Metribuzin. Herbicide used on processed potatoes, including potato chips. Herbicide is applied on the raw agricultural commodity. The FDA tolerances are 3 ppm in processed potatoes and potato chips; 3 ppm in animal feed using wheat; 2 ppm in animal feed using tomato pomace; 0.3 ppm in animal feed using sugarcane molasses; and 0.5 ppm in animal feed using sugarcane bagasse. Toxic.

4-AMINO-3,5,6-TRICHLOROPICOLINIC ACID • Amdon Grazon. Borolin. Chloramp. An herbicide and defoliant used on barley, oats, and wheat. An experimental cancer-causing agent and teratogen. Moderately toxic by ingestion.

p-AMINOBENZOIC ACID • See para-Aminobenzoic Acid.

para-AMINOBENZOIC ACID • The colorless or yellowish acid found in vitamin B complex. Miscellaneous use. The FDA has said it should be used at less than thirty milligrams per day as a food additive. In an alcohol and water solution plus a little light perfume, it is sold under a wide variety of names as a sunscreen lotion. It is also used as a local anesthetic in sunburn products. It is used medicinally to treat arthritis. However, it can cause eczema *(see)* and a sensitivity to light in susceptible people whose skin may react to sunlight by erupting with a rash, sloughing, and/or swelling. GRAS.

AMINOBENZYLPENICILLIN • Acillin. Ado Bacillin. Alpen. Penbritin. Vicilin. Animal drug used in beef, milk, and pork. Under the EPA Genetic Toxicology Program. Moderately toxic by injection. Human systemic effects by ingestion: fever, agranulocytosis, and other blood effects. May be mutagenic.

6-AMINOCAPROIC ACID • *See* Amino Acids and Caproic Acid.

AMINOGLYCOSIDE 3′-PHOPHOTRANS FERASE II • There is reported use of the chemical; it has not yet been assigned for toxicology literature.

AMINOMETHYL PROPANEDIOL • Crystals made from nitrogen compounds that are soluble in alcohol and mixable with water. Used as an emulsifying ingredient in mineral oils. No known toxicity.

AMINOMETHYL PROPANOL • An alcohol made from nitrogen compounds; mixes with water. Soluble in alcohol and used as an emulsifying ingredient. Used in medicines that reduce body water. Prolonged skin exposure may cause irritation due to alkalinity, but in most commercial products the alkalinity is neutralized. It is used in cosmetics up to 10 percent.

AMINOPEPTIDASE FROM LACTOCOCCUS LACTIS • Enzyme used to make cheddar cheese and protein hydrolysates. There is reported use of the chemical; it has not yet been assigned for toxicology literature. GRAS.

AMITRAZ • A pesticide that is tolerated in 7 ppm in citrus pulp for use in animal feeds. The toleration in milk is 0.03 ppm and in the fat of cattle and hogs, 0.1 ppm. As residues in kidney and liver of hogs, 0.2 ppm, and in meat byproducts of cattle and hogs, 0.03 ppm.

AMMONIA • Liquid used in permanent wave (cold) and hair bleaches. Obtained by blowing steam through incandescent coke. Ammonia is also used in the manufacture of explosives and synthetic fabrics. It is extremely toxic when inhaled in concentrated vapors and is irritating to the eyes and mucous membranes. It may cause hair breakage when used in permanent waves and hair bleaches.

AMMONIATED GLYCYRRHIZIN • GRAS. *See* Licorice.

AMMONIUM ALGINATE • A stabilizer and water retainer. The report to the FDA of the Select Committee on GRAS Substances stated in 1980 that there is no evidence in the available information that it is a hazard to the public when used as it is now, and it should continue its GRAS status with limitation on amounts that can be added to food. *See* Alginates.

AMMONIUM BICARBONATE • An alkali used as a leavening agent in the production of baked goods, confections, and cacao products. Usually prepared by passing carbon dioxide gas through concentrated ammonia water. Shiny, hard, colorless, or white crystals; faint odor of ammonia. Used also in powder formulas in cooling baths. Used medicinally as an expectorant and to break up intestinal gas. Also used in compost heaps to accelerate decomposition. The final report to the FDA of the

Select Committee on GRAS Substances stated in 1980 that it should continue its GRAS status with no limitations other than good manufacturing practices.

AMMONIUM BITARTRATE • White crystals, soluble in water, derived from tartaric acid. Used in baking powder. No known toxicity.

AMMONIUM CARBONATE • A white solid alkali derived partly from ammonium bicarbonate *(see)* and used as a neutralizer and buffer in permanent wave solutions and creams. It decomposes when exposed to air. Also used in baking powders, for defatting woolens, in fire extinguishers and as an expectorant. Ammonium carbonate can cause skin rashes on the scalp, forehead, or hands. The final report to the FDA of the Select Committee on GRAS Substances stated in 1980 that it should continue its GRAS status with no limitations other than good manufacturing practices. *See* Ammonium Bicarbonate.

AMMONIUM CASEINATE • The ammonium salt of casein, a protein occurring in milk and cheese. It is used in standard foods, particularly bakery products. Therefore, it does not have to be listed on the label. *See* Casein.

AMMONIUM CHLORIDE • Ammonium salt that occurs naturally. Colorless, odorless crystals or white powder, saline in taste, and incompatible with alkalies. Used as a dough conditioner and a yeast food in bread, rolls, buns, and so on. Saline in taste. Also used as an acidifier in permanent wave solutions, eye lotions, and as a cooling and stimulating skin wash. Industrially employed in freezing mixtures, batteries, dyes, safety explosives, and in medicine as a urinary acidifier and diuretic. Keep snow from melting on ski slopes. If ingested, can cause nausea, vomiting, and acidosis in doses of 0.5 to 1 gram. Lethal as an intramuscular dose in rats and guinea pigs. As with any ammonia compound, concentrated solutions can be irritating to the skin. The final report to the FDA of the Select Committee on GRAS Substances stated in 1980 that it should continue GRAS status for packaging only with no limitations other than good manufacturing practices.

AMMONIUM CITRATE • The salt of citric acid *(see),* it is a natural constituent of plants and animals and dissolves easily in water, releasing free acid. Used as a sequestrant, flavor enhancer, and as a firming agent. The final report to the FDA of the Select Committee on GRAS Substances stated in 1980 that it should continue its GRAS status with no limitations other than good manufacturing practices.

AMMONIUM GLUCONATE • Prepared from gluconic acid with ammonia, it is used as an emulsifying agent for cheese and salad dressings. No known toxicity.

AMMONIUM HYDROXIDE • Ammonium Bicarbonate. Ammonia Water. A weak alkali formed when ammonia dissolves in water; exists only in solution. A clear colorless liquid with an extremely pungent odor. Used as a buffer and neutralizer in cocoa products and in animal feeds. Also used as an alkali *(see)* in metallic hair dyes, hair straighteners, and in protective skin creams. Also used in detergents and for removing stains. It is irritating to the eyes and mucous membranes. It may cause hair breakage. A human poison by ingestion. A severe eye irritant. The final report to the FDA of the Select Committee on GRAS Substances stated in 1980 that it should continue its GRAS status for packaging only, with no limitations other than good manufacturing practices. GRAS.

AMMONIUM ISOVALERATE • *See* Isovaleric Acid.

AMMONIUM OLEATE • The ammonium salt of oleic acid *(see)* used as an emulsifying agent.

AMMONIUM PERSULFATE • Ammonium Peroxydisulfate. Odorless crystals or white powder. Used as an oxidizer and bleacher and as a modifier for food starch. *See* Modified Starch.

AMMONIUM PHOSPHATE • Monobasic and Dibasic. Ammonium Salt. An odorless, white, or colorless crystalline powder with a cooling taste used in mouthwashes. It is used as acidic constituents of baking powder. They are used as buffers, leavening agents, and bread, roll, and bun improvers up to 10 percent of product. Used in brewing industry. They are also used in fireproofing textiles, paper, and wood, for purifying sugar, and in yeast cultures and fertilizers. Monobasic is used as baking powder with sodium bicarbonate. Medically used for their saline action. They have a diuretic effect (reducing body water) and they make urine more acid. No known toxicity. The final report to the FDA of the Select Committee on GRAS Substances stated in 1980 that it should continue its GRAS status with no limitations other than good manufacturing practices.

AMMONIUM POTASSIUM HYDROGEN • A stabilizer used in packaging.

AMMONIUM SACCHARIN • *See* Saccharin.

AMMONIUM SULFATE • Ammonium salt. A yeast food, dough conditioner, and buffer in bakery products. Colorless, odorless, white crystals or powder. A neutralizer in permanent wave lotions. Industrially used in freezing mixtures, fireproofing fabrics, and tanning. Used medicinally to prolong analgesia. No known toxicity when used cosmetically. Fatal to rats in large doses. The final report to the FDA of the Select Committee on GRAS Substances stated in 1980 that it should continue its GRAS status with no limitations other than good manufacturing practices. *See* uses for Ammonium Phosphate.

AMMONIUM SULFIDE • A salt derived from sulfur and ammonium used as a synthetic spice flavoring agent for baked foods and condiments. Also used as a neutralizer in permanent wave lotions, as a depilatory, to apply patina to bronze, and in film developers. May evolve into toxic hydrogen sulfide, and a fatality has been reported from ingestion of ammonium sulfide permanent-wave solution. Irritating to the skin when used in depilatories.

AMOXICILLIN TRIHYDRATE • An animal drug used in meat and milk. Tolerance is 0.01 ppm in milk and uncooked edible tissues of meat. Moderately toxic.

AMP • The abbreviation for aminomethyl propanol *(see)*.

AMPD • The abbreviation for aminomethyl propanediol *(see)*.

AMPHO • Means double or both.

AMPHOTERIC • A material that can display both acid and basic properties. Used primarily in surfactants *(see)* and contains betaines and imidazoles *(see both)*.

AMPICILLIN TRIHYDRATE • Amcill. Princillin. Vidopen. Animal drug used in meat. FDA tolerance is 0.01 ppm residue in uncooked tissue of cattle and swine and in milk.

AMPROLIUM • Crystals from methanol and ethanol *(see both)* used as an animal drug in beef, chicken, eggs, pheasants, and turkey. Limitation in chickens and turkeys of 1 ppm in liver and kidney, 0.5 ppm in muscle. Limitation of 8 ppm in egg yolks, 4 ppm in whole eggs.

AMYL • Prefix meaning derived from amyl alcohol *(see)*.

AMYL ACETATE • Banana Oil. Pear Oil. Obtained from amyl alcohol, with a strong fruity odor. Used in nail finishes and nail polish remover as a solvent, and as an artificial fruit essence in perfume. Also used in food and beverage flavoring and for perfuming shoe polish. Amyl acetate is a skin irritant and causes central nervous system depression when ingested. Exposure of 950 ppm for one hour has caused headache, fatigue, chest pain, and irritation of the mucous membranes.

AMYL ALCOHOL • A synthetic berry, chocolate, apple, banana, pineapple, liquor, and rum flavoring agent for beverages, ice cream, ices, candy, baked goods, gelatin desserts, and chewing gum. Used as a solvent in nail polish. It occurs naturally in cocoa and oranges and smells like camphor. Highly toxic and narcotic; ingestion of as little as 30 milligrams has killed humans. Inhalation causes violent coughing.

AMYL ALDEHYDE • *See* Valeraldehyde.

AMYL BUTYRATE • A synthetic flavoring agent, colorless, with a strong apricot odor. Occurs naturally in cocoa. Used in raspberry, strawberry, butter, butterscotch, fruit, apple, apricot, banana, cherry, grape, peach, pineapple, and vanilla flavorings for beverages, ice cream, ices, candy, baked goods, cherry syrup, and chewing gums. Used in some perfume formulas for its apricotlike odor.

AMYL CAPRATE • *See* Cognac Oil.

AMYL CINNAMIC ALDEHYDE • Liquid with a strong floral odor in perfumes and flavorings. *See* Cinnamic Acid.

AMYL DECANOATE • Approved as a synthetic flavoring, but there is no current reported use of the chemical, and therefore, although toxicology information may be available, it is not being updated by the FDA.

AMYL FORMATE • A synthetic flavoring.

AMYL 2-FUROATE • A synthetic rum and maple flavoring agent for beverages, candy, baked goods, and condiments.

AMYL GALLATE • An antioxidant obtained from nutgalls and from molds. *See* Gallates.

AMYL HEPTANOATE • A synthetic lemon, coconut, fruit, and nut flavoring agent for beverages, ice cream, ices, candy, baked goods, gelatin desserts, puddings, and chewing gum.

AMYL HEXANOATE • A synthetic citrus, chocolate, fruit, and liquor flavoring agent for beverages, ice cream, ices, candy, baked goods, and gelatin desserts.

2-AMYL-59 or 60-KETO-1, 4-DIOXANE • A synthetic fruit flavoring agent for beverages, ice cream, ices, candy, baked goods, and shortening.

AMYL OCTANOATE • Occurs naturally in apples. A synthetic chocolate, fruit, and liquor flavoring agent for beverages, ice cream, ices, candy, baked goods, and gelatin desserts.

a-**AMYL-B-PHENYL ACROLEIN BUXINE** • *See* a-Amylcinnamaldehyde.

AMYL PROPIONATE • Colorless liquid with a fruity, applelike odor used in perfumes, flavors, and in lacquers. When heated to decomposition it emits acrid smoke and irritating fumes.

AMYLASE (Bacterial) • *Aspergillus flavus, niger,* or *oryzae* or *Bacillus subtilis.* Enzymes from various fungi used as antibacterial agents.

AMYLASE (Swine) • An enzyme prepared from hog pancreas used in flour to break down starch into smaller sugar molecules. Then, in turn, the enzymes produced by yeast in the dough again split these sugar molecules to form carbon dioxide gas, which causes the dough to rise. It improves crumb softness and shelf life. Used as a texturizer in cosmetics, it is also used medically to combat inflammation. Nontoxic.

a-**AMYLCINNAMALDEHYDE** • A synthetic agent, yellow, with a strong floral odor of jasmine, used in strawberry, apple, apricot, peach, and walnut flavorings for beverages, ice cream, ices, candy, baked goods, gelatin desserts, and chewing gum. Moderately toxic by ingestion. A mild skin irritant. Susceptible to oxidation by air.

a-**AMYLCINNAMALDEHYDE DIMETHYL ACETAL** • A synthetic fruit flavoring agent for beverages, ice cream, candy, and baked goods. No known toxicity.

AMYLCINNAMATE • Colorless to pale yellow liquid with a cocoa odor. Used as a flavoring agent.

a-**AMYLCINNAMYL ACETATE** • A synthetic chocolate, fruit, and honey flavoring agent for beverages, ice cream, ices, candy, baked goods, and chewing gum. No known toxicity.

a-**AMYLCINNAMYL ALCOHOL** • A synthetic chocolate, fruit, and honey flavoring agent for beverages, ice cream, ices, candy, baked goods, and chewing gum. No known toxicity.

a-**AMYLCINNAMYL FORMATE** • A synthetic chocolate, fruit, nut, and maple flavoring agent for beverages, ice cream, ices, candy, baked goods, and chewing gum. No known toxicity.

a-**AMYLCINNAMYL ISOVALERATE** • A synthetic chocolate, fruit, grape, and nut flavoring agent for beverages, ice cream, ices, candy, baked goods, and chewing gum. No known toxicity.

AMYLOGLUCOSIDASE • A sweet enzyme derived from *Rhizopus niveus* with a growth-encouraging potential. Used in the production of gelatinized starch into sugars and in the production of distilled spirits and vinegar. No known toxicity.

AMYLOPECTIN • Amioca. Derived from starch, it is the almost insoluble outer portion of the starch granule. The gel constituent of starch. Forms a paste with water. Used as a texturizer in foods and cosmetics. Obtained from corn. Gives a red color when mixed with iodine and does not gel when mixed with water. No known toxicity.

AMYLOSE • Starches commonly processed from plants contain 18 to 27 percent amylose. It is the inner, relatively soluble portion of starch granules. Cornstarch solutions often form opaque gels after cooking and cooling; this is because of the presence of amylose. It is used as a dispersing and mixing agent for oleoresins. Nontoxic.

AMYRIS OIL • Sandalwood Oil. The volatile oil obtained from a gummy wood and used as a flavoring agent in chewing gum and candy. It is a clear, pale yellow, viscous liquid with a distinct odor of sandalwood.

ANCHUSIN EXTRACT • *See* Alkanet Root.

ANETHOLE • A flavoring agent used in fruit, honey, licorice, anise, liquor, nut, root beer, sarsaparilla, spice, vanilla, wintergreen, and birch beer flavorings for beverages, ice cream, ices, candy, baked goods, chewing gum (1,500 ppm), and liquors (1,400 ppm). Obtained from anise *(see)* oil, fennel, and other sources. Colorless or faintly yellow liquid with a sweet taste and a characteristic aniselike odor. Chief constituent of anise. Anethole is affected by light and caused irritation of the gums and throat when used in a denture cream. When applied to the skin, anethole may produce hives, scaling, and blisters. GRAS.

ANETHUM GRAVEOLENS L • *See* Dill.

ANGELIC ACID • *See* Angelica.

ANGELICA • Used in inexpensive fragrances, toothpastes, and mouthwashes. Grown in Europe and Asia, the aromatic seeds, leaves, stems, and roots have been used in medicine for flatus (gas), to increase sweating, and reduce body water. When perfume is applied, skin may break out with a rash and swell when exposed to sunlight. The *bark* is used medicinally as a purgative and emetic. The *root oil* is used in fruit, gin, and rum flavorings for beverages, ice cream, ices, candy, baked goods, gelatin desserts, chewing gum, and liquors. The *root extract* is used in berry, liquor, wine, maple, nut, walnut, and root beer flavorings for the same foods, up to baked goods, plus syrups. The *seed extract* is used in berry, fruit, walnut, maple, and spice flavorings for beverages, candy, baked goods, syrups, and condiments. The *seed oil* is used for fruit and gin flavoring for beverages, ice cream, ices, candy, baked goods, gelatin, desserts, and liquors. The *stem oil* is used for fruit flavoring for the same foods as seed oil, excepting liquors. Angelica can induce sensitivity to light. GRAS.

ANGOLA WEED • A weed from West Africa used as a flavoring agent in alcoholic beverages only.

ANGOSTURA • Cusparia Bark. Flavoring agent from the bark of trees, grown in Venezuela and Brazil. Unpleasant musty odor and bitter aromatic taste. The light yellow liquid extract is used in bitters, liquor, root beer, and spice flavorings for beverages and liquors (1,700 ppm). Formerly used to lessen fever. GRAS.

ANHYDRIDE • A residue resulting from water being removed from a compound. An oxide—combination of oxygen and an element—that can combine with water to form an acid, or that is derived from an acid by the abstraction of water. Acetic acid *(see)* is an example.

ANHYDROUS • Describes a substance that contains no water.

ANHYDROUS AMMONIA • Source of crude fiber and nonprotein nitrogen in animal feed. *See* Anhydrous and Ammonia.

ANILINE • A colorless to brown liquid that darkens with age. Slightly soluble in water, it is one of the most commonly used of the organic bases, the parent substance for many dyes and drugs. It is derived from nitrobenzene or chlorobenzene and is among the top five organic chemicals produced each year in the United States. It is used as a rubber accelerator to speed vulcanization, as an antioxidant to retard aging, and as an intermediate *(see);* it is also used in dyes, photographic chemicals, the manufacture of urethane foams, pharmaceuticals, explosives, petroleum refining, resins and adhesive products, paint removers, herbicides, and fungicides. Also used in crayons and shoe polishes. It is toxic when ingested, inhaled, or absorbed through the skin. It causes allergic reactions. It is a potential human cancer-causing ingredient. It caused cancer in mice when injected under the skin or administered orally. It can also cause contact dermatitis. In a 1991 report of a study of 1,749 workers at the Goodyear Tire & Rubber Company plant in Niagara Falls, N.Y., it was revealed that workers exposed directly to aniline had 6.5 times the rate of bladder cancer of the average state resident.

ANIMAL COLLAGEN AMINO ACIDS • The major protein of the white fibers of connective tissue, cartilage, and bone that is insoluble in water, but easily altered to gelatins by boiling in water, dilute acids, or alkalies. *See* Hydrolyzed Protein.

ANIMAL KERATIN AMINO ACIDS • A mixture of amino acids from the hydrolysis of keratin *(see)*. *See also* Hydrolyzed Keratin.

ANIMAL PROTEIN HYDROLYSATE • A source of animal protein.

***p*-ANISALDEHYDE** • A colorless oil with a hawthorn odor, it is used as a flavoring agent in various foods. Moderately toxic by ingestion. A skin irritant.

ANISE • Anise Seed. Dried ripe fruit of Asia, Europe, and the U.S. Used in licorice, anise, pepperoni sausage, spice, and vanilla flavorings for beverages, ice cream, ices, candy, baked goods, condiments (5,000 ppm), and meats (1,200 ppm). The oil is used for butter, caramel, licorice, anise, rum, sausage, nut, root beer, sarsaparilla, spice, vanilla, wintergreen, and birch beer flavorings for the same foods as above excepting condiments but including chewing gum (3,200 ppm) and liquors. Sometimes used to break up intestinal gas. Used in masculine-type perfumes, cleaners, and shampoos. Can cause contact dermatitis. GRAS. *See* Star Anise.

ANISOLE • A synthetic agent with a pleasant odor used in licorice, root beer, sarsaparilla, wintergreen, and birch beer flavorings for beverages, ice cream, ices, candy, and baked goods. Also used in perfumery.

ANISYL ACETATE • Colorless liquid with a lilac odor used in perfumery and flavorings. *See* Anise and Anisyl Alcohol.

ANISYL ALCOHOL • A synthetic berry, chocolate, cocoa, fruit, and vanilla flavoring agent for beverages, ice cream, ices, candy, baked goods, gelatin desserts, and chewing gum.

ANISYL BUTYRATE • A synthetic fruit and licorice-flavoring agent for beverages, ice cream, ices, candy, and baked goods.

ANISYL FORMATE • Formic Acid. A synthetic raspberry, fruit, licorice, and vanilla flavoring agent for beverages, ice cream, ices, baked goods, and gelatin desserts. Also used in perfumery. Found naturally in currant and vanilla. *See* Formic Acid for toxicity.

ANISYL PHENYLACETATE • A synthetic honey flavoring agent for beverages, ice cream, ices, candy, and baked goods.

ANISYL PROPIONATE • Occurs naturally in quince, apple, banana, cherry, peach, and pineapple. A raspberry, cherry, and licorice-flavoring agent for beverages, ice cream, ices, candy, baked goods, and gelatin desserts. No known toxicity.

ANNATTO • Extract and Seed. A vegetable dye from a tropical tree, yellow to pink, it is used in dairy products, baked goods, margarine, and breakfast cereals. It is also used to color such meat-product casings as bologna and frankfurters. A spice flavoring for beverages, ice cream, baked goods (2,000 ppm), margarine, breakfast cereals (2,000 ppm), and baked goods. Permanently listed in 1963 but certification not necessary for use (*see* Certified).

ANOXOMER • An antioxidant used up to 5,000 ppm.

ANTHOCYANINS • Intensely colored, water-soluble pigments responsible for nearly all the reds and blues of flowers and other plant parts. Such color, which is dissolved in plant sap, is markedly affected by the acidity and alkalinity of substances: red at low pH *(see)* and blue at higher pH values. There are about two hundred known anthocyanins, including those obtained from grapes, cranberries, cherries, and plums. They can be used to color acid compounds, such as wines and cranberry juice cocktail. The twenty anthocyanins in grapes are the major source of anthocyanin pigment for food color. No known toxicity.

ANTHRACITE COAL, SULFONATED • A resin for miscellaneous uses, according to the FDA.

ANTHRANILIC ACID • *o*-Aminobenzoic Acid. Yellowish crystals with a sweet taste used in flavorings, dyes, and perfumes. *See* Benzoic Acid.

ANTHRANILIC ACID, CINNAMYL ESTER • Reddish yellow powder with the odor of balsam used in baked goods, beverages, and candy as a flavoring agent. May be a cancer-causing agent.

ANTHRANILIC ACID, METHYL ESTER • A flavoring agent used in various foods. May cause tumors. Moderately toxic by ingestion. A skin irritant.

ANTIBIOTICS • For growth promotion and feed efficiency. *See* Bacitracin, Bambermycin, Chlortetracycline, Erythromycin, Lincomycin, Monensin, Oleandomycin Hydrochloride, Oxytetracycline, Tylosin, and Virginiamycin.

ANTIBODY • Protein in blood formed in response to invasion by a germ, virus, or other foreign body. In sensitive individuals, a special antibody, IgE *(see),* is responsible for the allergic reaction.

ANTICAKING AGENTS • These keep powders and salt free-flowing, such as with calcium phosphates *(see)* in instant breakfast drinks and other soft-drink mixes.

ANTIFOAMING AGENT • Defoaming Agent. A substance used to reduce foaming due to proteins, gases, or nitrogenous materials that may interfere with processing.

ANTIGEN • Any substance that provokes an immune response when introduced into the body.

ANTIOXIDANTS • Substances added to food to keep oxygen from changing the food's color or flavor. Apples, for instance, will turn brown when exposed to air, and fats will become rancid after exposure. Among the most widely used antioxidants are butylated hydroxyanisole (BHA) and butylated hydroxytoluene (BHT) *(see both)*. Vitamin E and vitamin C are natural antioxidants.

ANTIPROTOZOAL • A medication that combats single-celled parasites that are slightly bigger than bacterial. Many live in human and animal intestine and are harmless, but some cause a variety of ills including dysentery.

APPLE ACID • *See* Malic Acid.

APPLE ESSENCE, NATURAL • A flavoring.

b-APO-8′-CAROTENAL • A fine crystalline powder used as a color additive in orange beverages, cheese, desserts, and ice cream. *See* Carotene.

APRAMYCIN • Ambylan. An animal drug used in pork. FDA tolerance: 0.1–0.4 ppm in swine.

APRICOT • Fruit and Oil. Persic Oil. The tart orange-colored fruit is used as a natural cherry flavoring agent for beverages, ice cream, ices, candy, baked goods, and soups. The oil is used in brilliantine and in crushed fruit as a facial mask to soften the skin. No known toxicity. GRAS.

APRICOT KERNEL OIL • The oil from the kernel of *Prunus Armeniaca*. There is reported use of the chemical; it has not yet been assigned for toxicology literature.

ARABIC GUM • *See* Acacia.

ARABINOGALACTAN • A polysaccharide extracted with water from larch wood used in the minimum quantity required to be effective as an emulsifier, stabilizer, binder, or bodying agent in essential oils. Used in nonnutritive sweeteners, flavor bases, nonstandardized dressings, and pudding mixes.

L-ARABINOSE • A common vegetable gum, especially from gum Arabic. Used as a culture medium.

ARACHIDIC ACID • A fatty acid, also called eicosanoic acid, that is widely distributed in peanut oil fats and related compounds. It is used in lubricants, greases, waxes, and plastics. No known toxicity.

ARACHIDONIC ACID • A liquid unsaturated fatty acid that occurs in liver, brain, glands, and fat of animals and humans. The acid is generally isolated from animal liver. Used essentially for nutrition and to soothe eczema and rashes in skin creams and lotions. No known toxicity.

ARACHIDYL PROPIONATE • The ester of arachidyl alcohol and *n*-propionic acid used as a wax. *See* Arachidic Acid.

ARBUTIN • A diuretic and anti-infective derived from the dried leaves of the berry family, including blueberries, cranberries, bearberries, and most pear plants. This may explain why cranberry juice is reputed to ward off and/or treat urinary tract infections.

ARGININE • An essential amino acid *(see)*, strongly alkaline. The FDA has asked for further information on the nutrient, which plays an important role in urea excretion. It has been used for the treatment of liver disease. GRAS.

L-ARGININE • An essential amino acid *(see)*, strongly alkaline. It plays an important part in urea excretion. It has been used for the treatment of liver disease. Banned as not safe by the FDA, February 10, 1992, for use in over-the-counter diet pills.

ARHEOL • *See* Sandalwood Oil, Yellow.

ARNICA • Wolf's Bane. The dried flowerhead has long been used as an astringent to treat skin disorders. It is used as a flavoring in alcohol beverages only. Ingestion can lead to severe intestinal upset, nervous disturbances, irregular heartbeat, and collapse. Ingestion of one ounce has caused severe illness but no death. It should not be used on broken skin.

ARNOTTA EXTRACT and SEED • *See* Annatto.

AROMATIC • In the context of cosmetics, a chemical that has an aroma.

AROMATIC BITTERS • Usually made from the maceration of bitter herbs and used to intensify the aroma of perfume. The herbs selected for aromatic bitters must have a persistent fragrant aroma. Ginger and cinnamon are examples.

ARROWROOT STARCH • From the rhizome of *Maranta arundinacea,* a plant of tropical America. Used in the diet of babies and invalids because it is easy to digest. An ingredient in dusting powders and hair dyes made from the root starch of plants. Arrowroot was used by the American Indians to heal wounds from poisoned arrows. It is used as a culture medium and as a medicine. In cosmetics, it is used to help moisturizers penetrate the skin. The final report to the FDA of the Select Committee on GRAS Substances stated in 1980 that it should continue its GRAS status with no limitations other than good manufacturing practices. No known toxicity.

ARSANILIC ACID • Aminobenzene Arsonic Acid. Used in animal feed. Poison by ingestion and injection. A human cancer-causing agent. Arsenic and its compounds are on the Community Right-To-Know List *(see)*. Can cause blindness.

ARSENIC • Silvery black crystals used as an animal drug to promote growth for livestock and poultry. Tolerance set by the FDA of 0.5 ppm in muscle, 2 ppm in uncooked edible byproducts, 0.5 ppm in eggs from chickens and turkeys. Limitation of 2 ppm in liver. A human carcinogen. Poison by subcutaneous, intramuscular, and intraperitoneal routes. Human systemic skin and gastrointestinal effects by ingestion. May cause birth defects.

ARTEMISIA OIL • Mugwort. A shrub and herb, native to north and south temperate climate, having strongly scented foliage and small rayless flower heads. Used as a flavoring in alcoholic beverages. The FDA says there is no reported use of the extract and there is no toxicology information available. As for the oil, the FDA has not yet done a toxicology search. *See* Wormwood.

ARTICHOKE LEAVES • A tall herb that resembles a thistle. Used as a flavoring in alcoholic beverages only. There is reported use of the chemical; it has not yet been assigned for toxicology literature.

ARTIFICIAL • In foods, the term follows the standard meaning: a substance not duplicated in nature. A flavoring, for instance, may have all the natural ingredients but it must be called artificial if it has no counterpart in nature.

AS PACKAGED • Refers to the state of the product as it is marked for purchase, while *as prepared* refers to the product after it has been made ready for consumption (e.g., ingredients added per instructions and cooked, such as a cake mix that has been prepared and baked, or a condensed or dry soup that has been reconstituted).

ASAFOETIDA EXTRACT • Asafetida. Devil's Dung. A gum or resin obtained from the roots or rhizome of *Ferula asafoetida,* any of several plants grown in Iran, Turkestan, and Afghanistan. The soft lumps, or "tears," have a garlicky odor and are used as a natural flavoring. The fluid extract is used in sausage, onion, and spice flavorings for beverages, ice cream, ices, candy, baked goods, meat, condiments, and soups. The gum is used in onion and spice flavorings for beverages, ice cream, ices, candy, baked goods, and seasonings. The gums have also been used medicinally as an expectorant and to break up intestinal gas. The oil is used for spice flavoring in candy, baked goods, and condiments. Asafetida has a bitter taste, an offensive charcoal odor, and is used in India and Iran as a condiment. There is reported use of the chemical; it has not yet been assigned for toxicology literature search. GRAS.

ASCORBATE • Calcium and Sodium. Vitamin C salts. Antioxidants used in concentrated milk products, cooked, cured, or pulverized meat products, and in the pickle in which pork and beef products are cured or packed.

ASCORBIC ACID • Vitamin C. A preservative and antioxidant used in frozen fruit, particularly sliced peaches, frozen fish dip, dry milk, beer and ale, flavoring oils, apple juices, soft drinks, fluid milk, candy, artificially sweetened jellies and preserves, canned mushrooms, cooked, cured, pulverized meat food products, pickle in which beef or pork is cured or packed (seventy-five ounces of vitamin C per one hundred gallons). Vitamin C is necessary for normal teeth, bones, and blood vessels. The white or slightly yellow powder darkens upon exposure to air. Reasonably stable when it remains dry in air, but deteriorates rapidly when exposed to air while in solution. Nobel Laureate Linus Pauling caused a run on vitamin C in 1970 by endorsing it as a cold medicine. Although his theories were not widely accepted by the medical community, a great deal of work is now in progress studying vitamin C and immunity. Vitamin C is known to affect the excretion of medications such as barbiturates and to make them more toxic. Pharmaceutically incompatible with sodium salicylate, sodium nitrate, theobromine, and methenamine. The final report to the FDA of the Select Committee on GRAS Substances stated in 1980 that it should continue its GRAS status with no limitations other than good manufacturing practices.

ASCORBYL PALMITATE • A salt of ascorbic acid *(see),* it is used as a preservative and antioxidant for candy. Like ascorbic acid, prevents rancidity, browning of cut apples and other fruits, and is used in meat curing. Nontoxic.

ASEPTIC PROCESSING • Dates back to at least the mid-1940s but has yet to realize its full potential. The most widely used of these new technologies, aseptic processing involves sterilizing a food product in a continuous process through a heat exchanger and then filling that food in an aseptic filler. The aseptic filler is a highly specialized piece of equipment designed to sterilize the packaging material, fill the sterile product into its container in a sterile environment, and then seal the package.

ASPARAGINE • L Form. A nonessential amino acid *(see),* widely found in plants and animals both free and combined with proteins. It is used as a dietary supplement, a culture medium, and as a medicine. In cosmetics, it is used to help moisturizers penetrate the skin.

ASPARAGUS SEED and ROOT EXTRACT • *Asparagus officinalis.* Sparrow Grass. The root is used in Chinese medicine as a tonic. In India, it is used as a hormonal tonic for women to promote fertility, relieve menstrual pains, increase breast milk, and generally nourish and strengthen the female reproductive system. It is also used as a tonic for the lungs in consumptive diseases and for AIDS wasting. Asparagus contains glycosides, asparagine, sucrose, starch, and mucilage. In 1992, the FDA proposed a ban on asparagus in oral menstrual drug products because it has not been shown to be safe and effective for its stated claims. There is reported use of the chemical; it has not yet been assigned for toxicology literature search.

ASPARTAME • NutraSweet. A compound prepared from aspartic acid and phenylalanine *(see both),* with about two hundred times the sweetness of sugar, discovered during routine screening of drugs for the treatment of ulcers. The G. D. Searle Company sought FDA approval in 1973, and it was approved in 1974, but objections that aspartame might cause brain damage led to a stay, or legal postponement, of that approval. Another problem arose. An FDA investigation of records of animal studies conducted for Searle drug approvals and for aspartame raised questions. The FDA arranged for an independent audit, which took more than two years and concluded that the aspartame studies and results were authentic. The agency then organized an expert board of inquiry and the members concluded that the evidence did not support the charge that aspartame might kill clusters of brain cells or cause other damage. However, persons with phenylketonuria, or PKU, must avoid protein foods such as meat that contain phenylalanine—one of two components of aspartame. The board did, however, recommend that aspartame not be approved until further long-term animal testing could be conducted to rule out a possibility that aspartame might cause brain tumors. The FDA's Bureau of Foods reviewed the study data already available and concluded that the board's concern was unfounded. Aspartame was approved for use as a tabletop sweetener in certain dry foods on October 22, 1981. It was also approved for breath mints, hard and soft; as a flavor enhancer in chewing gum, hard candy, instant coffee and tea beverages, ready-to-serve nonalcoholic beverages, fruit juice–based beverages, concentrates, or syrup, for malt beverages containing less than 3 percent alcohol, and for frosting, toppings, fillings, glazes, and icings for precooked baked goods.

In 1984 news reports fueled by the announcement that the Arizona Department of Health Services was testing soft drinks containing aspartame to see if it deteriorated into toxic levels of methyl alcohol under storage conditions created alarm. The Arizona Health Department acted after the director of the Food Sciences and

Research Laboratory at Arizona State submitted a study alleging that higher than normal temperatures could lead to a dangerous breakdown in the chemical composition. The author of this dictionary checked with representatives of the Food and Drug Administration. They said that there are higher levels of methyl alcohol in regular fruit juices, and as far as the agency was concerned, the fears about decomposition products were unfounded.

Aspartame lowers the acidity of urine and therefore reportedly makes the urinary tract more susceptible to infection. In 1988, the Mexican government stopped soda and food processors from using *nutra* in the name because it was "misleading." The Mexicans also required labeling that carries the following warning: "This product should not be used by individuals who are allergic to phenylalanine. Consumption by pregnant women and children under 7 years is not recommended. Users should follow a balanced diet. Consumption by diabetics must be authorized by a physician."

ASPARTIC ACID • DL and L Forms. Aminosuccinate Acid. A nonessential amino acid *(see)* occurring in animals and plants, sugar cane, sugar beets, and molasses. It is usually synthesized for commercial purposes. No known toxicity.

ASPERGILLUS • A genus of fungi. It contains many species of molds and spores that produce the antibiotic aspergillic acid. An *Aspergillus flavus-oryzae* group of mold has been cleared by the U.S. Department of Agriculture's Meat Inspection Division to soften tissues of beef cuts, to wit: "Solutions containing water, salt, monosodium glutamate, and approved proteolytic enzymes applied or injected into cuts of beef shall not result in a gain of more than 3 percent above the weight of the untreated product." It is also used in bakery products such as bread, roll, and buns. Toxicity is unknown, but because of the use of the fungi antibiotics and monosodium glutamate, allergic reactions would certainly be possible. The FDA says that there is no current reported use of *Aspergillus niger* for fermentation production of citric acid, and therefore there is not toxicology information available.

ASTAXANTHIN • A yellow coloring found mostly in animal organisms, it is used in fish feed for salmon to increase their orange coloring. Limited to less than 8 mg per kg of finished feed. It is exempt from color certification. There is reported use of the chemical; it has not yet been assigned for toxicology literature.

ASTRINGENT • A substance that causes skin or mucous membranes to pucker and shrink by reducing their ability to absorb water. Often used in skin cleansers, and to help stop bleeding.

ATTAR OF ROSES • *See* Rose Bulgarian.

ATTENTION DEFICIT HYPERACTIVITY DISORDER (ADHD) • Commonly called *hyperactivity,* Attention Deficit Hyperactivity Disorder is a clinical diagnosis based on specific criteria. These include excessive motor activity, impulsiveness, short attention span, and low tolerance to frustration and onset before seven years of age.

ATOPIC DERMATITIS • A chronic, itching, inflammation of the skin also called eczema *(see)*.

AUBERPINE LIQUID • *See* p-Methoxybenzaldehyde.

AUTOLYZED YEAST • The concentrated, nonextracted, partially soluble digest obtained from food-grade yeasts. Solubilization *(see)* is accomplished with enzymes. Food-grade salts and enzymes may also be added. The additive is composed primarily of amino acids *(see)*, peptides *(see)*, proteins, carbohydrates, fats, and salts. Individual products may be in grains, powder, flake, or paste form. It is used as a flavoring agent or enhancer, a protein source, and as a binder. *See* Yeast.

AVERMECTIN B and DELTA • Broad-spectrum antiparasitic and antibiotics used on dried citrus pulp and cottonseeds. FDA tolerance 0.1 ppm on citrus pulp and 0.005 ppm on cottonseed. As a residue in or on tomato pompace 0.07; as residues in meat and meat byproducts, 0.02 ppm; as a residue in milk, 0.005.

AVOIDANCE • Measures taken to avoid contact with allergy-producing substances. Since there are no cures for allergies as of yet, avoiding allergens is the best way to combat them.

AZAPERONE • A tranquilizer and sedative used to treat swine.

AZINPHOS METHYL • Crystals or brown waxy solid used as an insecticide for citrus pulp, soybean oil, and sugarcane. Poison by inhalation, ingestion, skin contact, intravenous, intraperitoneal, and possibly other routes. May cause tumors and birth defects.

AZO DYES • A large category of colorings used in both the food and cosmetic industries, the dyes are characterized by the way they combine with nitrogen. Made from diazonium compounds and phenol, the dyes usually contain a mild acid, such as citric or tartaric acid. Among the foods in which they are used are "penny" candies, caramels and chews, Life Savers, fruit drops, filled chocolates (but not pure chocolate); soft drinks, fruit drinks, and ades; jellies, jams, marmalades, stewed fruit sauces, fruit gelatins, fruit yogurts; ice cream, pie fillings, vanilla, butterscotch, and chocolate puddings, caramel custard, whips, dessert sauces such as vanilla, and cream in powdered form; bakery goods (except plain rolls), crackers, cheese puffs, chips, cake and cookie mixes, waffle/pancake mixes, macaroni and spaghetti (certain brands); mayonnaise, salad dressings, catsup (certain brands), mustard, ready-made salads with dressings, remoulade, béarnaise, and hollandaise sauces, as well as sauces such as curry, fish, onion, tomato, and white cream; mashed rutabagas, purees, packaged soups and some canned soups; canned anchovies, herring, sardines, fish balls, caviar, cleaned shellfish. Azo dyes can cause allergic reactions, particularly hives. People who become sensitized to permanent hair dyes containing *p*-phenylenediamine *(see)* also develop a cross sensitivity to azo dyes. That is, a person who is allergic to permanent *p*-phenylenediamine dyes will also be allergic to azo dyes. Also used in nonpermanent hair rinses and tints. There are reports that azo dyes are absorbed through the skin.

AZODICARBONAMIDE • A bleaching and maturing agent for flour. Yellow to orange red, a crystalline powder, practically insoluble in water. Used in amounts up to 45 ppm. The FDA wants further study of this chemical for both short-term and long-term effects. Although allowed as a food additive, there is no current reported use of the chemical, and, therefore, although toxicology information may be available, it is not being updated.

B

BABASSU OIL • A nondrying edible oil expressed from the kernels of the babassu palm, which grows in Brazil. Used in foods and soaps but is expensive. No known toxicity.

BACITRACIN • An antibiotic. White to pale with a slight odor. Used as an animal drug in beef, chicken, eggs, milk, pheasant, pork, and turkey. Used to increase weight gain, improve feed efficiency, and treat bacterial infections in swine. Tolerance set by the FDA is 0.5 ppm in uncooked tissue of cattle, swine, chickens, turkeys, pheasants, quail, and in milk and eggs. Moderately toxic by ingestion and injection. Possibly mutagenic.

BACITRACIN METHYLENE DISALICYLATE and BACITRACIN ZINC • White to brownish-gray powder used as an animal feed drug that the FDA permits at a level not in excess of the amount reasonably required to accomplish the intended effect.

BACTERIA • Microscopic single-cell organisms. Bacteria are among the most common microorganisms responsible for diseases in humans. Many are harmless. Those from lactic acid and propionic acid are harmless and used to produce cheeses and margarine.

BACTERIAL CATALASE • A catalase is an enzyme in plant and animal tissues. It exerts a chemical reaction that converts hydrogen peroxide into water and oxygen. Derived from bacteria by a pure culture fermentation process, bacterial catalase may be used safely, according to the FDA, in destroying and removing the hydrogen peroxide that has been used in the manufacture of cheese—providing "the organism *Micrococcus lysodeikticus* from which the bacterial catalase is to be derived is demonstrated to be nontoxic and nonpathogenic." The organism is removed from the bacterial catalase prior to the use of the catalase, the catalase to be used in an amount not in excess of the minimum required to produce its intended effect.

BACTERIOCINS • Antibodies having bactericidal activity, such as nisin preparation *(see)*.

BAKER'S YEAST GLYCAN • Used as an emulsifier, thickeners, and stabilizer in frozen desserts, sour cream, cheese spread, cheese flavored, and flavored snack dips. *See* Baker's Yeast Protein.

BAKER'S YEAST PROTEIN • *Saccharomyces cerevisiae.* A yeast strain yielding high growth and used in leavening bakery products and as a dietary supplement.

BAKING POWDER • In baking, any powders used as a substitute for yeast, usually a mixture of sodium bicarbonate, starch, as a filler, and harmless acid such as tartaric. Cream of tartar is often used as the necessary acid. Nontoxic.

BAKING SODA • A common name for sodium bicarbonate *(see)*.

BALM, LEMON • *See* Lemon Balm. GRAS.

BALM OIL • *Melissa officinalis.* A natural fruit and liquor flavoring agent for beverages, ice cream, ices, candy, and baked goods. The balm leaves extract also is used in fruit flavors for beverages. The FDA has not yet done a search of the toxicology literature concerning this additive. GRAS.

BALSAM PERU • Obtained from Peruvian balsam in Central America near the Pacific Coast. A dark brown viscous liquid with a pleasant lingering odor and a warm bitter taste extracted from a variety of evergreens. Used in strawberry, chocolate, cherry, grape, brandy, rum, maple, walnut, coconut, spice, and vanilla flavoring for beverages, ice cream, ices, candy, baked goods, gelatin desserts, chewing gum, and syrups. The oil is used in berry, coconut, fruit, rum, maple, and vanilla flavoring for beverages, ice cream, ices, candy, and baked goods. *Balsam fir oil* is a natural pineapple, lime, and spice flavoring for beverages, ice cream, ices, candy, baked goods, and gelatin desserts. *Balsam fir oleoresin* is a natural fruit and spice flavoring for beverages, ice cream, ices, candy, and baked goods. Balsam fir is yellowish green, thick, transparently liquid, with a pinelike smell and a bitter aftertaste. It is also used in the manufacture of chocolate, in face masks, perfumes, cream hair rinses, and astringents. Mildly antiseptic and irritating to the skin and may cause contact dermatitis and a stuffy nose. It is one of the most common sensitizers and may cross-react with benzoin, rosin, benzoic acid, benzyl alcohol, cinnamic acid, essential oils, orange peel, eugenol, cinnamon, clove, tolu balsam, storax, benzyl benzoate, and wood tars.

BAMBERMYCINS • Antibiotics used as an antibacterial in feed for poultry, cattle, and swine. *See* Antibiotics.

BANTHIONINE • *See* Acimeton.

BARLEY FLOUR • A cereal grass cultivated since prehistoric times. Used in the manufacture of malt beverages, as a breakfast food, and as a demulcent *(see)* in cosmetics. No known toxicity.

BARRIER AGENT • A protective for hand creams and lotions, which acts as a barrier against irritating chemicals, including water and detergents. The water-repellent types deposit a film that acts as a barrier to water and water-soluble agents that irritate the skin; oil-repellent types act as barriers against oil and oil-soluble irritants. Silicones *(see)* are widely used as barrier agents. Other skin protective ingredients in barrier agents include petrolatum, paraffin, ozokerite, vegetables, beeswax, casein, various celluloses, alginic acid, zein, gum tragacanth, pectin, quince seed, bentonite, zinc oxide, zinc stearate, sodium silicate, talc, stearic acid, and titanium dioxide *(see all)*. Covering one's hands with Vaseline or zinc oxide ointment will protect them well and inexpensively.

BASES • Alkalies, such as ammonium hydroxide *(see)*, used to control the acidity-alkalinity balance of food products. *See* pH.

BASIL EXTRACT • Sweet Basil. The extract of the leaves and flowers of *Ocimum basilicum*, an herb having spikes of small white flowers and aromatic leaves used as a seasoning. A natural flavoring distilled from the flowering tops of the plant has a slightly yellowish color and a spicy odor. Used in sausage and spice flavorings for beverages, candy, ice cream, baked goods, condiments, and meats. The oleoresin is used in spice flavorings for baked goods and condiments. The oil is used in loganberry, strawberry, orange, rose, violet, cherry, honey, licorice, basil, muscatel, meat, and root beer flavorings for beverages, ice cream, ices, candy, baked goods. Moderately toxic by ingestion. A skin irritant. GRAS.

BAYBERRY BARK • Myrica Oil. A yellow essential oil used in rum and other flavorings and fragrances. GRAS.

BAY, SWEET • *Laurus nobilis.* A natural flavoring native to a Mediterranean plant with stiff, glossy, fragrant leaves. Used in vermouth, sausage, and spice flavorings for beverages, ice cream, ices, candy, baked goods, condiments, and meats.

BAY LEAVES • *Pimenta racemosa.* The West Indian extract is a natural flavoring used in vermouth and spice flavorings for beverages, ice cream, ices, candy, baked goods, meat, and soups. The *oil* is used in fruit, liquor, and bay flavorings for beverages, ice cream, ices, candy, baked goods, condiments, and meats. The *oleoresin (see)* is used in sausage flavoring for meats and soups. No known toxicity. GRAS.

BCD • *See* Beta-Cyclodextrin.

BEECHWOOD, CREOSOTE • *See* Creosote.

BEEF TALLOW • *See* Tallow Flakes. GRAS for packaging.

BEESWAX • From virgin bees and primarily used as an emulsifier. Practically insoluble in water. Yellow beeswax from the honeycomb is yellowish, soft to brittle, and has a honeylike odor. White beeswax is yellowish white and slightly different in taste but otherwise has the same properties as yellow beeswax. Used as a candy glaze and polish. Also used in many cosmetics including baby creams, brilliantine hair dressings, cold cream, emollient creams, wax depilatories, eye creams, eye shadow, foundation creams and makeup, lipstick, mascara, nail whiteners, protective creams, and paste rouge. Can cause contact dermatitis *(see).* The final report to the FDA of the Select Committee on GRAS Substances stated in 1980 that it should continue its GRAS status with no limitations other than good manufacturing practices. *See* Beeswax, Bleached.

BEESWAX, BLEACHED • White Wax. Yellow wax bleached and purified from the honeycomb of the bee. Remains yellowish white, is solid, somewhat translucent, and fairly insoluble in water. Differs slightly in taste from yellow beeswax. Used in fruit and honey flavorings for beverages, ice cream, ices, baked goods, and honey. *See* Yellow Beeswax for medicinal uses. Mild allergen. The final report to the FDA of the Select Committee on GRAS Substances stated in 1980 that it should continue its GRAS status with no limitations other than good manufacturing practices.

BEET • Juice and Powder. Vegetable dye used to color dairy products. Listed for food use in 1967. Exempt from color certification. No known toxicity.

BEETROOT JUICE POWDER • The powdered stem base of the beet used for its reddish color in powders and rouges. Exempt from color certification. No known toxicity.

BEHENIC ACID • Docosanoic acid. Colorless water, soluble, constituent of seed fats, animal fats, and marine animal oils. It is a fatty acid *(see)* used to opacify shampoos. No known toxicity.

BENOMYL • Methyl-1-(butyl carbamoyl)-2-benzimidazole-carbamate. Tersan 1991. Bonide. White crystalline solid, a carbamate *(see).* It is the generic name for a fungicide used on peaches, apples, and other fruits after they are picked. The

FDA tolerances for residues in animal feed are: 70 ppm in dried apple pomace resulting from application to apples as a residue; 125 ppm in dried grape pomace and raisin waste resulting from application to growing grapes; 50 ppm in raisins resulting from application to growing grapes; 50 ppm in dried citrus pulp when present therein as a result of application to the raw agricultural citrus fruits; 50 ppm in concentrated tomato products resulting from application to growing crop; and 50 ppm in rice hulls resulting from application to raw agricultural rice. It is also used as an oxidizer in sewage treatment. It is extremely toxic by ingestion. It may cause birth defects. It is a mild irritant to human skin.

BENSULFURON METHYL ESTER • Herbicide. Tolerance for residue in or on rice, 0.02 ppm.

BENTAZON • Herbicide. FDA residue tolerance is 4 ppm in or on mint hay used for feed resulting from application to growing mint.

BENTONITE • A colloidal clay (aluminum silicate) that has a high swelling capacity in water. Used as a food additive as a thickener and as a colorant in wine. Poison if given by vein, causing blood clots, and may cause tumors. GRAS.

BENZALDEHYDE • Artificial Almond Oil. A colorless liquid that occurs in the kernels of bitter almonds. Lime is used in its synthetic manufacture. As the artificial essential oil of almonds, it is used in berry, butter, coconut, apricot, cherry, peach, liquor, brandy, rum, almond, pecan, pistachio, spice, and vanilla flavoring. Occurs naturally in cherries, raspberries, tea, almonds, bitter oil, cajeput oil, and cassia bark. Used in beverages, ice cream, ices, candy, baked goods, chewing gum, and cordials. Also used in cosmetic creams and lotions, perfumes, soaps, and dyes. May cause allergic reactions. A skin irritant, contact may cause a rash. Highly toxic. Produces central nervous system depression and convulsions. Fatal dose is estimated to be two ounces. GRAS. See Benzyl Acetate.

BENZALDEHYDE DIMETHYL ACETAL • A synthetic agent used in fruit, cherry, nut, and almond flavorings for beverages, ice cream, ices, candy, baked goods, gelatin, and puddings. See Benzyl Acetate.

BENZALDEHYDE GLYCERYL ACETAL • A synthetic agent used in fruit, cherry, nut, and almond flavorings for beverages, ice cream, ices, candy, baked goods, and chewing gum. See Benzyl Acetate.

BENZALDEHYDE PROPYLENE GLYCOL ACETAL • A synthetic agent used in fruit, cherry, nut, and almond flavorings for beverages, ice cream, ices, candy, baked goods, and chewing gum. See Benzyl Acetate.

BENZALKONIUM CHLORIDE (BAK) • A widely used ammonium detergent. It is germicide with an aromatic odor and a very bitter taste. Soluble in water and alcohol but incompatible with most detergents and soaps. Used medicinally as a topical antiseptic and detergent. Allergic conjunctivitis has been reported when used in eye lotions. Lethal to frogs in concentrated oral doses. Highly toxic. The FDA proposed a ban in 1992 for the use of benzalkonium chloride to treat insect bites and stings and in astringent (see) drugs because it has not been shown to be safe and effective for stated claims in OTC products.

BENZATHINE CLOXACILLIN • A veterinary antibiotic. The FDA tolerance for residues in milk is 0.02 ppm.

BENZENE • A solvent obtained from coal and used in modified hop extract for beer regulated by the FDA at 1.0 ppm. Derived from toluene or gasoline, it is used in the manufacture of nail polish remover, detergents, nylon, artificial leather, as an antiknock in gasoline, in airplane fuel, dope, varnish, lacquer, and as a solvent for waxes, resins, and oils. Highly flammable. Poisonous when ingested and irritating to the mucous membranes. Harmful amounts may be absorbed through the skin. Also can cause sensitivity to light in which the skin may break out in a rash or swell. Inhalation of the fumes may be toxic. The Consumer Product Safety Commission voted unanimously in February 1978 to ban the use of benzene in the manufacture of many household products. The commission took the action in response to a petition filed by the Consumer Health Research Group, an organization affiliated with consumer advocate Ralph Nader. Earlier in the year, OSHA and the EPA both cited benzene as a threat to public health. For more than a century, scientists have known that benzene is a powerful bone-marrow poison, destroying the marrow's ability to produce blood cells, causing such conditions as aplastic anemia. In the past several decades evidence has been mounting that it also causes leukemia. Safety standards for cosmetic manufacturing workers and other workers have been set at 10 parts per million during an eight-hour day, but OSHA wants it reduced to 1 part per million. Although listed as a food additive, the FDA says there is no current reported use of the chemical in food and therefore it is not being updated in its data bank.

BENZENE ACETALDEHYDE • Oily, colorless liquid that grows thicker on standing. Has a hyacinth odor. Used as a flavoring agent in bakery products, beverages, chewing gum, confections, gelatin desserts, ice cream, maraschino cherries, and puddings. Moderately toxic by ingestion. Human skin irritant.

BENZENECARBONAL • *See* Benzaldehyde.

BENZENE CARBOXYLIC ACID • *See* Benzoic Acid.

BENZENE HEXACHLORIDE (BHC) • Hexachlorane. Hexylan. A pesticide widely used. Poison by ingestion and by subcutaneous injection. Moderately toxic by skin contact. An experimental cancer-causing and tumor-causing agent by ingestion and skin contact. Human systemic effects by inhalation; headache, nausea or vomiting, and fever. Implicated in aplastic anemia. Possible reproductive effects. It is persistent in the environment and accumulates in mammalian tissue.

BENZENE METHYLAL • *See* Benzaldehyde.

BENZIN • Dark straw-colored to colorless liquid made from coal and oil. Used to dilute color, as a solvent, and as a protective coating for eggshells, fresh fruits, and vegetables. A human poison if injected into the vein. Chronic exposure may cause headache, lack of appetite, dizziness, and other symptoms of intoxication. The FDA permits its use at a level not in excess of the amount reasonably required to accomplish intended use.

1,2-BENZISOTHIAZOL-3 (2H)-ONE-1,1-DIOXIDE • Benzosulfimide. Zaharina. Saccharina. Saccharin Acid. Sucrette. Saccarinose. White crystals or powder, odorless with a sweet taste. Used as a masticatory substance in chewing-gum base. A nonnutritive sweetener used in artificial sweetener, bacon, beverage mixes, beverages, chewing gum, desserts, fruit juice drinks, and jams. The FDA limits it to 12 mg per fluid ounce in beverages, fruit juice drinks, and beverage mixes. Limitation of 20 mg per teaspoon of sugar sweetening equivalent and 230 mg per designated size in processed foods. Sufficient evidence of carcinogenicity in animals but not in humans, although it is a possible human cancer-causing agent. Mild acute toxicity by ingestion.

BENZOATE OF SODA • *See* Sodium Benzoate.

BENZOATES • The salts of benzoic acid *(see)* used primarily as preservatives. The Joint FAO-WHO Expert Committee on Food Additives concluded in June 1998: "The potential exists for high consumers of benzoate to exceed the ADI [Acceptable Daily Intake], but the available data were insufficient to estimate the number of high consumers or the magnitude and duration of intake above the ADI." The Committee is reviewing this additive's level in cheeses, vegetables in vinegar or brine, fish products, liquid eggs, and carbonated water-based soft drinks.

1,2-BENZODIHYDROPYRONE • *See* Dihydrocoumarin.

BENZOE • *See* Benzoin.

BENZOEPIN • Brown crystals used as an insecticide in dried tea. Residue tolerance of 25 ppm in dried tea. Poison by ingestion, inhalation, and skin contact and other routes. Causes tumors in laboratory animals and birth defects. A central nervous system stimulant producing convulsions in humans. A highly toxic organochlorine pesticide that does not accumulate in human tissue. Absorption is normally slow, but is increased by alcohol, oil, and emulsifiers.

BENZOFUROLINE • 5-Benzyl-3-Furyl Methyl(+)-cis, trans-Chrysanthemate. A pesticide used in various food products. Poison by inhalation, ingestion, and intravenous routes. Moderately toxic by skin contact. When heated to decomposition, it emits acrid and irritating fumes.

BENZOIC ACID • A preservative that occurs in nature in cherry bark, raspberries, tea, anise, and cassia bark. First described in 1608 when it was found in gum benzoin. Used in chocolate, lemon, orange, cherry, fruit, nut, and tobacco flavorings for beverages, ice cream, ices, candy, baked goods, icings, and chewing gum. Also used in margarine and pickles. Also an antifungal agent. Used as a chemical preservative and a dietary supplement up to .1 percent. A mild irritant to the skin. It can cause allergic reactions such as asthma, red eyes, and skin rashes, especially in people sensitive to aspirin. Listed by the FDA as GRAS in a reevaluation of safety in 1976. The final report to the FDA of the Select Committee on GRAS Substances stated in 1980 that it should continue its GRAS status with no limitations other than good manufacturing practices.

BENZOIC ALDEHYDE • *See* Benzaldehyde.

BENZOIC RESIN • A flavor additive. *See* Benzoic Acid and Resins.

BENZOIN • Gum Benjamin. Gum Benzoin. Any of several resins containing benzoic acid *(see),* obtained as a gum from various trees. Used as a preserving ointment for fumigating, in perfumes and cosmetics as a compound tincture of benzoin, as a skin protectant and respiratory inhalant. The resin is used as a flavoring agent in chocolate, cherry, rum, spice, and vanilla for beverages, ice cream, ices, candy, baked goods, and chewing gum. Benzoin also is a natural flavoring agent for butterscotch, butter, fruit liquor, and rum. Nontoxic. It was tested by the National Cancer Institute and found not to be a cancer-causing agent in rats and mice but may be mutagenic.

BENZOPHENONES (1–12) • At least a dozen different benzophenones exist. Synthetic agents used in berry, butter, fruit, apricot, peach, nut, and vanilla for beverages, ice cream, ices, candy, and baked goods. They are used as fixatives *(see)* for heavy perfumes (geranium, for example) and soaps (the smell of "new mown hay"). Obtained as a white flaky solid with a delicate, persistent roselike odor, and soluble in most fixed oils and in mineral oil. Also used in the manufacture of hairsprays, and in sunscreens. They help prevent deterioration of ingredients that might be affected by the ultraviolet rays found in ordinary daylight. May produce hives and contact sensitivity. In sunscreens they may cause immediate hives as well as other photoallergic reactions. Toxic when injected.

BENZOPYRENE • A hydrocarbon found in coal tar, cigarette smoke, and in the atmosphere as a product of incomplete combustion. Highly toxic and a cancer-causing agent.

2,3-BENZOPYRROLE • *See* Indole.

BENZOYL EUGENOL • *See* Eugenyl Benzoate.

BENZOYL PEROXIDE • A bleaching agent for flours, blue cheese, Gorgonzola, and milk. A catalyst for hardening certain fiberglass resins. A drying agent in cosmetics. Toxic by inhalation. A skin allergen and irritant.

BENZYL ACETATE • A colorless liquid with a pear or flowerlike odor obtained from a number of plants, especially jasmine, for use in perfumery and soap. A synthetic raspberry, strawberry, butter, violet, apple, cherry, banana, and plum flavoring agent for beverages, ice cream, ices, candy, baked goods, chewing gum, and gelatin desserts. Can be irritating to the skin, eyes, and respiratory tract. Ingestion causes intestinal upset, including vomiting and diarrhea. The FAO-WHO Expert Committee on Food Additives has studied this additive a number of times. The Committee noted brain damage involving the cerebellum and/or hippocampus in rats and mice given benzyl acetate at a dose level of 5 percent in the diet for 13 weeks. No such effect was observed in the long-term toxicity-carcinogenicity studies in mice or rats at lower doses. In the long-term study in rats, no adverse effects were observed at levels of up to 550 mg per kg of body weight per day in the diet. In long-term study, treated males and female mice showed lower body weights than controls. The Committee has noted the absence of reproductive/birth defect studies for substances in this group, and has recommended that a full review of benzyl acetate, benzoic acid, the benzoate salts, benzaldehyde, and benzyl alcohol be performed to determine "whether these or other studies are required."

BENZYL ACETOACETATE • A synthetic berry and fruit flavoring agent for beverages, ice cream, ices, candy, baked goods, gelatin desserts, and chewing gum. *See* Benzyl Acetate for toxicity.

BENZYL ACETYL ACETATE • *See* Benzyl Acetoacetate.

BENZYL ALCOHOL • A flavoring that is derived as a pure alcohol and is a constituent of jasmine, hyacinth, and other plants. It has a faint, sweet odor. Used in synthetic blueberry, loganberry, raspberry, orange, floral, rose, violet, fruit, cherry, grape, honey, liquor, muscatel, nut, walnut, root beer, and vanilla flavorings for beverages, ice cream, ices, candy, baked goods, gelatin desserts, and chewing gum. A solvent in perfumes and a preservative in hair dyes and a topical antiseptic. Irritating and corrosive to the skin and mucous membranes. Ingestion of large doses causes intestinal upsets. It may cross-react in the sensitive with balsam Peru *(see)*.

BENZYL BENZOATE • Plasticizer in nail polishes, solvent and fixative for perfumes. Occurs naturally in balsams Tolu and Peru and in various flower oils. Colorless, oily liquid or white crystals with a light floral scent and sharp burning taste.

BENZYL BUTYL ETHER • Synthetic fruit flavoring agent for beverages, ice cream, ices, candy, baked goods, gelatin desserts, and puddings.

BENZYL BUTYRATE • Butyric Acid. A synthetic flavoring agent, colorless, liquid, with a plumlike odor. Used in loganberry, raspberry, strawberry, butter, apricot, peach, pear, liquor, muscatel, cheese, and nut flavorings for beverages, ice cream, ices, candy, baked goods, chewing gum, and gelatin desserts.

BENZYL CARBINOL • *See* Phenethyl Alcohol.

BENZYL CINNAMATE • Sweet Odor of Balsam. Colorless prisms, used to give artificial fruit scents to perfumes. A synthetic flavoring agent found in balsams of Peru, Tolu, styrax, copaiba, and others. Used in raspberry, chocolate, apricot, cherry, peach, pineapple, plum, prune, honey, liquor, and rum for beverages, ice cream, ices, candy, baked goods, chewing gum, and gelatin desserts. Moderately toxic by ingestion. A mild allergen and skin irritant. *See* Balsam Peru for toxicity.

BENZYL DIMETHYL CARBINYL ACETATE • *See* a,a,-Dimethylphenethyl Acetate.

BENZYL DIMETHYL CARBINYL BUTYRATE • *See* a,a,-Dimethylphenethyl Butyrate.

BENZYL DIMETHYL CARBINYL FORMATE • *See* a,a,-Dimethylphenethyl Formate.

BENZYL 2,3-DIMETHYLCROTONATE • A synthetic fruit and spice flavoring agent for beverages, ice cream, ices, candy, and baked goods.

BENZYLDIMETHYLDODECYLAMMONIUM CHLORIDE • Benzyl Ammonium Chloride. An antimicrobial agent used in beets and sugarcane. A skin and eye irritant.

BENZYL DI PROPYL KETONE • *See* 3-Benzyl-4-Heptanone.

BENZYL DISULFIDE • A synthetic fruit flavoring agent for beverages, ice cream, ices, and candy.

BENZYL ETHYL ETHER • Colorless, oily liquid, aromatic odor, insoluble in water, miscible in alcohol. Used in flavoring for beverages, ice cream, ices, candy, and baked goods. Narcotic in high concentrations. May be a skin irritant.

BENZYL FORMATE • Formic Acid. A synthetic chocolate, apricot, cherry, peach, pineapple, plum, prune, honey, and liquor flavoring agent for beverages, ice cream, ices, candy, baked goods, and chewing gum. Pleasant fruity odor. Practically insoluble in water. There is no specific data for toxicity, but it is believed to be narcotic in high concentrations.

3-BENZYL-4-HEPTANONE • Synthetic fruit flavoring for beverages ice cream, ices, candy, and baked goods.

BENZYL o-HYDROXYBENZOATE • *See* Benzyl Salicylate.

BENZYL ISOAMYL ALCOHOL • *See a*-Isobutylphenethyl Alcohol.

BENZYL ISOBUTYL CARBINOL • *See a*-Isobutylphenethyl Alcohol.

BENZYL ISOBUTYRATE • A synthetic strawberry and fruit flavoring for beverages, ice cream, ices, candy, and baked goods.

BENZYL ISOEUGENOL • A synthetic spice flavoring for beverages, ice cream, ices, candy, and baked goods. No known toxicity.

BENZYL ISOVALERATE • A synthetic raspberry, apple, apricot, banana, cherry, pineapple, walnut, and cheese flavoring agent for beverages, ice cream, ices, candy, baked goods, gelatin desserts, and chewing gum.

BENZYL MERCAPTAN • A synthetic coffee-flavoring agent used for beverages, ice cream, ices, candy, and baked goods.

BENZYL METHOXYETHYL ACETAL • Synthetic fruit and cherry flavoring agent for beverages, ice cream, ices, candy, and baked goods.

BENZYL PHENYLACETATE • A synthetic butter, caramel, fruit, and honey flavoring agent for beverages, ice cream, ices, candy, baked goods, and toppings. A colorless liquid with a sweet floral odor; occurs naturally in honey.

BENZYL B-PHENYL ACRYLATE • *See* Benzyl Cinnamate.

BENZYL PROPIONATE • A synthetic flavoring substance, colorless liquid, with a sweet fruity odor. Used in berry, apple, banana, grape, pear, and pineapple flavorings for beverages, ice cream, ices, candy, baked goods, chewing gum, and icings.

BENZYL SALICYLATE • Salicylic Acid. Used in floral and peach flavorings for beverages, ice cream, ices, candy, and baked goods. A fixative in perfumes and a solvent in sunscreen lotions. It is a thick liquid with a light, pleasant odor, it is mixed with alcohol or ether. As with other salicylates it may interact adversely with such medications as antidepressants and anticoagulants, and may cause skin to break out with a rash and swell when exposed to sunlight. *See* Salicylates.

BENZYL ACETIC ACID • *See* Cinnamic Acid.

BENZYL ACETONE • *See* 4-Phenyl-3-Buten-2-One.

BENZYETHYL ALCOHOL • *See* Benzyl Alcohol.

1-BENZYLOXY (B-METHOXY) ETHOXY ETHANE • *See* Benzyl Methoxy-ethyl Acetal.

BENZYL PROPYL ACETATE • *See a,a*-Dimethylphenethyl Acetate.

BENZYL PROPYL ALCOHOL • *See a,a*-Dimethylphenethyl Acetate.

BENZYL PROPYL CARBINOL • *See a*-Propylphenethyl Alcohol.

BENZYL THIOL • *See* Benzyl Mercaptan.

BERGAMOL • *See* Linalyl Acetate.

BERGAMOT • Bergamot Orange or Red. Oswego Tea. An orange flavoring extracted from a pear-shaped fruit, whose rind yields a greenish brown oil much used in perfumery and brilliantine hairdressings. Used in strawberry, lemon, orange, tangerine, cola, floral, banana, grape, peach, pear, pineapple, liquor, spice, and vanilla flavorings for beverages, ice cream, ices, candy, baked goods, gelatin desserts, chewing gum, and icings. The oil can cause brown skin stains (berloque) when exposed to sunlight and is considered a prime photosensitizer (sensitivity to light). *See* Berloque Dermatitis. GRAS.

BERLOQUE DERMATITIS • Some perfumes, which contain oil of bergamot *(see)* and other photosensitizers, may produce increased pigmentation (brown spots) in the area where the perfume has been applied, especially when it is immediately exposed to sunlight. There is no effective treatment and the pigmentation generally persists for some time.

BETA-APO-8′-CAROTENAL • Orange coloring agent for solid or semisolid foods. Limited to 15 mg per pound of solid or semisolid food. Does not require certification. Nontoxic.

BETA-CAROTENE • Provitamin A. Beta Carotene. Found in all plants and in many animal tissues. It is the chief yellow coloring matter of carrots, butter, and egg yolk. Extracted as red crystals or crystalline powder, it is used as a coloring in food and cosmetics and as a direct food additive. It is exempt from certification. Also used in the manufacture of vitamin A. Too much carotene in the blood can lead to carotenemia, a pale yellow red pigmentation of the skin that may be mistaken for jaundice. It is a benign condition, and withdrawal of carotene from the diet cures it. Beta-carotene has less serious side effects than vitamin A and was given to 22,000 physicians as part of a five-year study to determine whether aspirin could protect against heart disease and beta carotene against tumors. It is nontoxic. The FAO-WHO Expert Committee on Food Additives concluded that there was no objection to the use of vegetable extracts as coloring agents provided the level of use did not exceed the level normally present in vegetables. Implicit in this conclusion, the Committee notes, is that the extracts should not be made toxic by virtues of the concentrations of toxic compounds (including toxicants naturally occurring in the vegetables) or by the generation of reaction products or residues of a nature or in such amounts as to be toxicologically significant. The past specifications for carotenes (vegetables) were revised to include material derived from carrots, alfalfa, and palm oil, which are known to be used commercially. GRAS.

BETA-CITRAURIN • Excellent raw material for the extraction of carotinoids (*see* Carotene), or orange coloring. Found in tangerine and orange peels. Soluble in alcohol.

BETA-CYCLODEXTRIN (BCD) • A naturally occurring substance from the action of enzymes on starch. A white, odorless, fine crystalline solid or powder having a sweet taste. It is used as an encapsulating agent, processing aid, or stabilizer in foods. No known toxicity.

BETA-GLUCANS • Polysaccharides *(see)* that yield sugars (glucose) on hydrolysis when exposed to water treatment. Beta-glucan is in cellulose and is found in edibles such as oat fiber and barley.

BETAINE • Used as a coloring and as a dietary supplement. Occurs in common beets and in many vegetables as well as animal substances. Used in resins. Has been employed to treat muscle weakness medically. No known toxicity.

BETAINE, ANHYDROUS • Betaine *(see)* with the water removed.

BETULA • Obtained from the European white birch and a source of asphalt and tar. Used in hair tonics; it reddens the scalp and creates a warm feeling due to an increased flow of blood to the area. Also used in moisturizing creams and astringents. Betula leaves were formerly used to treat rheumatism. *See* Salicylates.

BHA • *See* Butylated Hydroxyanisole.

BHT • *See* Butylated Hydroxytoluene.

BIACETYL • *See* Diacetyl.

BICARBONATE OF SODA • A buffer and neutralizing agent used in self-rising cornmeal. GRAS. *See* Sodium Bicarbonate.

BIFENTHRIN • A synthetic pyrethroid pesticide. Used to combat insects and mites. FDA tolerances are 0.02 ppm in milk, 0.10 ppm in fat, meat, and meat byproducts of cattle, goats, hogs, and sheep, and 0.50 as a residue in cottonseed. Lower toxicity than most pesticides.

BILBERRY EXTRACT • The extract of *Vaccinum myrtillus,* a plant found in North America and the Alps that differ from the typical blueberries in having single flowers or very small buds.

BILE SALTS and OX BILE EXTRACT • *See* Ox Bile.

BINDER • Substances such as gum arabic, gum tragacanth, glycerin, and sorbitol *(see all)* that dispense, swell, or absorb water, increase consistency, and hold ingredients together. For example, binders are used to make powders in women's compacts retain their shape; binders in toothpaste provide for the smooth dispensing of the paste.

BIOCHEMICAL • A substance that is produced by a chemical reaction in a living organism. Some can also be made in the laboratory.

BIOFLAVONOIDS • Vitamin P Complex. Citrus-flavored compounds needed to maintain healthy blood vessel walls. Needed to maintain healthy blood vessel walls. Widely distributed among plants, especially citrus fruits and rose hips. Usually taken from orange and lemon rinds and used as a reducing agent *(see)*. No known toxicity. Any claim for special dietary use, according to FDA regulations, renders the food misbranded.

BIOTECHNOLOGY • The use of living cells or parts of cells to perform procedures and to make products.

BIOTIN • Vitamin H. Vitamin B Factor. A whitish crystalline powder used as a texturizer in cosmetic creams. Present in minute amounts in every living cell and in larger amounts in yeast and milk. Vital to growth, it acts as a coenzyme in the formation of certain essential fatlike substances and plays a part in reactions involving carbon dioxide. It is needed by humans for healthy circulation and red blood cells. There is reported use of the chemical; it has not yet been assigned for toxicology literature.

BIPHENYL • Derived from benzene. Used as a fungistat in packaging of citrus fruits and in manufacturing processes.

BIRCH FAMILY • *Betulaceae.* Sweet Oil and Tar Oil A flavoring agent from the bark and wood of deciduous trees common in the Northern Hemisphere. The oils are obtained by distillation. It is a clear, dark brown liquid with a strong leatherlike odor. Birch sweet oil is used in synthetic strawberry, pineapple, maple, nut, root beer, sarsaparilla, spice, wintergreen, and birch beer flavorings for beverages, ice cream, ices, candy, baked goods, gelatins, puddings (4,300 ppm), and syrups. Birch tar oil, which is refined, is used in chewing gum and has also been used for preserving leather. Used as an astringent in creams and shampoos, it is an ancient remedy. The medicinal properties of the plant tend to vary, depending upon which part of the tree is used. It has been used as a laxative, as an aid for gout, to treat rheumatism and dropsy, and to dissolve kidney stones. It is supposedly good for bathing skin eruptions. The oil is used in food flavorings. There is reported use of the chemical, it has not yet been assigned for toxicology literature. *See* Betula.

BIS- • A prefix meaning twice.

BISABOLENE • A colorless oily sesquiterpene found in many essential oils such as oil of bisabol and lime oil. Used as a flavoring.

BIS(2-CARBOXYETHYL) SULFIDE • Thiodipropionic Acid. TDPA. An antioxidant used in packaging material. Poisonous by injection. Moderately toxic by ingestion. A skin and eye irritant.

3,6-BIS(2-CHLORPHENYL)-1,2,4,5 TETRAZINE • A pesticide with a tolerance of 20 ppm in apple pomace as a result of application to apples.

1,1-BIS(p-CHLOROPHENYL)-2,2,2-TRICHLOROETHANOL • Acarin. Decofol. An insecticide used on dried tea. Poison by ingestion and skin contact. May cause cancer and mutations in humans.

2,4-BIS(ETHYLAMINO)-6-CHLORO-s-TRIAZINE • Aktinit S. Aquazine. Zeapur. An herbicide used in animal feed, molasses, potable water, sugarcane byproducts, sugarcane syrups. The FDA's residue tolerances are 1 ppm in sugarcane by products, molasses, and syrup, and 0.01 ppm in potable water. Limitation of 1 ppm sugarcane byproduct molasses when used for animal feed. It is in the EPA Genetic Toxicology Program *(see)*. Poison by intravenous route. Causes tumors in experimental animals. A skin and eye irritant in humans.

BIS(2-ETHYL HEXYL)PHTHALATE • BEHP. Witcizer 312. A plasticizer used in packaging materials for foods of high water content. Suspected human cancer-causing agent and teratogen. Affects the human gastrointestinal tract. A mild skin and eye irritant. *See* Phthalates.

N,N-BIS(2-HYDROXYETHYL)DODECAN AMIDE • Lauryl Diethanolamide. Lauric Acid Diethanolamide. Antistatic agent used in packaging materials and limited to 0.5 percent in polyethylene containers.

BIS(8-OXYQUINOLINE) COPPER • Bioquin. Quinondo. Furitdo. A preservative for wood. Copper and its compounds are on the Community Right-To-Know List *(see)*.

BIS(TRIS[BETA, BETA-DIMETHYLPHENETHYL]TIN)OXIDE • Bendex. An insecticide used in animal feed, dried apples, dried citrus pulp, dried grapes, dried prunes, and raisins. The FDA's tolerances are 20.0 ppm in prunes, 20 ppm in raisins. Limitations of 75.0 ppm in dried apple pomace, 35.0 ppm in dried citrus pulp, 100 ppm in dried grape pomace, 20 ppm in raisin waste when used for animal feed. Moderately toxic by ingestion and skin contact.

BITTER ALMOND OIL • Almond Oil. Sweet Almond Oil. Expressed Almond Oil. A colorless to pale yellow, bland, nearly odorless, essential and expressed oil from the ripe seed of the small sweet almond grown in Italy, Spain, and France. It has a strong almond odor and a mild taste. Used as a flavoring and in the manufacture of perfumes and as an oil in hair creams, nail whiteners, nail polish remover, eye creams, emollients, soaps, and perfumes. Many users are allergic to cosmetics with almond oil. It causes stuffy nose and skin rashes. GRAS when free of prussic acid.

BITTER ASH EXTRACT • *See* Quassia Extract.

BITTER ORANGE OIL • The pale yellow volatile oil expressed from the fresh peel of a species of citrus and used in perfumes and flavorings. May cause skin irritation and allergic reactions.

BITTER PRINCIPLES • A group of chemicals in plants that are bitter tasting. They differ chemically but most belong to the iris or pine families. Bitter principles reputedly stimulate the secretion of digestive juices and stimulate the liver. They are being investigated scientifically today as antifungals and antibiotics as well as anticancer agents. The bitter principle in mallow plants is being investigated as a male contraceptive. Other bitter principles in herbs are used to combat coughs and as sedatives.

BITTER WOOD EXTRACT • *See* Quassia Extract.

BIURET • A nutrient in animal feed for ruminants except for those producing milk for human consumption. *See* Urea.

BIXIN • Norbixin. The active ingredients of annatto, both carotenoidlike compounds, but with five times the coloring power of carotene, and with better stability. They impart a yellow coloring to food. *See* Annatto.

BIX ORELLANA • A solvent extraction of *Bixa orellana* seeds. A yellow carotenoid *(see)* solution or powder, it is a color additive in ink used for marking foods, and is used in oleomargarine, poultry, sausage casings, and shortening. May cause contact dermatitis.

BLACK COHOSH • *Cimicifuga racemosa.* Cimicifuga. Snakeroot. Bugbane. Black Snakeroot. Rattleroot. Used in astringents, perennial herb with a flower that is supposedly distasteful to insects. Grown from Canada to North Carolina and Kansas. Has a reputation for curing snakebites. It is used in ginger ale flavoring. A tonic and antispasmodic. No known toxicity. The root contains various glycosides *(see)* including estrogenic substances and tannins. Herbalists have used it to relieve nerve pains, menstrual pains, and the pain of childbirth; also used to speed delivery and reduce blood pressure. Black cohosh is believed to have sedative properties. In 1992, the FDA proposed a ban on black cohosh in oral menstrual drug products because it had not been shown to be safe and effective as claimed.

BLACK CURRANT EXTRACT • The extract of the fruit of *Ribes nigrum,* a European plant that produces hanging yellow flowers and black aromatic fruit.

BLACK CUTCH EXTRACT • *See* Catechu Extract.

BLACK PEPPER OIL • From steam distillation of dried fruit of *Piper nigrum.* An odorless to greenish liquid with the odor and taste of pepper. A flavoring agent used in meat, salads, soups, and vegetables. A moderate skin irritant.

BLACK WALNUT EXTRACT • Extract of the leaves or bark of the black walnut tree, *Juglans nigra,* found in eastern North America. It produces nuts with a thick oil and is used as a black coloring.

BLACKBERRY BARK EXTRACT • *Rubus fruiticosus.* A natural flavoring agent extracted from the woody plant. Used in berry, pineapple, grenadine, root beer, sarsaparilla, wintergreen, and birch beer flavorings for beverages, ice cream, ices, candy, baked goods, and liquor. The berries, leaves, and root bark are also used to treat fevers, colds, sore throats, vaginal discharge, diarrhea, and dysentery. The berries contain isocitric and malic acids, sugars, pectin, monoglycoside of cyanidin, vitamins C and A. The leaves and bark are said to lower fever, are astringent, and stop bleeding. The leaves are used for a soothing bath.

BLACKTHORN BERRIES • *See* Sloe Berries.

BLEACHING AGENTS • Used by many industries, particularly flour milling, to make dough rise faster. Certain chemical qualities, which pastry chefs call "gluten characteristics," are needed to make an elastic, stable dough. Such qualities are acquired during aging, but in the process flour oxidizes, that is, combines with oxygen, and loses its natural gold color. Although mature flour is white, it possesses the qualities bakers want. But proper aging costs money and makes the flour more susceptible to insects and rodents, according to food manufacturers. Hence, the widespread use of bleaching and maturing agents.

BLOOM INHIBITOR • Bloom is an "undesirable effect" caused by the migration of cocoa fat from the cocoa fibers to the chocolate's surface. Chocolate that has bloomed has a gray-white appearance. Nonbloomed chocolate has a bright, shiny surface, with a rich appearance. The blood inhibitor—a surfactant *(see)* such as sorbitan or lecithin *(see both)*—controls the size of the chocolate crystals and reduces the tendency of the fat to mobilize.

BLUE • *See* FD and C Blue.

BLUE NO. 1 • *See* FD and C Blue No. 1.

BOILER WATER ADDITIVES • Most are used in food processing as cleaning agents. Those regulated by the FDA include ammonium alginate, cobalt sulfate, lignosulfonic acid, monbutyl ether of polyoxyethylene glycol or potassium tripolyphosphate, sodium carboxymethyl cellulose, sodium glucoheptonate, sodium humate, sodium meta silicate, sodium metabisulfite, polyoxypropylene glycol, polyoxyethylene glycol, potassium carbonate, sodium acetate, sodium alginate, sodium aluminate, sodium carbonate, sodium hexametaphosphate, sodium hydroxide, sodium lignosulfonate, sodium nitrate, sodium phosphate (mono-, di-, and tri-). sodium poly acrylate, sodium poly methacrylate, sodium silicate, sodium sulfate, sodium sulfite, sodium tripolyphosphate, tannin, tetraodium EDTA, tetrasodium pyrophosphate, 1-hydroxy-ethylidene-1,1-diphosphonic acid and its sodium, and potassium salt. Hydrazine *(see)* must be zero in steam contacting food; Acrylamide-sodium acrylate resin is restricted to 0.05 percent of acrylamide monomer in steam contact food. Cyclohexylamine or morpholine must be less than 10 ppm in steam contact food except milk and milk products. Octadecylamine must be less than 3 ppm; diethylaminoethanol must be less than 15 ppm; trisodium nitrilotriacetate must be less than 5 ppm in feed water; polymaleic acid and/or its sodium salt must be less than 1 ppm in feed water and in steam-contacting food.

BOIS DE ROSE OIL • A fragrance from the chipped wood of the tropical rosewood tree obtained through steam distillation. The volatile oil is colorless, pale yellow, with a light camphor odor. Used in citrus, floral, fruit, meat, and spice flavorings for beverages, ice cream, ices, candy, baked goods, and chewing gum. There is reported use of the chemical; it has not yet been assigned for toxicology literature. GRAS.

BOLDUS LEAVES • Flavoring from a Chilean fir tree with a sweet edible fruit used in alcoholic beverages only. There is no reported use of the chemical and there is no toxicology information available.

BOLETIC ACID • *See* Fumaric Acid.

BORAGE EXTRACT • The extract of the herb *Borago officinalis*. Contains potassium and calcium and has emollient properties and is used in a "tea" for sore eyes.

BORAX • Illegal for use in foods including wax coating for fruits and vegetables. It is permitted for use in export meats.

BORIC ACID • An antiseptic with bactericidal and fungicidal properties used as a fungus control on citrus fruit (FDA tolerance 8 ppm boron residues). Also used in baby powders, bath powders, eye creams, liquid powders, mouthwashes, protective creams, after-shave lotions, soaps, and skin fresheners. It is still widely used despite repeated warnings from the American Medical Association of possible toxicity. Severe poisonings have followed both ingestion and topical application to abraded skin. There is reported use of the chemical, it has not yet been assigned for toxicology literature.

BORNEO CAMPHOR • *See* Borneol.

BORNEOL • A flavoring agent with a peppery odor and a burning taste. Occurs naturally in coriander, ginger oil, oil of lime, rosemary, strawberries, thyme, citronella, and nutmeg. Toxicity is similar to camphor oil *(see)*. Used as a synthetic nut or spice flavoring for beverages, syrups, ice cream, ices, candy, baked goods, chewing gum. Used in perfumery. Can cause nausea, vomiting, convulsions, confusion, and dizziness. It has a toxicity similar to camphor.

BORNYL ACETATE • It may be obtained from various pine needle oils. Strong piney odor. As a yarrow herb and iva herb extract, it is used as synthetic fruit and spice flavorings for beverages, ice cream, ices, candy, baked goods, chewing gum, and syrups. Colorless liquid derived from borneol *(see)* is also used in perfumery and as a solvent.

BORNYL FORMATE • Formic Acid. A synthetic fruit flavoring agent for beverages, ice cream, ices, candy, baked goods, and syrups. Used in perfumes, soaps, and as a disinfectant. *See* Borneol.

BORNYL ISOVALERATE • A synthetic fruit flavoring agent with a camphorlike smell used for beverages, ice cream, ices, candy, baked goods, and syrups. Used in perfumes, soaps, and as a disinfectant. Also used medicinally as a sedative. *See* Borneol.

BORNYL VALERATE • A synthetic fruit flavoring agent for beverages, ice cream, ices, candy, and baked goods. *See* Borneol.

BORNYVAL • *See* Bornyl Isovalerate.

BORON SOURCES • Boric Acid. Sodium Borate. Boron occurs in the earth's crust (in the form of its compounds, not the metal) and borates are widely used as antiseptics even though toxicologists warn about possible adverse reactions. Used in modified hop extract. Boric acid and sodium borate are astringents and antiseptics. Borates are absorbed by the mucous membranes and can cause symptoms such as gastrointestinal bleeding, skin rash, central nervous system stimulation. The adult lethal dose is 30 grams (1 ounce). Infants and young children are more susceptible. Boron is used as a dietary supplement up to 1 milligram per day. Cleared for use by the FDA in modified hops extract up to 310 ppm.

BORONIA, ABSOLUTE • A synthetic violet and fruit-flavoring agent extracted from a plant. Used as a flavoring for beverages, ice cream, ices, and baked goods. There is reported use of the chemical; it has not yet been assigned for toxicology literature.

BOSWELLIA SPECIES • *See* Olibanum Extract.

BOULLION • Vegetable Smoke. There is reported use of the chemical; it has not yet been assigned for toxicology literature.

BOURBONENE • *See* Ethyl Vanillin.

BOVINE SOMATOTROPIN (BST) • Bovine growth hormone (BGH) is a natural protein produced by the pituitary gland of all cattle. It is a protein hormone and is not structurally or functionally related to steroid hormones. Biotechnology has enabled scientists to produce a recombinant form of this protein called BST. They have found that supplementing cows' natural levels of BST improves their efficiency as milk producers. The mammary glands of such dairy cows take in more nutrients from the bloodstream and produce more milk. Introduced on the market in 1994, the producers of the hormone, the FDA, and some other experts claim that there is no difference in the milk of cows given the hormone since cow's milk naturally contains the hormone anyway. Consumer groups, some scientists, small farmers, and a number of dairy product producers are against the use of the hormone. Among the reasons: it increases inflammation of the udder in cows, has unknown potential effects on humans, and is unnecessary because the U.S. government already support milk prices because there is an overabundance of milk on the market. Certain states have enacted laws that direct farmers who use BST or BGH to say that the cows have or have not been treated. They are Maine, Minnesota, West Virginia, and Wisconsin. You can obtain more information about the addition of the hormone to milk by contacting:

Office of Consumer Affairs
U.S. Food & Drug Administration
HFE88/Room 16-63
5600 Fishers Lane
Rockville, MD 30857

National Center for Nutrition and Dietetics
American Dietetic Association
216 West Jackson Blvd.
Chicago, IL 60606
312-899-4953

BRAN • The outer indigestible shell of cereal grain that is usually removed before the grain is ground into flour. It provides bulk and fiber.

BRASSICA ALBA • *See* Mustard.

BREWER'S YEAST • Originally used by beer brewers, it is a good source of B vitamins and protein. It can cause allergic reactions.

BRILLIANT BLUE • *See* FD and C Blue No. 1.

BROMATED • Combined or saturated with bromine, a nonmetallic, reddish, volatile liquid element. *See* Bromates.

BROMATES • Calcium bromate is a maturing agent and dough conditioner in bromated flours and bromated whole-wheat flour. Potassium bromate is a bread improver. Sugar contaminated with potassium bromate caused a food poisoning outbreak in New Zealand. The lethal dose is not certain but two to four ounces of a 2 percent solution causes serious poisoning in children. Death in animals and man apparently is due to kidney failure, but central nervous system problems have been reported. Also used in permanent wave neutralizers. Topical application to abraded skin. Has also caused poisoning. Bromates may also cause skin eruptions.

BROMELIN • Bromelain. A protein-digesting and milk-clotting enzyme found in pineapple. Used for tenderizing meat, chill-proofing beer, and as an anti-inflammatory medication. "Solutions consisting of water, salt, monosodium glutamate, and approved proteolytic enzymes applied or injected into cuts of beef shall not result in a gain of more than 3 percent of the weight of the untreated product."

BROMIC ACID, POTASSIUM SALT • White crystals used as a dough conditioner and maturing agent in baked goods, beverages, and confectionery products. A poison by ingestion. An experimental carcinogen. A powerful oxidizer. An irritant to skin, eyes, and mucous membranes.

BROMIDES, INORGANIC • Potassium and Sodium. Used as fumigants. Bromides can cause skin rashes; large doses can cause central nervous system depression, and prolonged intake may cause mental deterioration.

BROMINATED VEGETABLE OIL • Bromine, a heavy, volatile, corrosive, nonmetallic liquid element, added to vegetable oil or other oils. Dark brown or pale yellow, with a bland or fruity odor. These high-density oils are blended with low-density essential oils to make them easier to emulsify. Used largely in soft drinks, citrus-flavored beverages, ice cream, ices, and baked goods. The FDA has them on the "suspect list." "Less than 15 ppm in fruit flavored beverages are not precluded by a standard," according to the FDA. *See* Bromates for toxicity.

0-(4-BROMO-2-CHLOROPHENYL)-O-ETHYL-S-PROPYL PHOSPHORO-THIOATE • Curacron. Profenofos. Selecron. An insecticide used in animal feed, and cottonseed hulls. Poison by ingestion and skin contact.

BROMOMETHANE • A colorless, volatile liquid that is used as a fumigant in animal feed, apples, barley, cereal grains, corn, cracked rice, fava beans, fermented malt beverages, flour, grain sorghum, kiwi fruit, lentils, macadamia nuts, oats, pistachio nuts, rice, rye, sweet potatoes, and wheat. FDA residue tolerances include 125 ppm in cereal grain, 25 ppm in fermented malt beverages, 400 ppm in dog food, 125 ppm in barley, corn, grain sorghum, oats, rice, rye, and wheat when used for animal feed. Extremely hazardous, especially by inhalation. Death following acute poisoning is usually caused by lung irritation. In chronic poisoning, death is due to injury to the central nervous system.

BROOM EXTRACT • *See* Genet, Absolute.

BRYONIA • A small herb used for flavoring in alcoholic beverages only.

BST • Abbreviation for Bovine Somatotropin *(see)* Hormone.

BUCHU LEAF OIL • A natural flavoring agent from a South African plant used in berry, fruit, chocolate, mint, and spice flavorings for beverages, ice cream, ices, candy, baked goods, liquors, and condiments. Has been used as a urinary antiseptic and mild diuretic.

BUCHA LEAVES OIL • *See* Bucha Leaf Oil.

BUCKBEAN LEAVES • Flavoring in alcoholic beverages only.

BUCKTHORN • Frangula. A shrub or tree grown on the Mediterranean Coast of Africa, it has thorny branches and often contains a purgative in the bark or sap. Its fruits are used as a source of yellow and green dyes. No known toxicity.

BUFFER • Usually a solution with a relatively constant acidity-alkalinity ration, which is unaffected by the addition of comparatively large amounts of acid or alkali. A typical buffer solution would be hydrochloric acid *(see)* and sodium hydroxide *(see)*.

BUQUINOLATE • An animal drug used in chicken feed to combat parasites. FDA limitations are 0.4 ppm in uncooked liver, kidney, and skin of chickens and 0.1 ppm in uncooked chicken muscle. Limitation of 0.5 ppm in egg yoke and 0.2 ppm in whole eggs.

BUTADIENE-STYRENE COPOLYMER • A component for a chewing-gum base. Butadiene is produced largely from petroleum gases and is used in the manufacture of synthetic rubber. It may be irritating to the skin and mucous membranes and narcotic in high concentrations. Styrene, obtained from ethyl benzene, is an oily liquid with a penetrating odor. It has the same uses and toxicity. Under study by NTP *(see)* as a carcinogen.

BUTADIENE-STYRENE RUBBER • Latex. A chewing-gum base. No known toxicity.

BUTANAL • *See* Butyraldehyde.

BUTANDIONE • *See* Diacetyl.

BUTANE • N-butane. Methylsulfonal. Bioxiran. Dibutadiene Dioxide. A flammable, easily liquefiable gas derived from petroleum. A solvent, refrigerant, and food additive. Also used as a propellant or aerosol in cosmetics. The principal hazard is that of fire and explosion, but it may be narcotic in high doses and cause asphyxiation. It has been determined by the National Institute of Occupational Safety and Health to be an animal carcinogen. GRAS.

1,4-BUTANE DICARBOXYLIC ACID • *See* Adipic Acid.

1,3-BUTANEDIOL • A thick liquid used as a flavoring agent and solvent for flavorings. Mildly toxic by ingestion. An eye irritant.

2,3-BUTANEDIONE • A greenish yellow liquid with a strong odor used as a flavoring agent with margarine. Moderately toxic by ingestion. A skin irritant. GRAS.

BUTANOIC ACID • *See* Butyric Acid.

1-BUTANOL • *See* Butyl Alcohol.

4-BUTANOLIDE • A colorless liquid with a caramel odor, it is used as a flavoring agent in candy and soy milk. Moderately toxic by ingestion. May cause skin tumors. GRAS.

2,3-BUTANOLONE • *See* Acetoin.

2-BUTANONE • Colorless liquid with an acetonelike odor used as a flavoring agent in various foods. On the Community Right-To-Know List and in the EPA Genetic Toxicology Program *(see both)*. Moderately toxic by ingestion, skin contact, and injection.

BUTAN-3-ONE-2YL BUTYRATE • White to yellow liquid used as a flavoring agent in various foods. GRAS.

(trans)-BUTANEDIOIC ACID • *See* Fumaric Acid.

BUTOXYPOLYETHYLENE • A synthetic antifoaming agent used in beet sugar manufacture. No known toxicity.

BUTYRIC ACID • A clear, colorless liquid present in butter at 4 to 5 percent. It has a strong, rancid butter odor and is used in butterscotch, caramel, and fruit flavorings. It is also used in chewing gums, and margarines, as well as cosmetics. It is found naturally in apples, geraniums, rose oil, grapes, strawberries, and wormseed oil. It has a low toxicity but can be a mild irritation. GRAS.

BUTTER FAT • The oily portions of the milk of mammals. Cow's milk contains about 4 percent butterfat.

BUTTERMILK • The fluid remaining after butter has been formed from churned cream. It can also be made from sweet milk by the addition of certain organic cultures. Used as an astringent right from the bottle. Apply liberally and let dry about 10 minutes. Rinse off with cool water.

BUTTERS • Acids, Esters, and Distillate. *Butter acids* are synthetic butter and cheese flavoring agents for beverages, ice cream, ices, candy (2,800 ppm), baked goods. *Butter esters* are synthetic butter, caramel, and chocolate flavoring agents for beverages, ice cream, ices, baked goods, toppings, and popcorn (1,200 ppm). *Butter starter distillate* is a synthetic butter flavoring agent for ice cream, ices, baked goods, and shortening (12,000 ppm). In cosmetology, substances that are solid at room temperature but that melt at body temperature are called butters. Cocoa butter is one of the most frequently used in both foods and cosmetics. Newer butters are made from natural fats by hydrogenation *(see),* which increases the butter's melting point or alters its plasticity. Butters may be used in stick or molded cosmetics such as lipsticks or to give the proper texture to a variety of finished percents. Nontoxic.

BUTTER STARTER DISTILLATE • A flavoring. GRAS.

BUTYL ACETATE • Acetic Acid. Butyl Ester. A synthetic flavoring agent, a clear liquid with a strong fruit odor, prepared from acetic acid and butyl alcohol. Used in raspberry, strawberry, butter, banana, and pineapple flavorings for beverages, ice cream, ices, candy, baked goods, chewing gum, and gelatin desserts. Used in perfumery, nail polish, and nail polish remover. Also used in the manufacture of lacquer, artificial leather, plastics, and safety glass. It is an irritant and may cause eye irritation (conjunctivitis). It is a narcotic in high concentrations, and toxic to man when inhaled at 200 ppm.

BUTYL ACETOACETATE • A synthetic berry and fruit flavoring agent for beverages, ice cream, candy, and baked goods.

BUTYL ACETYL RICINOLEATE • *See* Ricinoleate.

BUTYL ALCOHOL • A synthetic butter, cream, fruit, liquor, rum, and whiskey flavoring agent for beverages, ice cream, ices, candy, baked goods, cordials, and cream. A colorless liquid, with an unpleasant odor it occurs naturally in apples and raspberries. Used as a clarifying agent *(see)* in shampoos; also a solvent for waxes, fats, resins, and shellac. It may cause irritation of the mucous membranes, headache, dizziness, and drowsiness when ingested. Inhalation of as little as 25 ppm causes pulmonary problems in man. It can also cause contact dermatitis when applied to the skin.

t-**BUTYL ALCOHOL** • *See* Butyl Alcohol.

BUTYL ALDEHYDE • *See* Butyraldehyde.

BUTYLAMINE • Colorless, volatile liquid with an ammonia odor derived from butanol or butyl chloride with ammonia. Used as an intermediate for emulsifying agents, insecticides, and dyes.

sec-BUTYLAMINE • Tutane. A fungicide used in animal feed, citrus molasses, and dried citrus pulp. Limitations of 90 ppm in citrus molasses and dried citrus pulp when used for cattle feed. Poisonous by ingestion. A powerful irritant. Moderately toxic by skin contact.

BUTYL ANTHRANILATE • A synthetic grape, mandarin, and pineapple flavoring agent for beverages, ice cream, ices, candy, and baked goods.

n-**BUTYL** *n*-**BUTANOATE** • Colorless liquid with pineapple odor used as a flavoring agent in various foods. Mildly toxic by ingestion. Moderately irritating to eyes, skin, and mucous membranes by inhalation. Narcotic in high concentrations.

BUTYL BUTYROLLACTATE • Colorless liquid with a buttery, creamlike odor used as a flavoring agent in baked goods and candy. A skin irritant.

BUTYL BUTYRATE • A colorless liquid used as a flavoring. It is an irritant and narcotic.

BUTYL BUTYRYLLACTATE • A colorless, synthetic flavoring agent from butyl alcohol, with a fruity odor. Used in berry, butter, apple, banana, peach, pineapple, liquor, scotch, and nut flavoring for beverages, ice cream, ices, candy, baked goods, chewing gum, and gelatin desserts.

BUTYL CARBOBUTOXYMETHYL PHTHALATE • A plasticizer used in packaging material. Mildly toxic via injection. Causes birth defects in laboratory animals. An eye irritant in humans.

a-BUTYL CINNAMALDEHYDE • A synthetic fruit, nut, spice, and cinnamon flavoring agent for beverages, ice cream, ices, candy, and baked goods.

BUTYL CINNAMATE • A synthetic chocolate, cocoa, and fruit flavoring for beverages, ice cream, ices, candy, baked goods, and liquor.

BUTYL 2-DECENOATE • A synthetic apricot and peach flavoring agent for beverages, ice cream, ices, candy, baked goods, chewing gum (2,000 ppm).

BUTYL DECYLENATE • *See* Butyl 2-Decanoate.

BUTYL DODECANOATE • *See* Butyl Laurate.

BUTYL ETHYL MALONATE • A synthetic fruit and apple flavoring for beverages, ice cream, ices, candy, and baked goods.

BUTYL FORMATE • Formic Acid. A synthetic fruit, plum, liquor, and rum flavoring for beverages, ice cream, ices, candy, and baked goods. *See* Formic Acid for toxicity.

BUTYL HEPTANOATE • A synthetic fruit and liquor flavoring for beverages, ice cream, ices, candy, and baked goods.

BUTYL HEXANOATE • A synthetic butter, butterscotch, pineapple, and rum flavoring agent for beverages, ice cream, ices, candy, and baked goods.

Tert-BUTYL HYDROQUINONE (TBHQ) • White crystalline solid used as an antioxidant in beef products, dry cereals, edible fats, margarine, meat, pizza toppings, pork, potato chips, poultry, sausage, and vegetable oils. Moderately toxic by ingestion. May be mutagenic. The Joint FAO-WHO Expert Committee on Food Additives concluded in June 1998, "The potential exists for high consumers of TBHQ to exceed the ADI [Acceptable Daily Intake], but the available data were insufficient to estimate the number of high consumers or the magnitude and duration of intake above the ADI." The Committee is reviewing this additive's level in edible fats and oils, fish and fish products, and carbonated water-based soft drinks.

BUTYL *p*-HYDROXYBENZOATE • Butyl Paraben. Butyl p-Oxybenzoate. Almost odorless, small colorless crystals or a white powder used as an antimicrobial preservative.

BUTYL ISOBUTYRATE • A synthetic raspberry, strawberry, butter, banana, and cherry flavoring agent for beverages, ice cream, ices, candy, baked goods, and chewing gum (2000 ppm).

BUTYL ISOVALERATE • A synthetic chocolate and fruit flavoring for beverages, ice cream, ices, candy, puddings, and gelatin desserts. No known toxicity.

2-BUTYL-5 (or 6)-KETO-1, 4-DIOXANE • A synthetic fruit and spice flavoring for beverages, ice cream, ices, candy, baked goods, and shortenings. No known toxicity.

BUTYL LACTATE • A synthetic butter, butterscotch, caramel, and fruit flavoring agent for beverages, ice cream, ices, candy, baked goods. No known toxicity.

BUTYL LAURATE • A synthetic fruit flavoring for beverages, ice cream, ices, candy, and baked goods. No known toxicity.

BUTYL LEVULINATE • A synthetic butter, fruit, and rum flavoring agent for beverages, ice cream, ices, candy, baked goods. No known toxicity.

BUTYL PARASEPT • *See* Butyl *p*-Hydroxybenzoate.

BUTYL PHENYLACETATE • Synthetic butter, honey, caramel, chocolate, rose, fruit, and nut flavoring agent for beverages, ice cream, ices, candy, baked goods, gelatin desserts, and puddings. No known toxicity.

BUTYL PHOSPHOROTRITHIOATE • Butifos. A defoliant used in animal feed and cottonseed hulls. A poison by ingestion, skin contact, and possibly other routes. Caused mutations in animals and affect nerve transmission. FDA limitations of 6 ppm in cottonseed hulls when used for animal feed.

BUTYL PROPIONATE • A synthetic butter, rum butter, fruit, and rum flavoring agent for beverages, ice cream, ices, candy, and baked goods. May be an irritant.

BUTYL RUBBER • A synthetic rubber used as a chewing-gum base component. No known toxicity.

BUTYL SEBACATE • *See* Dibutyl Sebacate.

BUTYL STEARATE • A synthetic antifoaming agent used in the production of beet sugar. Also a synthetic banana, butter, and liquor for beverages, ice cream, ices, candy, baked goods, chewing gum, and liqueurs.

BUTYL SULFIDE • A synthetic floral, violet, and fruit flavoring for beverages, ice cream, ices, candy, and baked goods.

BUTYL 10-UNDECENOATE • A synthetic butter, apricot, cognac, and nut flavoring agent for beverages, ice cream, ices, candy, baked goods, chewing gum, icing, and liquor.

BUTYL VALERATE • A synthetic butter, fruit, and chocolate flavoring agent for beverages, ice cream, ices, candy, baked goods, puddings, and gelatin desserts.

BUTYLATED HYDROXYANISOLE (BHA) • A preservative, stabilizer, and antioxidant in many products, including beverages, ice cream, ices, candy, baked goods, chewing gum, gelatin desserts, soup bases, potatoes, glacéed fruits, potato flakes, sweet potato flakes, dry breakfast cereals, dry yeast, dry mixes for desserts, lard, shortening, unsmoked dry sausage, and in emulsions for stabilizers for shortenings. It is a white or slightly yellow, waxy solid with a faint, characteristic odor.

Insoluble in water. Total content of antioxidants is not to exceed .02 percent of fat or oil content of food; allowed up to 1,000 ppm in dry yeast; 200 ppm in shortenings; 50 ppm in potato flakes; and 50 ppm with BHT (butylated hydroxytoluene) in dry cereals. Can cause allergic reactions. BHA affects the liver and kidney functions (the liver detoxifies it). BHA may be more rapidly metabolized than BHT *(see)* and in experiments at Michigan State University it appeared to be less toxic to the kidneys of living animals than BHT. It is also used as a flavoring agent and to treat mastitis for dairy cattle. Can cause allergic reactions. The final report to the FDA of the Select Committee on GRAS Substances stated in 1980 that while no evidence in the available information demonstrates a hazard to the public at current use levels, uncertainties exist, requiring that additional studies be conducted. The FDA said in 1980 that GRAS status should continue while tests on BHA are being completed and evaluated. As of this writing, nothing further has been reported. In *The 1990 Annual Review of Pharmacology and Toxicology,* scientists from the United Kingdom and the United States reviewed Japanese reports of a high incidence of cancerous and benign tumors in the forestomach of rats fed BHA. The reviewers concluded that because we humans don't have forestomachs and because the doses of BHA administered to the rats were so high, there was nothing to be alarmed about. In November 1990, Glenn Scott, MD, a Cincinnati physician, filed a petition with the FDA asking the agency to prohibit the use of BHA in food. Before acting on Scott's petition, however, the FDA asked the Federation of American Societies for Experimental Biology (FASEB) to reexamine the scientific data on BHA and make a report by March 1992. The joint FAO-WHO Expert Committee on Food Additives concluded in June 1998, "The potential exists for high consumers of BHA to exceed the ADI [Acceptable Daily Intake], but the available data were insufficient to estimate the number of high consumers or the magnitude and duration of intake above the ADI." The Committee is reviewing this additive's level in edible fats and oils, dried vegetables, cocoa products, processed meat, frozen fish, ready-to-eat soup and broth, and food supplements.

BUTYLATED HYDROXYMETHYLPHENOL • A new antioxidant, a nearly white crystalline solid with a faint characteristic odor. Insoluble in water and propylene glycol; soluble in alcohol. No known toxicity, but the formula, 4-hydroxymethyl-2, 6-di-tert-butyl phenol, contains phenol, which is very toxic.

BUTYLATED HYDROXYTOLUENE (BHT) • A preservative, stabilizer, and antioxidant employed in many foods. Used as a chewing-gum base, added to potato and sweet potato flakes and dry breakfast cereals, an emulsion stabilizer for shortenings used in enriched rice, animal fats, and shortenings containing animal fats. White crystalline solid with a faint characteristic odor. Insoluble in water. Total content of antioxidants in fat or oils not to exceed .02 percent. Allowed up to 200 ppm in emulsions stabilizes for shortenings, 50 ppm in dry breakfast cereals and potato flakes. Used also as an antioxidant to retard rancidity in frozen fresh pork sausage and freeze-dried meats up to .01 percent based on fat content. It is also used as a flavoring agent and to treat mastitis in dairy cattle. Can cause allergic reactions. Loyola University scientists reported on April 14, 1972, that pregnant mice fed a diet consisting of one half of one percent of BHT (or BHA, butylated hydroxyanisole) gave birth to offspring that frequently had chemical changes in the brain and subsequently abnormal behavior patterns. BHT and BHA are chemically similar, but BHT may be more toxic to the kidney than BHA *(see),* according to researchers at Michigan State University. The Select Committee of the American Societies for Experimental Biology, which advises the FDA on food additives, recommended further studies to determine "the effects of BHT at levels now present in foods under conditions where steroid hormones or oral contraceptives are being ingested." They said the possibility that BHT may convert other ingested substances into toxic or cancer-causing agents should be investigated. BHT is prohibited as a food additive in England. The FDA is pursuing further study of BHT. GRAS. Prohibited as a food additive in England. Chemically similar to BHA, it can cause allergic reactions. The joint FAO-WHO Expert Committee on Food Additives concluded in June 1998, "The potential exists for high consumers of BHT to exceed the ADI [Acceptable Daily Intake], but the available data were insufficient to estimate the number of high consumers or the magnitude and duration of intake above the ADI." The Committee is reviewing this additive's levels in edible fats and oils, chewing gum, and fish and fish products.

1,3-BUTYLENE GLYCOL • A clear, colorless, viscous liquid with a slight taste. A solvent and humectant most resistant to high humidity and thus valuable in foods and cosmetics. It retains scents and preserves against spoilage. It has a similar toxicity to ethylene glycol *(see),* which when ingested may cause transient stimulation of the central nervous system, then depression, vomiting, drowsiness, coma, respiratory failure, and convulsions; renal damage may proceed to uremia and death. One of the few humectants not on the GRAS list, although efforts to place it there have been made through the years.

BUTYLPARABEN • Widely used in food and cosmetics as an antifungal preservative, it is the ester of butyl alcohol and *p*-hydroxybenzoic acid *(see both).* No known toxicity.

BUTYRALDEHYDE • A synthetic flavoring agent found naturally in coffee and strawberries. Used in butter, caramel, fruit, liquor, brandy, and nut flavorings for beverages, ice cream, ices, candy, baked goods, alcoholic beverages, and icings. Used also in the manufacture of rubber, gas accelerators, synthetic resins, and plasticizers. May be an irritant and a narcotic.

BUTYRIC ACID • *n*-Butyric Acid. Butanoic Acid. A clear, colorless liquid present in butter at 4 to 5 percent with a strong penetrating rancid-butter odor. Butter, butterscotch, caramel, fruit, and nut flavoring agent for beverages, ice cream, ices, candy, baked goods, gelatin desserts, puddings, chewing gum, and margarine. Found naturally in apples, butter acids, geranium rose oil, grapes, strawberries and wormseed oil. It has a low toxicity but can be a mild irritant. GRAS.

BUTYRIC ALDEHYDE • *See* Butyraldehyde.

BUTYRIN • *See* (tri-)Butyrin.

(tri-)BUTYRIN • A synthetic flavoring agent found naturally in butter. Butter flavoring for beverages, ice cream, ices, candy (1,000 ppm), baked goods, margarine, and puddings. No known toxicity.

BUTYROIN • *See* 5-Hydroxy-4-Octanone.

BUTYROLACTONE • Butanolide. Liquid lactone used chiefly as a solvent for resins. It is also an intermediate *(see)* in the manufacture of polyvinylpyrrolidone *(see)* and as a solvent for nail polish. Human toxicity is unknown.

BUTYRONE • *See* 4-Heptanone.

BUXINE • *See* a-Amyl Cinnamaldehyde.

BUXINOL • *See* a-Amylcinnamyl Alcohol.

C

CACAO SHELL • Cocoa shells of the seeds of trees grown in Brazil, Central America, and most tropical countries. Weak chocolatelike odor and taste, thin and peppery, with a reddish brown color. Used in the manufacture of caffeine *(see)* and theobromine, which occurs in chocolate products and is used as a diuretic and nerve stimulant. Occasionally causes allergic reactions from handling. GRAS.

CACHOU EXTRACT • *See* Catechu Extract.

CACTUS ROOT EXTRACT • *See* Yucca Extract.

CADINENE • A general fixative that occurs naturally in juniper oil and pepper oil. It has a faint, pleasant smell. Used in candy, baked goods (1,200 ppm), and chewing gum (1,000 ppm).

CADMIUM • A naturally occurring metal used to control molds, and diseases that attack home lawns, golf courses, and other grasses. However, less than 0.1 percent of the annual U.S. consumption of twelve million pounds of cadmium is used in pesticides—most of it in industries. Cadmium in drinking water has been correlated with cancer of the pharynx, esophagus, intestines, larynx, lungs, and bladder. Cadmium is believed to cause mutations. It is poisonous when ingested and is also a potential cancer-causing agent. It has an extremely long biological clearance in humans and accumulates in body tissues, particularly in the liver and kidney. There are no available chelating agents to enhance cadmium excretion. The FAO-WHO Expert Committee on Food Additives allocated a Provisional Tolerable Weekly Intake (PTWI) of 400–500 nanograms of cadmium per person. The average dietary intake, according to the United Nations, is approximately 10 to 50 nanograms per day in areas of normal exposure. The Committee noted there was a question about how much biologically active cadmium was available from various foods, such as rice or grains. For example, in a study in New Zealand, the blood concentration and urinary excretion of cadmium were found to be "surprisingly low" in a population with a high dietary intake of New Zealand oysters, which contain high levels of cadmium. The Committee maintains the current PTWI of 7 nanograms per kilogram of body weight pending future research. The

FDA, which previously allowed cadmium as a colorant in polystyrenes, no longer allows its use. Being reviewed by NTP *(see)* as a carcinogen.

CAFFEINE • Guaranine. Methyltheobromine. Theine. Trimethylxanthine. An odorless white powder with a bitter taste that occurs naturally in the coffee, cola, guarana paste, tea, and kola nuts. Caffeine is the number one psychoactive drug. Obtained as a byproduct of caffeine-free coffee. Used as a flavor in root beer beverages and other foods. It is a central nervous system, heart, and respiratory system stimulant. Caffeine can alter blood sugar release and cross the placental barrier. It can cause nervousness, insomnia, irregular heartbeat, noises in ears, and, in high doses, convulsions. It has been linked to spontaneous panic attacks in persons sensitive to caffeine. It has been found to be addictive. It also causes increases in calcium excretion. Because of its capability to cause birth defects in rats, the FDA proposed regulations to request new safety studies and to encourage the manufacture and sale of caffeine-free colas. One regulation would make the food industry's continued use of caffeine as an added ingredient in soft drinks and other foods conditional upon its funding of studies of caffeine's effects on children and the unborn. A University of Montreal study published in the *Journal of the American Medical Association,* December 22, 1993, said that women who consume the amount of caffeine in one and a half to three cups of coffee a day may nearly double their risk of miscarriage. Under present regulations, a soft drink, except one artificially sweetened, must contain caffeine if it is to be labeled as *cola* or *pepper,* and the FDA wants soda producers to be able to use this name when caffeine is not used. The FDA has asked for studies on the long-term effects of the additive to determine whether it may cause cancer or birth defects. The final report to the FDA of the Select Committee on GRAS Substances stated in 1980 that while no evidence in the available information on it demonstrates a hazard to the public at current use levels, uncertainties exist, requiring that additional studies be conducted. GRAS status continues while tests are being conducted.

CAJEPUT OIL • A spice flavoring from the cajeput tree native to Australia. The leaves yield an aromatic oil. Used for beverages, ice cream, ices, candy, and baked goods.

CAJEPUTENE • *See* Limonene.

CAJEPUTOL • *See* Eucalyptol.

CALAMUS • Sweet Flag. Sweet Sedge. *Acorus calamus.* The rhizome contains essential oil, mucilage, glycosides, amino acid, and tannins. The oil is obtained by steam distillation of the stem or root and is used as a flavoring agent and in perfumery. Calamus root is an ancient Indian and Chinese herbal medicine used to treat stomach acid, irregular heart rhythm, low blood pressure, coughs, and lack of mental focus. Native Americans would chew the root to enable them to run long distances with increased stamina. Externally, it was used to induce a state of tranquility. Banned as a food additive by the FDA.

CALCIUM ACETATE • Brown Acetate of Lime. A white amorphous powder that has been used medicinally as a source of calcium. It is used in the manufacture of acetic acid and acetone and in dyeing, tanning, and curing skins as well as a corrosion inhibitor in metal containers. Used cosmetically for solidifying fragrances and as an emulsifier and firming agent. Low oral toxicity. The final report to the FDA of the Select Committee on GRAS Substances stated in 1980 that it should continue its GRAS status with no limitations other than good manufacturing practices.

CALCIUM ACID PHOSPHATE • *See* Calcium Phosphate.

CALCIUM ALGINATE • A stabilizer, thickener, gelling agent, and texturizer. Also used as a solvent and vehicle for flavorings. Found in ice cream and popsicles, soft and cottage cheeses, cheese snacks, dressings and spreads, fruit drinks, beverages, and instant desserts. *See* Alginates. GRAS.

CALCIUM ASCORBATE • A preservative and antioxidant prepared from ascorbic acid (vitamin C) and calcium carbonate *(see)*. Used in concentrated milk products; in cooked, cured, or pulverized meat products; in pickles in which pork and beef products are cured and packed (up to 75 ounces per 100 gallons). *See* Ascorbic Acid for toxicity. The final report to the FDA of the Select Committee on GRAS Substances stated in 1980 that it should continue its GRAS status with no limitations other than good manufacturing practices.

CALCIUM BENZOATE • *See* Benzoic Acid.

CALCIUM BROMATE • A maturing agent and dough conditioner used in bromated flours. The FDA allows 0.0075 part per 100 parts by weight of flour used. *See* Bromate.

CALCIUM CARBONATE • Chalk. Absorbent that removes shine from talc. A tasteless, odorless powder that occurs naturally in limestone, marble, and coral. Used as a white food dye and alkali to reduce acidity in wine up to 2.5 percent, a neutralizer for ice cream and in cream syrups up to .25 percent, in confections up to .25 percent, and in baking powder up to 50 percent. Employed as a carrier for bleaches. Once widely used as a white coloring in foods and cosmetics, the authorization by the FDA was withdrawn in 1988. Calcium carbonate is also used as an alkali to reduce acidity, a neutralizer, and firming agent. Also used in dentifrices as a tooth polisher, in deodorants as a filler, in depilatories as a filler, and in face powder as a buffer. A gastric antacid and antidiarrhea medicine, it may cause constipation. Female mice were bred after a week on diets supplemented with calcium carbonate at 220 and 880 times the human intake of this additive. At all dosage levels, the first and second litters of newly weaned mice were lower in weight and number, and mortality was increased. The highest level caused heart enlargement. Supplementing the maternal diet with iron prevents this, so the side effects were attributed to mineral imbalance due to excessive calcium intake. In humans, 500 milligrams per kilograms of body weight was fed to ulcer victims for three weeks. The amount ingested was 145 times the normal amount ingested as an additive. Some patients developed an excess of calcium in the blood and suffered nausea, weakness, and dizziness. Calcium carbonate can cause constipation. GRAS.

CALCIUM CARBONATE CUDEAR • Log wood, chips, and extract. Purple coloring from lichens. It is the source of litmus. Previously commonly used as a coloring in food, the FDA no longer authorizes its use.

CALCIUM CARRAGEENAN • *See* Carrageenan.

CALCIUM CASEINATE • Used as a nutrient supplement for frozen desserts (except water ices) and in creamed cottage cheese. *See* Casein.

CALCIUM CHLORIDE • The chloride salt of calcium. White, hard, odorless fragments, granules, powder, or as a solution. It absorbs water. Used in its anhydrous *(see)* form as a drying agent for organic liquids and gases. Used as a firming agent for sliced apples and other fruits, in apple pie mix, as a jelly ingredient, in certain cheeses to aid coagulation, in artificially sweetened fruit jelly, and in canned tomatoes. It is also used to treat mastitis in dairy animals. An emulsifier and texturizer in cosmetics and an antiseptic in eye lotions. Also used in fire extinguishers, to preserve wood, and to melt ice and snow. Employed medicinally as a diuretic and a urinary acidifier. Ingestion can cause stomach and heart disturbances. The final report to the FDA of the Select Committee on GRAS Substances stated in 1980 that it should continue its GRAS status with no limitations other than good manufacturing practices.

CALCIUM CITRATE • A fine, white odorless powder prepared from citrus fruit. Used as a buffer to neutralize acids in confections, jellies, jams, and in saccharine at the rate of three ounces per one hundred pounds of the artificial sweetener. It is also used to improve the baking properties of flour. *See* Citrate Salts for toxicity. The final report to the FDA of the Select Committee on GRAS Substances stated in 1980 that it should continue its GRAS status with no limitations other than good manufacturing practices.

CALCIUM DIACETATE • A sequestrant used in cereal. *See* Calcium Acetate. GRAS.

CALCIUM DI-L-GLUTAMATE • The salt of glutamic acid *(see)*. A flavor enhancer and salt substitute. Almost odorless white powder. The FDA says that it needs further study. As of this writing, nothing has been reported.

CALCIUM DIOXIDE • Used in cereal flours. *See* Calcium Peroxide.

CALCIUM DISODIUM EDTA • Edetate Calcium Disodium. Calcium Disodium Ethylenediamine Tetraacetic Acid. A preservative and sequestrant, white, odorless powder with a faint salty taste. Used as a food additive to prevent crystal formation and to retard color loss. Used in canned and carbonated soft drinks for flavor retention; in canned white potatoes and cooked canned clams for color retention; in crabmeat to retard struvite (crystal formation); in dressings as a preservative; in cooked and canned dried lima beans for color retention; in fermented malt beverages to prevent gushing; in mayonnaise and oleomargarine as a preservative; in processed dried pinto beans for color retention; and in sandwich spreads as a preservative. Residue tolerances set by the FDA for this additive are: cereal flours, 25 ppm; fermented malt beverages, 25 ppm; spice extractives 60 ppm; pecan pie filling, 100 ppm; clams (cooked-canned) to promote color retention, 340 ppm; lima beans to promote color, 310 ppm; crabmeat (cooked-canned) to retard struvite formation, 275 ppm; shrimp (cooked-canned) to retard struvite and to promote color retention, 250 ppm; carbonated soft drinks to promote flavor, 33 ppm; canned white potatoes to promote color retention, 110 ppm; canned mushrooms, 200 ppm; pickled cucumbers or pickled cabbage to promote color, flavor, and texture retention, 220 ppm; artificially colored lemon and orange-flavored spreads, 100 ppm; potato salad preservative, 100 ppm; French dressing, mayonnaise, and salad dressing; nonstandardized dressings and sauces, preservative, 75 ppm; sandwich spread as a preservative, 100 ppm; by weight of egg yolk portion, 200 ppm; distilled alcoholic beverages to promote stability of color, flavor, and or product clarity; oleomargarine as a preservative, 75 ppm. Promotes stability of color. Used medically as a chelating agent to detoxify poisoning by lead and other heavy metals. May cause intestinal upsets, muscle cramps, kidney damage, and blood in urine. On the FDA priority list of food additives to be studied for mutagenic, teratogenic, subacute, and reproductive effects.

CALCIUM GLUCONATE • Odorless, tasteless, white crystalline granules, stale in air. Used as a buffer, firming agent, sequestrant in jelly and preserves. Also used in animal feeds. It is soluble in water. May cause gastrointestinal and cardiac disturbances. The final report to the FDA of the Select Committee on GRAS Substances stated in 1980 that it should continue its GRAS status with no limitations other than good manufacturing practices.

CALCIUM GLYCEROPHOSPHATE • A fine, white, odorless, nearly tasteless powder used in dentifrices, baking powder, and as a food stabilizer and dietary supplement. A component of many over-the-counter nerve-tonic foods. Administered medicinally for numbness and debility. The final report to the FDA of the Select Committee on GRAS Substances stated in 1980 that it should continue its GRAS status with no limitations other than good manufacturing practices. *See* Calcium Sources.

CALCIUM 5′-GUANYLATE • Flavor potentiator. Odorless white crystals or powder having a characteristic taste. *See* Flavor Potentiators.

CALCIUM HEXAMETAPHOSPHATE • An emulsifier, sequestering agent, and texturizer used in breakfast cereals, angel food cake, flaked fish (prevents struvite), ice cream, ices, milk, bottled beer, reconstituted lemon juice, puddings, processed cheeses, artificially sweetened jellies and preserves, potable water supplies to prevent scale formation and corrosion and in pickle for curing hams. The final report to the FDA of the Select Committee on GRAS Substances stated in 1980 that it should continue but at this writing, its GRAS status is under review.

CALCIUM HYDROXIDE • Slaked Lime. Calcium Hydrate. Limewater. Lye. An alkali, a white powder with a slightly bitter taste. Used as a firming agent for various fruit products, canned peas, as an egg preservative, in water treatment, in animal feeds, and for dehairing hides. Used in cream depilatories; also in mortar, plaster, cement, pesticides, and fireproofing. Accidental ingestion can cause burns of the throat and esophagus; also death from shock and asphyxia due to swelling of the glottis and infection. Calcium hydroxide also can cause burns of the skin and eyes. The final report to the FDA of the Select Committee on GRAS Substances stated in 1980 that it should continue its GRAS status with no limitations other than good manufacturing practices.

CALCIUM HYPOCHLORITE • A germicide and sterilizing agent, the active ingredient of chlorinated lime, used in the curd washing of cottage cheese, in sugar refining, as an oxidizing and bleaching agent, and as an algae killer, bactericide, deodorant, disinfectant, and fungicide. Sterilizes fruits and vegetables by washing in a 50 percent solution. Under various names, dilute hypochlorite is found in homes as laundry bleach and household bleach. Occasionally cases of poisoning occur when people mix household hypochlorite solution with various other household chemicals, which causes the release of poisonous chlorine gas. As with other corrosive agents, calcium hypochlorite's toxicity depends upon its concentrations. It is highly corrosive to skin and mucous membranes. Ingestion may cause pain and inflammation of the mouth, pharynx, esophagus, and stomach, with erosion particularly of the mucous membranes of the stomach.

CALCIUM HYPOPHOSPHITE • Crystals of powder, slightly acid in solution, and practically insoluble in alcohol. It is a corrosion inhibitor and has been used as a dietary supplement in veterinary medicine. The final report to the FDA of the Select Committee on GRAS Substances stated in 1980 that it should continue its GRAS status with no limitations other than good manufacturing practices. There is no reported use of the chemical and there is no toxicology information available, according to the FDA.

CALCIUM 5'-INOSINATE • *See* Inosinate.

CALCIUM IODATE • White odorless or nearly odorless powder used as a dough conditioner and oxidizing agent in bread, rolls, and buns. It is a nutritional source of iodine in foods such as table salt, and used also in a topical disinfectant and as a deodorant. Low toxicity, but may cause allergic reactions. GRAS.

CALCIUM IODOBEHENATE • Dietary supplement used in animal feed as a source of iodine *(see)*. GRAS.

CALCIUM LACTATE • White, almost odorless crystals or powder used as a buffer and as such is a constituent of baking powders and is employed in confections; also used in dentifrices and as a yeast food and dough conditioner. It improves crispness in canned bean sprouts. Also used in animal feeds. In medical use, given for calcium deficiency; may cause gastrointestinal and cardiac disturbances. The final report to the FDA of the Select Committee on GRAS Substances stated in 1980 that it should continue its GRAS status with no limitations other than good manufacturing practices.

CALCIUM LACTOBIONATE • A firming agent in dry pudding mixes. *See* Calcium Lactate.

CALCIUM LIGNOSULFONATE • A brown, amorphous substance obtained from the pulp of wood mixed with calcium and sodium salts. It may contain up to 30 percent sugars. It is used as a dispersing agent and stabilizer for pesticides used on bananas. It is also employed in molasses fed to animals. *See* Calcium Sources.

CALCIUM METASILICATE • White powder, insoluble in water, used as an absorbent, antacid, filler for paper coatings, and as a food additive. Use in food restricted to 5 percent in baking powder and 2 percent in table salt. Irritating dust.

CALCIUM ORTHOPHOSPHATE • Buffer and neutralizing agent used in non-carbonated beverages. No known toxicity. GRAS.

CALCIUM OXIDE • Quicklime. Burnt Lime. A hard, white or grayish white, odorless mass or powder that is used as a yeast food and dough conditioner for bread, rolls, and buns. It is also an alkali for neutralizing dairy products (including ice cream mixes) and alkalizes sour cream, butter, and confections, and is used in the processing of tripe. Industrial uses are for bricks, plaster, mortar, stucco, dehairing hides, fungicides, insecticides, and for clarification of beet and cane sugar juices. A strong caustic, it may severely damage skin and mucous membranes. *See* Calcium Sources. The final report to the FDA of the Select Committee on GRAS Substances stated in 1980 that it should continue its GRAS status with no limitations other than good manufacturing practices.

CALCIUM PANTOTHENATE • Pantothenic Acid Calcium Salt. A B-complex vitamin, pantothenate is a white odorless powder with a sweetish taste and bitter aftertaste. Pantothenic acid occurs everywhere in plant and animal tissue, and the richest common source is liver; jelly of the queen bee contains six times as much. Rice bran and molasses are other good sources. Acid derivatives sold commercially are synthesized. *See* d-Pantothenamide. Biochemical defects from lack of calcium pantothenate may exist undetected for some time but eventually manifest themselves as tissue failures. The calcium chloride double salt of calcium pantothenate has been cleared for use in foods for special dietary uses. Moderately toxic by ingestion. The final report to the FDA of the Select Committee on GRAS Substances stated in 1980 that it should continue its GRAS status with no limitations other than good manufacturing practices.

CALCIUM PERIODATE • A nutrient source of iodine in salt for livestock.

CALCIUM PEROXIDE • White or yellowish, odorless, almost tasteless powder that is derived from an interaction of a calcium salt and sodium peroxide with subsequent crystallization. Used in bakery products as a dough conditioner, bleaching of oils, modification of starches, and as a seed disinfectant. Irritating to the skin.

CALCIUM PHOSPHATE • Dibasic, Monobasic, and Tribasic. White, odorless powders used as yeast foods, dough conditioners, and firming agents. *Tribasic* is an anticaking agent used in table salt, powdered sugar, malted milk powder, condiments, puddings, meat, dry-curing mixtures, cereal flours, and vanilla powder. It is tasteless. Used as a gastric antacid mineral supplement and a clarifying agent for sugars and syrups. *Dibasic* is used to improve bread, rolls, buns, cereal flours; a carrier for bleaching; used as a mineral supplement in cereals, in dental products, and in fertilizers. *Monobasic* is used in bread, rolls, and buns, artificially sweetened fruit jelly, canned potatoes, canned sweet peppers, canned tomatoes, and as a jelling ingredient. Employed as a fertilizer, as an acidulant, in baking powders, and in wheat flours as a mineral supplement. Skin and eye irritant. The final report to the FDA of the Select Committee on GRAS Substances stated in 1980 that it should continue its GRAS status with no limitations other than good manufacturing practices.

CALCIUM PHYTATE • Used as a sequestering agent *(see)*. When 300 milligrams per kilogram of body weight was fed to rats as a diet supplement, it successfully provided calcium for bone deposition, and the animals remained healthy. The final report to the FDA of the Select Committee on GRAS Substances stated in 1980 that it should continue its GRAS status with no limitations other than good manufacturing practices. There is no reported use of the chemical and there is no toxicology information available, according to the FDA.

CALCIUM PROPIONATE • Propanoic Acid. Calcium Salt. White crystals or crystalline solid with the faint odor of propionic acid. A mold and rope inhibitor in breads, rolls, and poultry stuffing, it is used in processed cheese, chocolate products, cakes, cupcakes, and artificially sweetened fruit jelly. It is used as a preservative in cosmetics and as an antifungal medication for the skin. GRAS.

CALCIUM PYROPHOSPHATE • A fine, white, odorless, tasteless powder used as a nutrient, an abrasive in dentifrices, a buffer, and as a neutralizing agent in foodstuffs. No known toxicity. The final report to the FDA of the Select Committee on GRAS Substances stated in 1980 that it should continue its GRAS status with no limitations other than good manufacturing practices. *See* Calcium Sources.

CALCIUM RESINATE • Yellowish white powder or lumps used to dilute color eggshells. No residue is permitted.

CALCIUM 5'-RIBONUCLEOTIDES • Flavor potentiators *(see)*, in odorless white crystals or powder, with a characteristic taste. *See* Inosinates.

CALCIUM SACCHARIN • *See* Saccharin.

CALCIUM SALTS • Acetate, Chloride, Citrate, Diacetate, Gluconate, Phosphate (monobasic), Phytate, Sulfate. Emulsifier salts used in evaporated milk and frozen desserts, also in enriched bread. Firming agent in potatoes and canned tomatoes. May be gastric irritants, but they have little oral toxicity. *See* Calcium Sulfate and Calcium Phosphate.

CALCIUM SALTS OF FATTY ACIDS • Used as binders, emulsifiers, and anti-caking agent in foods.

CALCIUM SALTS OF PARTIALLY DIMERIZED ROSIN • Used as a coating on free citrus fruits. *See* Calcium Salts.

CALCIUM SILICATE • Okenite. An anticaking agent, white or slightly cream-colored, free-flowing powder. It is used up to 5 percent in baking powder and 2 percent of table salts. Also used in vanilla powder. Absorbs water. Used in face powders because it has extremely fine particles and good water absorption. Also used as a coloring agent. Constituent of lime glass and cement, used in road construction. Practically nontoxic orally, except inhalation may cause irritation of the respiratory tract. On the FDA list of additives that need further study for mutagenic, teratogenic, subacute, and reproductive effects.

CALCIUM SORBATE • A preservative and fungus preventative used in beverages, baked goods, chocolate syrups, soda-fountain syrups, fresh fruit cocktail, tangerine puree (sherbet base), salads (potato, macaroni, cole slaw, gelatin), cheesecake, pie fillings, cake, cheese in consumer-size packages, and artificially sweetened jellies and preserves. No known toxicity. The final report to the FDA of the Select Committee on GRAS Substances stated in 1980 that it should continue its GRAS status with no limitations other than good manufacturing practices.

CALCIUM SOURCES • Harmless calcium salts: Carbonate, Citrate, Glycero-phosphate, Oxide, Phosphate, Pyrophosphate, Sulfate. Calcium is a mineral sup-plement for breakfast cereals, white corn meal, infant dietary formula, enriched flour, enriched bromated flour (*see* Bromates), enriched macaroni, noodle prod-ucts, self-rising flours, enriched farina, corn meal and corn grits, and enriched bread and rolls. Calcium is a major mineral in the body. It is incompletely absorbed from the gastrointestinal tract when in the diet so its absorption is enhanced by calcium normally present in intestinal secretions. Vitamin D is also required for efficient absorption of calcium. Recommended daily requirements for adult females is 1.5 grams, for adult males 1.2 grams, and for children 0.8 gram. Calcium and phosphorus are the major constituents of teeth and bones. The ratio of calcium to phosphorus in cow's milk is approximately 1.2 to 1. In human milk the ratio is 2 to 1. The final report to the FDA of the Select Committee on GRAS Substances stated in 1980 that it should continue its GRAS status with no limita-tions other than good manufacturing practices.

CALCIUM STEARATE • Vanilla powder used in beet sugar and yeast. Prepared from lime water (*see*), it is an emulsifier, a coloring agent, and is used in water-proofing. It is used as an emulsifier in hair-grooming products and in paints and printing ink. Nontoxic. The final report to the FDA of the Select Committee on GRAS Substances stated in 1980 that it should continue its GRAS status with no limitations other than good manufacturing practices.

CALCIUM STEAROYL LACTYLATE • *See* Calcium Stearoyl-2-Lactylate.

CALCIUM STEAROYL-2-LACTYLATE • The calcium salt of the stearic acid ester of lactyl lactate. A free-flowing, white powder dough conditioner in yeast-leavened bakery products and prepared mixes for yeast-leavened bakery products. Also a whipping agent in dried, liquid, and frozen egg whites. On the FDA list of additives requiring further safety information since 1980.

CALCIUM SULFATE • Plaster of Paris. A fine, white to slightly yellow, odor-less, tasteless powder used as a firming agent and yeast food and dough condi-tioner. Utilized in brewing and other fermentation industries, in Spanish-type sherry, as a jelling ingredient, in cereal flours, as a carrier for bleaching agent, in bread, rolls, and buns, in blue cheese and Gorgonzola cheese, artificially sweet-ened fruit, jelly, canned potatoes, canned sweet peppers, and canned tomatoes. Used also in creamed cottage cheese as an alkali. Also used in toothpaste and tooth powders as an abrasive and firming agent. Also used as a coloring agent in cos-metics. Employed industrially in cement, wall plaster, and insecticides. Because it absorbs moisture and hardens quickly, its ingestion may result in intestinal obstruction. Mixed with flour, it has been used to kill rodents. GRAS.

CALCIUM TARTRATE • White crystals soluble in acids derived from cream of tartar. Used as a food preservative and antacid. No known toxicity.

CALENDULA • Dried flowers of pot marigolds grown in gardens everywhere. Used as a natural flavoring agent. *See* Marigold, Pot, for foods in which it is used. Formerly used to soothe inflammation of skin and mucous membranes, now used in "natural" creams, oils, and powders for babies. GRAS.

CALORIE • A unit used to express the heat output of an organism and the fuel or energy value of food. The amount of heat required to raise the temperature of one gram of water from 14.5 to 15.5°C at atmospheric pressure. When a caloric value for a serving of a food is less than 5 calories, the FDA allows the label to read "zero calories." If a fat calorie is less than 0.5 grams, it can also be listed as "calories from fat zero."

CALUMBA ROOT • Flavoring used in alcoholic beverage only.

CAMOMILE • *See* Chamomile.

2-CAMPHANOL • *See* Borneol.

CAMPHENE • A synthetic spice and nutmeg flavoring agent for beverages, ice cream, ices, candy, and baked goods. Occurs naturally in calamus oil, citronella, ginger, lemon oil, mandarin oil, myrtle, petitgrain oil, and juniper berries. May be mutagenic.

CAMPHOR OIL • Japanese White Oil. Camphor Tree. Distilled from trees at least fifty years old grown in China, Japan, Formosa, Brazil, and Sumatra. Camphor tree is used in spice flavorings for beverages, baked goods, and condiments. Must be safrole *(see)*. Used in emollient creams, hair tonics, eye lotions, preshave lotions, after-shave lotions, and skin fresheners as a preservative and to give a cool feeling to the skin. It is also used in horn-rimmed glasses, as a drug preservative, in embalming fluid, in the manufacture of explosives, in lacquers, as a moth repellent, and topically in liniments, cold medications, and anesthetics. It can cause contact dermatitis. In 1980, the FDA banned camphorated oil as a liniment for colds and sore muscles because of reports of poisonings through skin absorption and because of accidental ingestion. A New Jersey pharmacist had collected case reports and testified before the FDA Advisory Review Panel on Over-the-Counter Drugs in 1980. Camphor is readily absorbed through all sites of administration. Ingestion of 2 grams generally produces dangerous effects in an adult. Ingestion by pregnant women has caused fetal deaths. As of this writing, nothing new to report. There is reported use of the chemical; it has not yet been assigned for toxicology literature search.

CANANGA OIL • A natural flavor extract obtained by distillation from the flowers of the tree. Light to deep yellow liquid with a harsh, floral odor. Used in cola, fruit, spice, and ginger ale flavoring for beverages, ice cream, ices, candy, baked goods. May cause allergic reactions. No known toxicity. GRAS. There is reported use of the chemical; it has not yet been assigned for toxicology literature.

CANDELILLA WAX • Obtained from candelilla plants. Brownish to yellow brown, hard, brittle, easily pulverized partially insoluble in water. Hardens other waxes. Used as a coating for foods. GRAS. There is reported use of the chemical; it has not yet been assigned for toxicology literature.

CANDIDIA GUILLIERMONDII • An enzyme derived from *Candidia guillermondii;* used as a production aid in citric acid. No known toxicity.

CANDIDA LIPOLYTICA • Derived from *Candida lypolytica;* used as a fermentation organism in the production of citric acid. No known toxicity.

CANE SUGAR • *See* Sucrose.

CANOLA OIL • A low erucic acid rapeseed oil *(see)* used in salad oils because it contains 50 percent less saturated oils than other popular oils. GRAS.

CANTHAXANTHIN • A color additive derived from edible mushrooms, crustaceans, trout, and salmon, and tropical birds. It produces a pink color when used in foods. FAO-WHO Expert Committee on Food Additives said that up to twenty-five milligrams per kilogram of body weight is acceptable. Permanently listed in 1969 for human food and permanently listed in 1985 in chicken feed to enhance the yellow color of chicken skin. It is exempt from certification. Oral intake may cause loss of night vision.

CAPERS • A natural flavoring from the spiny shrub. The picked flower bud is used as a condiment for sauces and salads. GRAS.

CAPRALDEHYDE • *See* Decanal.

CAPRENIN • A five-calorie per gram fat substitute for cocoa butter in candy bars. Made of capric acid and caprylic acid, two fatty acids found in coconut and palm kernel oil. The other half is made of behenic acid, a poorly digested fat taken from hydrogenated rapeseed oil *(see)*. Developed by Procter & Gamble, it was introduced in Milky Way II candy bars. GRAS.

CAPRIC ACID • Obtained from a large group of American plants. Solid crystalline mass with a rancid odor used in the manufacture of artificial fruit flavors. Also used to flavor lipsticks. No known toxicity. *See* Decanoic Acid.

CAPRIC ALDEHYDE • *See* Decanal.

CAPRINALDEHYDE • *See* Decanal.

CAPROALDEHYDE • *See* Hexanal.

CAPROIC ACID • Hexanoic Acid. Occurs as glyceride in natural oils. Derived from coconut oil fatty acids, it is used in fruit flavors and as an intermediate for food-grade additives. It is also used in peeling solutions for fruits and vegetables.

CAPRYLAMINE OXIDE • *See* Caprylic Acid and Capric Acid.

CAPRYL BETAINE • *See* Caprylic Acid and Betaine.

CAPRYLIC ACID • An oily liquid that occurs naturally as a fatty acid in sweat, fusel oil, in the milk of cows and goats, and in palm and coconut oil. Cleared for use as a synthetic flavoring. No known toxicity. The final report to the FDA of the Select Committee on GRAS Substances stated in 1980 that it should continue its GRAS status with no limitations other than good manufacturing practices.

CAPRYLIC ALCOHOL • *See* 1-Octanol.

CAPSICUM • African Chilies. Cayenne Pepper. Tabasco Pepper. The dried fruit of a tropical plant used as a natural spice and ginger ale flavoring for beverages, ice cream, ices, candy, baked goods, chewing gum, meats, and sauces. The oleoresin form is used in sausage, spice, ginger ale, and cinnamon flavorings for beverages, ice cream, ices, candy, baked goods, chewing gum, meats, and condiments. Used internally as a digestive stimulant. Irritating to the mucous membranes, it can produce severe diarrhea and gastritis. May cause a "hot" sensation and sweating. *See* Cayenne Pepper for toxicity. GRAS.

CAPSORUBIN • Coloring from paprika *(see)*.

CAPTAN • Agrosol. Merpan. Orthocide. Osocide. Vanguard. Vanicide. White-to creamy-colored powder, practically insoluble in water, derived from tetrahy-drophthalmide and trichloromethylmercaptan. Used to treat seeds, to preserve fruit, and as a fungicide on almonds, animal feed, apples, beans, beef, beets, broc-coli, cabbage, carrots, corn, garlic, kale, lettuce, peaches, peas, pork, potatoes, raisins, spinach, and strawberries. The FDA permits residues of up to 50 ppm in raisins, 100 ppm on corn seed for cattle and hog feed. It is a fungicide of lower toxicity than most, but in large doses can cause diarrhea and weight loss. A skin and lung irritant, and a suspected cause of human birth defects. Pregnant women should avoid exposure to it. Also suspected of causing cancer. Moderately toxic to humans by ingestion.

CARAMEL • A chemically ill-defined group of material produced by heating car-bohydrates. Burnt sugar with a pleasant, slightly bitter taste. Made by heating sugar or glucose and adding small quantities of alkali or a trace mineral acid dur-ing heating. Caramel color prepared by ammonia process has been associated with blood toxicity in rats. Because of this, the joint FAO-WHO Expert Committee on Food Additives temporarily removed the acceptable daily intake for ammonia-made caramel. It was found to inhibit the metabolism of B_6 in rabbits. Caramel is widely used as a brown coloring in ice cream, baked goods, soft drinks, and con-fections. As a flavoring, it is used in strawberry, butter, butterscotch, caramel, chocolate, cocoa, cola, fruit, cherry, grape, birch beer, liquor, rum, brandy, maple, black walnut, walnut, root beer, spice, ginger, ginger ale, vanilla, and cream soda beverages (2,200 ppm), ice cream, candy, baked goods, syrups (2,800 ppm), and meats (2,100 ppm). Used as a coloring in cosmetics and a soothing agent in skin lotions. The FDA has given caramel priority for testing its mutagenic, teratogenic subacute, and reproductive effects as a food additive. Sulfite ammonia caramels tested on humans produced soft to liquid stools and increased bowel movements. The final report to the FDA of the Select Committee on GRAS Substances stated in 1980 that it should continue its GRAS status with no limitations other than good manufacturing practices. Permanently listed in 1963 as a coloring. Certification not required.

CARAMEL COLOR III • Used as a color additive in beers and a variety of foods. Beer is the most important single source of this additive in the diet although con-sumption of dark beers has been decreasing in recent years. The FAO-WHO Expert Committee on Food Additives has established an ADI *(see)* of 200 per kilo-gram of body weight per day. The safety of caramel color III has been questioned during recent years following feeding studies in the rat that were associated with reduced white cells and lymphocyte counts. In studies at Hazelton Laboratories America, Madison, Wisconsin, rats given caramel color III had soft feces and lower food and fluid consumption. No other toxicity was noted.

CARAWAY SEED and OIL • The dried ripe seeds of a plant common to Europe and Asia and cultivated in England, Russia, and the U.S. A volatile, colorless to pale yellow liquid, it is used in liquor flavorings for beverages, ice cream, baked goods, and condiments; also used as a spice in baking. The oil is used in grape licorice, anisette, kümmel, liver, sausage, mint, caraway, and rye flavorings for beverages, ice cream, ices, candy, baked goods, chewing gum, meats, condiments, and liquors. The oil is used to perfume soap. Can cause contact dermatitis. A mild carminative, from one to two grams breaks up intestinal gas. Moderately toxic by ingestion and skin contact. A skin irritant. May be mutagenic. GRAS.

CARAZOLOL • A beta-blocker that lowers blood pressure, chest pain, and irregular heartbeat. It is used for the treatment of stress in pigs.

CARBADOX • Mecadox. Fortigro. An antibacterial used in animal feed for swine. The FAO-WHO Expert Committee on Food Additives would not set an ADI or NOEL *(see both)* for this drug since it is a cancer-causing agent. FDA tolerance for carbadox residues in swine is zero. On January 4, 1994, the FDA was notified by a Quincy, Illinois, company that twenty-five dairy cows at a small Wisconsin farm had been accidentally fed for several months with swine feed containing carbadox. The agency was also notified that milk from these cows had been shipped to Wisconsin dairies for processing into mozzarella cheese, butter, and whey. The whey, in turn, had been further processed into lactose, which was used in infant formula and other products. Carbadox is approved for use in pig feed to treat swine dysentery. Studies have indicated that the drug can cause liver tumors in rodents when fed at high levels over their entire lifetime. Research reportedly had "found no significant adverse effects associated with short-term carbadox exposure in animals." Analyses by FDA, state, and other experts indicated that any carbadox residue in any of the suspect products would have been so "minuscule that it would not pose a risk to public health." A study of milk from a cow fed with carbadox-treated feed showed the amount of carbadox in the milk was less than one percent of the amount that was fed to the animals. Metabolism studies of carbadox in animal species show the drug can be converted to less toxic compounds. The FDA said it is likely that much of the carbadox fed to the cows was converted to less toxic compounds. In addition, any milk used that contained carbadox would have been mixed with milk from many other sources, and therefore diluted.

CARBAMATE • A compound based on carbamic acid which is used only in the form of its numerous derivatives and salts. Carbamates are used in pesticides. Among the carbamate pesticides are aldicarb, 4-benzothienyl-N-methyl carbamate, bufencarb (BUX), carbaryl, carbofuran, isolan, 2-isopropyl phenyl-N-methyl carbamate, 3-isopropyl phenylmethyl carbamate, maneb, propoxur, thiram, Zectran, zineb, and ziram. Carbamic acid, which is colorless and odorless, causes depression of bone marrow and degeneration of the brain, nausea, vomiting. It is moderately toxic by many routes.

N-CARBAMOYL ARSANILIC ACID • White, nearly odorless powder added to animal feed as a growth stimulant. It is an arsenic *(see)* compound that is on the Community Right-To-Know List *(see)*. Poison by ingestion. Has caused tumors in laboratory animals.

CARBARSONE • An antiamebic and antihistomonad used in turkey and chicken feed. FDA residue tolerance is 0.025 percent to 0.0375 percent in the feed, 2 ppm in residue in edible byproducts of chicken and turkeys, and 0.5 ppm as residue in muscle meat of chickens and turkeys and in eggs.

CARBARYL • Sevin. Pesticide used on corn and other vegetables and fruits. FDA residue tolerances are for pineapple bran for feed, 20 ppm; as residues in or on pineapples, 2.0 ppm; as residue in eggs, 0.25 ppm; as residue in fat, meat, meat byproducts from layer chickens, 0.05 ppm; as residues in kidney and liver of cattle, goats, horses, sheep, and swine, 1.0 ppm; as residue in fat, meat, and meat byproducts of cattle, swine, goats, horses, and shrimp, 0.1 ppm; as a residue in various raw agricultural conditions, 0.2–100 ppm. Causes nausea, vomiting, diarrhea, lung damage, blurred vision, excessive salivation, muscle twitching, cyanosis, convulsions, coma, and death. It is a poison via oral and skin absorption. It is an eye and skin irritant. Absorption through skin is slow. It does not accumulate in the tissues and is much less toxic than parathion *(see)*.

CARBETHOXY MALATHION • Malathion. Vegru Malatox. Vetiol. Zithiol. Malacide. Carbophos. A brown to yellow liquid used as an insecticide on animal feed, citrus pulp, grapes, nonmedicated cattle-feed concentrate blocks, packaging material, and safflower oil. FDA permits a residue of up to 12 ppm in grapes, 0.6 ppm in safflower oil, 50 ppm in dehydrated citrus pulp, 10 ppm in nonmedicated cattle-feed concentrate blocks. A human poison by ingestion. May be mutagenic. Has caused allergic skin reactions. It can interfere with nerve transmission.

CARBOFURAN • A pesticide used in animal feed. FDA residue tolerances are in various raw agricultural commodities, 2 ppm; on dried grape pomace, 6 ppm; soybean soap stock, 6 ppm; in raisin waste, 6 ppm; peanut soap stock, 24 ppm.

CARBOHYDRASE, ASPERGILLUS • An enzyme from fermentation of *Aspergillus oryzae* used as a production aid and tenderizing agent in alcoholic beverages, ale, bakery products, beer, dairy products, meats, poultry, and starch syrups. Used in the production of dextrose. The FDA says that solutions of water and this enzyme applied or injected into raw meat cuts shall not result in a gain of more than 3 percent above the weight of the treated product. When heated to decomposition it emits acrid smoke and irritating fumes.

CARBOHYDRASE and CELLULASE • Derived from *Aspergillus niger,* this enzyme permits easy shucking of clams and peeling of shrimp. The FDA permits use at a level not in excess of the amount reasonably required to accomplish the intended effect. When heated to decomposition it emits acrid smoke and irritating fumes.

CARBOHYDRASE and PROTEASE • An enzyme from the controlled fermentation of *Bacillus licheniformus,* it is a brown powder or liquid used in beer, alcoholic beverages, candy, dextrose, fish meal, nutritive sweeteners, protein hydrolysates, and starch syrups. When heated to decomposition it emits acrid smoke and irritating fumes. GRAS. There is reported use of the chemical, it has not yet been assigned for toxicology literature.

CARBOHYDRASE, RHIZOPUS • An enzyme derived from *Rhizopus oryzae* used in processing dextrose *(see)*. When heated to decomposition, it emits acrid smoke and irritating fumes.

CARBOHYDRATES • Starches and sugars contain a high proportion of carbohydrates. Carbohydrates are chemicals that contain carbon, hydrogen, and oxygen, and they are widely available in plants. In the body, however, carbohydrates in the blood supply are held at an almost constant level of about 0.05 to 0.1 percent. Carbohydrates are the fuel of life. Each gram of carbohydrate provides about four calories of energy—the same as protein but less than fat. Following digestion and absorption, available carbohydrates may be used to meet immediate energy needs of tissue cells, converted to glycogen, the storage form of glucose in liver and muscle for later energy needs, or converted to fat as a reserve for energy. It is possible that relatively pure carbohydrate solutions have different effects in young and elderly individuals. Carbohydrates can act as a supplemental fuel source during exercise. The ability of carbohydrate supplements to prolong endurance during exercising is related to preventing fatigue in a physiological sense in both body and mind. The effect of carbohydrate in increasing the tryptophan ratio in blood is considered to be a possible mechanism.

CARBOMYCIN • Deltamycin. An animal antibiotic used on chicken. It is also used in combination with oxytetracycline *(see)*. The FDA allows no residue in cooked edible tissues of chicken. Poison by subcutaneous route. Moderately toxic by vein and injection into the muscle. When heated to decomposition it emits toxic fumes.

CARBON BLACK • Several forms of artificially prepared carbon or charcoal, including animal charcoal, furnace black, channel (gas) black, lamp black, activated charcoal, and ferric sulfate. Animal charcoal is used as a black coloring in confectionery. Activated charcoal is used as an antidote for ingested poisons, and as an adsorbent in diarrhea. The others have industrial uses. Carbon black, which was not subject to certification *(see)* by the FDA was reevaluated and then banned in 1976. It was found in tests to contain a cancer-causing byproduct that was released during dye manufacture. It can no longer be used in candies such as licorice and jellybeans or in drugs or cosmetics.

CARBON DIOXIDE • Colorless, odorless, noncombustible gas with a faint acid taste. Used as a pressure-dispensing agent in gassed creams. Also used in the carbonation of beverages and as dry ice for refrigeration in the frozen food industry. Used onstage to produce harmless smoke or fumes. Under pressure of about fifty-nine atmospheres it may be condensed into a liquid, a portion of which forms a white solid (dry ice). May cause shortness of breath, vomiting, high blood pressure, and disorientation if inhaled in sufficient amounts. GRAS.

CARBON DISULFIDE • A clear, colorless liquid used as a fumigant for cereal grains. Extremely hazardous. A human poison by ingestion. Mildly toxic to humans by inhalation.

CARBON TETRACHLORIDE • Carbon Tet. Tetrachloromethane. Perchlormethane. A colorless, clear, heavy, nonflammable liquid obtained from carbon disulfide and chlorine. It is used as a fumigant on cereal grains. Poisonous by inhalation, ingestion, or skin absorption. Acute poisoning causes nausea, diarrhea, headache, stupor, kidney damage, and can be fatal. Chronic poisoning involves liver damage, but can also cause kidney damage. It has caused cancer in animals. Because it is so toxic, the FDA banned its use in products for the home in 1970.

CARBONYL IRON • Iron that has been processed with carbon and oxygen. Used as a coloring. The final report to the FDA of the Select Committee on GRAS

Substances stated in 1980 that there is no evidence in the available information that it is a hazard to the public when used as it is now and it should continue its GRAS status with limitations on the amounts that can be added to food.

CARBOPHENOTHION • A pesticide used on citrus meal fed to cattle. FDA tolerance is 10 ppm. *See* Organophosphates.

CARBOXINE • Vitavax. Carboxin. A fungicide used on barley, beans, corn, oats, peanut hulls, rice, sorghum, and wheat for animal feeds. Poison by ingestion. Moderately toxic by skin contact.

CARBOXYMETHYL CELLULOSE • Sodium. GRAS. *See* Cellulose Gums.

CARDAMOM OIL • Grains of Paradise. A natural flavoring and aromatic agent from the dried ripe seeds of trees common to India, Ceylon, and Guatemala. Used in butter, chocolate, liquor, spice and vanilla flavorings for beverages, ice cream, ices, candy, baked goods (1,700 ppm), meats, and condiments. The seed oil is used in chocolate, cocoa, coffee, cherry liquor, liver, sausage, root beer, sarsaparilla, cardamom, ginger ale, vanilla, and cream soda flavorings for beverages, ice cream, ices, candy, baked goods, chewing gum, liquor, pickles, curry powder, and condiments. Used also in perfumes and soaps. As a medicine, it breaks up intestinal gas. May be mutagenic. GRAS. There is reported use of the chemical; it has not yet been assigned for toxicology literature.

CARMINE • Cochineal. A crimson pigment derived from a Mexican and Central American species of a scaly female insect that feeds on various cacti. Carmine and Cochineal extracts are permanently listed, but cochineal alone is not authorized for use. The colorings are used in red applesauce, confections, baked goods, meats, and spices. Cochineal was involved in an outbreak of salmonellosis (an intestinal infection) that killed one infant in a Boston hospital and made twenty-two patients seriously ill. Carmine, used in the diagnostic solution to test the digestive organs, was found to be the infecting agent. Also used in cosmetics. University of Michigan medical researchers said this color additive extracted from dried bugs and used in candy, yogurt, fruit drinks, and other foods can cause life-threatening allergic reactions. It is often just listed as a "natural" ingredient on the label. A paper on the subject was published in 1997 in the November issue of *Annals of Allergy, Asthma & Immunology*. There is reported use of the chemical; it has not yet been assigned for toxicology literature.

CARMINIC ACID • Natural Red No. 4. Used in mascaras, liquid rouge, paste rouge, and red eye shadows. It is the glucosidal coloring matter from a scaly insect (*see* Carmine). Color is deep red in water and violet to yellow in acids. May cause allergic reactions. Not subject to certification by the FDA.

CARNAUBA WAX • The exudate from the leaves of the Brazilian wax palm tree used as a candy glaze and polish. The crude wax is yellow or dirty green, brittle, and very hard. It is used in many polishes and varnishes, and when mixed with other waxes makes them harder and gives them more luster. Used as a texturizer in foundation makeups, mascara, cream rouge, lipsticks, liquid powders, depilatories, and deodorant sticks. It rarely causes allergic reactions. It is on the FDA list for further study for mutagenic, teratogenic, subacute, and reproductive effects. The final report to the FDA of the Select Committee on GRAS Substances stated in 1980 that there were insufficient relevant biological and other studies upon which to base an evaluation of it when it is used as a food ingredient. GRAS.

I-CARNITINE • Levocarnitine Carnitor. Vitacarn. A B-vitamin factor found in muscle, liver, and meat extracts. Used for patients born with systemic carnitine deficiency. It is a thyroid inhibitor. It enables fatty acids to produce energy in persons who are carnitine deficient. Potential adverse reactions include nausea, vomiting, cramps, diarrhea, and body odor. There is reported use of the chemical; it has not yet been assigned for toxicology literature.

CAROB BEAN • Essential Oil. GRAS. *See* Locust Bean Gum.

CAROPHYLLENE ALCOHOL • A flavoring that occurs in essential oils, especially in clove oil. Colorless, oily, with a clovelike odor. Used as a synthetic mushroom flavoring for baked goods and condiments.

CAROTENE • Provitamin A. Beta-carotene. Found in all plants and many animal tissues, it is the chief yellow coloring matter of carrots, butter, and egg yolk. Extracted as red crystals or crystalline powder, it is used as a vegetable dye in butter, margarine, shortening, skimmed milk, buttermilk, and cottage cheese. It is also used to manufacture vitamin A and is a nutrient added to skimmed milk, vegetable shortening, and margarine at the rate of 5,000 to 13,000 IU per pound. Insoluble in water, acids, and alkalies. Too much carotene in the blood (exceeding 200 micrograms per 100 milliliters of blood) can lead to carotinemia—a pale yellow-red pigmentation of the skin that may be mistaken for jaundice. It is a benign condition and withdrawal of carotene from the diet cures it. The final report to the FDA of the Select Committee on GRAS Substances stated in 1980 that it should continue its GRAS status with no limitations other than good manufacturing practices. Beta-carotene has been permanently listed as a coloring since 1964.

CAROTENOID • Any of several pigments that give fruits and vegetables yellow, orange, or red coloring.

CARRAGEENAN • Chondrus Extract. Irish Moss. A stabilizer and emulsifier, seaweedlike in odor, derived from Irish moss, used in oils in cosmetics and foods. It is used as an emulsifier in chocolate products, chocolate-flavored drinks, chocolate milk, gassed cream (pressure-dispensed whipped cream), syrups for frozen products, confections, evaporated milk, cheese spreads and cheese foods, ice cream, frozen custard, sherbets, ices, French dressing, artificially sweetened jellies and jams. Completely soluble in hot water and not coagulated by acids. Salts of carrageenan, such as calcium, ammonium, potassium, or sodium, are used as a demulcent to soothe mucous membrane irritation. With polysorbate 80 at 500 ppm in final food containing the additives, it is used for producing gels. Carrageenan is on the FDA list for further study. Carrageenan stimulated the formation of fibrous tissue when subcutaneously injected into the guinea pig. When a single dose of it dissolved in saline was injected under the skin of the rat, it caused sarcomas after approximately two years. Its cancer-causing ability may be that of a foreign body irritant, because upon administration to rats and mice at high levels in their diet, it did not appear to induce tumors, although survival of the animals for this period was not good. Its use as a food additive is being studied. The final report to the FDA of the Select Committee on GRAS Substances stated in 1980 that while no evidence in the available information it demonstrates a hazard to the public at current use levels, uncertainties exist, requiring that additional studies be conducted. GRAS status continues while tests are being completed and evaluated. As of this writing, nothing has been reported. The FAO-WHO Expert Committee on Food Additives requested in June 1998 that "clarification of the significance of the promotion of colon cancer observed in experiments in rats" is needed for evaluation in 2001.

CARROT JUICE POWDER • *See* Carrot Oil.

CARROT OIL • Either of two oils from the seeds of carrots. A light yellow essential oil that has a spicy odor and is used in liqueurs, flavorings, and perfumes. It is used as a violet, fruit, rum, and spice flavoring for beverages, ice cream, ices, candy, baked goods, gelatin desserts, puddings, condiments, and soups. Rich in vitamin A, it is also used as a coloring and has been permanently listed since 1964. A skin irritant. When heated to decomposition it emits acrid smoke and irritating fumes. GRAS.

CARROT SEED EXTRACT • Extract of the seeds of *Daucus carota sativa*. *See* Carrot Oil.

CARVACROL • A colorless to pale yellow liquid with a pungent, spicy odor related to thymol but more toxic. It is found naturally in oil of origanum, dittany-of-crete oil, oregano, lavage oil, marjoram, and savory. It is a synthetic flavoring used in citrus, fruit, mint, and spice flavorings for beverages, ice cream, ices, candy, baked goods, and condiments. It is used as a disinfectant and is corrosive; one gram by mouth can cause respiratory and circulatory depression and cardiac failure leading to death.

CARVACRYL ETHYL ETHER • A synthetic spice-flavoring agent for beverages, ice cream, ices, candy, and baked goods. Found naturally in caraway and grapefruit.

CARVEOL • A synthetic mint, spearmint, spice, and caraway flavoring agent for beverages, ice cream, ices, candy, and baked goods. Found naturally in caraway and grape, baked fruit.

CARVOL • *See d*-Carvone.

4-CARVOMENTHENOL • A synthetic citrus and spice flavoring for beverages, ice cream, ices, candy, and baked goods. Occurs naturally in cardamom oil, juniper berries.

(*d*- or *l*-)CARVONE • Oil of Caraway. *d*-Carvone is usually prepared by distillation from caraway seed and dill seed oil. It is colorless to light yellow with an odor of caraway. *l*-Carvone occurs in several essential oils. It may be isolated from spearmint oil or synthesized commercially from *d*-limonene. It is colorless to pale yellow with the odor of spearmint. Carvol is a synthetic liquor, mint, and spice flavoring agent for beverages, ice cream, ices, candy, and baked goods. Also used in perfumery and soaps. It breaks up intestinal gas and is used as a stimulant. GRAS.

CARVYL ACETATE • A synthetic mint flavoring for beverages, ice cream, ices, candy, and baked goods.

CARVYLOPHYLLENE ACETATE • A general fixative that occurs in many essential oils, especially in clove oil. Colorless, oily, with a clovelike odor. Used for beverages, ice cream, ices, candy, baked goods, and chewing gum. Practically insoluble in alcohol. No known toxicity.

CARVYL PROPIONATE • A synthetic mint flavoring for beverages, ice cream, ices, candy, and baked goods.

***b*-CARYOPHYLLENE** • A synthetic spice flavoring. Occurs naturally in cloves, black currant buds, yarrow herb, grapefruit, allspice, and black pepper. The liquid smells like oil of cloves and turpentine. Used in beverages, ice cream, ices, candy, baked goods, chewing gum, and condiments. A skin irritant.

CASCARA, BITTERLESS EXTRACT • A natural flavoring derived from the dried bark of a plant grown from northern Idaho to northern California. Cathartic. Used in butter, maple, caramel, and vanilla flavoring for beverages, ice cream, ices, and baked goods. Also used as a laxative. The freshly dried bark causes vomiting, so it must be dried for a year before use, when the side effect has disappeared. It has a bitter taste and its laxative effect is due to its ability to irritate the mucosa of the large intestine.

CASCARILLA BARK • A natural flavoring agent obtained from the bark of a tree grown in Haiti, the Bahamas, and Cuba. The dried extract is added to smoking tobacco for flavoring and is used in bitters and spice flavorings for beverages. The oil, obtained by distillation, is light yellow to amber, with a spicy odor. It is used in cola, fruit, root beer, and spice flavorings for beverages, ice cream, ices, candy, baked goods, and condiments. No known toxicity. GRAS.

CASEIN • Ammonium Caseinate. Calcium Caseinate. Potassium Caseinate. Sodium Caseinate. The principal protein of cow's milk. It is a white, water-absorbing powder without noticeable odor. Used as a texturizer for ice cream, frozen custard, ice milk, fruit sherbets, and in special diet preparations. Also used in protective cream and as the "protein" in hair preparations to make the hair thicker and more manageable. It is also used to make depilatories less irritating, as a film-former in beauty masks, and an emulsifier in many cosmetics and in special diet preparations. Nontoxic. The final report to the FDA of the Select Committee on GRAS Substances stated in 1980 that it should continue its GRAS status with no limitations other than good manufacturing practices.

CASHOO EXTRACT • *See* Catechu Extract.

CASSIA BARK • Padang or Batavia. GRAS. *See* Cassia Bark, Chinese.

CASSIA BARK, CHINESE • A natural flavoring extract from cultivated trees. Used in cola, root beer, and spice flavorings for beverages, ice cream, candy, and baked goods. The bark oil is used in berry, chocolate, lemon, coffee, cola, cherry, peach, rum, peppermint, pecan, root beer, cassia, ginger ale, and cinnamon flavorings for beverages, ice cream, ices, candy, baked goods, chewing gum, meats, and condiments. The buds are used in spice flavorings for beverages. Cassia bark can cause inflammation and erosion of the gastrointestinal tract. GRAS.

CASSIA FLOWERS • Flavoring. *See* Cassia Oil.

CASSIA OIL • Cloves. Chinese Oil of Cinnamon. Darker, less agreeable, and heavier than true cinnamon. Obtained from a tropical Asian tree, it is used in bitters, fruit, liquor, meat, root beer, sarsaparilla, and spice flavorings for beverages, ice cream, candy, and baked goods (3,000 ppm). It is also used in perfumes, poultices, and as a laxative. It can cause irritation and allergy, such as a stuffy nose.

CASSIE FLOWERS • A natural flavoring from the flowers of the acacia plant. Used in blackberry, violet, vermouth, and fruit flavorings for beverages, ice cream, ices, candy, baked goods, and gelatin desserts. No known toxicity.

CASSIS • *See* Currant Buds, Absolute.

CASTOR OIL • Palm Christi Oil. Tang Tang Oil. Ricinus Oil. Palm Cristi Oil. The seed of the castor oil plant. After the oil is expressed from the beans, a residual castor pomace remains, which contains a potent allergen. This may be incorporated in fertilizer, which is the main source of exposure, but people who live near a castor bean–processing factory may also be sensitized. A flavoring, pale yellow and viscous, it has a slightly acrid, sometimes nauseating taste. Used in butter and nut flavorings for beverages, ice cream, ices, candy, and baked goods. Also an antisticking agent in hard-candy products and a component of protective coatings, drying oil, and releasing agent *(see)*. The raw material is a constituent of embalming fluid and a cathartic. It is also used in bath oils, nail polish removers, solid perfumes, face masks, shaving creams, lipsticks, and many men's hairdressings. It is also used as a plasticizer in nail polish; it forms a tough shiny film when dried. More than 50 percent of the lipsticks in the United States use a substantial amount of castor oil. Ingestion of large amounts may cause pelvic congestion and induce abortions. Soothing to the skin.

CASTOREUM EXTRACT • Castor. Used in perfumes as a fixative *(see)*. A creamy, orange-brown substance with strong penetrating odor and bitter taste that consists of the dried perineal glands of the beaver and their secretion. The glands and secretions are taken from the area between the vulva and anus in the female beaver and from the scrotum and anus in the male beaver. Professional trappers use castor to scent bait. There is reported use of the chemical; it has not yet been assigned for toxicology literature.

CATALASE • An enzyme from bovine liver used in milk, for making cheese, and for the elimination of peroxide. It is used also in combination with glucose oxidase for treatment of food wrappers to prevent oxidative deterioration of food. There is reported use of the chemical; it has not yet been assigned for toxicology literature.

CATALYST • A substance that causes or speeds up a chemical reaction but does not itself change.

CATECHU EXTRACT • Black Cutch Extract. Cachou Extract. Cashoo Extract. Pegu Catechu Extract. A preparation from the heartwood of the acacia catechu (*see* Acacia) grown in India, Sri Lanka, and Jamaica. Used in bitters, fruit, and rum flavorings for beverages, ice cream, ices, candy, baked goods, and chewing gum. Used also in toilet preparations and for brown and black colorings. The powder is used in fruit, rum, and spice flavorings for beverages, ice cream, candy, baked goods, and chewing gum. Incompatible with iron compounds, gelatin, limewater and zinc. Used as an astringent in diarrhea. May cause allergic reactions. There is reported use of the chemical; it has not yet been assigned for toxicology literature.

CAYENNE PEPPER • Red Pepper. A condiment made from the pungent fruit of the plant. Used in sausage and pepper flavorings for beverages, ice cream, ices, candy, meats (910 ppm), soups, and condiments. Reported to retard growth of Mexicans, South Americans, and Spaniards who eat a great deal of these peppers. Rats fed the ingredient of pepper, a reddish-brown liquid called capsaicin, used in flavoring and pickles, were stunted in growth. A report by F. M. Gannett of the Eppley Institute for Research Institute, University of Nebraska Medical Center, Omaha, at the 1988 American Chemical Society meeting, Toronto, Canada, said that capsaicin, the substance that makes these peppers hot, is not a low-level mutagen as earlier believed but is actually antimutagenic. GRAS.

CEDAR • Cedar Wood Oil. The oil from white, red, or various cedars obtained by distillation from fresh leaves and branches. A colorless to yellow liquid, it is used in fruit and spice flavorings for beverages, ice cream, ices, candy, baked goods, chewing gum, and liquors. It is often used in perfumes, soaps, and sachets for its warm woodsy scent. Used frequently as a substitute for oil of lavender. There is usually a strong camphor odor that repels insects. Cedar oil can be a photosensitizer, causing skin reactions when the skin is exposed to light. Similar toxicity to camphor oil *(see)*. Finished food should be thujone-free. Thujone is a toxic substance found in oils such as cedar, tansy, thuja, wormwood, and sage.

CEDAR WOOD OIL • *See* Cedar.

CEDRO OIL • *See* Lemon Oil.

CEDRYL ACETATE • Colorless liquid having a light cedar odor. Used in fragrances.

CEFTIOFUR • An animal drug used in beef. The FDA limits residues to 3 ppm in muscle, 9 ppm in kidney, 6 ppm in liver, and 12 ppm in fat of cattle. When heated to decomposition it emits acrid smoke and irritating fumes.

CELERY SEED • A yellowish to greenish brown liquid, having a pleasant aromatic odor, distilled from the dried ripe fruit of the plant grown in southern Europe. Celery seed is used in sausage and celery flavorings for beverages (1,000 ppm), baked goods, condiments (2,500 ppm), soups, meats, and pickles. Celery seed solid extract is used in celery, meat, and spice flavorings for beverages, ice cream, ices, candy, baked goods, condiments, and maple syrup. Celery seed oil is used in fruit, honey, maple, sausage, nut, root beer, spice, vanilla, and cream soda flavorings for beverages, ice cream, ices, candy, baked goods, chewing gum, meats, soup, pickles, and condiments. Celery seed may cause a sensitivity to light. GRAS.

CELLULASE ENZYME • Derived from *Aspergillus niger*. An enzyme for removal of visceral mass in clam processing and shell from shrimp.

CELLULOSE • Chief constituent of the fiber of plants. Cotton contains about 90 percent. It is the basic material for cellulose gums *(see)*. Used as an emulsifier in cosmetic creams. There is reported use of the chemical, it has not yet been assigned for toxicology literature search.

CELLULOSE GUMS • Sodium Carboxymethylcellulose. CMC. Modified Cellulose. Occurs as a white- to cream-colored powder or granules. It absorbs water. Fibrous substances consisting of the chief part of the cell walls of plants. Made from cotton byproducts, it occurs as a white powder or in granules. A synthetic gum, it is used as a stabilizer in ice cream, beverages, and other foods. Cellulose acetate is obtained by treating cellulose with food starch modifier; it is insoluble in water, alcohol, and ether. Used in the manufacture of rubber and celluloid substitutes, airplane dopes, varnishes, and lacquer. *Ethylcellulose* is a film-former in lipstick. *Methylcellulose* (Methocel) and *hydroxyethylcellulose* (Cellosize) are used as emulsifiers in hand creams and lotions. They are resistant to bacterial decomposition and give uniform viscosity to products. No known toxicity, but it has been shown to cause cancer in animals when ingested. The final report to the FDA of the Select Committee on GRAS Substances stated in 1980 that it should continue its GRAS status for packaging only with no limitations other than good manufacturing practices.

CENTAURY (CENTRUIUM) HERB • Flavoring in alcoholic beverages only.

CEPHARPIRIN • An animal drug used in beef and milk. The FDA limits residue to 0.02 ppm in milk and 0.1 ppm in uncooked edible tissues of dairy cattle. Moderately toxic by injection into the vein. When heated to decomposition it emits toxic fumes.

CERESIN • Ceresine. Earth Wax. Used in protective creams. It is a white or yellow, hard, brittle wax made by purifying ozokerite *(see),* found in Ukraine, Utah, and Texas. It is used as a substitute for beeswax and paraffin wax *(see both);* also used to wax paper and cloth, as a polish, and in dentistry for taking wax impressions. May cause allergic reactions.

CERTIFIED • Each batch of coal tar or petrochemical colors, with the exception of those used in food and the FDA must certify cosmetic dyes as "harmless and suitable for use." The manufacturer must submit samples of every batch for testing and the lot test number accompanies the colors thorough all subsequent packaging.

CETONE D • *See* Methyl *b*-Naphthyl Ketone.

CETONE V • *See* Allyl *a*-Ionone.

CETYL • Means derived from cetyl alcohol *(see).*

CETYL ALCOHOL • An emollient and emulsion stabilizer used in many foods and cosmetics preparations including baby lotion, brilliantine hairdressings, deodorants and antiperspirants, cream depilatories, eyelash creams and oils, foundation creams, hair lacquers, hair straighteners, hand lotions, lipsticks, liquid powders, mascaras, nail polish removers, nail whiteners, cream rouge, and shampoos. Cetyl alcohol is waxy, crystalline, and solid, and found in spermaceti *(see).* It has a low toxicity for both skin and ingestion and is sometimes used as a laxative. Can cause hives. *See* Fatty Alcohols.

CETYL ARACHIDATE • An ester produced by the reaction of cetyl alcohol and arachidic acid. The acid is found in fish oils and vegetables, particularly peanut oil. A fatty compound used as an emulsifier. Nontoxic.

CETYL ESTERS • Synthetic spermaceti *(see)*.

CETYLIC ACID • *See* Palmitic Acid.

CEYLON CINNAMON • *See* Cinnamon.

CEYLON CINNAMON LEAF OIL • *See* Cinnamon Leaf Oil.

CF-3 • Preempt. A blend of twenty-nine beneficial microbes found in the gastrointestinal tract of mature, healthy chickens that can reduce salmonella *(see)* colonization. A single spray of bacterial suspension will be administered to newly hatched chicks at a dose of approximately 0.25-milliliter per chick. The bacteria on the chick's feathers are subsequently ingested through normal grooming (preening) behavior. It is essentially replacing the mother hen. Before the advent of large modern poultry farms, hens would pass the good microbes—and disease resistance—on to their chicks. On March 13, 1998, the FDA approved this first *competitive exclusion (CE)* product for animals in the U.S. CE products are made up of live bacteria that can be given to animals to establish normal gut-microflora, thereby helping to reduce or prevent the colonization of undesirable bacteria. By populating the gut with normal microflora, thereby excluding undesirable bacteria, CE products may help reduce carcass contamination and the incidence of food-borne illness in humans. Reduction of salmonella colonization in chickens is an important step in reducing salmonella contamination in processed poultry products. While salmonella colonization is generally not a problem for the chickens, it is a problem for humans who may develop salmonellosis through the ingestion of improperly cooked or handled Salmonella-contaminated chicken. While the use of Preempt will help reduce one type of contamination, poultry must be properly handled and cooked to be safe. This CE culture product was originally developed and tested by a USDA-Agricultural Research Service team at College Station, Texas. This specific culture is produced as Preempt under an exclusive licensing agreement between the USDA and MS BioScience. During clinical studies, no adverse effects were observed in the chicks following Preempt administration. In addition since Preempt is a suspension of bacteria, there are no concerns regarding chemical residues in edible tissue from treated chickens. However, since this product consists of live bacteria, using antimicrobials in feed or drinking water along with Preempt would inhibit the survival and ultimate establishment of these organisms in the gut.

CHACONINE • An alkaloid in plants of the *Solanaceae* family such as potatoes and tomatoes. In laboratory animals, it causes birth defects but the World Health Organization said that the amount in potatoes is not significant.

CHAMOMILE • Roman, English, and Hungarian Chamomile. The daisylike white and yellow heads of these flowers provide a coloring agent known as apigenin. The essential oil distilled from the flower heads is pale blue and is added to shampoos to impart the odor of chamomile. Powdered flowers are used to bring out a bright yellow color in the hair. Also used in rinses and skin fresheners. *Roman Chamomile* is used in berry, fruit, vermouth, maple, spice, and vanilla flavorings. *English chamomile* is used as a flavoring in chocolate, fruit, and liquor flavorings for beverages, ice cream, ices, candy, and baked goods. *Roman chamomile* oil is used in chocolate, fruit, vermouth, and spice flavorings for beverages, ice cream, ices, candy, baked goods, gelatin desserts, and liquors. *Hungarian chamomile* oil is used in chocolate, fruit, and liquor flavorings for beverages, ice cream, ices, candy, baked goods, chewing gum, and liquors. Chamomile contains sesquiterpene lactones that may cause allergic contact dermatitis and stomach upsets. GRAS. There is reported use of the chemical; it has not yet been assigned for toxicology literature.

CHARCOAL • Formerly widely used as a black coloring; the FDA no longer authorizes its use.

CHAR SMOKE FLAVOR • A flavoring. There is reported use of the chemical; it has not yet been assigned for toxicology literature.

CHECKERBERRY EXTRACT • *See* Wintergreen Oil.

CHECKERBERRY OIL • *See* Wintergreen Oil.

CHELATING AGENT • Any compound, usually one that binds and precipitates metals, such as ethylenediamine tetraacetic acid (EDTA), which removes trace metals. *See* Sequestering Agent.

CHEMICALS USED IN WASHING FRUITS and VEGETABLES • Polyacrylamide, potassium bromide, sodium dodecylbenzenesulfonate, sodium hypochlorite, sodium 2-ethyl-1-hexylsulfate, sodium *n*-alkylbenzene sulfonate, sodium mono- and dimethyl-naphthalene sulfonates; alkylene oxide adducts of alkyl alcohols, and phosphate esters of alkylene oxides. Adducts of alkyl alcohols mixtures. Uses of such chemicals followed by rinsing to remove residues. Some individual chemicals remain in limited amounts in wash water, according to the FDA.

CHERRY BARK (WILD) EXTRACT • A natural flavoring extracted from the pits of sweet and sour cherries used in cherry flavoring for beverages, ice cream, and ices. GRAS.

CHERRY LAUREL LEAVES • *Prunus Laurocerasus.* A flavoring.

CHERRY PIT OIL • A natural flavoring and fragrance extracted from the pits of sweet and sour cherries. Also a cherry flavoring for beverages, ice cream, and condiments.

CHERRY PLUM • Source of purplish red color. *See* Anthocyanins.

CHERVIL • A natural flavoring extracted from an aromatic Eurasian plant and used in spice flavorings for beverages, ice cream, ices, candy, baked goods, and condiments. A chewing-gum base. GRAS.

CHESTNUT • *Castanea dentata.* Nuts from a European tree used as a remedy for piles, backaches, and for coughs. An astringent, the bark and leaves were used to make a tonic, which was also reportedly useful in the treatment of upper respiratory ailments such as coughs, particularly whopping cough. The bark of Spanish chestnut contains tannins *(see)*. There is reported use of the chemical; it has not yet been assigned for toxicology literature.

CHEWING-GUM BASE • Chicle, chiquibal, crown gum, gutta hang kang, massaranduba balata, massaranduba chocolate, nispero lechi caspi, pendare, perillo, rosidinha, Venezuelan chicle, liche devaca, Niger gutta, tuno, chilte, natural rubber, glycerol ester of tall oil resin.

CHICLE • The gummy milky resin obtained from trees grown in Mexico and

Central America. Rubberlike and quite soft at moderate temperatures. Used in the manufacture of chewing gum, insulation, and waterproofing.

CHICORY EXTRACT • A natural flavor extract from a plant, usually with blue flowers and leaves. Used in butter, caramel, chocolate, coffee, maple, nut, root-beer, sarsaparilla, vanilla, wintergreen, and birch beer flavorings for beverages, ice cream, ices, candy, and baked goods. The root of the plant is dried roasted and ground for mixing with coffee. GRAS.

CHILI • *Capsicum fastigatum.* Chili is the dried pod of a species of capsicum *(see)* or red pepper. The small pods have been used for dyspepsia *(see)* and dilated blood vessels arising from drunkenness. A capsicum poultice has been used with caution for the relief of aches and pains. Modern herbalists use it in liniments and gargles.

CHILTE • A chewing-gum base component of vegetable origin. No known toxicity.

CHINA BARK EXTRACT • *See* Quillaja Extract.

CHINESE CINNAMON • *See* Cinnamon.

CHINESE CINNAMON LEAF OIL • *See* Cinnamon Leaf Oil.

CHINESE RESTAURANT SYNDROME • Manifested by anxiety, flushed face, and pressure in the chest, has been shown to be caused by eating large amounts of the flavor enhancer MSG. Sulfite preservatives are now known to have the potential to cause a serious attack of asthma and even death.

CHIQUIBUL • *Manilkara zapotilla.* A composition in chewing-gum bases.

CHIRATA (CHIRETTA, EAST INDIAN BOLONONG) and HERB EXTRACT • Flavoring used in alcoholic beverages only. There is reported use of the chemical; it has not yet been assigned for toxicology literature search.

CHIVES • A member of the onion family, native to Eurasia. The leaves are used for a seasoning. GRAS.

CHLORAMPHENICOL • Drug in any form may no longer be used in food-producing animals (meat, milk, and egg). Once widely used in animals. In the EPA Genetic Toxicology Program *(see)*. Poison by intraperitoneal, intravenous, and subcutaneous routes. Moderately toxic by ingestion. A human carcinogen that causes leukemia, aplastic anemia, and other bone marrow changes by ingestion.

CHLORDANE • An organochlorine pesticide introduced in 1945 that was among the first to be developed for insect control. Because of its persistence in the environment, most of its uses were suspended by order of the EPA in 1975. Several specified uses are still permitted, including pest control on pineapple, strawberries, and Florida citrus crops. It also can be used to remedy a number of other pest-control problems that plague certain areas of the United States. Chlordane causes cancer of the liver in mice. It is less toxic than other similar pesticides, but acute exposure has the effect of stimulating the central nervous system. It has also been implicated in acute blood dyscrasia (abnormalities) such as aplastic anemia. Can be absorbed through the skin.

CHLORDIMEFORM • Colorless crystals derived from ethyl formate and ammonia; it is a fumigant, an insecticide, and miticide. It also kills insect eggs. It is sold for use on cotton and vegetable crops. It is less toxic than organophosphates and is biodegradable. It is used in dried apple pomace, cottonseed hulls, and in dried prunes as a residue resulting from application to growing plums. In animal feed the tolerance is up to 25 ppm. In prunes it is 15 ppm.

CHLORETHEPHON • Water-absorbing needles from benzene used as a plant-growth regulator used in animal feed, barley, raisin waste, sugarcane molasses, and wheat-milling fractions (except flour). The FDA permits a residue of 5.0 ppm in barley and wheat-milling fractions (except flour), 1.5 ppm in sugarcane molasses, and 65.0 ppm in raisin waste when used for animal feed. Moderately toxic by ingestion. Mildly toxic by skin contact. May be irritating to exposed skin and eyes or if inhaled.

CHLORHEXIDINE DIHYDROCHLORIDE • A veterinarian drug used for cattle. The FDA tolerance residue in edible tissue of calves is zero.

CHLORIMURON • A pesticide and herbicide used in soybeans, peanuts, peanut hulls. FDA tolerance residues are from 0.02 to 0.05 ppm.

CHLORINE DIOXIDE • Flour bleacher and oxidizing agent. A yellow to reddish yellow gas, with an unpleasant odor, highly irritating and corrosive to the skin and mucous membranes of respiratory tract. Reacts violently with organic materials. It can kill. There is reported use of the chemical; it has not yet been assigned for toxicology literature.

CHLORINE GAS • Flour-bleaching and aging and oxidizing agent. Also used in water purification. Found in the earth's crust, it is a greenish yellow gas with a suffocating odor. A powerful irritant, dangerous to inhale, and lethal. Thirty ppm will cause coughing. The chlorine used in drinking water often contains carcinogenic carbon tetrachloride, a contaminant formed during the production process. Chlorination has also been found to sometimes form undesirable "ring" compounds in water, such as toluene, xylene, and the suspected carcinogen styrene—they have been observed in both the drinking water and wastewater plants in the Midwest.

CHLORITE • *See* Calcium Hypochlorite.

CHLORMETHYLATED AMINATED STYRENE DI-VINYLBENZENE RESIN • Used to clarify *(see)* sugar liquor up to 500 ppm.

CHLOROACETIC ACID • Used in packaging adhesives and as a preservative. Not permitted in alcoholic beverages or foods. In EPA Genetic Toxicology Program *(see)* and considered an extremely hazardous substance.

CHLOROBUTANOL • Tetramethylene Chlorohydrin. An animal drug used to treat mastitis in cows. The FDA does not permit any residue in milk. Moderately toxic by ingestion and may be mutagenic.

CHLOROFLUOROCARBONS • Any of several compounds comprised of carbon, fluorine, chlorine, and hydrogen, the best known of which are trichloromethane and dichlorodifluoromethane. Their use was prohibited in 1979 except for a few specialized items because of their depleting effect on stratospheric ozone. The FDA permits it for use in cooling or freezing chickens.

2-CHLORO-4-NITROENZMIDE • A feed additive. *See* Aklomide.

CHLOROPHENAMIDINE • Acaron. Fundex. A pesticide used in animal feed, apple pomace (dried) cottonseed hulls, prunes (dried). FDA residue tolerance of

15 ppm on dried prunes, 25 ppm in dried apple pomace, 10 ppm in cottonseed hulls when used for animal feed. Poison by ingestion, skin contact, and injection. Possible cancer-causing agent and mutagen. Eye and skin irritant.

1-(4-CHLOROPHENOXY)-3,3-DIMETHYL-1-(1,2,3-TRIAZOL-1-YL)-2-BUTAN-2-ONE • Amiral. MEB 6447. Triadimefon. A fungicide used on barley (except flour) and wheat (except flour). FDA residue tolerance is 4 ppm in barley and wheat, milled fractions (except flour). Poisonous by ingestion.

1-(4-CHLOROPHENYL)-3-(2,6-DIFLUOROBENZOYL) UREA • Difluon. Dimilin. An insecticide used in animal feed, soybean hulls, and soybean soap stock when used for animal feed. EPA Genetic Toxicology Program *(see)*. Moderately toxic by skin contact. Mildly toxic by ingestion. May be mutagenic.

1-(4-CHLOROPHENOXY)-3-3-DIMETHYL-1-(IH-1,2,4-TRIAZOL-1-YL)-2-BUTANONE • A fungicide used in animal feed. FDA residue tolerances are residues on grape pomace, 3 ppm; on apple pomace, 4 ppm; on raisin waste, 7 ppm.

p-CHLOROPHENYL-2,4,5-TRICHLOROPHENYL SULFONE • Tetradifon. Akaritox. A pesticide used in dried figs, dried hops, and dried tea. FDA residue tolerance is 120 ppm in dried hops, 10 ppm in dried figs, and 8 ppm in dried tea. Moderately toxic by ingestion. Mildly toxic by skin contact. May cause birth defects.

CHLOROPHYLL • The green coloring matter of plants, which plays an essential part in the plant's photosynthesis process. Used in antiperspirants, dentifrices, deodorants, and mouthwashes as a deodorizing agent. It imparts a greenish color to certain fats and oils, notably olive oil and soybean. Can cause a sensitivity to light. There is reported use of the chemical; it has not yet been assigned for toxicology literature.

CHLOROPROPANOLS • Certain chlorinated propanols used as insecticides and herbicides contaminate hydrolyzed vegetable proteins *(see)*. The two substances considered by the FAO-WHO Expert Committee on Food Additives were 3-chloro-1,2-propanediol and 1,30dichloro-2-propanol, neither of which had been previously evaluated. During traditional processing of vegetable proteins with hydrochloric acid, "significant amounts" of these two contaminants have been found. With newer methods, the level of propanediol compound has been reduced to less than 2 mg per kg and the propanol compound to less than 0.02 mg per kg in hydrolyzed vegetable protein. In monkeys, the propanediol compound induced anemia, increased white blood cell count and other blood changes following ingestion of 30 mg per kg of body weight a day for six weeks. It also reduced fertility in male rats and caused malignant and gene-damaging effects in cells in laboratory dishes. The propanediol also did the same in mouse cells in laboratory dishes. In more recent experiments in which rats were fed 1.1 to 28 mg per kg of body weight per day of either one of the compounds, the animals developed cancers of the testes, breast, and tongue among others. The Committee concluded that these substances are "undesirable contaminants in food" and expressed the opinion that their levels in hydrolyzed vegetable proteins should be reduced as far as "technically possible."

CHLORPENTAFLUOROETHANE • Alone or with carbon dioxide. Used as propellant and aerating agent in foods. *See* Chlorofluorocarbons.

2(m-CHLOROPHENOXY) PROPIONIC ACID • A growth regulator used in pineapple bran. FDA residue tolerance is 3 ppm.

CHLORPROMAZINE • Ormazine. Thorazine. Thor-Pram. An antipsychotic and antinausea medication introduced in the 1950s, it is also used for intractable hiccups and mild alcohol withdrawal. It is used to tranquilize pigs on their way to market. Potential adverse reactions to the medication in humans include a drop in white blood cells, sedation, uncontrolled movements, Parkinsonism-like symptoms, dizziness, a drop in blood pressure when rising from a seated or prone position, vision changes, dry mouth, constipation, urine retention, male breast enlargement, inhibited ejaculation, liver dysfunction, weight gain, increased appetite, fever, photosensitivity, irregular heartbeat, and sweating. Tardive dyskinesia *(see)* may occur after prolonged use. Alcohol and other central nervous system depressants may increase central nervous system depression. Drugs used to treat Parkinsonism and antidepressants may increase chlorpromazine's nerve-suppressing activity. Blood pressure medications that act on the brain may be less effective. Oral blood thinners may be less effective and propranolol can increase the levels of both propranolol and chlorpromazine. Contraindicated in central nervous system depression, bone marrow suppression, brain damage, Reye's syndrome, and coma. Also contraindicated with the use of spinal or epidural anesthetic; in arteries, cardiovascular disease, or respiratory disorders, glaucoma, and enlarged prostate, and in acutely ill or dehydrated children. The ingested drug may take effect in thirty to sixty minutes and may last up to three weeks after stopping the drug.

CHLORPYRIFOS • O,O-Dimethyl-0-(3,5,6-Trichloro-2-Pyridyl) Phosphorothioate. Dursban. Lorsban. White granular powder used as an insecticide and acaricide on corn and other vegetables. Poison by ingestion. A skin irritant. FDA residue tolerance is 90 ppm in barley milling fractions (except flour), 130 ppm in oats milling fractions (except flour), 90 ppm in sorghum milling fractions (except flour), 30 ppm in rice-milling fractions (except flour), 30 ppm in wheat-milling fractions (except flour). The FDA tolerance as residues in milk fat is 1.25 ppm and 0.5 ppm as residues in fat, meat, and meat byproducts of cattle, goats, hogs, poultry, and sheep. As a residue in barley, oat, rice, and wheat grain, the tolerance is 6 ppm.

CHLORSULON • Curatrem. An animal drug used to treat worms. The FDA tolerance is 1 ppm in uncooked edible muscle tissue of cattle; 2 ppm as residue in uncooked liver; 3.0 ppm as residue in kidney; 4 ppm as residue in uncooked cattle fat.

CHLORTETRACYCLINE • Aureomycin. Biomycin. Biomitsin. PfiClor. A preservative, an antibiotic, used in dip and feed to improve feed efficiency and increase weight gain. The FDA permits 4 ppm residue in uncooked kidneys of chickens and turkeys; 1 ppm in uncooked muscle, liver, fat, and skin of chickens and turkeys, and zero residue in eggs. The residues permitted in uncooked swine liver is 2 ppm, 0.2 ppm in uncooked fat of calves, 4 ppm in uncooked liver and kidneys of calves, 0.1 ppm in uncooked muscle and fat of calves, uncooked liver, and kidneys of beef cattle and non-lactating dairy cows. Residue in milk is supposed to be zero. One of the reasons for increased resistance to antibiotics in patients is believed to be the widespread use of antibiotics in food animals. In 1969, the British restricted the veterinary use of antibiotics. In 1972, the FDA-appointed committee to study the use of antibiotics in animals recommended curbs on use. Many strains of bacteria are known to be resistant to tetracycline. The use of this antibiotic has caused discoloration of permanent teeth in children given the drug prior to the eruption of the second teeth. The drug can also cause skin rash, gastrointestinal upsets, and inflammations in the ano-genital area.

CHOLECALCIFEROL • Vitamin D_3. White crystals used as a dietary supplement and nutrient. In breakfast cereals, grain products, margarine, milk, milk products, and pasta. Poison by ingestion and may cause birth defects. GRAS.

CHOLEST • Listing on labels for cholesterol *(see)*.

CHOLESTEROL (DIETARY) • Cholesterol is not fat, but rather a fatlike substance classified as a lipid. Cholesterol is vital to life and is found in all cell membranes. It is necessary for the production of bile acids and steroid hormones. Dietary cholesterol is found only in animal foods. Abundant in organ meats and egg yolks, cholesterol is also contained in meats, chicken, and shellfish. Vegetable oils and shortenings are cholesterol-free.

CHOLESTEROL (SERUM or BLOOD) • High blood cholesterol is a risk factor in the development of coronary heart disease. Most of the cholesterol that is found in the blood is manufactured by the body at a rate of about 800 to 1,500 milligrams a day. By comparison, the average American consumes 300 to 450 milligrams daily in foods. Cholesterol travels through the blood via particles called lipoproteins—combinations of lipids and proteins. Too much cholesterol can build up in the blood and accumulate in the walls of the blood vessels, a condition known as atherosclerosis. This can ultimately reduce the flow of blood in major arteries, leading to heart attack. Blood cholesterol reflects the amount of three major classes of lipoproteins: very low-density lipoprotein (VLDL); low-density lipoprotein (LDL), which contains most of the cholesterol found in the blood; and high-density lipoprotein (HDL). LDL seems to be the culprit in coronary heart disease and is popularly known as the "bad cholesterol." By contrast, HDL is increasingly considered desirable and known as the "good cholesterol." Diet is just one factor influencing blood cholesterol levels. For some people at risk, heredity is a stronger predictor of cholesterol levels than diet. Age, race, and gender are other risk factors for high cholesterol levels.

CHOLIC ACID • A colorless or white crystalline powder that occurs in the bile of most vertebrates and is used as an emulsifying agent in dried egg whites and as a choleretic to regulate the secretion of bile. Bitter taste; sweetish aftertaste. No known toxicity. The final report to the FDA of the Select Committee on GRAS Substances stated in 1980 that it should continue its GRAS status with no limitations other than good manufacturing practices.

CHOLINE • Found in most animal tissues, either free or in combinations such as lecithin or acetylcholine. Choline is being actively studied for its effects on brain neurotransmission and memory.

CHOLINE BITARTRATE • A dietary supplement included in the B complex and found in the form of a thick syrupy liquid in most animal tissue. It is necessary to nerve function and fat metabolism and can be manufactured in the body but not at a sufficient rate to meet health requirements. Dietary choline protects against poor growth, fatty liver, and renal damage in many animals. Choline deficiency has not been demonstrated in man but the National Academy of Sciences lists 500 to 900 milligrams per day as sufficient for the average man. The final report to the FDA of the Select Committee on GRAS Substances stated in 1980 that it should continue its GRAS status with no limitations other than good manufacturing practices.

CHOLINE CHLORIDE • Ferric Choline Citrate. A dietary supplement with the same function as choline bitartrate *(see)*. The final report to the FDA of the Select Committee on GRAS Substances stated in 1980 that it should continue its GRAS status with no limitations other than good manufacturing practices.

CHOLINE HYDROCHLORIDE • Colorless to white, water-absorbing crystals used as a fungicide on various feeds. It is listed in the Community Right-to-Know List *(see)*. Moderately toxic to humans by ingestion. May be mutagenic.

CHOLINE XANTHATE • A feed additive for poultry, swine, and ruminants.

CHONDRUS • *See* Carrageenan.

CHROMIUM • Occurs in the earth's crust and plays a vital role in the activities of some human enzymes. It is involved in the breakdown of sugar for conversion into energy and in the manufacture of certain fats. It works together with insulin and is essential to the body's ability to use sugar. Traces of chromium are widely available in food. However, chromium deficiency may frequently occur because the soil in the United States contains low levels. Those who are deficient may show symptoms similar to diabetes such as tiredness, mental confusion, and numbness or tingling of the hands and feet. Deficiency may worsen preexisting diabetes, depress growth in children, or contribute to the development of narrowing of the arteries.

Chromium-rich diet may prevent Type II diabetes, the non-insulin dependent form of the disease that starts in adulthood. Richard A. Anderson, a biochemist at the USDA Human Nutrition Research Center in Beltsville, Maryland, has shown that diets high in simple sugars such as glucose and fructose rob the body of chromium, while those high in complex carbohydrates such as pasta preserve it. The new research builds on data from Anderson's lab showing that chromium supplementation in rats improves glucose tolerance—the ability to transport blood glucose into cells.

Chromium is poisonous in large amounts. Ingestion can result in violent gastrointestinal irritation. Foods that contain chromium include fruits, beers, oysters, liver, egg yolk, potatoes with skin, mushrooms, brewer's yeast, and wines. Not always absorbed—for example, much of the chromium in potatoes never gets incorporated into the body cells. Simple sugars, furthermore, cause the body to excrete large amounts of the mineral. An attempt was made to permit chromium to be listed on a food label as reducing the risk of high blood sugar in adults. The FDA denied the claim because it said the statements submitted as the basis of it were not "authoritative."

CHROMOSOME • One or more small rod-shaped elements in a cell that contains genetic information.

CHYMOSIN • Enzyme prepared from calf stomach. Used as a stabilizer and thickener. GRAS. There is reported use of the chemical; it has not yet been assigned for toxicology literature search.

CINCHONA EXTRACT • The extract of the bark of various species of cinchona cultivated in Java, India, and South America. A natural flavoring, *red cinchona bark* is used in bitters, fruit, rum, vermouth, and spice flavorings for beverages, ice cream, ices, candy, liquors, and bitters (1,000 ppm). *Yellow cinchona bark* is a natural flavoring from the bark of a species of South American tree used in bitters, fruit, and vermouth flavorings for liquors. The yellow extract is used as a bitters flavoring for beverages. Quinine is derived from it. Cinchona stimulates digestion. May rarely cause allergies and stomach upsets. There is reported use of the chemical; it has not yet been assigned for toxicology literature.

CINENE • *See d*-Limonene.

CINEOLE • *See* Eucalyptol.

CINNAMAL • *See* Cinnamaldehyde.

CINNAMALDEHYDE • Cinnamic Aldehyde. A synthetic yellowish oily liquid with a strong odor of cinnamon isolated from a wood-rotting fungus. Occurs naturally in cassia bark extract, cinnamon bark, and root oils. Used in cola, apple cherry, liquor, rum, nut, pecan, spice, cinnamon, vanilla, and cream soda flavorings for beverages, ice cream, ices, candy, baked goods, chewing gum (4,900 ppm), condiments, and meats. Also used in perfume industry, to flavor mouthwash and toothpaste, and to scent powder and hair tonic. It is irritating to the skin and mucous membranes, especially if undiluted. Can cause inflammation and erosion of the gastrointestinal tract. One of the most common allergens. GRAS.

CINNAMALDEHYDE ETHYLENE GLYCOL ACETAL • Cinncloval. Spice, cassia, cinnamon, and clove flavorings for beverages, ice cream, ices, candy, baked goods, chewing gum, and condiments. *See* Cinnamaldehyde for toxicity.

CINNAMEIN • *See* Benzyl Cinnamate.

CINNAMIC ACID • A cherry, honey, spice, cassia, and cinnamon flavoring agent for beverages, ice cream, ices, candy, baked goods, and chewing gum. Also used in suntan lotions and perfumes. Occurs in storax, balsam Peru, cinnamon leaves, and coca leaves. Usually isolated from wood-rotting fungus. Used mainly in the perfume industry. It may cause allergic skin rashes.

CINNAMIC ALCOHOL • Fragrance ingredient. One of the most common allergens in fragrances and flavorings. Used in mouthwashes, toilet soaps, toothpastes, and sanitary napkins. *See* Cinnamal.

CINNAMIC ALDEHYDE • Found in cinnamon oil, cassia oil, cinnamon powder, patchouli oil, favoring agents, toilet soaps, and perfumes. It cross-reacts with Balsam Peru and benzoin. May cause depigmentation and hives.

CINNAMON (CEYLON, CHINESE, SAIGON) • Obtained from the dried bark of cultivated trees. *See* Cinnamal for toxicity. Used in bitters, cola, apple, plum, vermouth, sausage, eggnog, cinnamon, and vanilla flavorings for beverages, ice cream, ices, candy (4,000 ppm), baked goods (1,900 ppm), condiments, meats, and apple butter. Used to flavor toothpaste and mouthwash and to scent hair tonic and powder. Extracts have been used to break up intestinal gas and to treat diarrhea, but can be irritating to the gastrointestinal system. GRAS.

CINNAMON BARK • Extract and Oil. From the dried bark of cultivated trees, the *extract* is used in cola, eggnog, root beer, cinnamon, and ginger ale for beverages, ice cream, baked goods, condiments, and meats. The oil is used in berry, cola, cherry, rum, root beer, cinnamon, and ginger ale flavorings for beverages, condiments, and meats. Can be a skin sensitizer in humans and cause mild sensitivity to light. GRAS.

CINNAMON LEAF OIL • Oil of Cassia. Chinese Cinnamon. Yellowish to brown volatile oil from the leaves and twigs of cultivated trees. About 80 to 90 percent cinnamal. It has the characteristic odor and taste of cassia cinnamon and darkens and thickens upon aging or exposure to air. Used in cola, apricot, rum, root beer, cinnamon, and ginger ale flavorings for beverages, ice cream, ices, candy, baked goods, chewing gum, gelatin desserts, condiments, pickles, and sliced fruits. Cinnamon oil is used to scent perfumes and as a flavoring in dentifrices. Can cause contact dermatitis.

CINNAMYL ACETATE • A synthetic flavoring, colorless to yellow liquid with a sweet floral odor. Occurs naturally in cassia bark. Used in apricot, cherry, grape, peach, pineapple, cinnamon, and vanilla flavorings for beverages, ice cream, ices, candy, baked goods, chewing gum, and condiments. Can cause allergic reactions.

CINNAMYL ALCOHOL • A synthetic flavoring, white to slightly yellow liquid with a balsamic odor. Occurs in storax, balsam Peru, cinnamon leaves, and hyacinth oil. Used in raspberry, strawberry, apricot, peach, plum, prune, grape, liquor, brandy, nut, black walnut, spice, and cinnamon flavorings for beverages, ice cream, ices, candy, baked goods, chewing gum, gelatin desserts, and brandy. Used also in synthetic perfumes and in deodorants. Can cause allergic reactions.

CINNAMYL ANTHRANILATE • A synthetic flavoring agent that has been banned by the FDA. The National Cancer Institute reported, December 20, 1980, that it caused liver cancer in male and female mice and caused both kidney and pancreatic cancers in male rats in feeding studies. Earlier studies showed it increased lung tumors in mice. The FDA banned the use of it in food in 1982. Most companies voluntarily stopped using it in cosmetics after publication of the NCI information. It has not been banned.

CINNAMYL BENZOATE • A synthetic butter, caramel, and fruit flavoring agent for beverages, ice cream, ices, candy, baked goods, condiments, and chewing gum.

CINNAMYL BUTYRATE • A synthetic citrus orange and fruit flavoring for beverages, ice cream, ices, candy, baked goods, and chewing gum.

CINNAMYL CINNAMATE • A synthetic fruit flavoring agent for beverages, ice cream, ices, candy, and baked goods.

CINNAMYL FORMATE • Formic Acid. A synthetic flavoring, colorless to yellow liquid with a faint cinnamon odor. Used in banana, cherry, pear, and spice flavorings for beverages, ice cream, ices, candy, baked goods, and chewing gum. *See* Formic Acid for toxicity.

CINNAMYL ISOBUTYRATE • A synthetic strawberry, citrus, apple, banana, grape, peach, pear, and pineapple flavoring agent for beverages, ice cream, ices, candy, baked goods, gelatin desserts, chewing gum, and toppings.

CINNAMYL ISOVALERATE • A synthetic flavoring, colorless to yellow liquid with a spicy, fruity, floral odor. Used in strawberry, chocolate, apple, apricot, cherry, grape, maple nut, nut, spice, peach, pineapple, and plum flavorings for beverages, ice cream, ices, candy, baked goods, chewing gum, and gelatin desserts.

CINNAMYL PHENYLACETATE • A synthetic flavoring, colorless to yellow liquid, with a fruity floral odor. Used in berry, apple, chocolate, currant, grape, peach, pear, and pineapple flavorings for beverages, ice cream, ices, candy, and baked goods.

CINNAMYL PROPIONATE • A synthetic flavoring, colorless to yellow liquid with a fruity floral odor. Used in berry, apple, chocolate, currant, grape, peach, pear, and pineapple flavorings for beverages, ice cream, ices, candy, baked goods, chewing gum, and gelatin desserts.

CINNCLOVAL • *See* Cinnamaldehyde Ethylene Glycol Acetal.

CINOXATE • *See* Cinnamic Acid.

CIRE D'ABEILLE ABSOLUTE • *See* Beeswax, Bleached.

CITRAL • A light, oily liquid that occurs naturally in grapefruit, orange, peach, ginger, grapefruit oil, oil of lemon, and oil of lime. Either isolated from citral oils or made synthetically. Used in strawberry, lemon, lime, orange, apple, cherry, grape, spice, ginger, and vanilla flavorings for beverages, ice cream, ices, candy, baked goods, and chewing gum. Used in perfumes, soaps, and colognes for its lemon and verbena scents. Also used in the synthesis of vitamin A. Causes discoloration of white soaps. Used in soaps and colognes for its lemon and verbena scents. Found also in detergents and furniture polish. The compound has been reported to inhibit wound healing and tumor rejection in animals. Vitamin A counteracts its toxicity, but in commercial products to which pure citral has been added vitamin A may not be present. GRAS.

CITRAL DIMETHYL ACETAL • A synthetic citrus, lemon, and fruit flavoring agent for beverages, ices, candy, and condiments.

CITRATE, CALCIUM • *See* Calcium Citrate.

CITRATE, ISOPROPYL • *See* Isopropyl Citrate.

CITRATE, MONOGLYCERIDE • *See* Monoglyceride Citrate.

CITRATE, SODIUM • *See* Sodium Citrate.

CITRATE, STEARYL • *See* Stearyl Citrate.

CITRATE SALTS • Softening agent for cheese spreads; emulsifier salts to blend pasteurized processed cheeses and cheese foods. Citrates may interfere with the results of laboratory tests including tests for pancreatic function, abnormal liver function, and blood alkalinity-acidity.

CITRIC ACID • One of the most widely used acids in the cosmetic industry, it is derived from citrus fruit by fermentation of crude sugars. It is also extracted from citrus fruits and occurs naturally in coffee and peaches. It is a flavoring for beverages (2,500 ppm), ice cream, ices, candy (4,300 ppm), baked goods, and chewing gum (3,600 ppm). Citric acid is used to neutralize lye employed in peeling vegetables, as an adjuster of acid-alkalinity in fruit juices, wines, jams, jellies, jelly candies, canned fruit, carbonated beverages, frozen fruit, canned vegetables, frozen dairy products, cheese spreads, sherbet, confections, canned figs, dried egg whites, mayonnaise, salad dressing, fruit butter, preserves, and fresh beef blood. Employed in curing meats, for firming peppers, potatoes, tomatoes, and lima beans and to prevent off-flavors in fried potatoes. Removes trace metals and brightens color in various commercial products. Employed as a preservative, sequestering agent *(see),* to adjust acid-alkali balance, as a foam inhibitor and plasticizer in cosmetics, and also used as an astringent alone or in astringent compounds. Among the cosmetic products in which it is frequently found are freckle and nail bleaches, bath preparations, skin fresheners, cleansing creams, depilatories, eye lotions, hair colorings, hair rinses, and hair-waving preparations. The clear, crystalline, water-absorbing chemicals are also used to prevent scurvy, a deficiency disease, and as a refreshing drink with water and sugar added. It has been used to dissolve urinary bladder stones. No known toxicity. The final report to the FDA of the Select Committee on GRAS Substances stated in 1980 that it should continue its GRAS status with no limitations other than good manufacturing practices.

CITRIDIC ACID • *See* Aconitic Acid.

CITROFLEX A-4 • *See* Tributyl Acetylcitrate.

CITRONELLA OIL • A natural food flavoring extract from fresh grass grown in Asia. It consists of about 60 percent geraniol *(see),* 15 percent citronellol *(see),* and 10 to 15 percent camphene *(see).* Almost colorless with a pleasant odor. Used in citrus, fruit, and ginger ale flavorings for beverages, ice cream, ices, candy, and baked goods. Used in perfumes, toilet waters, and perfumed cosmetics; also an insect repellent. May cause allergic reactions such as stuffy nose, hay fever, asthma, and skin rash when used in cosmetics. Can cause vomiting when ingested, cyanosis, convulsions, damage to intestinal mucosa, and when taken in sufficient amounts, death. GRAS.

CITRONELLAL • A synthetic flavoring agent. The chief constituent of citronella oil *(see).* Also found in lemon and lemon grass oils. Colorless liquid with an intense lemon-rose odor. Used in citrus, lemon, cherry, and spice flavorings for beverages, ice cream, ices, candy, baked goods, chewing gum, and gelatin desserts. A milk irritant. *See* Citronella Oil for toxicity.

CITRONELLOL • A synthetic flavoring. Obtained from citronellal or geraniol, geranium rose oil, or citronella oil *(see all).* Colorless liquid with a roselike odor. The *d* form is oilier and is the major ingredient of rhodinol *(see).* Used in berry, citrus, cola, fruit, rose, and floral flavorings for beverages, ice cream, ices, candy, baked goods, chewing gum, and gelatin desserts. Used in perfumes. A mild irritant. *See* Citronella Oil. There is reported use of the chemical; it has not yet been assigned for toxicology literature.

CITRONELLOXY ACETALDEHYDE • A synthetic floral, rose, and fruit flavoring agent for beverages, ice cream, ices, candy, and baked goods. *See* Citronella Oil for toxicity.

CITRONELLYL ACETATE • A synthetic flavoring agent, colorless liquid with a fruity odor. Used in lemon, rose, apricot, banana, grape, pear, and raisin flavorings for beverages, ice cream, ices, candy, baked goods, chewing gum, and gelatin desserts. A major ingredient of rhodinyl acetate *(see)*.

CITRONELLYL BUTYRATE • A synthetic flavoring agent, colorless liquid, with a strong rose-fruit odor. Used in cola, floral, rose, apple, pineapple, plum, prune, and honey flavorings for beverages, ice cream, ices, candy, baked goods, chewing gum, and gelatin desserts. A major ingredient of rhodinyl acetate *(see)*.

CITRONELLYL FORMATE • Formic Acid. A synthetic flavoring agent, colorless liquid, with a strong fruity odor. Used in orange, apple, apricot, peach, plum, and honey flavorings for beverages, ice cream, ices, candy, baked goods. A major ingredient of rhodinyl acetate *(see)*. *See* Formic Acid for toxicity.

CITRONELLYL ISOBUTYRATE • A synthetic flavoring agent, colorless liquid, with a fruit-rose odor. Used in raspberry, strawberry, floral, rose, and grape flavorings for beverages, ice cream, ices, candy, baked goods, and gelatin desserts. A major ingredient of rhodinyl acetate *(see)*.

CITRONELLYL PHENYLACETATE • A synthetic butter, caramel, rose, fruit, and honey flavoring agent for beverages, ice cream, ices, candy, and baked goods. A major ingredient of rhodinyl acetate *(see)*.

CITRONELLYL PROPIONATE • A synthetic flavoring agent, colorless liquid, with a rose-fruit odor. Used in lemon and fruit flavorings for beverages, ice cream, ices, candy, baked goods, and chewing gum. A major ingredient of rhodinyl acetate *(see)*.

CITRONELLYL VALERATE • A synthetic flavoring agent for beverages, ice cream, ices, candy, and baked goods.

CITRUS BIOFLAVONOIDS • Vitamin P complex nutrient supplement up to one gram per day. Occurs naturally in plant coloring and in the tonka bean; also in lemon juice. High concentrates can be obtained from all citrus fruits, rose hips, and black currants. Commercial methods extract rinds of oranges, tangerines, lemons, limes, kumquats, and grapefruit. P vitamin is related to healthy blood vessels and skin. At one time it was thought to prevent colds. Any claim for bioflavonoids renders the product illegal, according to FDA rules.

CITRUS OILS • Eugenol. Eucalyptol. Anethole, *a*-irone, orris, and menthol *(see all)*. Used in flavoring food products and cosmetics and as odorants in special soaps.

CITRUS PEEL EXTRACT • A natural flavor extract from the peel or rind of grapefruit, lemon, lime, orange, and tangerine. Color, odor, and taste characteristic of source. Used as flavoring agents in bitters, lemon, lime, orange, vermouth, beer, and ginger ale flavorings for beverages, ice cream, ices, candy, and baked goods. GRAS.

CITRUS RED NO. 2 • Monoazo. Used only for coloring orange skins that are not intended for processing and that meet minimum maturity standards established by or under laws of the states in which the oranges are grown. Used to color Florida but not California oranges. Oranges colored with Citrus Red No. 2 are not supposed to bear more than 2 ppm of the color additive calculated on the weight of the whole fruit. Citrus Red No. 2 toxicity is far from determined even though, theoretically, consumers would not ingest the dye because they peel the orange before eating. The 2-naphthol constituent of the dye if ingested in quantity can cause eye lens clouding, kidney damage, vomiting, and circulatory collapse. May cause allergic reactions and cross-react with clothing, hair dyes, and with sulfanilimides. Application to the skin can cause peeling and deaths have been reported after application to the skin. *See* FD and C Colors.

CIVET, ABSOLUTE • Zibeth. Zibet. Zibetum. Essential oil used as a flavoring. Derived from the unctuous secretions from the receptacles between the anus and genitalia of both the male and female civet cat. Semisolid, yellowish to brown mass, with an unpleasant odor. Used in raspberry, butter, caramel, grape, and rum flavorings for beverages, ice cream, ices, candy, baked goods, gelatin desserts, and chewing gum. A fixative in perfumery. GRAS. There is reported use of the chemical; it has not yet been assigned for toxicology literature.

CLARIFICATION • Removal from liquid of small amounts of suspended matter; for example, the removal of particles and traces of copper and iron from vinegar and certain beverages.

CLARIFYING AGENT • A substance that removes from liquids small amounts of suspended matter. Butyl alcohol, for instance, is a clarifying agent for clear shampoos.

CLARY • Clary Sage. A well-known spice in food and beverages. A fixative *(see)* for perfumes. A natural extract of an aromatic herb grown in southern Europe and cultivated widely in England. The herb is a vermouth and spice flavoring agent in vermouth (500 ppm). Clary oil is used in butter, black cherry, grape, licorice, vermouth, wine, root beer, birch beer, spice, vanilla, and cream soda flavorings for beverages, ice cream, ices, candy, baked goods, condiments, and vermouth. GRAS. There is reported use of the chemical; it has not yet been assigned for toxicology literature.

CLAYS • Kaolin. China Clay. Used to clarify liquids (*see* Clarification) and as a filler for paper. Also used in the manufacture of porcelain and pottery, as an emollient, and as a poultice and gastrointestinal adsorbent. Nontoxic. The final report to the FDA of the Select Committee on GRAS Substances stated in 1980 that it should continue its GRAS status with no limitations other than good manufacturing practices.

CLOPIDOL • Additive used in chicken and turkey feeds to combat parasites.

The FDA tolerance for residues in milk is 0.02; for cereal, grains, vegetables, fruits, meat of cattle, sheep, and goats, and in edible tissue of swine, it is 0.2 ppm. The tolerance is 1.5 ppm in liver of cattle, sheep, and goats; 5 ppm in muscle of chicken and turkeys; 5 ppm in liver and kidneys of chickens and turkeys.

CLOPROSTENOL • Estrumate. An animal drug used to treat infertility in sows and to synchronize estrus in cows.

CLOPYRALID • An herbicide used in animal feed, barley (milled, except flour), oats (except flour), and wheat (milled, except flour). FDA residue limits are 12.0 ppm in barley, oats, and wheat (except in their flours) when used for animal feed. The tolerance for residues in fat, meat, byproducts of sheep is 2 ppm and 0.2 ppm for the fat, kidneys, and meat of hogs and poultry.

CLOVE BUD EXTRACT • A natural flavor extract from the pungent, fragrant, reddish brown dried flower buds of a tropical tree. Used in berry, fruit, meat, root beer, and spice flavorings for beverages, ice cream, candy, baked goods, condiments, and meats. Cloves are used also as a dental analgesic and germicide. They may cause intestinal upsets. Rats poisoned with clove oil have shown paralysis of hind legs and jaws, with prostration and eventually death. The FDA gave toxicity studies of clove additives top priority in 1980. As of this writing, nothing new has been reported. GRAS.

CLOVE BUD OIL • The volatile, colorless or pale yellow oil obtained by steam distillation from the dried flower buds of a tropical tree. A characteristic clove odor and taste. Used in raspberry, coffee, cola, banana, cherry, peach, plum, rum, sausage, eggnog, pecan, root beer flavorings for beverages, ice cream, ices, candy, baked goods, chewing gum (1,800 ppm), gelatin desserts, meats, liquors, spiced fruit (830 ppm), jelly, condiments. Used as an antiseptic and flavoring in tooth powders and as a scent in hair tonics and to flavor postage stamp glue, as a toothache treatment, as a condiment, and as a flavoring in chewing gum. It is 82 to 87 percent eugenol *(see)* and has the characteristic clove oil odor and taste. It is strongly irritating to the skin and can cause allergic skin rashes. Its use in perfumes and cosmetics is frowned upon, although in very diluted forms it is innocuous. The final report to the FDA of the Select Committee on GRAS Substances stated in 1980 that it should continue its GRAS status with no limitations other than good manufacturing practices.

CLOVE BUD OLEORESIN • A natural resinous, viscous flavoring extract from the tree that produces clove buds. Used in fruit, meat, and spice flavorings for meat.

CLOVE LEAF OIL • The volatile pale yellow oil obtained by steam distillation of the leaves of the tropical tree that produces clove buds. Used in loganberry, cherry, root beer, sarsaparilla, and cinnamon flavorings for beverages, ice cream, ices, candy, baked goods, chewing gum, gelatin desserts, meats, pickles, apple butter, and condiments. *See* Clove Bud Extract for toxicity. The final report to the FDA of the Select Committee on GRAS Substances stated in 1980 that it should continue its GRAS status with no limitations other than good manufacturing practices.

CLOVE STEM OIL • The volatile, yellow to light brown oil obtained by steam distillation from the dried stems of the tropical tree that produces clove buds.

Characteristic odor and taste of cloves. Used in berry, cherry, root beer, ginger ale, and ginger beer flavorings for beverages, ice cream, ices, candy, baked goods, and condiments. *See* Clove Bud Extract for toxicity. The final report to the FDA of the Select Committee on GRAS Substances stated in 1980 that it should continue its GRAS status with no limitations other than good manufacturing practices.

CLOVER • An herb, a natural flavoring extract from a plant characterized by three leaves and flower in dense heads. Used in fruit flavorings for beverages, ice cream, ices, candy, and baked goods. May cause sensitivity to light. GRAS. There is reported use of the chemical; it has not yet been assigned for toxicology literature.

CLOVER BLOSSOM EXTRACT • Trifolium Extract. The extract of the flowers of *Trifolium pratense*. Used in fruit flavorings. May cause sensitivity to light.

CLOVERLEAF OIL • Eugenia Caryophyllus Leaf Oil. The volatile oil obtained by steam distillation of the leaves of *Eugenia caryophyllus*. It consists mostly of eugenol *(see)*.

CLOVES • *Eugenia caryophyllata*. An evergreen tree, the clove is native to the Spice Islands and the Philippines and is cultivated in India, South America, the West Indies, and other tropical areas. The oldest medical use was in China, where it was taken for various ailments as early as 240 B.C. Medicinally, herbalists use cloves to treat flatulence, diarrhea, and for liver, stomach, and bowel ailments. It is also used as a stimulant for nerves. Clove oil is still sold in modern drugstores as a treatment for toothaches. Clove tea with mace is used in a tea for nausea. In 1992, the FDA proposed a ban on clove oil in astringent *(see)* drug products because it has not been shown to be safe and effective for its stated claims.

CLOXACILLIN • Alcloxa. Apo-Cloxi. Austrastaph. Bactopen. Cloxapen. Novo-cloxin. Orbenin. Orbenin Injection. Tegopen. A penicillin antibiotic introduced in 1962 for systemic infections caused by penicillinase-producing staphylococci (*see* Staphybiotic). It is used in cattle. The FDA says residues in cattle meat should not exceed 0.1 ppm. In humans, it may cause lung problems (eosinophilia), nausea, vomiting, gastric distress, diarrhea, hypersensitivity including potentially fatal allergic reaction, liver problems, and overgrowth of nonsusceptible organisms.

CMC • *See* Cellulose Gums.

COAL TAR • Used in adhesives, creosotes, insecticides, phenols, woodworking, preservation of food, synthetic flavors, and dyes to makes colors used in cosmetics, including hair dyes. Thick liquid or semisolid tar obtained from bituminous coal, it contains many constituents including benzene, xylenes, naphthalene, pyridine, quinolineoline, phenol, and cresol. The main concern about coal tar derivatives is that they cause cancer in animals, but they are also frequent sources of allergic reactions, particularly skin rashes and hives.

COBALT SALTS • Acetate, Chloride, and Sulfate. Illegal for use. In 1960, it was discovered that cobalt salts added to beer to maintain the head caused serious heart problems in beer drinkers. Cobalt sulfate has been banned.

COBALT SOURCES • Acetate, Carbonate, Chloride, Oxide, and Sulfate. Cobalt is a metal occurring in the earth's crust; gray, hard, and magnetic. All here are used as a mineral supplement at the rate of one milligram per day. Used as a nutrient in animal feed. Excess administration can result in an overproduction of red blood cells and gastrointestinal upset. GRAS.

COCA LEAF EXTRACT (DECOCAINIZED) • Flavoring from the dried leaves of cocaine-containing plants grown in Bolivia, Brazil, Peru, and Java. Used in bitters and cola flavoring for beverages, ice cream, ices, and candy. Once a central nervous system stimulant. GRAS.

COCCIDIOSIS • A group of diseases due to coccidia, one-celled animals that cause serious infections in many species of animals. It is rare in humans except in persons suffering from AIDS.

COCCIDIOSTAT • A drug generally added to animal feed to partially inhibit or delay the development of coccidiosis *(see)*.

COCHINEAL • *See* Carmine.

COCOA • A powder prepared from the roasted and cured kernels of ripe seeds of *Theobroma cacao* and other species of *Theobroma*. A brownish powder with a chocolate odor, it is used as a flavoring. May cause wheezing, rash, and other symptoms of allergy, particularly in children.

COCOA BUTTER SUBSTITUTE FROM PALM KERNEL OIL, COCONUT OIL, or BOTH • Coating material for vitamins, citric acid, succinic acid, and spices. In lieu of cocoa butter in sweets. There is reported use of the chemical; it has not yet been assigned for toxicology literature. GRAS.

COCOA EXTRACT • Extract of *Theobroma cacao*. *See* Cocoa Butter.

COCOAMPHOCARBOXYPROPIONIC ACID • *See* Coconut Oil.

COCOAMPHODIACETATE • Widely used in cosmetics in the manufacture of toilet soaps, creams, lubricants, chocolate, and suppositories. *See* Coconut Oil.

COCOAMPHODIPRIOPIONATE • *See* Coconut Oil.

COCONUT ACIDS • *See* Coconut Oil.

COCONUT ALCOHOLS • *See* Coconut Oil.

COCONUT OIL • The white, semisolid, highly saturated fat expressed from the kernels of the coconut. Used in chocolate, candies, in baking, instead of lard, and in self-basting turkeys. A saturated fat that is not recommended for those worried about fat-clogged arteries. No known toxicity. Used in the manufacture of baby soaps, shampoos, shaving lathers, cuticle removers, preshaving lotions, hairdressings, soaps, ointment bases, and massage creams. Stable when exposed to air. Lathers readily and is a fine skin cleaner. Usually blended with other fats. May cause allergic skin rashes. The final report to the FDA of the Select Committee on GRAS Substances stated in 1980 that it should continue its GRAS status with no limitations other than good manufacturing practices.

COD-LIVER OIL • The fixed oil expressed from fresh cod livers used in skin ointments and special skin creams to promote healing. Pale yellow, with a bland, slightly fishy odor. Contains vitamins A and D, which promote healing of wounds and abscesses. No known toxicity.

COFFEE • Coffee beans. Dry, unroasted seeds of *Coffea arabica*. Contains caffeine *(see)*. An essential oil used as a flavoring. GRAS.

COGNAC OIL • Wine Yeast Oil. The volatile oil obtained from distillation of wine, with the characteristic aroma of cognac. Green cognac oil is used as a flavoring for beverages, ice cream, ices, candy, baked goods, chewing gum, liquors, and condiments. White cognac oil, which has the same constituents as green oil, is used in berry, cherry, grape, brandy, and rum flavorings for beverages, ice cream, ices, candy, baked goods, and gelatin desserts. No known toxicity. GRAS.

COLA NUT • Essential oil used for flavoring. GRAS.

COLISTIMETHATE SODIUM • First Guard Sterile Powder. Used on one- to three-day-old chickens for control of early mortality due to *Escherichia coli* organisms. It is injected into the neck of chicks.

COLLAGEN • Protein substance found in connective tissue. In cosmetics, it is usually derived from animal tissue. Allergic reactions are not infrequent.

COLLOIDAL SILICON DIOXIDE • Practically insoluble in water. A free-flowing agent in salt, seasoned salt, and sodium bicarbonate. Also included in vitamin products, dietary products, spices, meat-curing compounds, flavoring powders, dehydrated honey, dehydrated molasses, and dehydrated nondiastatic malt. Percentages range from 1 percent in salt to dehydrated nondiastatic malt. Percentages range from 1 percent in salt to 2 percent in dehydrated products. Prolonged inhalation of the silicon dust can cause fibrosis of the lungs. Increases susceptibility to tuberculosis. Chemically and biologically inert when ingested. *See* Silicon Dioxide.

COLORING • More than 90 percent of the food colorings now in use are manufactured, frequently from coal-tar colors. The coal-tar derivatives need to be certified, which means that batches of the dyes are chemically tested and approved by the FDA. As more and more food colors are banned, interest has grown in color derived from natural sources such as carotene *(see)* from carrots, which is used to color margarine, and beet juice, which provides a red color for some foods. For information on the synthetics now in use, *see* FD & C Colors.

COLORS • *See* FD and C Colors.

COMMUNITY RIGHT-TO-KNOW LIST • Manufacturers that employ toxic chemicals while making products must respond, under the law, to inquiries from employees and citizens in the area. Cyanide, which is used in the manufacture of pesticides and some food additives is an example of a chemical on this list compiled by the U.S. Environmental Protection Agency.

COMPETITIVE MICROBIAL INHIBITION • Relies on the fact that many harmless bacteria, notably lactic acid bacteria, can inhibit the growth of both spoilage bacteria and pathogens. Inhibitory strains of lactic acid bacteria can be selected for use in dairy cultures or added to refrigerated foods to extend shelf life and enhance safety.

CONCRETE • A semisolid mixture of essential oil and fatty, waxy material that is obtained by the solvent extraction of flowers or plants followed by solvent removal.

CONDENSED ANIMAL PROTEIN HYDROLYSATE • A feed used for poultry and cattle.

CONTACT DERMATITIS • *See* Allergic Contact Dermatitis.

COPAIBA OIL • Jesuit's Balsam. From steam distillation of South American balsam, *Copaifera l.* It is a yellow liquid with an aromatic odor and slightly bitter taste. It is used as a flavoring agent in various food. There is reported use of the chemical; it has not yet been assigned for toxicology literature.

COPALS, MANILA • A resin obtained as a fossil or as an exudate from various species of tropical plants. Must be heated in alcohol or other solvents. May cause allergic reactions, particularly skin rashes.

COPOLYMER • Result of polymerization (*see* Polymer), which includes at least two different molecules, each of which is capable of polymerizing alone. Together they form a new, distinct molecule. They are used in the manufacture of nail enamels and face masks.

COPOLYMER CONDENSATES OF ETHYLENE OXIDE and PROPYLENE OXIDE • Stabilizers in flavor concentrates, processing and wetting agents in yeast-leavened bakery products, dough conditioners, surfactants, defoaming agents, and nutrient supplements in animal feed. No known toxicity.

COPPER • One of the earliest known metals. An essential nutrient for all mammals. Naturally occurring or experimentally produced copper deficiency in animals leads to a variety of abnormalities including anemia, skeletal defects, and muscle degeneration. Copper deficiency is extremely rare in man. The body of an adult contains from 75 to 150 milligrams of copper. Concentrations are highest in the brain and liver and heart. A copper intake of 2 milligrams per day appears to maintain a balance in adults. An ordinary diet provides 2 to 5 milligrams daily. Copper compounds are used as a pesticide to control aquatic plants in sources of potable water.

COPPER DISODIUM EDTA • Used as an injection for cattle. *See* Copper and Copper Salts.

COPPER SALTS • Used as nutrient supplements in animal feed. Copper itself is nontoxic, but soluble copper salts, notably copper sulfate, are highly irritating to the skin and mucous membranes, and when ingested cause serious vomiting. Copper salts include copper carbonate, chloride, gluconate, hydroxide, orthophosphate, oxide, pyrophosphate, and sulfate. The final report to the FDA of the Select Committee on GRAS Substances stated in 1980 that it should continue its GRAS status with no limitations other than good manufacturing practices.

COPRA OIL • From the kernel of the fruit of the coconut palm *Cocos nucifera.* Fatty solid or liquid with a sweet, nutty taste. Used as a coating agent, emulsifying agent, and as a texturizer in baked goods, candy, desserts, and margarine. Nontoxic. GRAS.

CORIANDER OIL • The colorless or pale yellow volatile oil from the dried ripe fruit of a plant grown in Asia and Europe. Used as a flavoring agent in raspberry, bitters, fruit, meat, spice, ginger ale, and vanilla flavorings for beverages, ice cream, ices, candy, baked goods (880 ppm), chewing gum, meats (1,300 ppm), liquors (1,000 ppm), and condiments. Used to flavor dentifrices. The oil is used in blackberry, raspberry, chocolate, coffee, cola, fruit, liquor, sausage, root beer, spice, ginger ale, and vanilla flavorings for beverages, ice cream, ices, candy, baked goods, chewing gum, condiments, meats, and liquors. Can cause allergic reactions, particularly of the skin. Coriander is used as a weak medication (up to 1 gram) to break up intestinal gas. GRAS. There is reported use of the chemical; it has not yet been assigned for toxicology literature search.

CORK, OAK • Flavoring in alcoholic beverages only. There is reported use of the chemical; it has not yet been assigned for toxicology literature.

CORN • Corn Sugar. Dextrose. Used in maple, nut, and root beer flavorings for beverages, ice cream, ices, candy, and baked goods. The oil is used in emollient creams and toothpastes. The syrup is used as a texturizer and carrying agent in cosmetics. It is also used for envelopes, paper, stamps, sticker tapes, ale, aspirin, bacon, baking mixes, and powders, beers, bourbon, breads, cheeses, cereals, chop suey, chow mein, confectioners' sugar, cream puffs, fish products, ginger ale, hams, jellies, processed meats, peanut butters, canned peas, plastic food wrappers, sherbets, whiskeys, and American wines. It may also be found in capsules, lozenges, ointments, suppositories, vitamins, fritters, Fritos, frostings, canned or frozen fruit, graham crackers, gravies, grits, gum, monosodium glutamate, Nescafé, oleomargarine, bologna, pablum, tortillas, vinegar, yeasts, frying fats, fruit juices, laxatives. May cause allergic reactions including skin rashes and asthma.

CORN ACID • *See* Corn Oil.

CORN COB MEAL • The milled powder prepared from the cobs of *Zea mays*.

CORN DEXTRIN • Dextri-Maltose. A white or yellow powder obtained by enzymatic action of barley malt on corn flours and used as a modifier or thickening agent in milk and milk products. Nontoxic. The final report to the FDA of the Select Committee on GRAS Substances stated in 1980 that it should continue its GRAS status with no limitations other than good manufacturing practices.

CORN ENDOSPERM OIL • For use in chicken feed to enhance yellow color of chicken skin and eggs. Permanently listed since 1967.

CORN FLOUR • A finely ground powder. Used in face and bath powder. *See* Corn Oil.

CORN GERM EXTRACT • The extract of the germ of *Zea mays*.

CORN GLUTEN • A nutrient supplement for various foods.

CORN OIL • Light yellow, clear, oily liquid used as a coating agent, emulsifying agent, and texturizer in bakery products, margarine, mayonnaise, and salad oil. Also used in emollient creams and toothpastes. Obtained as a byproduct by wet-milling the grain for use in the manufacture of cornstarch, dextrins, and yellow oil. It has a faint characteristic odor and taste and thickens upon exposure to air. Human skin irritant and allergen. Has caused birth defects in experimental animals. GRAS.

CORN POPPY EXTRACT • The extract obtained from the petals of the *Papaver rhoeas*.

CORN SILK • Used as a natural flavoring extract in baked goods, baking mixes, beverages, soft candies, and frozen dairy desserts. The final report to the FDA of the Select Committee on GRAS Substances stated in 1980 that there were insufficient relevant biological and other studies upon which to base an evaluation of it when it is used as a food ingredient. It remains GRAS. There is reported use of the chemical; it has not yet been assigned for toxicology literature.

CORN SUGAR • Nutrient. GRAS. *See* Corn Syrup.

CORN SYRUP • Corn Sugar. Dextrose. A sweet syrup prepared from cornstarch. Used in maple, nut, and root beer flavorings for beverages, ice cream, ices, candy, and baked goods. Also used for envelopes, stamps, sticking tapes, aspirin, and many food products including bacon, baking mixes, powders, beer, bourbon, breads, breakfast cereals, pastries, candy, carbonated beverages, catsups, cheeses, cereals, chop suey, chow mein, confectioners' sugar, cream puffs, fish products, ginger ale, hams, jellies, processed meats, peanut butter, canned peas, plastic food wraps, sherbet, whiskey, and American wines. May cause allergic reactions. The final report to the FDA of the Select Committee on GRAS Substances stated in 1980 that there is no evidence in the available information that it is a hazard to the public when used as it is now, and it should continue in GRAS status with no limitations on amounts that can be added to food.

CORNSTARCH • Many containers are powdered with cornstarch to prevent sticking. The dietetic grade is marketed as Maizena and Mondamin. It is an absorbent dusting powder and a demulcent for irritated colons. May cause allergic reactions, including skin rashes and asthma. The final report to the FDA of the Select Committee on GRAS Substances stated in 1980 that it should continue its GRAS status with no limitations other than good manufacturing practices.

CORPS PRALINE • *See* Maltol.

COSTMARY • Virgin Mary. A natural flavoring derived from an herb native to Asia. Its yellow aromatic flowers are shaped like buttons. Used as a pot herb and salad plant. Infrequently used today as a flavoring in beer and ale. Regarded as sacred to the Virgin Mary.

COSTUS ROOT OIL • The volatile oil is obtained by steam distillation from dried roots of an herb. Light yellow to brown viscous liquid, with a persistent violetlike odor. A natural fruit and vanilla flavoring for beverages, ice cream, ices, candy, baked goods, chewing gum, and gelatin desserts. There is reported use of the chemical; it has not yet been assigned for toxicology literature search.

COTTONSEED FLOUR • Cooked, partly defatted, and toasted flour used for pale yellow coloring. Sometimes used to make gin. The oil is used in most salad oils, oleomargarines, mayonnaises, and salad dressings. Lard compounds and lard substitutes are made with cottonseed oil. Sardines and other smoked seafood may be packed in it. Most commercial fried products such as potato chips and doughnuts are fried in cottonseed oil, and restaurants almost universally use it for cooking. Candies, particularly chocolates, often contain this oil and it is used to polish fruits at stands. It is permanently listed as a coloring. It is known to cause allergies, and because it is used in a wide variety of products without notice, it may be hard to avoid. More often, exposures to the allergens arise from the use of *cottonseed meal,* which may be found in fertilizers and as a constituent of feed for cattle, hogs, poultry, and dogs. Symptoms usually result from inhalation but allergic reactions also can occur from ingesting cottonseed meal used in pan-greasing compounds and in foods such as some fried cakes, fig bars, and cookies.

COTTONSEED OIL • The fixed oil from the seeds of the cultivated varieties of the plant. Pale yellow, oily, odorless liquid used in the manufacture of soaps, creams, baby creams, nail polish removers, and lubricants. The oil is used in most salad oils, oleomargarines, mayonnaises, and salad dressings. Lard compounds and lard substitutes are made with cottonseed oil. Sardines may be packed in it. Most commercial fried products such as potato chips and doughnuts are fried in cottonseed oil, and restaurants use it for cooking. Candies, particularly chocolates often contain this oil and it is used to polish fruits at stands. It is used in baby creams, soaps, creams, nail polish removers, and lubricants. It is also used in cotton wadding or batting in cushions, comforters, mattresses, and upholstery, varnishes, fertilizers, and in animal feeds. Known to cause many allergic reactions, but because of its wide use in cosmetics, foods, and other products, it is hard to avoid.

COTTONSEED and SOYBEAN FATTY ACIDS • Used as a lubricant, binder, defoaming agent, and component in manufacture of other food-grade additives.

COUCHGRASS • *See* Dog Grass Extract.

COUMAPHOS • Agridip. Asunthol. Baymix 50. Used in cattle and chicken feed as an insecticide and to counteract worms. Poison by ingestion, skin contact, inhalation, and injection. May be a mutagen. The FDA tolerance in meat and meat byproducts of cattle, goats, hogs, horses, poultry, and sheep is 1.0 ppm. In eggs and milk it is zero.

COUMARIN • Tonka Bean. Cumarin. A fragrant ingredient of tonka beans, sweet woodruff, cramp bark, and many other plants. It is made synthetically as well. Coumarin is prohibited in foods because it is toxic by ingestion and carcinogenic.

COUMARONE-IDENE RESIN • Coating for fruit. FDA limits it to 200 ppm on fresh-weight basis.

COUNTERIRRITANT • An ingredient applied locally to produce superficial inflammation with the object of reducing existing inflammation in deeper adjacent structures. Iodine *(see)* is an example of a counterirritant.

CRANBERRY JUICE CONCENTRATE • Bright red coloring from the juice of the red acid berry, produced by any of several plants of the genus *Vaccinium,* grown in the United States and Europe. Food manufacturers may substitute this natural coloring for the synthetic reds that were banned. No known toxicity.

CRANBERRY POMACE • Source of natural red coloring. *See* Anthocyanins.

CREAM OF TARTAR • A white crystalline salt in tartars from wine making, prepared especially from argols and also synthetically from tartaric acid *(see)*. Has a pleasant acid taste. Used as a thickening agent and in certain treatment of metals.

CREOSOL • *See* 2-Methoxy-4-Methylphenol.

CREOSOTE • Obtain from wood tar, either almost colorless or yellowish. Used locally as an antiseptic, internally as an expectorant. It has a smoky odor and a caustic, burning taste. Large doses internally may cause stomach irritation, heart problems, and death. It is also used as a mild insect repellent.

p-CRESOL • A synthetic nut and vanilla flavoring agent. Obtained from coal tar. It occurs naturally in tea and is used for beverages, ice cream, ices, candy, and baked goods. It is more powerful than phenol and less toxic. Phenol is an extremely toxic acid obtained from coal tar that has many industrial uses, including as a disinfectant for toilets and as an anesthetic.

4-CRESOL • *See p*-Cresol.

o-**CRESYL ACETATE** • *See o*-Tolyl Acetate.

p-**CRESYL ACETATE** • *See p*-Tolyl Acetate.

CRETAN DITTANY • *See* Dittany of Crete.

CROCETIN • Yellow coloring from saffron *(see)*.

CROCUS EXTRACT • *See* Saffron.

CROSS-REACTIVITY • When the body mistakes one compound for another of similar chemical composition.

CROWN GUM • Catalyst. There is reported use of the chemical; it has not yet been assigned for toxicology literature.

CRUCIFEROUS VEGETABLES • A family of plants characterized by flowers and fruits that bear a cross in the center. The genus being studied intensively for health properties are the Brassica, which include brussels sprouts, cauliflower, and broccoli. These vegetables contain large quantities of some substances that have been shown to inhibit chemically induced cancers in animals.

CRUFOMATE • An antiworm insecticide from petroleum used on cattle, goats, and sheep. FDA residue tolerance is 1.0 ppm in meat, fat, and byproducts.

CRYOLITE (SODIUM ALUMINUM FLUORIDE) • A mineral used as an insecticide. The FDA tolerance on fruits and vegetables is 0.7 ppm.

CRYPTOXANTHIN • A natural yellow coloring from corn and marigolds. *See* Xanthophyll.

CRYSTALLINE FRUCTOSE • Used in baked goods, frozen foods, beverages, tabletop sweeteners. It has about 1 to 2 times the sweetness of sugar and has calories. *See* Fructose.

CUBEBS • *Piper Cubeba.* Tailed Pepper. Java Pepper. The mature, unripe, sun-dried fruit of a perennial vine grown in South Asia, Java, Sumatra, the Indies, and Sri Lanka. It has a strong, spicy odor and is used in fruit flavoring for beverages (800 ppm). The volatile oil is obtained by steam distillation from the fruit and is colorless to light green with a characteristic spicy odor and a slightly acrid taste. It is used in berry, fruit, and ginger flavorings for beverages, ice cream, ices, candy, baked goods, meats, and condiments. Java pepper was formerly used to stimulate healing of mucous membranes. The fruit has been used as a stimulant and diuretic and sometimes is smoked in cigarettes.

CUCUMBER JUICE • From the succulent fruit of the vine and used as an astringent by many "natural" cosmetic fans. It has a pleasant aroma and imparts a cool feeling to the skin. Nontoxic.

CUMALDEHYDE • *See* Cuminaldehyde.

CUMENEALDEHYDE • Colorless liquid with a floral odor used as a flavoring agent in various foods. Moderately toxic by ingestion. Narcotic in high doses.

CUMIN • Cummin. A natural flavoring obtained from the seeds of an Old World plant. Used in spice and sausage flavorings for baked goods (2,500 ppm), condiments (3,900 ppm), and meats. A *volatile oil,* light yellow to brown, with a strong, disagreeable odor, is distilled from the plant. It is used in berry, fruit, sausage, and spice flavorings for beverages, ice cream, ices, candy, chewing gum, baked goods, meats, pickles, and condiments. Moderately toxic by ingestion and skin contact. A skin irritant. May be mutagenic. GRAS.

CUMINAL • *See* Cuminaldehyde.

CUMINALDEHYDE • A constituent of eucalyptus, myrrh, cassia, cumin, and other essential oils, but often made synthetically. Colorless to yellowish, oily, with a strong, lasting odor. It is used as a synthetic flavoring in berry, fruit, and spice flavorings for beverages, ice cream, ices, candy, baked goods, chewing gum, and condiments. Used in perfumery. No known toxicity.

CUMINIC ALDEHYDE • *See* Cuminaldehyde.

CUPRIC ACETATE • The copper salts of acetic acid and copper *(see both).*

CUPRIC CHLORIDE • Copper Chloride. A copper salt used in hair dye. A yellow to brown water-absorbing powder that is soluble in diluted acids. Also used in pigments for glass and ceramics and as a feed additive, disinfectant, and wood preservative. Irritating to the skin and mucous membranes. Irritating when ingested, causing vomiting. *See* Copper.

CUPRIC OXIDE • *See* Copper.

CUPRIC SULFATE • Copper sulfate occurs in nature as hydrocyanite. Grayish white to greenish white crystals. Used as agricultural fungicide, herbicide, and in the preparation of azo dyes *(see).* Used in hair dyes as coloring. Very irritating if ingested. No known toxicity on the skin and is used medicinally as a skin fungicide. *See* Copper.

CUPROUS IODIDE • A source of dietary iodide. The final report to the FDA of the Select Committee on GRAS Substances stated in 1980 that it should continue its GRAS status with no limitations other than good manufacturing practices. *See* Iodine Sources.

CURACAO PEEL EXTRACT • A natural flavoring extracted from a plant native to the Caribbean island. Used in orange and liquor flavorings for beverages (1,700 ppm). GRAS.

CURACAO PEEL OIL • A natural flavoring extracted from a plant native to the Caribbean island. Used in berry, lime, and liquor flavorings for beverages, ice cream, ices, candy, and baked goods. No known toxicity.

CURCUMIN • Orange-yellow colorant derived from turmeric *(see)* and used as a natural food coloring. It does not require certification because it is a natural product, but the Expert Committee on Food Additives of the FDA recommended that the acceptable daily intake of curcumin (and turmeric) be limited to 0 to 0.5 milligrams per kilogram of body weight. Moderately toxic by injection. A skin irritant. The FAO-WHO Expert Committee on Food Additives, however, concluded in June 1998 that reproductive toxicity studies and more information concerning the solvents used in the manufacturing processes of this additive are needed for evaluation in 2001.

CURDLAN • Pureglucan. Received approval from the FDA. It is the first direct food additive completely developed and petitioned by a Japanese company. An enzyme that processes starch.

CURING AGENTS • These include salt, nitrites *(see),* and other compounds used to stabilize color, give flavor, and/or preserve.

CURRANT, BLACK, BUDS and LEAVES • *See* Currant Buds, Absolute.

CURRANT BUDS, ABSOLUTE • A natural flavoring from a variety of small raisins grown principally in Greece. Used in fruit, berry, and raspberry flavorings for beverages, ice cream, ices, candy, and baked goods. No known toxicity. There is reported use of the chemical; it has not yet been assigned for toxicology literature.

CUSPARIA BARK • Essential oil from the bark of Angostura used as a flavoring. *See* Angostura. GRAS.

CYANAMIDE • Water-absorbing crystals used as fumigant for uncooked bacon, cereal flours, cereals that are cooked before being eaten, cocoa, uncooked ham, and uncooked sausage. FDA residue tolerances are 125 ppm in cereal flours, 90 ppm in cereals that are cooked before being eaten, and 50 ppm in uncooked bacon, ham, and sausage, and 200 ppm in cocoa. Cyanide and its compounds are on the Community Right-To-Know List *(see).* Poison by ingestion, inhalation, and intraperitoneal route. Moderately toxic by skin contact. A severe eye irritant.

CYANIDE • Prussic Acid. Hydrocyanic Acid. An inorganic salt, it is one of the most rapid poisons known. Poisoning may occur when any compound releases cyanide. Cyanide is used as a fungistat, insecticide, and rodenticide and is in metal polishes, especially for silver, electroplating solutions, art materials, photographic processes, and metallurgy. It has been reported to reduce oxygen availability in the blood even in low doses.

CYANIDIN • Usually isolated from bananas or cherries, it is used as a coloring in foods. It has also been used to treat night blindness.

CYANO-, CYAN- • From the Greek *kaynos,* meaning a dark blue. The prefix is commonly used to signify compounds containing the cyanide group CN. If the cyanide is not released from the compound, its presence is presumed not harmful.

CYANO(4-FLURO-3-PHENOXYPHENYL)METHYL-3-(2,2-DICHLORO-ETHENYL)-2,2-DIMETHYL-PROPANECARBOXYLATE • An insecticide used in animal feed. *See* Cyanamide.

CYANO(3-PHENOXY PHENYL)-METHYL-4-CHLORO-ALPHA-(1-METHYL ETHYL)BENZENEACETATE • A pesticide used in apple pomace to be used in animal feeds up to 20 ppm. The tolerance is 10 ppm in tomato pomace in animal feed and 1.0 ppm in peanut hulls to be used in animal feeds.

CYANOCOBALAMIN • *See* Vitamin B_{12}.

CYANODITHIOIMIDOCARBONATE, DISODIUM • Bacteria-killing component in the processing of sugarcane. Many organic cyano compounds are decomposed in the body to yield highly toxic cyanide.

CYANOGENS • Substances in almonds, peach, and apricot pits that can cause headache and heart palpitations.

CYCLAMATES • Sodium and Calcium. Artificial sweetening agent about thirty times as sweet as refined sugar, removed from the food market on September 1,

1969, because they were found to cause bladder cancer in rats. At that time 175 million Americans were swallowing cyclamates in significant doses in many products ranging from chewing gum to soft drinks. There has been a concerted effort to bring cyclamates back to the market, but as of this writing, they have not been approved. The FDA's Cancer Assessment Committee's review of all the evidence reportedly indicates that neither cyclamate nor its major metabolic end product, cyclohexylamine, cause cancer.

CYCLAMEN ALDEHYDE • Colorless liquid with a strong floral odor used as a flavoring agent in various food products. Moderately toxic by ingestion. A human skin irritant. GRAS.

CYCLAMIC ACID • Fairly strong acid with a sweet taste. It is the acid from which cyclamates were derived *(see)*.

CYCLODEXTRINS • Enzymatically modified starches shaped like doughnuts. The cavity of the molecule repels water and organic compounds can fill the cavity. As a result, caffeine can be removed from tea and coffee, bitter components can be removed from citrus fruits, flavor oils can be extracted from onion, garlic, and other plants, and cyclodextrins can be recovered and reused. The FAO-WHO Expert Committee on Food Additives *(see)* evaluated the data on β-cyclodextrin. The members found that it is poorly absorbed in the upper gastrointestinal tract in humans and is largely utilized following breakdown by the microflora in the lower gut. A small proportion may be absorbed intact. A number of acute and short-term toxicity studies were reviewed that indicated low toxicity by the oral root. Despite its low toxicity, the Committee was concerned about its possible effect on fat absorbed nutrients and drugs. The experts set a temporary ADI *(see)* of 0–6 mg per kg of body weight and recommended further study of its effects on fat-absorbed nutrients. They also asked for more information on production methods. The FAO-WHO Expert Committee on Food Additives requested in June 1998 that a study of human tolerance be revived in 1999 "in order to confirm the absence of adverse gastrointestinal symptoms at normal levels of intake of gamma-cyclodextrin."

CYCLOHEXANE • Hexamethylene. A hydrocarbon *(see)* solvent widely used in industry in the manufacture of nylon, cellulose fats, oils, waxes, resins, paint and varnish removers, glass substitutes, and fungicides. Colorless liquid with a pungent odor. It is also used to dilute colors in food. Poison by intravenous route. Moderately toxic by ingestion. A systemic irritant by inhalation and ingestion. A skin irritant. May cause mutations.

CYCLOHEXANE ETHYL ACETATE • A synthetic fruit and honey flavoring for beverages, ice cream, ices, candy, and baked goods. *See* Cyclohexaneacetic Acid for toxicity.

CYCLOHEXANEACETIC ACID • A synthetic butter and fruit flavoring for beverages, ice cream, ices, candy, and baked goods. Cyclohexane in high concentrations may act as a narcotic and skin irritant.

CYCLOHEXYL ANTHRANILATE • A synthetic apple, banana, and grape flavoring for beverages, ice cream, ices, candy, baked goods, and gelatin desserts. Some cyclohexyl compounds are irritating to the skin.

CYCLOHEXYL CINNAMATE • A synthetic apple, apricot, peach, and prune flavoring for beverages, ice cream, ices, candy, and baked goods. Some cyclohexyl compounds are irritating to the skin.

CYCLOHEXYL FORMATE • Formic Acid. A synthetic cherry flavoring for beverages, ice cream, ices, candy, and baked goods. Some cyclohexyl compounds are irritating to the skin.

CYCLOHEXYL ISOVALERATE • A synthetic strawberry and apple flavoring for beverages, ice cream, ices, candy, and baked goods. Some cyclohexyl compounds are irritating to the skin.

CYCLOHEXYL PROPIONATE • A synthetic fruit flavoring for beverages, ice cream, ices, candy, and baked goods. Some cyclohexyl compounds are irritating to the skin.

CYCLOPENADECANOLIDE • *See* Pentadecalactone.

CYFLUTHRIN • An insecticide used on cattle, goats, hogs, and sheep. The FDA residues in meat are 0.05 ppm. Residues in milk 0.1 ppm.

CYHEXATIN • An insecticide used in animal feed. FDA residue in apple pomace and citrus pulp is 8 ppm.

*o***-CYMEN-3-OL** • *See p*-Cymene.

*p***-CYMENE** • A synthetic flavoring, a volatile hydrocarbon solvent that occurs naturally in star anise, coriander, cumin, mace oil, oil of mandarin, and origanum oil. Used in fragrances, also in citrus and spice flavorings for beverages, ice cream, candies, and baked goods. Its ingestion pure may cause a burning sensation in the mouth, nausea, salivation, headache, giddiness, vertigo, confusion, and coma. Contact with the pure liquid may cause blisters of the skin and inflammation of mucous membranes.

CYMOL • *See p*-Cymene.

CYMOPHENOL • *See* Carvacrol.

CYNARON • *See* Acimeton.

CYROMAZINE • A pesticide used in poultry feed. The FDA tolerance residue in fat, meat, and meat byproducts of poultry are 0.05 ppm; as residue in eggs, 0.25 ppm.

CYSTEINE • L-Form. An essential amino acid *(see)*, it is derived from hair and used in hair products and creams. Soluble in water, it is used in bakery products as a nutrient. It has been used to promote wound healing. On the list of FDA additives to be studied. As of this writing, no new evaluation has been made public. GRAS.

CYSTINE • A nonessential amino acid *(see)* found in urine and in horsehair. Colorless, practically odorless, white crystals, it is used as a nutrient supplement and in emollients. On the FDA list for further study. May have reproductive effects. As of this writing, no new evaluation has been made public. GRAS.

D

2,4-D. (2,4-DICHLOROPHENOXY) ACETIC ACID • Prepared from phenol and chloroacetic acid, it is an herbicide that belongs to the same class as dioxin *(see)* and is widely used by home gardeners and farmers. The FDA permits it in milled fractions (except flour) derived from barley, oats, rye, and wheat to be ingested as food or converted into food or feed as a residue. The FDA tolerances for residues are 2 ppm in milled fractions, 1 ppm in potable water in western United States, and 5 ppm in processed feeds using sugarcane bagasse or molasses. 2,4-D does not cause acute toxicity, but its long-term effects are a matter of controversy and it has been linked to cancer. An excess of non-Hodgkin's lymphoma among farmers has been strongly associated with its use. It does cause eye irritation and gastrointestinal upsets.

DAILY VALUE (DV) • Substituted for the percentage of U.S. Recommended Dietary Allowances *(see)*. It is a guideline based on the daily needs of the general population. The percentages are supposed to help you compare the nutrients in a particular food with dietary recommendations that help reduce risk for some chronic diseases.

DAIRY-LO • A fat replacer containing whey protein concentrate *(see)*. It can be used in other foods including reduced-fat versions of butter, sour cream, cheese, yogurt, salad dressing, margarine, mayonnaise, and baked goods, coffee creamers, soups, and sauces. GRAS.

DALAPON • 2,2-Dichloropropanoic Acid. Used as a herbicide in citrus pulp for cattle feed. FDA tolerance is 20 ppm.

DAMIANA LEAVES • The dried leaves of a California and Texas plant used as a flavoring. Formerly used as a tonic and aphrodisiac. Now used as a flavoring. There is reported use of the chemical; it has not yet been assigned for toxicology literature.

DAMINOZIDE • Alar. Butanedioic Acid Mono (2,2-dimethyl hydrazide). An apple growth regulator was a particular focus of alarm in 1988–89 when its residues were reported to be hazardous to children. The FDA residue tolerances were 10 ppm in dried tomato pomace, 90 ppm in residues of peanut meal (both for animal feed), 0.2 ppm in fat, meat, or meat byproducts of cattle, goats, hogs, poultry, and sheep, 0.02 ppm residues in milk, 0.2 ppm as residues in eggs, 20.0 as residues in apples, and 30.0 as residues in cherries, nectarines, and peaches. Probable human carcinogen. Causes multiple tumors in animals. Diaminozide was removed from the market in 1989 and is now permitted for use only on flowerbeds.

DAMMAR • Resin used to produce a gloss and adhesion in nail lacquer. It is a yellowish white, semitransparent exudate from a plant grown in the East Indies and the Philippines. Comes in varying degrees of hardness. It has a bitter taste. Also used for preserving animal and vegetable specimens for science laboratories. May cause allergic contact dermatitis.

DANDELION LEAF and ROOT • Lion's Tooth. Used as a skin-refreshing bath additive. Obtained from *Taraxacum* plants that grow abundantly in the United States. The Indians used the common dandelion weed, eaten as a salad green, for heartburn. Rich in vitamins A and C, it is also used as a flavoring. Dandelion coffee is made from the dried roots of the plant. The *root extract* is used in bitters, butter, caramel, floral, fruit, root beer, and vanilla flavorings for beverages, ice cream, ices, candy, and baked goods. The *fluid extract* is used in butter, caramel, fruit, maple, and vanilla flavorings for beverages, ice cream, ices, candy, and baked goods. GRAS. There is reported use of the chemical; it has not yet been assigned for toxicology literature.

DAUCUS CAROTA • *See* Carrot Oil.

DAVANA OIL • A plant extract used in fruit flavoring for beverages, ice cream, ices, candy, baked goods, and chewing gum. There is reported use of the chemical; it has not yet been assigned for toxicology literature.

DDE • Dichlorodiphenyldichlorethylene. It is a degradation product of DDT found as an impurity in DDT residues. It is believed to be an estrogen disrupter and is being studied by an EPA expert committee.

DDM • Dialkyl Dihexadecyl Malonate. A fat-based substance that is not absorbed into the body and can be used for frying and baking. It is not yet on the market as of this writing.

DDVP • *See* Dichlorvos.

o-DECALACTONE • A synthetic flavoring agent. Occurs naturally in butter, cream, and milk. Colorless with a fruity odor. Used in coconut and fruit flavorings for beverages, ice cream, ices, candy, baked goods, oleomargarine (10 ppm), and toppings.

γ-DECALACTONE • A synthetic flavoring agent, colorless, with a fruity odor, used in citrus, orange, coconut, and fruit flavorings for beverages, ice cream, ices, candy, baked goods, and gelatin desserts.

DECANAL • A synthetic flavoring agent. Occurs naturally in sweet orange peel, sweet mandarin oil, grapefruit oil, orris, and coriander. Colorless to light yellow, with a definite fatlike odor that becomes floral-like when diluted. Used in berry, citrus, lemon, orange, fruit, and honey flavorings for beverages, ice cream, ices, candy, baked goods, chewing gum, and gelatin desserts. Moderately toxic by ingestion. A severe skin irritant. GRAS.

DECANAL DIMETHYL ACETAL • A synthetic flavoring agent. Occurs naturally in anise, butter acid, oil of lemon, and oil of lime. Used in butter, coconut, fruit, liquor, whiskey, and cheese flavorings for beverages, ice cream, ices, candy, baked goods, chewing gum, and gelatin desserts. No known toxicity. GRAS.

DECANOIC ACID • A synthetic flavoring agent that occurs naturally in anise, butter acids, oil of lemon, and oil of lime and is used to flavor butter, coconut, fruit, liquor, and cheese flavorings for beverages, ice cream, ices, candy, baked goods, chewing gum, gelatin desserts, puddings, and shortenings. Also used for coating fruits and vegetables and in defoaming agents and fatty acids. Poisonous by intravenous route. A skin irritant. May be mutagenic.

1-DECANOL • A synthetic fatty acid flavoring agent. Occurs naturally in orange and ambrette seed. Used in butter, lemon, orange, coconut, and fruit flavorings for beverages, ice cream, ices, candy, baked goods, and chewing gum.

DECANYL ACETATE • *See* Decyl Acetate.

2-DECENAL • A synthetic fruit flavoring for beverages, ice cream, ices, candy, and baked goods. Moderately toxic by skin contact and mildly toxic by ingestion. A severe skin irritant.

DECENALDEHYDE • *See* 2-Decenal.

DECOQUINATE • Decox. An animal antifungal drug used in beef, chicken, and goat. FDA residues are 2 ppm in uncooked edible tissues other than muscle and 1 ppm in skeletal muscle of chickens, cattle, and goats.

DECYL ACETATE • A synthetic berry, orange, apple, peach, plum, and honey flavoring agent for beverages, ice cream, ices, candy, baked goods, and chewing gum. No known toxicity.

DECYL ALCOHOL • A synthetic fatty acid. An intermediate *(see)* for surface-active agents, an antifoam agent, and a fixative in perfumes. Occurs naturally in sweet orange and ambrette seed. Derived commercially from liquid paraffin wax *(see)*. Colorless to light yellow liquid. Used also for synthetic lubricants and as a synthetic fruit flavoring. Moderately toxic by skin contact. Mildly toxic by ingestion, inhalation, and possibly other routes. Has caused tumors in animals. A severe human skin and eye irritant.

DECYL BENZENE SODIUM SULFONATE • Defoaming agent and dispersing aid used on fresh citrus fruit. Poison by intravenous route. Moderately toxic by ingestion. A severe eye irritant.

DECYL BUTYRATE • A synthetic citrus and fruit flavoring agent for beverages, ice cream, ices, candy, and baked goods. No known toxicity.

DECYL PROPIONATE • A synthetic citrus and fruit flavoring agent for beverages, ice cream, ices, candy, and baked goods. No known toxicity.

DECYLIC ACID • *See* Decanoic Acid.

DECYLIC ALCOHOL • *See* 1-Decanol.

DEER'S TONGUE • Liatris wild vanilla. Vanilla plant. The extract of *Trilisa odoratissima* found from Virginia to Florida and Louisiana. Contains the volatile oil coumarin *(see)*. Used in perfumery and to make tobacco smell better. Once was on the GRAS list but removed because of coumarin.

DEFATTED • Meaning the fat has been partly or totally removed from a product. If partly removed there is no minimum percentage set by the FDA.

DEFATTED COTTONSEED OIL • From cottonseed flour *(see)* with the fat removed.

DEFOAMING AGENT • Antifoamer. Foam Inhibitor. Any number of surface-active agents *(see)*, such as liquid glycerides *(see)*, which are used to control the amount of foam produced in the processing of baked goods, coffee, whiteners, candies, milk products, jams, jellies, and fruit juices. They remove the head from processed drinks, such as orange and pineapple juice. Among the defoamers used are dimethylpolysiloxane, polyoxyethylene 40 monostearate, polysorbate 60, propylene glycol alginate, silicon dioxide, sorbitan monostearate, aluminum stearate, butyl stearate, fatty acids, hydroxylated lecithin, isopropyl alcohol, magnesium stearate, mineral oil, petrolatum, petroleum waxes, polyethylene glycol, polysorbate 80, potassium stearate, hydrogenated tallow alcohol, sodium poly-acrylate, synthetic petroleum wax, oleic acid from tall oil and fatty acids.

DEHYDRATED • With the water removed.

DEHYDRATED BEETS • Used for coloring and flavoring.

DEHYDROACETIC ACID • DHA. Sodium Dehydroacetate. A weak acid that forms a white, odorless powder with an acrid taste. Used as a preservative in cut or peeled squash. Used as an antienzyme agent in toothpaste to prevent tooth decay and as a preservative for shampoos. Also used as a fungi and bacteria-destroying agent in cosmetics. The presence of organic matter decreases its effectiveness. Not irritating or allergy causing, but it is a kidney-blocking agent and can cause impaired kidney function. Large doses can cause vomiting, imbalance, and convulsions.

DELANEY AMENDMENT • Written by Congressman James Delaney, the amendment was part of the 1958 law requested by the Food and Drug Administration. The law stated that food and chemical manufacturers had to test additives before they were put on the market and the results had to be submitted to the FDA. Delaney's amendment specifically states that no additive may be permitted in any amount if tests show that it produces cancer when fed to man or animals or other appropriate tests. Ever since it was enacted, the food and chemical industries have tried to get it repealed. Efforts have been made to substitute a negligible-risk standard to processed food. Up until 1996, the EPA observed different safety standards for raw and processed foods. For the latter, it used the zero-risk standard established by the Delaney clause. That standard, however, had proved to be impractical and even counterproductive, according to the EPA and manufacturers. It prohibited foods from carrying minute traces of carcinogenic compounds, while exempting many toxic chemicals that were registered before the clause was enacted. As a result, regulators were forced to allow the use of toxic chemicals while barring safer alternatives. Congress repealed the Delaney clause in the Food Quality Protection Act of 1996 for pesticides substituting the negligible-risk standard that had long been used to set tolerances for raw foods. This standard allows residues of potentially carcinogenic pesticides as long as there is a "reasonable certainty of no harm" to consumers. In practice, regulators will approve a pesticide application only if it will cause no more than one additional cancer case per million people who consume it over a lifetime. Some coal tar colors, nitrites, and nitrates that are considered cancer-causing agents are permitted in foods.

DELAYED HYPERSENSITIVITY • Manifested primarily as contact dermatitis due to chemicals such as neomycin sulfate or to parabens *(see both)*, a common preservative in food products. Certain multiple allergic reactions to chemicals added to food, directly or indirectly, may also cause delayed hypersensitivity, especially the antibiotics.

DELTAMETHRIN • A pesticide that contains cyanide used for tomato products. The FDA permits a residue of 1 ppm.

DEMETON-S • An organophosphate *(see)* pesticide used in animal feed. FDA residue limits of 5 ppm in dehydrated sugar beet pulp when used for animal feed. Poison by ingestion and other routes.

DEMULCENT • A soothing, usually thick, oily or creamy substance used to relieve pain in inflamed or irritated mucous surfaces. The gum acacia, for instance, is used as a demulcent.

DENATURANT • A substance that changes another substance's natural qualities or characteristics. For example, denatonium benzoate is added to the alcoholic content in cosmetics to make it undrinkable.

DERMATITIS • Inflammation of the skin.

DESOXYCHOLIC ACID • An emulsifying agent, white, crystalline, powdered, almost insoluble in water. Used in dried egg whites up to 0.1 percent. No known toxicity. The final report to the FDA of the Select Committee on GRAS Substances stated in 1980 that it should continue its GRAS status with no limitations other than good manufacturing practices. Moderately toxic by ingestion. Has caused tumors in animals.

DEXTRAN • A term applied to polysaccharides produced by bacteria growing on sugar. Used as a foam stabilizer for beer, in soft-center confections, and as a substitute for barley malt. It has also been used as a plasma expander for emergency treatment of shock. Has caused cancer in rats. The final report to the FDA of the Select Committee on GRAS Substances stated in 1980 that there is no evidence in the available information that it is a hazard to the public when used as it is now and it should continue its GRAS status with limitations on amounts that can be added to food.

DEXTRIN • British Gum. Starch Gum. White or yellow powder produced from starch and used as a foam stabilizer for beer, a diluting agent for dry extracts and pills, in polishing cereals, for preparing emulsions and dry bandages, for thickening industrial dye pastes, and in matches, fireworks, and explosives. Also used as a thickener in cream and liquid cosmetics. May cause an allergic reaction. The final report to the FDA of the Select Committee on GRAS Substances stated in 1980 that it should continue its GRAS status with no limitations other than good manufacturing practices.

DEXTROSE • The final report to the FDA of the Select Committee on GRAS Substances stated in 1980 that there is no evidence in the available information that it is a hazard to the public when used as it is now and it should continue its GRAS status with no limitations other than good manufacturing practices. *See* Corn Syrup.

DHC • *See* Dihydrochalcone.

DI-(BUTAN-3-ONE-YL) SULFIDE • Used in the manufacture of flavorings.

1,2(DI [1'-ETHOXY] ETHOXY) PROPANE • A gas. *See* Propane.

DI-(2-ETHYLHEXYL)ADIPATE • Light-colored, oily liquid used as a plasticizer, usually in processing polyvinyl and other polymers.

DI-(2-ETHYLHEXYL)PHTHALATE • A light-colored, odorless liquid used as a plasticizer for many resins.

DI-(2-ETHYLHEXYL)SODIUM SULFOSUCCINATE • White, waxy solid widely used as an emulsifier and as a processing aid. Used in beverage mixes, cocoa, eggs, fruit juice drinks, gelatin desserts, hog carcasses, milk, molasses, and poultry. FDA limits from 9 ppm in finished foods to 25 ppm in molasses.

DI-N-ALKYL (C8-C18 FROM COCONUT OIL) DIMETHYL AMMONIUM-CHLORIDE • Pesticide. FDA tolerance 5 percent by weight.

DIACETIN • A mixture of the diesters *(see)* of glycerin *(see)* and acetic acid *(see)*, used as a plasticizer, softening agent, or as a solvent for cellulose derivatives, resins, and shellacs. No known toxicity.

DIACETYL • Occurs naturally in cheese, cocoa, pears, coffee, raspberries, strawberries, and cooked chicken, but is usually prepared by a special fermentation of glucose. It is a yellowish green liquid. Also used as a carrier of aroma of butter, vinegar, and coffee. Also used in blueberry, raspberry, strawberry, butter, buttermilk, butterscotch, caramel, chocolate, coffee, fruit, cheese, cherry, liquor, rum, wine, nut, almond, spice, ginger ale, vanilla, and cream soda flavorings for beverages, ice cream, ices, candy, baked goods, gelatin desserts, chewing gum, and shortening. Cleared by U.S. Department of Agriculture (Meat Inspection Division) to flavor oleomargarine in "amount sufficient for the purpose." Diacetyl compounds have been associated with cancer when ingested by experimental animals. GRAS.

DIACETYL TARTARIC OF MONOGLYCERIDES and DIGLYCERIDES • An emulsifying agent used to improve volume and uniformity in bakery products up to 20 percent by weight of the combination such as preparation and the shortening. The final report to the FDA of the Select Committee on GRAS Substances stated in 1980 that it should continue its GRAS status with no limitations other than good manufacturing practices.

DIALKANOLAMIDE • A combination of methyl laurate and diethanolamine *(see both)* used to wash sugar beets prior to slicing operation. *See* Diethanolamine for potential cancer hazard.

DIALIFOR • Torak. An insecticide used in animal feed, apple pomace, dried citrus pulp, dried grape pomace, raisin waste, and raisins. FDA allows tolerances of up to 2 ppm in raisins, 40 ppm in dried apple pomace, 20 ppm in dried grape pomace, 115 ppm in dried citrus pulp, and 10 ppm in raisin waste when used for animal feed. Poison by ingestion and skin contact. Had adverse reproductive effects in experimental animals.

DIALLYL POLYSULFIDES • Used in the manufacture of flavors.

DIALLYL TRISULFIDES • Used in the manufacture of flavors.

2,4-DIAMINO-5 (6-METHYLVERATRYL) PYRIMIDINE • A feed additive. *See* Ormetoprim.

DIAMMONIUM PHOSPHATE • Used in animal feed as a source of non-protein nitrogen and phosphorous for ruminants.

1,4-DIANILINOANTHRAQUINONE • *See* Coal Tar.

DIASMOL • *See* 1,3-Nonanediol Acetate (mixed esters).

DIATASE • A mixture of enzymes from malt. It converts at least fifty times its weight of potato starch into sugars in thirty minutes. Used to convert starch into sugar. In 1992 diastase and diastase malt aluminum hydroxide were not shown to be safe and effective as claimed in OTC digestive-aid products.

DIATOMACEOUS EARTH • Kieselguhr. A porous and relatively pure form of silica formed from fossil remains of diatoms—one-celled algae with shells. Inert when ingested. Used in dentifrices, as a clarifying agent, and as an absorbent for liquids because it can absorb about four times its weight in water. Used as a buffer for acid-proofing food packaging and as an insecticide. Also used in nail polishes, face powders, as a clarifying agent, and as an absorbent for liquids. The dust can cause lung damage after long exposure to high concentrations. Not recommended for use on teeth or skin because of its abrasiveness. The final report to the FDA of the Select Committee on GRAS Substances stated in 1980 that it should continue its GRAS status with no limitations other than good manufacturing practices.

DIAZIDE • Alfa-Tox. Liquid with a faint esterlike odor widely used as an insecticide in animal feed. FDA permits 1 percent to 2 percent in animal feed. Poison by ingestion, skin contact, and other routes, except for inhalation during which it is mildly toxic. Human systemic effects by ingestion include changes in movement, muscle weakness, and sweating. Caused birth defects in animals. It is a severe skin and eye irritant in humans and emits toxic fumes when heated.

DIAZINON • A pesticide used in feed-handling establishments for crack and spot treatment in building floors and walls.

DIAZO- • A compound containing two nitrogen atoms such as diazolidinyl urea *(see)*, one of the newer preservatives, or diazepam, a popular muscle relaxant.

DIAZOLIDINYL UREA • Oxymethurea. 1,3-Bis(hydroxymethyl) Urea. Crystals from alcohol, soluble in water. Used in the textile industry in cotton, as a pesticide, and in cosmetics as an antiseptic. May release formaldehyde *(see)*.

DIBENZYL ETHER • A synthetic fruit and spice flavoring agent for beverages, ice cream, ices, candy, baked goods, and chewing gum. The Flavor and Extract Manufacturers Association evaluated the safety of this additive. High-dose female rats had increased liver weights. A no-effect level was achieved at 196 mg/kg/day. In a 60 kg human (about 132 pounds), this would be equivalent to approximately 11.8 grams a day.

a,a-DIBROMO-a-CYANOACETAMIDE • DBNPA. An antimicrobial agent used in beets and sugarcane. FDA limits are up to 10 ppm and not less than 2 ppm based on weight of raw sugarcane or raw beets. Poison by ingestion. A severe skin and eye irritation. Cyanide and its compounds are on the Community Right-To-Know List.

2,2-DIBROMO-3-NITRILOPROPIONAMIDE • Preservative used alone for control of microorganisms in raw sugarcane and beet sugar mills (2–10 ppm).

4,4-DIBUTYL-y-BUTYROLACTONE • A synthetic butter, coconut, and nut flavoring agent for ice cream, ices, candy, and baked goods.

DIBUTYL SEBACATE • Sebacic Acid. A synthetic fruit flavoring usually obtained from castor oil and used for beverages, ice cream, and baked goods. Also used for sealing food packages. Used in fruit-fragrance cosmetics. Mildly toxic by ingestion. Oral doses in rats cause reproductive effects.

DIBUTYL SULFIDE • *See* Butyl Sulfide.

DIBUTYLENE TETRAFURFURAL • Derived from bran, rice hulls, or corn cobs, it is used in the manufacture of medicinals and as a solvent and flavoring in cosmetics and food. Toxic when absorbed by the skin. Irritating to the eye.

DICALCIUM PHOSPHATE • A nutrient. *See* Calcium.

DICAMBA • A herbicide in or on sugarcane molasses.

DICHLORODIFLUOROMETHANE • Colorless, odorless gas used to freeze foods by direct contact and for chilling cocktail glasses. Narcotic in high doses. In EPA Genetic Toxicology Program *(see)*.

3,4-DICHLORO-2,6-DIMETHYL-4-PYRIDINOL • *See* Clopidol.

DICHLOROETHANE • Colorless, clear liquid with a pleasant odor and sweet taste. A human poison by ingestion. FAO-WHO Committee found it causes birth defects and that it causes cancer in mice and rats when administered orally. The Committee expressed the opinion that 1,2-dichloroethane should not be used in food. *See* Ethylene Dichloride.

DICHLOROMETHANE • *See* Methylene Chloride.

DICHLOROPHENOXYACETIC ACID • A widely used herbicide on milled barley, oats, rye, wheat (except their milled flour fractions), and sugarcane. FDA residue limits are up to 5 ppm in sugarcane molasses, 2 ppm in milled fractions (except flour) in barley, oats, and wheat, and 0.1 ppm in potable water. Poison by ingestion and other routes. Moderately toxic by skin contact. A suspected human cancer-causing agent. Human systemic effects by ingestion include sleepiness, convulsions, coma, and nausea or vomiting. Can cause liver and kidney injury. A skin and severe eye irritant. Human mutagenic data. Experimental reproductive effects. When heated to decomposition it emits toxic fumes.

3-(3,4-DICHLOROPHENYL)-1,1-DIMETHYL UREA • Marmer. Telvar Diuron Weed Killer. Vonduron. A widely used herbicide employed on animal feed. FDA limitation of 4 ppm in dried citrus pulp when used for livestock feed. In EPA Genetic Toxicology Program *(see)*. Chlorophenol compounds are on the Community Right-To-Know List *(see)*. Caused tumors and birth defects in laboratory animals.

a,a-**DICHLOROPRIONIC ACID, SODIUM SALT** • *See* Dichloropropionic Acid.

DICHLOROPROPIONANILIDE • Propanil. Supernox. A herbicide used on animal feed, rice, rice bran, rice hulls, and rice polishings. FDA limitations are 10 ppm in rice bran, rice hulls, and rice polishings when used for animal feed. In EPA Genetic Toxicology Program *(see)*. Poison by ingestion. Mildly toxic by skin contact.

DICHLOROPROPIONIC ACID • Basinex. Crisapon. Revenge. Unipon. An herbicide used in animal feed, citrus pulp, and potable water. FDA residue allowances are 0.2 ppm in potable water and 20 ppm in citrus pulp used as animal feed. Moderately toxic by ingestion. Corrosive. A skin irritant.

DICHLORVOS • Dimethyl Dichlorovinyl Phosphate. Apavap. Chlorvinphos. DDVF. VPON. 2,2-Dichlorovinyl. An organophosphate *(see)* insecticide with contact and vapor action. It has been widely used for control of agricultural, industrial, and domestic pests since the 1950s. It is used in pet flea collars and flea sprays. DDVP is available in oil solutions, emulsifiable concentration, and aerosol formulations. Its topical (skin) application has been approved for beef and dairy cattle, goats, sheep, swine, and chickens to control fleas, flies, and mites. It is also used in tomato greenhouses and applied to mushrooms, lettuce, and radishes. Aerosols and strips are used domestically for control of ants, bedbugs, ticks, cockroaches, and other pests. Nerve gases used in wars include organophosphates. It is suspected of causing cancer and birth defects. Heat decomposition causes highly toxic fumes to be emitted. In the last edition of this dictionary, the EPA was moving to have the use of dichlorvos on food packaging banned because it poses "more than a negligible risk." It is in at least 350 products. As of this writing, the EPA says that currently dichlorvos is undergoing a special review "on grounds that exposure to individuals by this compound from registered uses may pose an unreasonable risk of cancer and an inadequate margin of safety for cholinesterase inhibition [central nervous system effects]. Affected persons may include the general population from consuming foods with residues of dichlorvos, applicators, agriculture workers entering treated areas, residents/occupants of treated areas, and persons exposed to pets treated with this compound. As a result of the special review, the EPA expects to issue a proposed determination to cancel its use. It may take years to get this pesticide off the market.

3,5-DICHOLO-2,6-DIMETHYL-4-PYRIDINOL • *See* Clopidol.

DICYCLOHEXYL DISULFIDE • *See* Sulfides.

DIESTER • A compound containing two ester groupings. An ester is formed from an alcohol and an acid by eliminating water and is usually employed in fragrant liquids for artificial fruit perfumes and flavors.

DIETARY FOOD SUPPLEMENT • Any food product to which enough vitamins and minerals have been added to furnish more than 50 percent of the recommended daily allowance in a single serving, according to the FDA. Such foods must, of course, have ingredients identified on the label.

DIETHANOLAMINE (DEA) • Colorless liquid or crystalline fatty acid from soybeans or coconut oils. It is used as a solvent, emulsifying agent, and detergent. Also employed in emollients for its softening properties and as a dispersing agent and humectant in other cosmetic products. It may be irritating to the skin and mucous membranes. FDA became aware of a National Toxicology Program (NTP) study showing an association between the topical application of diethanolamine and certain DEA-related ingredients and cancer in laboratory animals. For the DEA-related ingredients, the NTP study suggests that the cancer response is linked to possible residual levels of DEA. Although DEA itself may be used in few products, DEA-related ingredients such as oleamide DEA, lauramide DEA, cocamide DEA, are widely used as emulsifiers or foaming agents, generally at levels of 1 to 5 percent. The FDA is studying the problem and is going to consider legal options at this writing. *See* Ethanolamines.

DIETHYL ACETALDEHYDE • Ethyl Butyraldehyde. A flavoring agent used in many foods. Moderately toxic by ingestion. A skin irritant.

DIETHYL ACETIC ACID • Colorless, volatile liquid with a rancid odor used as a flavoring in a variety of foods. Moderately toxic by ingestion and skin contact.

DIETHYL ASPARTATE • The diester of ethyl alcohol and aspartic acid *(see both)*.

DIETHYL DICARBONATE • Viscous liquid with a fruity odor used as a fermentation inhibitor and fungicide. Prohibited in the United States but permitted in wine in other countries. Poison by ingestion.

DIETHYL GLUTAMATE • *See* Glutamate.

DIETHYL MALATE • Malic Acid. A synthetic apple and rum flavoring agent for beverages, ice cream, ices, candy, baked goods, gelatin, and puddings.

DIETHYL MALONATE • A synthetic berry, fruit, apple, grape, peach, and pear flavoring for beverages, ice cream, ices, candy, and baked goods.

DIETHYL PALMITOYL ASPARTATE • *See* Aspartic Acid.

DIETHYL-*o*-PHTHALATE • Clear, colorless liquid used as a plasticizer in packaging material. Moderately toxic by ingestion. Has caused adverse effects in experimental animals.

DIETHYL PYROCARBONATE (DEP) • A fermentation inhibitor in still wines, beer, and orange juice added before or during bottling at a level not to exceed 200 to 500 parts per million. DEP was widely used because it supposedly did its job of preserving and then decomposed within twenty-four hours. However, instead of disappearing, it reacted with the ammonia in beverages to form urethane, according to University of Stockholm researchers. They said that DEP caused urethane concentration of 0.1 to 0.2 milligrams per liter in orange juice and approximately 1 milligram per liter in white wine and beer. Since 1943 urethane has been identified as a cancer-causing agent. The FDA had not required listing of DEP on the label and therefore did not know how many beverages were actually treated with this additive. The FDA banned the use of DEP in 1976.

DIETHYL SEBACATE • Sebacic Acid. A synthetic butter, coconut, apple, melon, peach, and nut flavoring for beverages, ice cream, ices, candy, baked goods, chewing gum, and gelatin desserts. Mildly toxic by ingestion. A skin irritant.

DIETHYL SUCCINATE • A synthetic raspberry, butter, orange, and grape flavoring for beverages, ice cream, ices, candy, and baked goods. No known toxicity.

DIETHYL TARTRATE • *See* Tartaric Acid.

DIETHYLAMINOETHANOL • Colorless, water-absorbing liquid with the properties of ammonia and alcohol. Toxic by ingestion. Used to obtain fatty acid derivatives, as an emulsifying agent, and as a curing agent for resin.

0,0-DIETHYL S-2 (ETHYTHIO)ETHYL PHOSPHORODITHIOATE(DI-SYSTON) • A pesticide applied to crops. The FDA tolerance is 5 ppm alone or with demeton-s *(see)* in dehydrated sugar beet pulp or pineapple bran for livestock feed.

DIETHYLENE GLYCOL DISTEARATE • White, waxlike solid with a faint fatty odor. Used as an emulsifying agent for oils, solvents, and waxes, a lubricating agent for paper and cardboard, and as a thickening agent.

DIETHYLENETRIAMINE • Yellow liquid with an ammonia odor, strongly alkaline. Used as a solvent.

DIETHYLPYRAZINE • Derived from ethyl bromide or chloride, it is used as a corrosion inhibitor and insecticide.

DIETHYLSTILBESTEROL (DES) • Stilbestrol. A synthetic estrogen fed to cattle and poultry to fatten them. A proven carcinogen, hormonal in nature, according to the FDA, which has given top priority to the study of the safety of DES. The FDA stipulates a zero tolerance for the compound after a proper withdrawal period. In 1971, three Harvard scientists linked DES to a rare form of vaginal cancer in the daughters of women who had taken DES during pregnancy. An estimated 100,000 to 150,000 head of cattle containing residues of the hormone are apparently getting to market. The European Union has forbidden the use of DES in cattle.

2,5-DIETHYLTETRAHYDROFURAN • A solvent used in processing resins.

DIFLUBENZURON • An insecticide used on soybean crops. It is limited by the FDA to 0.5 ppm as a residue on soybean hulls for use in animal feeds.

DIFURURYL ETHER • Used in the manufacture of food additives.

DIGLYCERIDES • Emulsifiers. *See* Glycerides.

DIHYDROANETHOLE • *See p*-Propyl Anisole.

DIHYDROCARVEOL • A synthetic flavoring agent occurring naturally in black pepper. Colorless oily liquid with a spearmint odor, it is used in liquor, mint, spice, and caraway flavorings for beverages, ice cream, ices, candy, baked goods, and alcoholic beverages. A moderate skin and eye irritant.

DIHYDROCARVONE • Colorless liquid with a spearmintlike odor used as a flavoring agent in various foods. Moderately toxic when injected under the skin.

DIHYDROCHALCONES (DHC) • A new class of intensely sweet compounds—about fifteen hundred times sweeter than sugar—obtained by a simple chemical modification of naturally occurring bioflavonoids *(see)*. Hydrogenation *(see)* of naringin and neohesperidin (the predominant bitter constituents in grapefruit and Seville orange rind) provides the intensely sweet dihydrochalcones. DHCs are seemingly safe. There have not been any reports, thus far, of side effects in either multigenerational feeding studies or in long-term feeding trials. The disadvantage is that they cannot be easily reproduced in the laboratory so supplies are dependent upon natural sources. A more serious problem is that the intense, pleasant sweetness of DHCs is slow in onset, with considerable lingering taste, which renders them unsuitable for many food uses. Approval to use DHCs in toothpaste and chewing gum is pending. Food scientists are now trying to find derivatives and analogs of DHCs to overcome the slow onset and lingering factor in the natural compounds.

DIHYDROCHOLESTEROL • *See* Cholesterol.

DIHYDROCHOLESTERYL OCTYLDECAOATE • *See* Cholesterol and Octadecanoic Acid.

DIHYDROCOUMARIN • A synthetic flavoring agent occurring naturally in tonka bean, oil of lavender, and sweet clovers. Used in butter, caramel, coconut, floral, fruit, cherry, liquor, rum, nut, root beer, spice, cinnamon, vanilla, cream soda, and tonka bean flavorings for beverages, ice cream, ices, candy, baked goods, chewing gum, gelatin desserts, and puddings. Prolonged feeding has revealed a possible trend toward liver injury.

5,6-DIHYDROL-2-(2,6-XYLIDINO)-4H1, 3-THIAZINE • Bay. Xylazine. An animal drug used in meat. Poison by ingestion.

5,7-DIHYDRO-2-METHYLTHIENO(3,4-D)PYRIMIDINE • Derived from organic matter used in the manufacture of food additives.

2,3-DIHYDRO-3-OXO-BENZISOSULFONAZOLE • *See* Saccharin.

1,2-DIHYDROPRYRIDAZINE-3,6-DIONE • A pesticide used on potato chips. FDA residue tolerance is 160 ppm. Moderately toxic by ingestion. Can cause chronic liver damage and acute central nervous system effects. Being studied as a possible cancer-causing agent.

DIHYDROSTREPTOMYCIN • An antibiotic used in beef and milk. FDA tolerance is zero in uncooked edible tissues of calves and in milk. May cause birth defects in humans. May be a mutagen.

DIHYDROXYACETOPHENONE • Light, tan crystals that absorb ultraviolet light. It is used in plastics, dyes, fungicides, and plant-growth promoters.

DIIODOSALYCYLIC ACID • A dietary supplement for animals. GRAS. (*See* Salicylic Acid.)

DIISOBUTYL ADIPATE • Diba. Isobutyl Adipate. A plasticizer used in packaging materials. Mildly toxic by ingestion.

DIISOPROPANOLAMINE. DIPA • White crystalline solid that is used as an emulsifying agent for polishes, textile specialties, leather compounds, insecticides, cutting oils, and water paints. *See* Propyl Alcohol.

2,3-DIKETOBUTANE • *See* Diacetyl.

DILAURYL CITRATE • *See* Lauryl Alcohol and Citric Acid.

DILAURYL THIODIPROPIONATE • An antioxidant. White crystalline flakes with a sweet odor, in general food use to extend shelf life. In fat or oil up to .02 percent. The final report to the FDA of the Select Committee on GRAS Substances stated in 1980 that there is no evidence in the available information that it is a hazard to the public when used as it is now and it should continue its GRAS status with no limitations other than good manufacturing practices.

DILINOLEATE • Dimer Acid. Widely used as an emulsifier, it is derived from Linoleic Acid *(see)*.

DILINOLEIC ACID • *See* Linoleic Acid.

DILL • *Anethum graveolens*. A natural flavoring agent from a European herb bearing a seedlike fruit. Used in sausage and spice flavorings for baked goods (4,800 ppm), meats, and pickles (8,200 ppm). Also used in medicine. Can cause sensitivity to light. The final report to the FDA of the Select Committee on GRAS Substances stated in 1980 that it should continue its GRAS status with no limitations other than good manufacturing practices.

DILL OIL • The volatile oil obtained from the crushed, dried seeds or fruits of the herb. Slightly yellow, with a caraway odor and flavor. Used in strawberry, fruit, sausage, and dill flavorings for beverages, ice cream, ices, baked goods, gelatin desserts, chewing gum, meat, liquors, pickles, and condiments. The final report to the FDA of the Select Committee on GRAS Substances stated in 1980 that it should continue its GRAS status with no limitations other than good manufacturing practices. *See* Dill for toxicity.

DILLSEED • Indian Dill. The volatile oil from a variety of dill herbs. Obtained by steam distillation. Light yellow, with a harsh carawaylike odor. Used in rye flavorings for baked goods, condiments, and meats. The final report to the FDA of the Select Committee on GRAS Substances stated in 1980 that it should continue its GRAS status with no limitations other than good manufacturing practices.

DILUENT • Any component of a color additive mixture that is not of itself a color additive and has been intentionally mixed in to facilitate the uses of the mixture in coloring cosmetics or in coloring the human body, food, and drugs. The diluent may service another functional purpose in cosmetics, as, for example, emulsifying or stabilizing. Ethylcellulose is an example.

DIMETHICONE • *See* Dimethyl Polysiloxane.

DIMETHIPIN • A growth regulator in animals. The FDA permits residues of 0.02 ppm as residues in meat, meat byproducts, and fat of cattle, goats, hogs, and sheep. The tolerance for residue in and on cottonseed hulls used in animal feed is 0.7 ppm.

DIMETHOATE • A pesticide permitted at 5 ppm in dried citrus pulp for cattle feed. The tolerance for meat, fat, and meat byproducts of cattle as a residue is 0.01 ppm and 0.001 ppm in milk.

***m*-DIMETHOXYBENZENE** • Resorcinol. A synthetic fruit, nut, and vanilla flavoring for beverages, ice cream, ices, candy, and baked goods. Used on the skin as a bactericidal and fungicidal ointment. Has the same toxicity as phenol (extremely toxic), but causes more severe convulsions.

***p*-DIMETHOXYBENZENE** • A synthetic raspberry, fruit, nut, hazelnut, root beer, and vanilla flavoring agent for beverages, ice cream, ices, candy, and baked goods. *See* above for toxicity.

3,4-DIMETHOXYBENZENECARBONAL • *See* Veratraldehyde.

1,1-DIMETHOXYETHANE • *See* Ethylene Glycol.

2,6-DIMETHOXYPHENOL • *See* Phenol.

1-([2,5-DIMETHOXYPHENYL] AZO)-2-NAPHTHOL • A coloring used on oranges with an FDA limit of 2 ppm by weight calculated on the basis of the whole fruit. Causes cancer in animals and is under International Agency for Cancer Research review.

3-(DIMETHOXYPHOSPHINYLOXY) n-METHYL-cis-CROTONAMIDE • Apadrin. Bilobran. A reddish brown solid with a mild odor widely used as an insecticide in tomato products. The FDA tolerance is 2 ppm in concentrated tomato products. In the EPA Genetic Toxicology Program *(see)*. The EPA considers it extremely hazardous. It is poisonous by ingestion, inhalation, and skin contact.

1,4-DIMETHYL-4-ACETYL-1-CYCLOHEXENE • Prepared from acetylaldehyde and methanol *(see both)* it is used in processing food additives.

DIMETHYL BENZYL CARBINOL and CARBINYL • Flavoring agents used in various foods. Moderately toxic by ingestion. *See a,a*-Dimethylphenethyl Alcohol.

DIMETHYL DIALKYL AMMONIUM CHLORIDE • Used as a decoloring agent in the manufacture of sugar. *See* Quaternary Ammonium Compounds.

DIMETHYL-0-(1,2-DIBROMO-2,2-DICHLOROETHYL)PHOSPHATE • Widely used insecticide on various foods. Poison by ingestion and inhalation. Moderately toxic by skin injection. *See* Organophosphates.

DIMETHYL DICARBONATE • A fungicide used in wine to inhibit yeast growth. The FDA set the tolerance of residues at 200 ppm. In ready-to-drink teas, the tolerance is 250 ppm.

DIMETHYL DICHLOROVINYL PHOSPHATE • *See* Dichlorvos.

DIMETHYL ETHER RESORCINOL • A benzene derivative originally obtained from certain resins but now usually synthesized. *See* m-Dimethoxybenzene.

DIMETHYL ETHERPROTOCATECHUALDHYDE • *See* Verataldehyde.

2,6-DIMETHYL-5-HEPTENAL • A synthetic fruit flavoring for ice cream, ices, candy, baked goods, gelatin desserts, and chewing gum.

3,7-DIMETHYL-7-HYDROXYOCTANAL • *See* Hydroxycitronellal.

DIMETHYL KETONE • *See* Diacetyl.

0,0-DIMETHYL METHYLCARBAMOYLMETHYL PHOSPHORODITHIO-ATE • A widely used insecticide in animal feed, citrus pulp. FDA limits are 5 ppm in dried citrus pulp when used for animal feed. Poison by ingestion, skin contact, and other routes. May cause cancer and birth defects.

N′,N′-DIMETHYL-N-([METHYL CARBAMOYL] OXY)-1-METHYLTHIOOXA-MIMIDIC ACID • Widely used insecticide in animal feed, pineapple bran, and pineapples. Limitations of 6 ppm in pineapple bran when used for animal feed. Poison by ingestion and inhalation. Moderately toxic by skin contact. On the EPA Extremely Hazardous Substances List.

3,7-DIMETHYL-2,6-OCTADIENAL • Pale yellow liquid with a strong lemon odor used as a flavoring agent in baked goods, candy, and ice cream. Mildly toxic by ingestion. A human skin irritant. *See* Citral.

3,7-DIMETHYL-(E)-2,6-OCTADIEN-1-OL • *See* Geraniol.

3,7-DIMETHYL-1-OCTANOL • A synthetic flavoring, colorless, with a sweet roselike odor. Used in floral, rose, and fruit flavorings for beverages, ice cream, ices, candy, and baked goods.

2,6-DIMETHYL-1-OCTEN-8-OL • *See* Rhodinol.

DIMETHYL PHOSPHATE OF 3-HYDROZY-N-METHYL-CISCROTON-AMIDE • A pesticide. The FDA tolerance is 2 ppm in concentrated tomato products when present as a result of application of the insecticide to growing tomatoes.

DIMETHYL POLYSILOXANE • Dimethicone. Antifoam A. An antifoaming agent for use in processing foods in "amounts reasonably required to inhibit foaming." Used as a chewing-gum base, in molasses, soft drinks, sugar distillation, skimmed milk, wine fermentation, syrups, soups, rendered fats, and curing solutions. Not to exceed 10 ppm in nonalcoholic beverages. Zero tolerance in milk; 250 ppm in salt for cooking and in other foods, 10 ppm in foods ready for consumption. Used to combat flatulence. Very low toxicity.

DIMETHYL PYRAZINE • *See* Piperazine.

2,5-DIMETHYL PYRROLE • A colorless to yellow oily liquid that was used as a flavoring agent in various foods. GRAS. Although allowed as a food additive, there is no current reported use of the chemical, and, therefore, although toxicology information may be available, it is not being updated, according to the FDA.

DIMETHYL RESORCINOL • *See m-*Dimethoxybenzene.

DIMETHYL SUCCINATE • Succinic Acid. A synthetic fruit flavoring agent for beverages, ice cream, ices, candy, baked goods, and chewing gum.

DIMETHYL SULFATE • Sulfuric Acid. Dimethyl Ester. Colorless, oily liquid used as a methylating agent (to add methyl) in the manufacture of cosmetic dyes, perfumes, and flavorings. Methyl salicylate is an example *(see)*. Extremely hazardous, dimethyl sulfate has delayed lethal qualities. Liquid produces severe blistering, necrosis of the skin. Sufficient skin absorption can result in serious poisoning. Vapors hurt the eyes. Ingestion can cause paralysis, coma, prostration, kidney damage, and death.

DIMETHYL SULFIDE • *See* Methyl Sulfide.

2,4-DIMETHYLACETOPHENONE • Colorless liquid with the odor of mimosa, it is used as a synthetic grape, vanilla, and cream soda flavoring agent for beverages, ice cream, ices, candy, and baked goods, and liquor. It is also used in perfumery.

2,4-DIMETHYLBENZALDEHYDE • *See* Benzyl Acetate.

DIMETHYLAMINE • A gas with an ammonia odor derived from ammonia and methanol. It was used in the processing of food additives, pesticides, surfactants, and many other products. There is no reported use of the chemical and there is no toxicology information available.

3,4-DIMETHOXY-1-VINYLBENZENE • *See* Benzene and Vinyl.

2,3-DIMETHYLBENZOFURAN • *See* Furfural and Benzene.

DIMETHYLBENZYL ALCOHOL • A constituent of the essential oil from *Curcuma long* and related plants. It smells like menthol. It is used as a flavoring and scent.

a,a-DIMETHYLBENZYL ISOBUTYRATE • A synthetic fruit flavoring agent for beverages, ice cream, ices, candy, and baked goods.

0,0-DIMETHYL(O-3METHYL-4-METHYLTHIO-M-TOLYL)PHOSPHOROTHIONATE • A pesticide. The FDA tolerance for residue in meat of cattle is 0.05 ppm.

DIMETHYL-3-METHYL-4-NITROPHENYLPHOSPHOROTHIONATE • Accothion. A widely used insecticide on wheat gluten. FDA tolerance for residue is 30 ppm in wheat gluten. In the EPA Genetic Toxicology Program and on the EPA Extremely Hazardous List *(see both)*. Poisonous by ingestion. inhalation, and other routes. Moderately toxic by skin contact. Human systemic effects upon ingestion include overactivity, diarrhea, nausea, or vomiting, and shortness of breath.

a,a-DIMETHYLPHENYETHYL ACETATE • Acetic Acid. A colorless liquid with a floral-fruity odor. A synthetic cherry and honey flavoring agent for beverages, ice cream, ices, candy, and baked goods, and chewing gum.

0,0-DIMETHYL-0-(3,5,6-TRICHLORO-2-PYRIDYL)PHOSPHOROTHIOATE • *See* Chlorpyrifos.

1,1-DIMETHYL-3-(a,a,a-TRIFLUORO-m-TOLYL)UREA • Cottonex. Herbicide used in animal feed. FDA limit of 0.2 ppm in sugarcane when used for animal feed. In EPA Genetic Toxicology Program *(see)* and under review by the IARC *(see)*. Moderately toxic by ingestion. May be mutagenic.

DIMETHYLGLYOXAL • *See* Diacetyl.

DIMETHYLKETOL • *See* Acetoin.

DIMETHYLOCTADECYLBENZYLAMMONIUM CHLORIDE • Quaternol 1. Varisoft SDC. An antimicrobial agent used in beets, sugarcane, and raw sugarcane juice. FDA residues limits are 1.5–6 ppm and .05 ppm based on weight of raw sugarcane or raw beets. Moderately toxic by ingestion. A human skin irritant and severe eye irritant.

DIMETHYLOCTANOL • Pelargol. Colorless liquid with a sweet rose odor used as a flavoring agent in bakery products, beverages, chewing gum, confections, ice cream, and pickles. Moderately toxic by skin contact.

a,a-DIMETHYLPHENYETHYL ALCOHOL • A synthetic fruit flavoring agent for beverages, ice cream, ices, candy, chewing gum, jellies, gelatin desserts, and baked goods.

a,a-DIMETHYLPHENYETHYL BUTYRATE • Butyric Acid. A synthetic fruit flavoring agent for beverages, ice cream, ices, candy, and baked goods.

a,a-DIMETHYLPHENYETHYL FORMATE • Formic Acid. A synthetic spice flavoring agent for beverages, ice cream, ices, and candy.

DIMETHYLPYRAZINE • Flavoring agent with a nutty or potatolike taste and coffee odor used in various foods. Moderately toxic by ingestion and is an experimental mutagen. GRAS.

DIMETRIDAZOLE • A feed additive. Not legal for animal use.

3,5-DINITROBENZAMIDE • A feed additive that the FDA says is supposed to be zero in edible tissues and byproducts of chickens.

2,6-DINITRO-N,N-DIPROPYL-4-(TRIFLUOROMETHYL)BENZENEAMINE • Agreflan. Crisalin. Widely used herbicide on barley, carrots, peppermint oil, soybeans, spearmint oil, and wheat. Residue tolerance set by FDA is 2 ppm in peppermint oil and spearmint oil. EPA Genetic Toxicology Program. Community Right-To-Know List *(see both)*. Moderately toxic by ingestion. Caused cancer, tumors, and birth defects in experimental animals.

DINKUM OIL • *See* Eucalyptus Oil.

2,7-DINITROSOS-1-NAPHTHOL • Used in the manufacture of dyes. *See* Coal Tar.

2,4-DINTRO-6-OCTYLPHENYL CROTONATE+2,6-DINTRO-4-OCTYL-PHENYL CROTONATE • Fungicide on dried apple pomace as a result of application to growing apples as residue. FDA allows residue tolerance of 0.3 ppm. Derived from crotonic acid, which is obtained from crotonaldehyde, which is used in chemical warfare.

DI-n-BUTYL PHTHALATE • An insect repellent. Used for the impregnation of clothing. May cause estrogenlike effects in humans. One of the chemicals being studied by the EPA's expert committee on environmental estrogen disrupters.

DIOCTYL- • Containing two octyl groups. Octyl is obtained from octane, a liquid paraffin found in petroleum.

DIOCTYL ADIPATE • *See* Adipic Acid.

DIOCTYL DILINOLEATE • *See* Dilinoleic Acid.

DIOCTYL MALEATE • *See* Malic Acid.

DIOCTYL SODIUM SULFOSUCCINATE • Docusate Sodium. A waxlike solid that is very soluble in water. It is used as a dispersing and solubilizing agent in foods, drugs, and cosmetics. In foods and beverages it is used as a dispersing and solubilizing agent for gums, cocoa, and various hard-to-wet materials. Also a wetting agent in the cleaning of fruits, vegetables, and leafy plant material. Used in nonalcoholic beverages and sherbets at a rate not to exceed 0.5 percent of the weight of such ingredients. Finished cocoa beverages can have 75 ppm in the finished products. It is a stool softener in laxatives. Eye irritation may result from use in eye preparations.

DIOXATHION • A widely used pesticide in animal feed and dehydrated citrus pulp. Poisonous by ingestion. *See* Organophosphates.

DIOXIN • The commonly used name for TCDD. 2,3,7,8-tetrachlorodibenzo-*p*-dioxin. It is a halogenated aromatic hydrocarbon, and it causes mutagenic and carcinogenic changes in animals. It is a byproduct of agent orange (2,4-D and 2,4,5-T). It is the most toxic of chlorine-containing dioxin compounds. The long-term human consequences of exposure to this compound are controversial but it certainly would be wise to avoid exposure to it. It is a suspected cancer-causing agent. Research at the University of Maryland has shown that children exposed to dioxins and PCBs *(see)* prenatally or during infancy can suffer behavioral, memory, and learning problems. The Maryland investigators suggest that the underlying mechanism may be thyroid hormone disruption. Even moderate impairment of thyroid hormone function has been associated with various problems in behavior and intellectual development, and certain thyroid diseases are associated with attention deficit hyperactivity disorder and language disorders. Studies of adults exposed to dioxin and PCBs show no marked neurological effects. The Maryland research was funded by the University and by the American Thyroid Association. Being removed by NTP *(see)* as a human carcinogen.

DIOXYMETHYLENE PROTOCATECHUICALDEHYDE • *See* Piperonal.

DIPA • The abbreviation for Diisopropanolamine *(see)*.

DIPENTENE • *See* Limonene.

DIPHENYL ETHER • Colorless crystals with the odor of geranium. Used in perfumery. Toxic by inhalation. Also as an intermediate in processing.

DIPHENYLKETONE • *See* Benzophenone.

1,3-DIPHENYL-2-PROPANONE • A synthetic fruit, honey, and nut flavoring for beverages, ice cream, ices, candy, and baked goods.

DIPHENYLAMINE • Big Dipper. An insecticide used on various products. Poison by ingestion. Has caused birth defects in experimental animals.

DIPOTASSIUM EDTA • *See* Ethylenediamine Tetraacetic Acid (EDTA).

DIPOTASSIUM GLYCYRRHIZATE • The dipotassium salt of glycyrrhizic acid *(see)*.

DIPOTASSIUM PERSULFATE • White, odorless crystals used as a defoaming agent and a dispersing agent *(see both)* in fresh citrus fruit and in poultry. Moderately toxic and a skin irritant.

DIPOTASSIUM PHOSPHATE • A sequestrant. A white grain, very soluble in water. Used as a buffering agent to control the degree of acidity in solutions. It is used in the preparation of nondairy powdered coffee creams and in cheeses up to 3 percent by weight of cheese. It is used medicinally as a saline cathartic. No known toxicity. GRAS.

DIPROPYL DISULFIDE • A synthetic flavoring agent. Colorless, insoluble in water. Occurs naturally in onions. Used in imitation onion flavoring for pickle products and in baked goods. No known toxicity.

DIPROPYL KETONE • *See* 4-Heptanone.

DIPROPYL TRISULFIDE • *See* Sulfides.

DIQUAT DIBROMIDE • Yellow crystals used as an herbicide in animal feed, potable water, potato chips, potato wastes, and processed potatoes. FDA residue tolerance for it is 0.01 ppm in potable water, 0.5 ppm in processed potatoes including potato chips, and 1.0 ppm in dried potato wastes when used for animal feed. EPA Genetic Toxicology Program *(see)*. Poison by ingestion and other routes. Poisoning complications include vomiting, mucosal ulcers, diarrhea, and other intestinal tract problems. Heart damage and irregular beats occur in severe poisonings. Causes birth defects in experimental animals. A skin and eye irritant.

DISODIUM ADENOSINE TRIPHOSPHATE • A preservative derived from adenylic acid. *See* Adenosine Triphosphate.

DISODIUM CITRATE • White granular powder or crystals used as a buffer, nutrient for cultured buttermilk and as a sequestrant *(see)*. It is used in cured beef, carbonated beverages, nondairy creamers, cured meat products, margarine, evaporated milk, oleomargarine, and cured and fresh pork. FDA says it is not to exceed 500 ppm or 1.8 mg/square inch of surface. Moderately toxic if injected under the skin. *See also* Sodium Citrate.

DISODIUM CYANODITHIOMIDOCARBONATE • Bacteria-killing component in the processing of sugarcane. Any substance that releases the cyanide ion can cause poisoning. Sodium cyanide is one of the swiftest poisons known. The FDA residue tolerance is less than 2.9 ppm in raw cane or sugar beets.

DISODIUM EDTA • White, crystalline powder, soluble in water, used as a food preservative and sequestering agent. Promotes color retention in frozen white potatoes (100 ppm), canned potatoes (110 ppm), cooked chick peas (165 ppm), dried banana cereal (315 ppm), canned strawberry pie filling (500 ppm), gefilte fish (50 ppm), and salad dressing (75 ppm.) *See* Ethylenediamine Tetraacetic Acid (EDTA).

DISODIUM EDTA-COPPER • Cooper Versenate. Used as a sequestering agent. *See* Ethylene Tetraacetic Acid for toxicity.

DISODIUM ETHYLENE-1, 2-DISODIUM ETHYLENE-1, 2-BISDITHIO-CARBAMATE • Chem Bam. Spring-Bak. An antimicrobial agent used on beets and sugarcane. FDA limits use to 3 ppm based on weight of raw sugarcane or raw beets. EPA Genetic Toxicology Program *(see)*. Poison by ingestion. Caused birth defects and mutations in experimental animals.

DISODIUM GUANYLATE • A flavor intensifier believed to be more effective than sodium inosinate and sodium glutamate. It is the disodium salt of 5'-guanylic acid, widely distributed in nature as a precursor of RNA and DNA. Can be isolated from certain mushrooms and is used in canned vegetables. Changes in dietary purine intake over the past decade resulting from the use of guanylate and inosinate *(see)* as flavor enhancers are no greater than those due to variability in the consumption of major dietary contributors of purines. Exposure to purines is low—approximately 4 mg per person per day, according to the FAO-WHO Expert Committee on Food Additives. The Committee concluded that on the basis of available data, the combined total daily intake of disodium 5'-guanylate and disodium 5'-inosinate is not of toxicological significance. The Committee decided there was no reason to recommend that foods to which these substances have been added should be labeled and withdrew its previous recommendation for labeling. Persons suffering from gout or uric acid kidney stones should limit their dietary sources of purines *(see)*.

DISODIUM INDIGO-5,5-DISULFONATE • Blue No. 2. Acid Blue W. Blue-brown powder used as a color additive used on various products. EPA Genetic Toxicology Program *(see)*. Moderately toxic by ingestion. Caused tumors in experimental animals. *See* Colors.

DISODIUM 5'-INOSINATE • Flavor potentiator *(see)*, odorless and colorless, or white crystal or powder, with a characteristic taste. Used in canned vegetables. *See* Inosinate.

DISODIUM PHOSPHATE (DIBASIC) • A sequestrant *(see)* used in evaporated milk, up to 0.1 percent by weight of finished product; in macaroni and noodle products at not less than 0.5 percent nor more than 1 percent. It is used as an emulsifier up to 3 percent by weight in specified cheeses. Cleared by the U.S. Department of Agriculture's Meat Inspection department to prevent cooked-out juices in cured hams, pork shoulders, and loins, canned hams, chopped hams, and bacon (5 percent in the pickling and 5 percent injected into the product). Used as a buffer to adjust acidity in chocolate products, beverages, sauces, and toppings, and enriched farina. Incompatible with alkaloids. It is a mild saline cathartic and has been used in phosphorous-deficiency treatment. It may cause mild irritation to the skin and mucous membranes, and can cause purging. GRAS.

DISODIUM PYROPHOSPHATE • Sodium Pyrophosphate. An emulsifier and texturizer used to decrease the loss of fluid from a compound. It is GRAS for use in foods as a sequestrant. *See* Sodium Pyrophosphate.

DISODIUM SUCCINATE • *See* Succinic Acid and Sodium.

DISOYAMINE • *See* Soybean Oil.

DISPERSANT • A dispersing agent, such as polyphosphate, for promoting the formation and stabilization of a dispersion of one substance in another. An emulsion, for instance, would consist of a dispersed substance and the medium in which it is dispersed.

DISTARCH PHOSPHATE • A combination of starch and sodium metaphosphate. It is a water softener, sequestering agent, and texturizer. A modified starch once commonly used in baby foods. It is used in dandruff shampoos. The final report to the FDA of the Select Committee on GRAS Substances stated in 1980 that there is no evidence in the available information that it is a hazard to the public when used as it is now and it should continue its GRAS status with no limitations other than good manufacturing practices.

DISTARCH PROPANOL • A modified starch. The final report to the FDA of the Select Committee on GRAS Substances stated in 1980 that while there is no evidence in the available information that it demonstrates a hazard to the public at current use levels, uncertainties exist, requiring that additional studies be conducted. The FDA allowed GRAS status to continue while tests were being completed and evaluated. Since 1980, however, nothing new has been reported.

DISTEARYL THIODIPROPIONATE • Antioxidant used in packaging materials. FDA limits it to 0.005 percent migrating from food packages.

DISTILLATE • The volatile material recovered by condensing the vapors of an extract or fruits material that is heated to its boiling point in a still.

DISTILLED • The result of evaporation and subsequent condensation of a liquid, as when water is boiled and steam is condensed.

DISTILLED ACETYLATED MONOGLYCERIDES • Food emulsifiers and binders in nutrient capsules and tablets to make them palatable; also food-coating agents. Use is "at level not in excess of the amount reasonably required to produce the intended effect." Cleared by the USDA Meat Inspection Department as an emulsifier for shortening. No known toxicity.

DITTANY OF CRETE • *Origanum dictamnus*. A natural flavoring extracted from a small herb grown in Crete. Employed in spice flavorings for beverages and baked goods.

DIURON • A preemergent herbicide in dried citrus pulp used as animal feed as a result of application during growing. Repeated doses produce anemia in rats.

DNA (DEOXYRIBONUCLEIC ACID) • The complex substance that makes up genes. It contains the genetic information for all organisms.

o-DODECALACTONE • A synthetic flavoring. Occurs naturally in butter, cream, and milk. Used in butter, fruit, and pear flavorings for candy, baked goods, oleomargarine, and toppings. Not to exceed 20 ppm in oleomargarine.

y-DODECALACTONE • A synthetic flavoring, colorless, with a coconut odor that becomes butterlike in low concentrations. Used in butter, butterscotch, coconut, fruit, maple, and nut flavorings for beverages, ice cream, ices, candy, baked goods, gelatin desserts, puddings, and jellies.

1-DODECANAL • Lauryl Aldehyde. Found in pine needles, lime, orange, and other essential oils. It is colorless to light yellow with a fatty odor. It is used as a flavoring agent in various products. Mildly toxic by ingestion.

DODECANOIC ACID • *See* Lauric Acid.

DODECYL ALCOHOL • *See* Lauryl Alcohol.

DODECYL GALLATE • An antioxidant. The FAO-WHO Expert Committee on Food Additives found that it caused a reduction in spleen weight and pathological changes in the liver, kidney, and spleen in a 150-day study in rats in which the substance was administered by gavage. In addition the study with dodecyl gallate revealed a no-observed-effect level (NOEL) that was ten-fold lower than the dietary NOEL for propyl gallate *(see)*. The Committee decided that this additive was "unlikely to be carcinogenic or genotoxic" and therefore recommended a temporary acceptable daily intake (ADI) for this additive at 0–0.5 mg per kg of body weight. *See* Gallates.

a-(p-DODECYL PHENYL)-1,1-DIMETHYL UREA • A pesticide.

N-DODECYL SARCOSINE SODIUM SALT • Antifogging agent, antistatic agent used in packaging material. When heated to decomposition it emits toxic fumes.

DODECYLBENZENESULFONIC ACID • A detergent used to sanitize glass containers for holding milk. FDA permits a residue of less than 400 ppm in solution. May cause skin irritation. If swallowed will cause vomiting.

DOG GRASS EXTRACT • A natural flavoring extract used in maple flavoring for beverages, ice cream, ices, candy, and baked goods. Derives its name from the fact that it is eaten by sick dogs. GRAS. There is reported use of the chemical; it has not yet been assigned for toxicology literature.

DOPAMIINE • 3-Hydroxytyramine. An intermediate in tyrosine metabolism and the precursor of norepinephrine and epinephrine. It is a brain chemical that initiates movement.

DOWCO 179 • *See* Chlorpyrifos.

DRACO RUBIN EXTRACT • *See* Dragon's Blood Extract.

DRAGON'S BLOOD EXTRACT • *Daemonorops* spp. The resinous secretion of the fruit of trees grown in Sumatra, Borneo, and India. Almost odorless and tasteless and available in the form of red sticks, pieces, or cakes. Makes a bright crimson powder. Used in bitters flavoring for beverages. Also used to color lacquers and varnishes.

DRIED SORGHUM GRAIN SYRUP • A corn syrup substitute produced from the starch of sorghum grain. *See* Sorghum.

DRIED YEAST • A dietary source of folic acid. Used to enrich farina, cornmeal, corn grits, and bakery products. Dried yeast is cleared for use in food provided the total folic acid content of the yeast does not exceed .04 milligrams per gram of yeast. Nontoxic.

DRY ICE • *See* Carbon Dioxide.

DRY MILK, NONFAT • *See* Nonfat Dry Milk.

DRYING AGENTS • *See* Rosin.

DULCAMARA EXTRACT • Bitter Sweet Nightshade. Extract of the dried stems of *Solanum dulcamara*. Belonging to the family of the nightshades, it is used as a preservative. The ripe berries are used for pies and jams. The unripened berries are deadly. It is made into an ointment by herbalists to treat skin cancers and burns. It induces sweating. *See also* Horse Nettle.

DULCIN • A nonnutritive sweetener that as of this writing is not legal in food.

DULSE • A natural flavoring extract from red seaweed. Used as a food condiment. No known toxicity. GRAS.

DV • Abbreviation for Daily Value *(see)*.

DYSPEPSIA • Indigestion.

E

EARTH WAX • General name for Ozocerite, Ceresin, and Montan Waxes. *See* Waxes.

ECHINACEA • *Echinacea angustifolia.* Snakeroot. Stoneflower. Coneflower. The roots and leaves of this herb served as a medicine for the Plains Indians. Said by herbalists to be a natural antibiotic and immune enhancer. Contains an antiseptic volatile oil, glycosides *(see),* and phenol, which is also an antiseptic. It was widely used by Dr. Wooster Beach, who in the mid-1800s founded Eclectic medicine, a blending of homeopathic and North American herbalism. Echinacea has been found to increase the ability of white blood cells to fight, destroy, and digest toxic organisms that invade the body. It is taken to combat colds, infections, and inflammations. The herb produces a numbing sensation when held in the mouth for a few minutes.

E. COLI (ESCHERICHIA COLI) • A type of bacteria normally found in the gut of most animals including humans. Much of the work scientists have done using recombinant DNA *(see)* techniques has used *E. coli* as a carrier because it is well understood. Some types of this bacteria class have been causing food poisoning, some of it fatal. Factory farming and overuse of antibiotics are believed to be contributing to the problem of resistant and dangerous types of *E. coli.*

ECZEMA • Inflammation of the skin.

EDTA • *See* Ethylenediamine Tetraacetic Acid.

EFROTOMYCIN • An antibiotic to improve swine-feed efficiency.

EGG • Particularly associated with eczema in children. May also cause reactions ranging from hives to anaphylaxis. Eggs may also be found in root beer, soups, sausage, coffee, and in cosmetics.

EICOSAPENTAENOIC ACID (EPA) • Found in fish oil *(see),* it reduces production of thromboxane, a clotting agent, in the blood, thus making the platelets less "sticky."

ELAIDIC ACID • *See* Oleic Acid.

ELDER FLOWERS • *Sambucus canadensis.* A natural flavoring from the small white flowers of a shrub or small tree. Used in fruit, wine, and spice flavorings for beverages, ice cream, ices, candy, baked goods, and wine. The leaves and bark can cause nausea, vomiting, and diarrhea. GRAS. There is reported use of the chemical; it has not yet been assigned for toxicology literature.

ELDER TREE LEAVES • Flavoring for use in alcoholic beverages only. There is no reported use of the chemical and there is no toxicology information available. *See* Elder Flowers.

ELDERBERRY JUICE POWDER • Dried powder from the juice of the edible berry of a North American elder tree. Used for red coloring. Nontoxic.

ELECAMPANE RHIZOME and ROOTS • Flavoring in alcoholic beverages only. From a large, coarse European herb having yellow ray flowers. There is no reported use of the chemical and there is no toxicology information available.

ELEMI • A soft, yellowish fragrant plastic resin from several Asiatic and Philippine trees. Slightly soluble in water but readily soluble in alcohol. An oily resin derived from the tropical trees. The *gum* is used in fruit flavoring for beverages, ice cream, ices, candy, and baked goods. The oil is used in citrus, fruit, vermouth, and spice flavorings for beverages, ice cream, ices, candy, baked goods, and soups. Used for gloss and adhesion in nail lacquer and to scent soaps and colognes. The resins are used industrially for making varnishes and inks. There is reported use of the chemical; it has not yet been assigned for toxicology literature.

EMULSIFIERS • Widely used additives to stabilize a mixture and to ensure consistency. They make chocolate more mixable with milk and keep puddings from separating. One of the most widely used emulsifiers is lecithin *(see)* and another is polysorbate 60 *(see)*. Di- and mono-glycerides *(see both)* are also used in many products. Among common emulsifiers in cosmetics are stearic acid soaps such as potassium and sodium stearates.

EMULSIFYING OIL • Soluble Oil. An oil, which when mixed with water, produces a milky emulsion. Sodium sulfonate is an example.

EMULSIFYING WAX • Waxes that are treated so that they mix more easily.

EMULSION • What is formed when two or more nonmixable liquids are shaken so thoroughly together that the mixture appears to be homogenized. Most oils form emulsions with water.

ENANTHIC ACID • Used in peeling solutions for fruits and vegetables. *See* Heptanoic Acid.

ENDOSULFAN • Thiodan. Brown crystals made from methane and benzene, related to the long banned but still environmentally present pesticide DDT, Endosulfan is used as an insecticide on fruits and vegetables and on growing tea. It is used especially on tomatoes, carrots, lettuce, and spinach. FDA residue limit on dried tea is 24 ppm. It is toxic by ingestion, inhalation, and skin absorption. Emerging evidence indicates that this insecticide and other chemicals that imitate the human reproductive hormone, estrogen, may be associated with instances of breast cancer, although definite proof is lacking.

ENDOTHAL • Aquathol. Endothall. An herbicide in potable water. FDA residue tolerance is 0.2 ppm potable water. Poisonous by ingestion. Very irritating to skin, eyes, and mucous membranes. Causes diarrhea.

ENTERIC NERVOUS SYSTEM • Our digestive systems are also chemical factories. In the linings of the esophagus, stomach, small intestine, and colon are millions of nerve cells that send out stop-and-go messages to our brains. The components of this digestive control center are lumped under the title "the enteric (from the Greek *entera* meaning bowels) nervous system." Current thinking among a number of scientists is that there is a "brain" in the gut, independent from the brain encased in the skull and that the enteric nervous system may be able to learn and remember independently of the central nervous system.

ENZYMATICALLY HYDROLYZED PROTEIN • Enzymes are used to break down the protein in solution. The final report to the FDA of the Select Committee on GRAS Substances stated in 1980 that it should continue its GRAS status with no limitations other than good manufacturing practices.

ENZYME • Any of a unique class of proteins that catalyze a broad spectrum of biochemical reactions. Enzymes are formed in living cells. One enzyme can cause a chemical process that no other enzyme can do. Among the enzymes used in foods are *Aspergillus niger* and *Aspergillus oryzae* for bakery products and, for milk clotting, *Endothis parasitica* or *Bacillus cerus*. Enzymes are used to remove visceral mass in clam processing, in bakery products, for making cheese, for flavorings, and many other food processing purposes. A number are recognized as GRAS and others have not yet been evaluated by the FDA.

ENZYME-MODIFIED FATS • Light to medium tan liquid, paste, or powder with strong fatty acid odor and flavor. Produced by enzyme action of fats obtained from milk, refined beef fat, or steam-rendered chicken fat. Enzyme-modified milkfat may be prepared from milk, concentrated milk, dry whole milk, cream; concentrated creams, dry cream, butter, butter oil, dried butter, or dried milkfat. Enzyme-modified milkfat may also be prepared from optional dairy ingredients including skim milk, nonfat dry milk, and buttermilk as well as dried whey. Enzymes such as lipase, for example, are used to break down fats that are used in the manufacture of cheese and similar foods. This type of additive is also used as a flavoring. No known toxicity.

ENZYME-MODIFIED SOY PROTEIN • A foaming agent in soda water. No known toxicity.

ENZYMES, CARBOHYDRASE, and CELLULASE FROM *ASPERGILLUS NIGER* • For the removal of visceral mass in clam processing.

ENZYMES from *ASPERGILLUS ORYZAE* • Used for browning in baking products.

ENZYMES (FOR MILK CLOTTING) FROM *ENDOTHIS PARASITICA* or *BACILLUS CEREUS* • For use in preparation of standardized cheese or cheese products, except enzyme from *B. cereus,* which is not suitable for cheese.

ENZYMES FROM PLANT and ANIMAL SOURCES • The following are considered GRAS: bromelin, catalase, ficin, lipase, malt extract, pancreatic extract, pepsin, and trypsin *(see all)*.

EPA EXTREMELY HAZARDOUS LIST • A list of highly toxic chemicals cited by the Environmental Protection Agency.

EPHEDRA • *Ephedra gerardiana. E. trifurca. E. sinica. E. Ephedra equisetina. E. helvetica.* Ma Huang. Mormon Tea. There are about forty species of this herb mentioned in ancient scriptures of India, and it was used by the Chinese for more than five thousand years. The stems contain alkaloids *(see)* including ephedrine *(see)*. Herbalists use the herb to treat arthritis, asthma, emphysema, bronchitis, hay fever, and hives. The Food and Drug Administration proposed in 1997 to reduce risks associated with dietary supplement products containing ephedrine alkaloids by limiting amount in products and requiring labeling and marketing measures that give adequate warning and information to consumers. Ephedrine alkaloids are amphetaminelike compounds with potentially powerful stimulant effects on the nervous system and heart. Hundreds of consumer illnesses and injuries associated with the use of these products have been reported.

The proposal would not ban dietary supplements that contain ephedrine alkaloids. "Consumers should be aware that just because a product is labeled 'natural' or from an herbal source it is not guaranteed to be safe," said Dr. Michael Friedman, deputy commissioner of the FDA. "The effects of ephedrine alkaloids are potentially powerful ones. We urge people to talk to their doctors before using dietary supplements containing ephedrine alkaloids, and to always use them with caution."

Because ephedrine alkaloids are heart and nervous system stimulants, certain individuals including those with hypertension, heart conditions, and neurologic disorders, should avoid their use. Pregnant women, too, should avoid the use of dietary supplements with ephedrine alkaloids.

The proposal would prohibit the marketing of dietary supplements containing 8 mg or more of ephedrine alkaloids per serving. Labeling that recommends or suggests conditions of use that would result in an intake of 8 mg or more in a 6-hour period or a total daily intake of 24 mg or more also would not be allowed. The proposal would also require label statements instructing consumers not to use the product for more than seven days, and would not allow label claims for uses for which long-term intake would be necessary to achieve the purported effect. These safety measures are based on the fact that long-term intake of ephedrine alkaloids increases the likelihood of serious adverse events.

Another measure in the proposal would apply to products with claims that encourage short-term excessive intake to enhance the claimed effect, such as energy enhancement. Such products would be required to bear a labeling statement that "taking more than the recommended serving may result in heart attack, stroke, seizure or death." The proposal would also prohibit the use of other stimulant ingredients such as botanical sources of caffeine with ephedrine alkaloids because the combination increases the stimulant effects of ephedrine alkaloids and the chance of consumer injury.

Dietary supplement products containing ephedrine alkaloids are currently sold for a variety of purposes including weight loss, increased energy, and body-building. Since 1994 the agency has received and investigated more than eight hundred reports of adverse events associated with the use of these products. Reported adverse events range from episodes of high blood pressure, irregularities in heart rate, insomnia, nervousness, tremors, and headaches to seizures, heart attacks, strokes, and death. Most events occurred in young to middle aged, otherwise healthy adults using the products for weight control and increased energy. Ephedrine alkaloids in dietary supplements are usually derived from one of several species of herbs of the genus *Ephedra*, sometimes called Ma

Huang, Chinese ephedra, and epitonin. Other botanical sources include *Sida cordifolia.*

The proposed measures were developed based on the FDA's review of its adverse event reports, the scientific literature, and public comments reviewed by the agency, including comments generated by an October 1995 advisory working group public meeting and an August 1996 public meeting of the FDA's Food Advisory Committee. These experts suggested a number of steps the agency might take to reduce injuries associated with use of dietary supplements containing ephedrine alkaloids. *See also* Ephedrine.

EPHEDRINE • The alkaloid ephedrine is derived from the plant *Ephedra equisetina* and others of the forty species of ephedra or produced synthetically. Ephedra has been used for more than five thousand years in Chinese medicine and has become more and more popular in Western medicine. It acts like epinephrine *(see)* and is used as a bronchodilator, nasal decongestant, to raise blood pressure, and topically to constrict blood vessels. *See also* Ephedra.

EPICHLOROHYDRIN • A colorless liquid with an odor resembling chloroform. It is soluble in water but mixes readily with alcohol and ether. A modifier for food starches that the FDA permits to be used up to level of 0.3 percent in starch. Used as a solvent for cosmetic resins and nitrocellulose *(see)* and in the manufacture of varnishes, lacquers, and cements for celluloid articles. A strong skin irritant and sensitizer. Daily administration of one milligram per kilogram of body weight to skin killed all of a group of rats in four days, indicating a cumulative potential. Chronic exposure is known to cause kidney damage. There may be fifty thousand workers exposed to epichlorohydrin, according to OSHA. A two-year study of workers who had been exposed to the substance for six months or more before January 1966 showed an increase in the incidence of cancer. Chronic exposure is known to cause kidney damage in humans. Germany regulates it as a known carcinogen. FDA residue tolerances are less than 0.1 percent with propylene and less than 5 ppm in food starch modified. There is no reported use of the chemical and there is no toxicology information available.

EPIGALLOCATECHIN GALLATE (EGCG) • A compound found in green tea that reportedly provides stronger damage protection of cells and their genetic material than vitamins E and C.

EPINEPHRINE • Adrenaline. The major hormone of the adrenal gland which increases heart rate and contractions, vasoconstriction or vasodilation, relaxation of the muscles in the lungs and intestinal smooth muscles, and the processing of sugar and fat.

EPOXY • Chemical term describing an oxygen atom bound to two linked carbon atoms. They are important chemical intermediates and the basis of epoxy resins *(see)*.

1,8-EPOXY-*p*-MENTHANE • *See* Eucalyptol.

EPOXY RESINS • The versatile epoxy resins are used widely in manufacturing for adhesive purposes and as films and durable coatings. When epoxy resins are used, the resin is combined with a curing agent. As the mixture "cures" it becomes hard. Epoxies are one of the most common causes of occupational health complaints. The Hazard Evaluation System and Information Service of California, for example, cites frequent effects of overexposure to the chemicals used in epoxy resins as eye, nose, throat, and skin irritations, allergies and asthma. Hardened epoxy products are practically nontoxic unless they are cut, sanded, or burned.

EXPOXIDIZED SOYBEAN OIL • Used as a stabilizer not to exceed one percent in brominated soybean oil.

EQUISETIC ACID • *See* Aconitic Acid.

ERGOCALCIFEROL • Vitamin D_2.

ERIGERON CANADENSIS • *See* Erigeron Oil.

ERIGERON OIL • *Erigeron canadensis.* Horseweed. Fleabane Oil. Derived from the leaves and tops of a plant grown in the northern and central United States. Used in fruit and spice flavorings for beverages, ice cream, ices, candy, baked goods, and sauces. There is no reported use of the chemical and there is no toxicology information available.

ERIODICTYON CALIFORNIUM • *See* Yerba Santa Fluid Extract.

ERUCIC ACID • Docosenoic Acid. An acid found in rapeseed, mustard seed, and wallflower seeds. It constitutes 40 to 50 percent of fatty acids of nasturtium seeds. No known toxicity.

ERYTHORBIC ACID • Isoascorbic Acid. Antioxidant. White, slightly yellow crystals, that darken on exposure to light. Isoascorbic acid contains one-twentieth the vitamin capacity of ascorbic acid *(see)*. Antioxidant used in pickling brine at a rate of 7.5 ounces per 100 gallons; in meat products at the rate of 0.75 ounces per hundred pounds; in beverages; baked goods; cured cuts and cured pulverized products to accelerate color fixing in curing, to 0.75 ounce per 100 pounds. Nontoxic. The final report to the FDA of the Select Committee on GRAS Substances stated in 1980 that it should continue its GRAS status with no limitations other than good manufacturing practices.

ERYTHROMYCIN • An antibacterial obtained from the strains of *Streptomyces erythraeus* found in the soil. Used to treat a wide range of bacterial infections in humans. It is used as a drug for beef, chicken eggs, pork, and turkey. FDA tolerances are 0.1 ppm in uncooked edible tissues of swine, zero in uncooked edible tissues of beef cattle and milk, 0.025 ppm in uncooked eggs, 0.125 ppm in uncooked edible residue of chickens and turkeys. EPA Genetic Toxicology Program *(see)*. Moderately toxic by ingestion. The use of antibiotics in animal feed is highly controversial because it could lead to resistance to the antibiotic in humans as well as allergic reactions.

ERYTHROSINE • Sodium or potassium salt of tetraiodofluorescein, a coal-tar derivative. A brown powder that becomes red in solution. FD & C Red No. 3 is an example. *See* Coal Tar for toxicity.

ERYTHROXYLON COCA • *See* Coca Leaf Extract (Decocainized).

ESCHERICHIA COLI • *E. coli.* A gram-negative *(see)* bacteria commonly found in fecal matter and in the human intestines, certain strains may cause intestinal and urinary tract infections. *See E. coli.*

ESSENCE • An extract of a substance that retains its fundamental or most desirable properties in concentrated form, such as a fragrance or flavoring.

ESSENTIAL OIL • The oily liquid obtained from plants through a variety of processes. The essential oil usually has the taste and smell of the original plant. Essential oils are called volatile because most of them are easily vaporized. The only theories for calling such oils essential are (1) the oils were believed essential to life and (2) they were the "essence" of the plant. The use of essential oils as preservatives is ancient. A large number of oils have antiseptic, germicidal, and preservative action; however, they are primarily used for fragrances and flavorings. No known toxicity when used on the skin. A teaspoon may cause illness in an adult and less than an ounce may kill.

ESTER • A compound formed from alcohol and acid by elimination of water, as ethyl acetate *(see).* Usually, fragrant liquids used for artificial fruit perfumes and flavors. Esterification of rosin, for example, reduces its allergy-causing properties. Toxicity depends on the ester.

ESTERASE-LIPASE • Derived from *Mucor miehei.* An enzyme used as a flavor enhancer in cheese, fats, oils, and milk products. There is no reported use of the chemical and there is no toxicology information available.

ESTRADIOL • Oestradiol. Estrace. Estinyl. Estra-L. Estraderm. depGynogen. Depo-Estradiol. Dura-Estrin. E-Cypionate. Estro-Cyp. Estrofem. Estroject-LA. Estronol-LA. Delestrogen. Dioval. Duragen 10. Estraval. Menaval. Valergen. Most potent of the natural estrogenic female hormones. In animals it is implanted in steers, heifers, and lambs. It is also implanted in combination with testosterone or progesterone, two other powerful sex hormones. The FDA permits zero tolerance in meat. Estradiol is given to humans by skin patch, tablets, injection, or vaginal cream and is used to treat menopausal symptoms, the effects of a hysterectomy, primary ovarian failure, atrophic vaginitis, postpartum breast engorgement, and inoperable prostate cancer. Potential adverse reactions include nausea, vomiting, depression, high blood pressure, dizziness, migraine, libido changes, blood clots, water retention, increased risk of stroke, blood clots to the lung, and heart attack. May also worsen nearsightedness, cause intolerance of contact lenses, and lead to loss of appetite, increased appetite, excessive thirst, pancreatitis, and bloating and abdominal cramps. Women may have breakthrough bleeding, altered menstrual flow, painful or absent menstruation, enlargement of benign tumors of the uterus, cervical erosion, abnormal secretions and vaginal candidiasis. In men there may be enlargement of the breast, testicular atrophy, and impotence. In both sexes there may be jaundice, high blood sugar, high calcium in the blood, folic acid deficiency, dark spots appearing on the skin, hives, acne, oily skin, hairiness or loss of hair, leg cramps, and hemorrhages into the skin. Contraindicated in persons with blood clot disorders, cancer of the breast, reproductive organs, or genitals, and in those with undiagnosed abnormal genital bleeding and in pregnancy. Should be used with caution in high blood pressure, asthma, mental depression, bone disease, blood problems, gallbladder disease, migraine, seizures, diabetes, absences of menstruation, heart failure, liver or kidney dysfunction, and a family history of breast or genital tract cancer. Estradiol's use as implants in animals is unnecessary and should be outlawed.

ESTRADIOL BENZOATE • White or slightly brownish crystalline hormone powder used as a growth promoter in beef and lamb. FDA tolerances are set at 120 parts per trillion in muscle; 480 ppt in fat; 360 ppt in kidney; 240 ppt in liver of heifers, steers, and calves. Tolerance of 120 ppm in muscles, 600 ppm in fat, kidney, and liver of lambs. Has caused cancer in experimental animals as well as birth defects. It is an estrogen used in human medication for birth control and post-menopausal symptoms and does cause side effects in humans as a medication. *See* Estradiol.

ESTRADIOL MONOPALMITATE • An estrogen used to promote growth in chickens. It has a zero tolerance in chickens for market. *See* Estradiol.

ESTRADIOL VALERATE • Used as an implant in combination with proges-terone. The FDA bans its use in veal calves.

ESTRAGOLE • A colorless to light yellow oily liquid occurring naturally in anise, anise star, basil, estragon oil, and pimento oil. Used as a synthetic fruit, licorice, anise, and spice flavorings for beverages, ice cream, ices, candy, baked goods, chewing gum, and condiments. GRAS.

ESTRAGON • Tarragon. A flavoring agent from the oil of leaves of a plant native to Eurasia and used in fruit, licorice, liquor, root beer, and spice flavorings for bev-erages, ice cream, ices, candy, baked goods, meats, liquor, and condiments. GRAS.

ESTROGEN • A hormone produced by the ovaries that is mainly responsible for female sexual characteristics. Estrogen influences bone mass by slowing or halt-ing bone loss, improving retention of calcium by the kidney, and improving the absorption of dietary calcium by the intestine. Estrogen is given to relieve menopausal symptoms, prevent or relieve aging changes in the vagina and ure-thra, and to help prevent osteoporosis *(see)*. *See* Estradiol.

ETHALFLURALIN • A herbicide. The FDA tolerance for residues in fat, meat, meat byproducts of cattle, hogs, goats, poultry, sheep, and milk is 0.05 ppm.

ETHANAL • *See* Acetaldehyde; Heptanal.

1,2-ETHANEDITHIOL • Derived from ethylene glycol, it is used as a chelating agent *(see)*. The vapors cause a severe headache and nausea.

ETHANOIC ACID • *See* Acetic Acid.

ETHANOL • Ethyl Alcohol. Rubbing Alcohol. Ordinary Alcohol. Used as a solvent in candy, candy glaze, beverages, ice cream, ices, baked goods, li-quors, sauces, and gelatin desserts. An antibacterial used in mouthwashes, nail enamel, astringents, liquid lip rouge, and many other cosmetic products. Clear, colorless, and very flammable, it is made by the fermentation of starch, sugar, and other carbohydrates. Used medicinally as a topical antiseptic, sedative, and blood vessel dilator. Ingestion of large amounts may cause nausea, vomiting, impaired perception, stupor, coma, and death. When it is deliberately denatured *(see* Denaturant), it is poisonous. GRAS.

ETHANOLAMINE DITHIODIGLYCOATE • *See* Ethanolamines.

ETHANOLAMINE THIOGLYCOLATE • *See* Ethanolamines.

ETHANOLAMINES • Three compounds—monoethanolamine, diethanolamine, and triethanolamine—with low melting points, colorless, and solid that readily absorb water and form viscous liquids and are soluble both in water and alcohol. They have an ammonia smell and are strong bases. Used in permanent-wave lotions as a preservative. Also form soaps with fatty acids (see) and are widely used as detergents and emulsifying agents. Very large quantities are required for a lethal oral dose in mice (2,140 milligrams per kilogram of body weight). They have been used medicinally as sclerosal agents for varicose veins. Can be irritating to skin if very alkaline. There is a big question about the safety of these compounds since they have been shown to be cancer-causing agents. See Diethanolamine.

ETHANTHALDEHYDE • See Heptanal.

ETHANTHIC ALCOHOL • See Heptyl Alcohol.

ETHANTHYL ALCOHOL • See Heptyl Alcohol.

ETHEPHON • A pesticide used in raisin water waste for use in animal feed. FDA residue tolerance is 65 ppm.

ETHER • An organic compound. Acetic ether (see Ethyl Acetate) is used in nail polishes as a solvent. Water insoluble, fat insoluble liquid with a characteristic odor. It is obtained chiefly by the distillation of alcohol with sulfuric acid and is used chiefly as a solvent. A mild skin irritant. Inhalation or ingestion causes central nervous system depression.

ETHION • An insecticide to kill mites. In fat of cattle it is permitted 2.5 ppm; in meat and byproducts of cattle as residue, 0.75 ppm, in milk, zero, and in animal feed from 4 to 10 ppm. It inhibits nerve signals. See Organophosphates.

ETHOFUMESATE • An herbicide with an FDA tolerance of 0.5 ppm as a residue in or on sugar beet molasses.

ETHOPABATE • Odorless white to pink crystals used as an animal drug in chickens. FDA limits residue to 1.5 ppm in uncooked liver and kidney, 0.5 ppm in uncooked muscles of chickens. Used to combat bacteria.

ETHOVAN • See Ethyl Vanillin.

p-ETHOXY BENZALDEHYDE • A synthetic fruit and vanilla flavoring for beverages, ice cream, ices, candy, and baked good. See Benzyl Acetate.

2-(1-[ETHOXY IMINO] BUTYL)-5-(2-[ETHYL THIO] PROPYL)-3-HYDROXY-2-CYCLOHEXENE-1-ONE • An herbicide used in animal feed flaxseed meal, potato pomace, sunflower meal, tomato products (concentrated), and peanut soap stock. FDA limitations of residue: 24 ppm in tomato products, concentrated; 15 ppm in cottonseed soap stock, 7 ppm in flaxseed meal, 75 ppm in peanut soap stock, and 20 ppm in sunflower meal used for animal feed.

ETHOXYLATE • An ethyl (see) and oxygen compound is added to an additive to make it less or more soluble in water, depending upon the mixture. Ethoxylate acts as an emulsifier.

ETHOXYLATED MONO- and DI-GLYCERIDES • Dough conditioners in bread used to increase the volume of the loaf (not to exceed 0.5 percent) of flour used. Also used as an emulsifier in pan-release agents for yeast-leavened bakery products. In solid, edible fat water emulsions as coffee creamer substitute. See Glycerides.

ETHOXYQUIN • 1,2-Dihydro-6-Ethoxy-2,2,4-Trimethylquinoline. An antioxidant *(see)* to preserve color in chili powder, paprika, and ground chili at levels not to exceed 100 ppm. The residues in or on edible products of animals are restricted to 5 ppm in or on the uncooked fat of meat from animals except poultry; 3 ppm in or on the uncooked liver and fat of poultry; and 0.5 ppm in or on the uncooked muscle meat of animals. There was a significant question about this additive in the late 1980s because its use in animal feed caused dogs to have symptoms from itchy skin and lethargy to thyroid and kidney problems. Reproductive disorders and cancer were also reported. It is used in both human and animal feed as an antioxidant. In 1995, there was a report in *Biochemical Pharmacology* by Mexican researchers that ethoxyquin affected the kidneys of rats. The FDA's toxicology program reported no adverse health effects from the additive. Then, in 1997, the FDA reduced the amount of ethoxyquin allowed in dog food. It is still permitted in human food. *See* Quinoline for toxicity. *See also* Santoquin.

ETHYL • Signifies a hydrocarbon derived from natural gas.

ETHYL ABIETATE • Amber-colored, thick liquid made from ethyl chloride and rosin. It is used in lacquers and coatings. Skin irritant. Although allowed as a food additive, there is no current reported use of the chemical, and therefore, although toxicology information may be available, it is not being updated, according to the FDA.

ETHYL ACETATE • A colorless liquid with a pleasant fruity odor that occurs naturally in apples, bananas, grape juice, pineapple, raspberries, and strawberries. It is employed as a synthetic flavoring agent in blackberry, raspberry, strawberry, butter, lemon, apple, banana, cherry, grape, peach, pineapple, brandy, muscatel, rum, whiskey, mint, almond, and cream soda flavoring for beverages, ice cream, ices, candy, baked goods, chewing gum, gelatins, puddings, and liquor. A useful solvent in nail enamels and nail polish remover. Also an artificial fruit essence for perfumes. It is a mild local irritant and central nervous system depressant. The vapors are irritating and prolonged inhalation may cause kidney and liver damage. Irritating to the skin. Its fat-solvent action produces drying and cracking and sets the stage for secondary infections. GRAS.

ETHYL ACETOACETATE • Acetoacetic Ester. A synthetic flavoring that occurs naturally in strawberries. Pleasant odor. Used in loganberry, strawberry, apple, apricot, cherry, peach, liquor, and muscatel flavorings for beverages, ice cream, ices, candy, baked goods, chewing gum, and gelatin desserts. Moderately irritating to skin and mucous membranes.

ETHYL ACETONE • *See* 2-Pentanone.

ETHYL 2-ACETYL-3-PHENYLPROPIONATE • A synthetic fruit flavoring for beverages, ice cream, ices, candy, baked goods, chewing gum, and gelatin desserts.

ETHYL ACONITATE • Aconitic Acid. A synthetic fruit, liquor, and rum flavoring for beverages, ice cream, ices, candy, baked goods, and gelatin desserts.

ETHYL ACRYLATE • A synthetic flavoring agent that occurs naturally in pineapple and raspberries. Used in fruit, liquor, and rum flavorings for beverages, ice cream, ices, candy, baked goods, and chewing gum. Also used in the manufacture of water-resistant paint, paper coating, and leather finishes. Highly irritating to the eyes, skin, and mucous membranes and may cause lethargy and convulsions if concentrated vapor is inhaled. The final report to the FDA of the Select Committee on GRAS Substances stated in 1980 that it should continue its GRAS status with no limitations other than good manufacturing practices.

ETHYL ALCOHOL • Contains ethanol *(see)*, grain alcohol, and neural spirits and is used as a solvent in candy glaze, beverages, ices, ice cream, candy, baked goods, liquors, sauces, gelatin desserts, and pizza crusts. It is rapidly absorbed through the gastric and intestinal mucosa. For ingestion within a few minutes, the fatal dose in adults is considered to be one and one-half to two pints of whiskey (40 to 55 percent ethyl alcohol). It was approved in 1976 for use in pizza crusts to extend handling and storage life. GRAS.

ETHYL *p*-ANISATE • A synthetic flavoring agent, colorless to light yellow liquid with a light fruity smell. Used in berry, fruit, grape, licorice, anise, liquor, rum, and vanilla flavorings for beverages, ice cream, ices, candy, and baked goods.

ETHYL ANTHRANILATE • Colorless liquid, fruit odor, soluble in alcohol and propylene glycol. A synthetic flavoring agent, clear, colorless to amber liquid with an odor of orange blossoms. Used in berry, mandarin, orange, floral, jasmine, neroli, fruit, grape, peach, and raisin flavorings for beverages, ice cream, ices, candy, baked goods, gelatin desserts, and chewing gum. Used in perfumery.

ETHYL ASPARTATE • The ester of ethyl alcohol and aspartic acid *(see both)*.

ETHYL BENZENECARBOXYLATE • *See* Ethyl Benzoate.

ETHYL BENZOATE • Essence de Niobe. Ethyl Benzenecarboxylate. An artificial fruit essence almost insoluble in water, with a pleasant odor. Used in currant, strawberry, fruit, cherry, grape, liquor, nut, walnut, vanilla, and raspberry flavorings for beverages, ice cream, ices, candy, baked goods, chewing gum, gelatin desserts, and liquors.

ETHYL BENZOYLACETATE • A synthetic fruit flavoring agent for beverages, ice cream, ices, candy, and baked goods. It becomes yellow when exposed to light. Pleasant odor.

ETHYL BENZYL ACETOACETATE • *See* Ethyl 2-Acetyl-3-Phenylpropionate.

ETHYL BENZYL BUTYRATE • A synthetic fruit flavoring for beverages, ice cream, ices, candy, and baked goods. Although allowed as a food additive, there is no current reported use of the chemical, and therefore, although toxicology information may be available, it is not being updated, according to the FDA.

ETHYL BUTYL ACETATE • A synthetic fruit flavoring for beverages, ice cream, ices, and candy.

ETHYL BUTYRATE • Butyric Acid. Pineapple Oil. Colorless, with a pineapple odor. It occurs naturally in apples and strawberries. In alcoholic solution it is known as pineapple oil. Used in blueberry, raspberry, strawberry, butter, caramel, cream, orange, banana, cherry, grape, peach, pineapple, rum, walnut, and eggnog flavorings for beverages, ice cream, ices, candy, baked goods, gelatins, puddings, and chewing gum (1,400 ppm). Mildly toxic by ingestion. A skin irritant. GRAS.

ETHYL CAPRATE • *See* Cognac Oil.

ETHYL CAPROATE • Colorless to yellowish liquid, pleasant odor, soluble in alcohol and ether. Used in artificial fruit essences. *See* Cognac Oil.

ETHYL CAPRYLATE • *See* Cognac Oil.

ETHYL CARBONATE • Carbonic Acid Diethyl Ester. Pleasant odor. Practically insoluble in water. Solvent for nail enamels. No known toxicity.

ETHYL CARVACROL • *See* Carvacryl Ethyl Ether.

ETHYL CELLULOSE • Cellulose Ether. White granules prepared from wood pulp or chemical cotton and used as a binder and filler in dry vitamin preparations up to 35 percent; chewing gum up to .025 percent, and in confectionery up to .012 percent. Also used in the manufacture of plastics and lacquers. Binding, dispersing, and emulsifying agent used in cosmetics, particularly nail polishes and liquid lip rouge. Also used as a diluent *(see)*. Not susceptible to bacterial or fungal decomposition. No known toxicity. GRAS.

ETHYL CINNAMATE • Cinnamic Acid. An almost colorless oily liquid with a faint cinnamon odor. Used as a synthetic flavoring in raspberry, strawberry, cherry, grape, peach, plum, spice, cinnamon, and vanilla flavorings for beverages, ice cream, ices, candy, baked goods, chewing gum, and gelatin desserts. Also used as a fixative for perfumes and to scent heavy oriental and floral perfumes in soaps, toilet waters, face powders, and perfumes. Insoluble in water. No known toxicity for the skin. Moderately toxic by ingestion.

ETHYL CITRATE • A bitter, oily sequestrant used in dried egg whites. No known toxicity. *See* Sequestrants.

ETHYL CYCLOHEXANEPROPIONATE • A synthetic pineapple flavoring agent for beverages, ice cream, ices, candy, and baked goods.

ETHYL DECANOATE • Decanoic Acid. A synthetic flavoring occurring naturally in green and white cognac oils. Used in strawberry, cherry, grape, pineapple, liquor, brandy, cognac, and rum flavorings for beverages, ice cream, ices, candy, baked goods, gelatin desserts, and liquors.

ETHYL 4,4′-DICHLOROBENZILATE • An insecticide for citrus fruits. The FDA allows a residue of 5 ppm in and on citrus fruits and 0.5 ppm as a residue in fat, meat, and meat byproducts of sheep and cattle.

ETHYL DIHYDROXYPROPYL • PABA. The ester of ethyl alcohol and *p*-dihydroxypropyl aminobenzoic acid. *See* Ethyl Alcohol and PABA.

ETHYL DIISOPROPYL CINNAMATE • *See* Cinnamic Acid.

2-ETHYL-3,5(6)-DIMETHYLPYRAZINE • A colorless to slightly yellow liquid with the smell of roasted cocoa used as a flavoring agent in various products. GRAS.

ETHYL DODECANOATE • *See* Ethyl Laurate.

ETHYL ESTER OF FATTY ACIDS • A compound for coating raisins. No known toxicity.

ETHYL FORMATE • Formic Acid. A colorless, flammable liquid with a distinct odor occurring naturally in apples and coffee extract. Used as a yeast and mold inhibitor and as a fumigant for bulk and packaged raisins and dried currants; fungicide for cashew nuts, cereals, tobacco, and dried fruits. Also a synthetic flavoring agent for blueberry, raspberry, strawberry, butter, butterscotch, apple, apricot, banana, cherry, grape, peach, plum, pineapple, tutti-frutti, brandy, rum, sherry, and whiskey flavorings for beverages, ice cream, ices, candy, baked goods, liquor, gelatin, and chewing gum. Irritating to the skin and mucous membranes, and in high concentrations it is narcotic. The final report to the FDA of the Select Committee on GRAS Substances stated in 1980 that it should continue its GRAS status with no limitations other than good manufacturing practices. *See* Formic Acid for further toxicity.

ETHYL FORMIC ACID • *See* Propionic Acid.

ETHYL 2-FURAN PROPIONATE • A synthetic raspberry, apple, cherry, and pineapple flavoring agent for beverages, ice cream, ices, candy, and baked goods.

ETHYL FURYLPROPIONATE • *See* Ethyl 2-Furan Propionate.

ETHYL GLUTAMATE • The ester of ethyl alcohol and glutamic acid. *See* Glutamate.

4-ETHYL GUAIACOL • A synthetic coffee and fruit flavoring agent for beverages, ice cream, ices, and gelatin desserts.

2-ETHYL-2-HEPTANAL • A synthetic pineapple flavoring agent for beverages and candy.

ETHYL HEPTANOATE • A synthetic flavoring agent, colorless, with a fruity, winelike odor and taste, and a burning aftertaste. Used in blueberry, strawberry, butter, butterscotch, coconut, apple, cherry, grape, melon, peach, pineapple, plum, vanilla, cheese, nut, rum, brandy, and cognac flavorings for beverages, ice cream, ices, candy, baked goods, gelatin desserts, chewing gum, and liqueurs.

ETHYL HEXADECANOATE • *See* Ethyl Palmitate.

ETHYL 2,4-HEXADIENOATE • *See* Ethyl Sorbate.

ETHYL HEXANEDIOL • *See* Sorbic Acid.

ETHYL HEXANOATE • A synthetic flavoring agent that occurs naturally in apples, pineapples, and strawberries. Used in fruit, rum, nut, and cheese flavorings for beverages, ice cream, ices, candy, baked goods, chewing gum, gelatin desserts, and jelly.

2-ETHYL-1-HEXANOL • A flavoring agent derived from alcohol. The FAO-WHO Expert Committee on Food Additives concluded that doses greater than about 350 mg per kg of body weight per day administered orally to rats and mice cause changes in the liver but did not result in cancer with long-term administration. In high doses it did cause birth defects in mice but at lower doses did not. On the basis of NOEL *(see)* of 50 mg per kg of body weight per day from the long term study in rats and a safety factor of 100, the Committee established an ADI *(see)* of 0–05 mg per kg of body weight for this additive.

ETHYL 3-HYDROXYBUTYRATE • Used as a stabilizer and antioxidant.

ETHYL HYDROXYMETHYL OLEYL OXAZOLINE • A synthetic wax. No known toxicity.

ETHYL a-HYDROXY PROPIONATE • *See* Ethyl Lactate.

ETHYL ISOBUTYRATE • Isobutyric Acid. A synthetic strawberry, fruit, cherry, and butter flavoring agent for flavorings for beverages, ice cream, ices, candy, baked goods, gelatin desserts, and toppings.

ETHYL ISOVALERATE • Colorless, oily liquid with a fruity odor derived from ethanol and valerate. A synthetic flavoring used in alcoholic solution for pineapple flavoring for beverages, ice cream, ices, candy, baked goods, chewing gum, and gelatin desserts. Used in essential oils and perfumery. *See* Valeric Acid.

ETHYL LACTATE • Colorless liquid with a mild odor. Derived from lactic acid with ethanol. Used as a solvent for nitrocellulose, lacquers, resins, and enamels. Used in strawberry, butter, butterscotch, coconut, grape, rum, maple, cheese, and nut flavorings for beverages, ice cream, ices, candy, baked goods, chewing gum (3,100 ppm), gelatin desserts, syrup, and brandy (1,000 ppm). *See* Lactic Acid.

ETHYL LAURATE • The ester of ethyl alcohol and lauric acid used as a synthetic flavoring agent. It is a colorless oil with a light, fruity odor. Insoluble in water, very soluble in alcohol. Used in berry, coconut, fruit, grape, liquor, cognac, rum, nut, spice, nutmeg, and cheese flavorings for beverages, ice cream, ices, candy, baked goods, chewing gum, and liqueurs. It is also used as a solvent.

ETHYL LEVULINATE • Levulinic Acid. Colorless liquid soluble in water. Used as a solvent for cellulose acetate and starch and flavorings. A synthetic apple flavoring for beverages, ice cream, ices, candy, and baked goods. *See* Levulinic Acid.

ETHYL LINOLEATE • Prepared from sunflower seed oil, it is used in the vitamin industry.

ETHYL MALATE • *See* Diethyl Malate.

ETHYL MALONATE • Colorless liquid, sweet ester odor. Insoluble in water. Used in certain pigments and flavoring. No known toxicity.

ETHYL MALTOL • White crystalline powder with a sweet fruity taste, it is used as a flavoring agent and processing aid in chocolate, desserts, and wine. Moderately toxic by injection.

4-ETHYL-2-METHOXYPHENOL • *See* 4-Ethyl Guaiacol.

ETHYL 3-METHYL BUTYRATE • A synthetic fruit flavoring agent for beverages, ice cream, ices, and candy.

ETHYL METHYLENE PHOSPHORODITHIOATE • A widely used insecticide in animal feed, citrus pulp, raisins, and dried tea. FDA allows residue tolerance of up to 10 ppm in dried tea, 4 ppm in raisins, and 10 ppm in dried citrus pulp when used for animal feed. Extremely hazardous substance. Poison by ingestion and skin contact. Human systemic effects by ingestion include paralysis, motor activity changes, fever, and interference with nerve transmission.

ETHYL-3-METHYL-4-(METHYL THIO) PHENYL(1-METHYL-ETHYL)PHOS-PHORAMIDATE • A pesticide allowed up to 1 ppm as residue in or on grape pomace; 2.5 in or on dried citrus pulp or citrus molasses that are fed to animals.

ETHYL METHYLPHENYLGLYCIDATE • Strawberry Aldehyde. Colorless to yellowish liquid having a strong odor suggestive of strawberry. A synthetic berry, loganberry, raspberry, strawberry, coconut, fruit, cherry, grape, pineapple, liquor, and wine flavoring for beverages, ice cream, ices, candy, baked goods, gelatin, pudding, and chewing gum. Used in perfumery. Caused growth retardation in rats, particularly males, and testicular atrophy. Females showed paralysis of hindquarters and deterioration of muscles. GRAS.

2-ETHYL-3-METHYLPYRAZINE • Colorless to slightly yellow liquid with a strong raw potato odor. Used as a flavoring agent in various foods. GRAS.

ETHYL MYRISTATE • The ester of ethyl alcohol and myristic acid *(see both)*. A synthetic coconut, fruit, honey, and cognac flavoring agent for beverages, ice cream, ices, candy, baked goods, and liqueurs.

ETHYL NITRITE • Sweet Spirit of Niter. Spirit of Nitrous Ether. A synthetic flavoring agent, colorless or yellowish liquid with a characteristic odor and a burning, sweetish taste. Used in strawberry, cherry, pineapple, liquor, brandy, and rum flavorings for beverages, ice cream, ices, candy, baked goods, chewing gum, syrups, and icings. It may cause hemoglobinemia, in which oxygen is diminished in the red blood cells, low blood pressure, and, when it is in high concentration, narcosis.

ETHYL NONANOATE • Nonanoic Acid. A synthetic fruit and rum flavoring agent for beverages, ice cream, ices, candy, baked goods, gelatin desserts, chewing gum, icings, and liqueurs. Mildly toxic by ingestion. A skin irritant.

ETHYL 2-NONYNOATE • A synthetic berry, fruit, and melon flavoring agent for beverages, ice cream, ices, candy, and baked goods.

ETHYL OCTANOATE • Octanoic Acid. A synthetic flavoring agent that occurs naturally in both cognac green and cognac white oils. Used in strawberry, butter, citrus, apple, pineapple, rum, nut, and cheese flavorings for beverages, ice cream, ices, candy, baked goods, gelatin desserts, and chewing gum. Mildly toxic by ingestion. A skin irritant.

ETHYL OCTYNE CARBONATE • *See* Ethyl 2-Nonynoate.

ETHYL OLEATE • Oleic Acid. A synthetic flavoring agent, yellowish, oily, insoluble in water. Used in butter and fruit flavorings for beverages, ice cream, ices, candy, baked goods, gelatin desserts, and puddings. An ingredient in nail polish remover. It is made from carbon, hydrogen, oxygen, and oleic acid *(see)*.

ETHYL 3-OXOBUTANOATE • *See* Ethyl Acetoacetate.

ETHYL OXYHYDRATE • *See* Rum Ether.

ETHYL PALMITATE • Ethyl Hexadecanoate. The ester of ethyl alcohol and palmitic acid *(see both)*. A synthetic flavoring agent, colorless or nearly colorless liquid, with a pleasant odor. Used in butter, honey, apricot, and cherry flavorings for beverages, ice cream, ices, candy, and baked goods.

ETHYLENE DICHLORIDE • A solvent used in the production of spices. Also used in processing animal byproducts for use in animal feeds and in pesticide compounds. The FDA's residue tolerances for spices is 30 ppm and 300 ppm in extracted byproducts.

ETHYLENE GLYCOL • A slightly viscous liquid with a sweet taste. Absorbs twice its weight in water. Used as an antifreeze and humectant *(see);* also as a solvent. Toxic when ingested, causing central nervous system depression, vomiting, drowsiness, coma, respiratory failure, kidney damage, and possibly death.

ETHYLPARABEN • *See* Propylparaben.

ETHYL PERSATE • Persic Oil Acid. Ethyl Ester. The ethyl ester of the fatty acids derived from either apricot kernel oil or peach kernel oil. *See* Apricot and Peach Kernel Oil.

ETHYL PHENYLACETATE • Phenylacetic Acid. A fixative for perfumes, colorless or nearly colorless liquid, with a sweet honey rose odor. Also a synthetic flavoring agent in honey, butter, apricot, and cherry flavorings for beverages, ice cream, ices, candy, baked goods, and syrups. Moderately toxic by ingestion.

ETHYL PHENYL ACRYLATE • *See* Ethyl Cinnamate.

ETHYL 3-PHENYL BUTYRATE • A synthetic berry, strawberry, fruit, and cherry flavoring agent for beverages, ice cream, ices, candy, baked goods, and gelatin desserts. No known toxicity.

ETHYL 4-PHENYL BUTYRATE • A synthetic fruit flavoring agent for beverages and candy.

ETHYL PHENYLGLYCIDATE • Colorless liquid with a strong strawberry odor used as a flavoring agent. Moderately toxic by ingestion. May be mutagenic.

ETHYL 3-PHENYLPROPIONATE • A synthetic fruit flavoring agent for beverages, ice cream, ices, candy, and baked goods. No known toxicity. *See* Ethyl Cinnamate.

ETHYL 1-PROPENE-1, 2,3-TRICARBOXYLATE • *See* Ethyl Aconitate.

ETHYL PROPIONATE • Propionic Acid. A synthetic flavoring agent, colorless, transparent liquid, with a fruit odor. Occurs naturally in apples. Used in butter, fruit, and rum flavorings for beverages, ice cream, gelatin desserts, baked goods, and chewing gum (1,100 ppm). Moderately toxic by ingestion. A skin irritant.

ETHYL PYRUVATE • Pyruvic Acid. A synthetic chocolate, fruit, rum, maple, and spice flavoring agent for beverages, ice cream, ices, candy, and baked goods.

ETHYL SALICYLATE • Salicylic Ether. Used in the manufacture of artificial perfumes. Occurs naturally in strawberries and has a pleasant odor. Used as a synthetic flavoring agent in fruit, root beer, sassafras, and wintergreen flavorings for beverages, ice cream, ices, candy, baked goods, chewing gum, gelatins, and puddings. At one time it was given medically to rheumatics. May interact with harmful results with medications such as anticoagulants, antidepressants, and medications for cancer such as Methotrexate. May cause allergic reaction in persons allergic to salicylates *(see)*. At one time it was used to treat rheumatics.

ETHYL SEBACATE • *See* Diethyl Sebacate.

ETHYL SORBATE • A synthetic fruit flavoring agent for beverages, ice cream, ices, candy, and baked goods.

ETHYL STEARATE • The ester of ethyl alcohol and stearic acid *(see both)*.

ETHYL TETRADECANOATE • *See* Ethyl Myristate.

ETHYL TIGLATE • Tiglic Acid. A synthetic raspberry, strawberry, pineapple, and rum flavoring agent for beverages, ice cream, ices, candy, and liquor.

ETHYL TRANS-2-METHYL-2-BUTENOATE • *See* Ethyl Tiglate.

ETHYL 10-UNDECENOATE • A synthetic coconut, fruit, cognac, and nut flavoring agent for beverages, ice cream, ices, candy, baked goods, and liquor.

ETHYL UROCANATE • The ester of ethyl alcohol and urocanic acid. *See* Imidazoline.

ETHYL VALERATE • Valeric Acid. A synthetic butter, apple, apricot, peach, and nut flavoring agent for beverages, ice cream, ices, candy, baked goods, gelatin desserts, and chewing gum.

ETHYL VANILLIN • An ingredient in perfumes. Colorless flakes, with an odor and flavor stronger than vanilla. Used as a synthetic flavoring agent in raspberry, strawberry, butter, butterscotch, caramel, rum, butter, chocolate, cocoa, citrus, coconut, macaroon, cola, fruit, cherry, grape, honey, liquor, muscatel, rum, maple, nut, pecan, root beer, vanilla, and cream soda for beverages, ice cream, ices, candy, baked goods, gelatin desserts, puddings, chewing gum, imitation vanilla extract (28,000 ppm), liquor, icings, and toppings. Caused mild skin irritation in humans. In rats, it produced a reduction in growth rate and heart, kidney, liver, lung, spleen, and stomach injuries. GRAS.

ETHYLACETIC ACID • *See* Butyric Acid.

2-ETHYLBUTRYIC ACID • A synthetic fruit, nut, and walnut flavoring agent for beverages, ice cream, ices, candy, and baked goods. No known toxicity.

ETHYLENE • The sixth-highest-volume chemical produced in the United States, it is a colorless gas with a sweet odor and taste. It is derived from heat-cracking hydrocarbon gases or from fluid removal of ethanol. It is used to make chemical compounds including those used to make plastics, refrigerants, anesthetics, and orchard sprays to accelerate fruit ripening. It is highly flammable and potentially explosive. It can asphyxiate.

ETHYLENE BRASSYLATE • *See* Erucic Acid.

1,2-ETHYLENE DIBROMIDE • A colorless, nonflammable liquid with a sweetish odor derived from bromine and ethylene. Used as a scavenger for lead in gasoline, as a fumigant, general solvent, and in waterproofing products. A cancer-causing agent, toxic by inhalation, ingestion, and skin absorption; a strong irritant to eyes and skin.

ETHYLENE DICHLORIDE (EDC) • Dutch Liquid. 1,2-Dichlorethane. Ethylene Chloride. The halogenate aliphatic hydrocarbon derived from the action of chlorine on ethylene. It is used in the manufacture of vinyl chloride *(see)*. Colorless, heavy liquid with a sweet odor, it is widely used as a fumigant for cereal grains, corn grits, cracked rice, and fermented malt beverages; as a solvent for fats, waxes, spices, and resins; as a lead scavenger in antiknock gasolines, in paint, varnish, and finish removers; as a wetting agent; as a penetrating agent; in organic synthesis; and in the making of polyvinyl chloride (PVC) *(see)*. EDC is also used as an ingredient in cosmetics and as a food additive. It is one of the highest volume chemicals produced. It can be highly toxic whether taken into the body by ingestion, inhalation, or skin absorption. It is irritating to the mucous membranes. In cancer testing, the National Cancer Institute found this compound caused stomach cancer, vascularized cancers of multiple organs, and cancers beneath the skin in male rats. Female rats exposed to EDC developed mammary cancers—in some high-dose animals as early as the twentieth week of the study. The chemical also caused breast cancers as well as uterine cancers in female mice and respiratory tract cancers in both sexes.

Deaths due to liver and kidney injury following ingestion of large amounts (30 to 70 grams) have been reported. Clouding of the eyes, hemorrhages, and destruction of the adrenal cortex have been reported in humans and dogs. Annual production in the United States is now estimated at about 10 billion pounds—the sixteenth largest of all chemicals. EDC has been found in human milk and in the exhaled breath of nursing mothers who were exposed to the chemical. FDA tolerances for residues are: 125 ppm in cereal grain; 25 ppm in fermented malt beverages. On the Community Right-To-Know List and under IARC Cancer Review *(see both)*. Human poison by ingestion. Skin irritant. Implicated in worker sterility. The FAO-WHO Committee found it causes birth defects and that it causes cancer in mice and rats when administered orally. The Committee expressed the opinion that this solvent (1,2-dichloroethane) should not be used in food.

ETHYLENE DIOLEAMIDE • *See* Fatty Acids.

ETHYLENE DISTEARAMIDE • *See* Fatty Acids.

ETHYLENE OXIDE • A fumigant used on ground spices and other processed natural seasonings. A colorless gas, liquid at 12°C. Derived from the oxidation of ethylene in air or oxygen with silver catalyst. Irritant to the eyes and skin. A suspected human carcinogen. On the Community Right-To-Know List and under IARC Cancer Review *(see both)*.

ETHYLENE OXIDE-METHYL FORMATE MIXTURE • A mold and yeast control agent in dried and glacéed fruits. Ethylene oxide is highly irritating to the mucous membranes and eyes. High concentrations may cause pulmonary edema. Inhalation of methyl formate vapor produces nasal and eye irritation, retching, narcosis, and death from pulmonary irritation. Exposure to 1 percent vapor for two and a half hours or 5 percent vapor for a half hour is lethal.

ETHYLENE OXIDE POLYMER • Used as a stabilizer in fermented malt beer (300 ppm by weight). *See* Ethylene Oxide and Polymers.

ETHYLENE UREA • *See* Urea.

ETHYLENEBUTYRALDEHYDE • A synthetic chocolate flavoring agent for beverages, ice cream, ices, candy, and baked goods. No known toxicity.

ETHYLENEDIAMINE • Colorless, clear, thick, and strongly alkaline. A component of a bacteria-killing component in processing sugarcane. Also used as a solvent for casein, albumin, and shellac. Has been used as a urinary acidifier. It can cause sensitization leading to asthma and allergic skin rashes.

ETHYLENEDIAMINE TETRAACETIC ACID (EDTA) • An important compound in cosmetics used primarily as a sequestering agent *(see)*, in carbonated beverages. EDTA salts are used in crabmeat (cooked and canned), to retard struvite (crystal) formation, and promote color retention. It is also used in nonstandardized dressings. It may be irritating to the skin and mucous membranes and cause allergies such as asthma and skin rashes. Also used as a sequestrant in carbonated beverages. When ingested, it may cause errors in a number of laboratory tests, including those for calcium, carbon dioxide, nitrogen, and muscular activity. It is on the FDA list of food additives to be studied for toxicity. It can cause kidney damage. The trisodium salt of EDTA was fed to rats and mice for nearly two years. According to a summary of the report, "Although a variety of tumors occurred among test and control animals of both species, the test did not indicate that any of the tumors observed in the test animals were attributed to EDTA. The tests were part of the National Cancer Institute's Carcinogenesis Bioassay Program."

trans-1,2-ETHYLENEDICARBOXYLIC ACID • *See* Fumaric Acid.

ETHYL4,4'-DICHLOROBENZILATE • An insecticide allowed up to 5 ppm as residue on or in citrus fruits and 0.5 ppm as residue in fat, meat, and meat byproducts of sheep and cattle.

ETHYL ESTER OF FATTY ACIDS • Compound used in coatings for raisins. *See* Fatty Acids.

O,O-ETHYL-S-2 (ETHYL THIO)ETHYL PHOSPHORODITHIOATE • Widely used insecticide on animal feed, pineapples, and dehydrated sugar beet pulp. FDA limitation of 5 ppm in dehydrated sugar beet pulp and pineapple bran when used for animal feed. Poisonous by ingestion, inhalation and skin contact. May cause mutations. EPA considers it extremely hazardous and it is on the EPA Genetic Toxicology Program *(See)*.

EUBATUS, RUBUS • *See* Blackberry Bark Extract.

EUCALYPTOL • Eucalyptus Oil. A chief constituent of eucalyptus and cajeput oils. Occurs naturally in allspice, star anise, bay, calamus, and peppermint oil. Eucalyptus oil is 70 to 80 percent active eucalyptol. Eucalyptol is used in mint flavorings for beverages, ice cream, ices, candy, baked goods, and chewing gum. An antiseptic, antispasmodic, and expectorant. Used to flavor toothpaste and mouthwash and to cover up malodors in depilatories. It is not used in hypoallergenic cosmetics. Fatalities followed ingestion of doses as small as 3 to 5 milliliters (about a teaspoon), and recovery has occurred after doses as large as 20 to 30 milliliters (about 4 to 5 teaspoons). Symptoms of poisoning are epigastric burning with nausea, weakness, water retention, and delirium.

EUCALYPTUS EXTRACT • *See* Eucalyptus Oil.

EUCALYPTUS GLOBULUS LEAVES • A flavoring. *See* Eucalyptus Oil.

EUCALYPTUS OIL • Dinkum Oil. The colorless to pale yellow volatile liquid from the fresh leaves of the eucalyptus tree. It is 70 to 80 percent eucalyptol and has a spicy cool taste and a characteristic aromatic, somewhat camphorlike odor. Used in fruit, mint, root beer, spice, and ginger ale flavorings for beverages, ice cream, ices, candy, baked goods, chewing gum, and liquor. Used as a local antiseptic. Has been used as an expectorant, vermifuge, and local antiseptic. Doses as small as 3 to 5 milliliters (about equal to a teaspoon) and about one milliliter has caused coma. Fatalities have followed doses as small as 3.5 milliliters. Symptoms include epigastric burning with nausea. Symptoms have been reported to occur as long as two hours after ingestion.

EUCHEUMA COTTONII **EXTRACT** • A flavoring. *See* Eucheuma Seaweed.

EUCHEUMA SEAWEED (PROCESSED) • Eucheuma Cottonii Extract. Eucheuma Spinosum Extract. A stabilizing and thickening agent derived from eucheuma seaweed used in dairy products to suspend particles and for gelling in foods. In a 90-day study in rats, processed eucheuma administered at 0.5 percent,

1.5 percent, and 5 percent in the diet produced "no effects of toxicological significance" according to the FAO-WHO Expert Committee on Food Additives. *See* Hydrogenation and Carrageenan.

EUCHEUMA SPINOSUM EXTRACT • An emulsifier and stabilizer. *See* Eucheuma Seaweed.

EUGENOL • An ingredient in perfumes and dentifrices obtained from clove oil. Occurs naturally in allspice, basil, bay leaves, calamus, pimento, and laurel leaves. It has a spicy, pungent taste. Used as a fixative in perfumes. Darkens and thickens upon exposure to air. Used as a defoamer in yeast production, in the manufacture of vanilla, and in perfumery. It is a synthetic fruit, nut, and spice flavoring for beverages, ice cream, ices, candy, baked goods, chewing gum, gelatin desserts, meats (2,000 ppm), and condiments. Eugenol also acts as a local antiseptic. When ingested, may cause vomiting and gastric irritation. Because of its potential as an allergen, it is left out of hypoallergenic cosmetics. Toxicity is similar to phenol, which is highly toxic. Death in laboratory animals given eugenol is due to vascular collapse. GRAS.

EUGENYL ACETATE • Acetic Acid. A synthetic berry, fruit, mint, spice, and vanilla flavoring agent for beverages, ice cream, ices, candy, baked goods, chewing gum, and condiments.

EUGENYL BENZOATE • A synthetic fruit and spice flavoring agent for beverages, ice cream, ices, candy, and baked goods.

EUGENYL FORMATE • Formic Acid. A synthetic spice flavoring agent used in condiments. *See* Formic Acid for toxicity.

EUGENYL METHYL ETHER • A synthetic raspberry, strawberry, fruit, spice, clove, and ginger flavoring agent for beverages, ice cream, ices, candy, baked goods, and jellies.

EVERNIA FURFURACEA • *See* Oakmoss, Absolute.

EVERNIA PRUNASTIC • *See* Oakmoss, Absolute.

EXATOLIDE • *See* Pentadecalactone.

EXCITOTOXICOLOGY • The study of chemicals that overstimulate and damage nerves. Glutamate *(see)* is considered an excitotoxin.

EXCITOTOXIN • *See* Excitotoxicology.

EXTRACT • The solution that results from passing alcohol or an alcohol-water mixture through a substance. Examples of extracts would be the alcohol-water mixture of vanillin, orange, or lemon extracts found among the spices and flavorings on the supermarket shelf. Extracts are not as strong as essential oils *(see)*.

EYE ALLERGY • There are many forms of allergy of the eye. The mucous membranes of the eye may be involved in allergic rhinitis. Such allergic conjunctivitis may also occur by itself without irritation of the nose. Another form, spring pinkeye, is probably due to allergens in the air. Dust, mold spores, foods, and eye medications may all cause conjunctivitis. There is also a less severe, chronic form of allergic conjunctivitis. Symptoms include prolonged photophobia, itching, burning, and a feeling of dryness. There may be a watery discharge and finding the source of allergy is often difficult.

F

FAMPHUR • 0,0-Dimethyl 0-P (Dimethylsulfo/amoyl) Phenyl Phosphoro-thioate. An insecticide to combat grubs in animal feed. The FDA residue tolerance is 0.1 ppm in meat, fat, and meat byproducts of cattle.

FANTESK • A fat replacer developed by the U.S. Department of Agriculture and licensed exclusively to Opta Food Ingredients. It is based on a combination of starches or gums with a small amount of oil. It has the taste and texture of regular fat but provides less than 0.5 grams of fat per serving.

FAO-WHO EXPERT COMMITTEE ON FOOD ADDITIVES • An international group of experts from the World Health Organization and the Food and Agriculture Organization of the United Nations. The members meet periodically to evaluate the safety of various food additives and contaminants with a view to recommending acceptable daily intakes for humans and to prepare specifications for the identity and purity of food additives. The preparatory work for toxicological evaluations of food additives and contaminants by the Joint FAO-WHO Expert Committee on Food Additives is actively supported by certain of the member states that contribute to the work of the International Program on Chemical Safety.

FARNESOL • A flavoring agent that occurs naturally in ambrette seed, star anise, cassia, linden flowers, oils of muskseed, citronella, rose, and balsam. Used in berry, apricot, banana, cherry, melon, peach, citrus, fruit, raspberry, and strawberry flavorings for beverages, ice cream, ices, candy, baked goods, and gelatin-desserts. Used in perfumery to emphasize the odor of sweet floral perfumes such as lilac. Mildly toxic when ingested. Caused mutations in laboratory animals.

FASEB • Abbreviation for the Federation of American Societies for Experimental Biology, members of which evaluate studies for the FDA.

FAT • The most concentrated source of food energy and very necessary to health. Fat deposits provide insulation and protection for body structure as well as a storehouse for energy. Food fats are carriers of fat-soluble vitamins and include certain essential unsaturated fatty acids *(see)*. Saturated fats contain only single-bond carbon linkages and are the least active chemically. They are usually solid at room temperature. Most animal fats are saturated. The common saturated fats are acetic, butyric, caproic, caprylic, capric, lauric, myristic, palmitic, stearic, arachidic, and behenic. Butterfat, coconut oil, and peanut oil are high in saturated fats. Unsaturated fats contain one or more double-bond carbon linkages and are usually liquid at room temperature. Vegetable oils and fish oils most frequently contain unsaturated fats. Among the unsaturated fats are caproleic, lauroleic, myristoleic, palmitoleic, oleic, petroselinic, vaccenic, linoleic, linolenic, elae-sosearic, gadoleic, arachidonic, and erucic.

FAT CAL • Listing on labels signifying calories from fat.

FAT FREE • Less than 0.5 grams per serving. However, manufacturers are permitted to "round down" and claim zero fat even if a product contains 0.6 grams of fat. Very few foods are actually complete fat free.

FATIGUE • Everyone's nose becomes "fatigued" when smelling a certain odor. No matter how much you like a fragrance, you can only smell it for a short interval. It is nature's way of protecting humans from overstimulation of the olfactory sense.

FAT REPLACERS • These additives are aimed at reducing a food's fat and calorie level while maintaining some of the desirable qualities of fat such as "mouth feel," texture, and flavor. Under FDA regulations, these additives usually fall into one of two categories: food additives or "generally recognized as safe" (GRAS) substances. Food additives must be evaluated for safety and approved by FDA before they can be marketed. They include substances with no proven track record of safety or with no known amount in food that may serve the purpose of fat replacement. Examples are polydextrose, carrageenan, and olestra *(see all)*, which are used as fat replacers. GRAS substances, on the other hand, are used in foods because they are generally recognized as safe by scientists because of their long history of use in foods. Examples of such fat replacers are cellulose gel, dextrins, guar gum, and gum arabic. Fat replacers may be carbohydrate, protein, or fat-based substances.

FATTY ACIDS • One of any mixture of liquid and solid acids, capric, caprylic, lauric, myristic, oleic, palmitic, and stearic. In combination with glycerin they form fat. Necessary for normal growth and skin. In foods they are used as emulsifiers, binders, and lubricants, and defoamer components in the processing of beet sugar and yeast. Polyglycerol esters of fatty acids are prepared from edible fats, oils, corn, cottonseed, palm, fruit, peanut, safflower, and soybean oils, lard, and tallow. Used as emulsifiers and defoaming agents in beet sugar and yeast production, and as lubricant binders and components in the manufacture of other food additives. Fatty acid salt (one or more of the aluminum, ammonium, calcium, magnesium potassium, and sodium salts of all the above fatty acids) are used as emulsifiers, binders, and anticaking agents. A free fatty acid (FFA) is the uncombined fatty acid present in a fat. Some raw oils may contain as much as 3 percent FFA. These are removed in the refining process and refined fats and oils ready for use as foods usually have extremely low FFA content. No known toxicity. *See* Stearic Acid.

FATTY ALCOHOLS • Hexyl, Octyl, Decyl, Cetyl, Steryl, Lauryl, Myristyl. Solid alcohols made from acids and widely used in cosmetics. Cetyl and stearyl alcohols form an occlusive film to keep skin moisture from evaporating and impart a velvety feel to the skin. Lauryl and myristyl are used in detergents and creams. In foods, synthetic fatty alcohols include hexyl, octyl, decyl, lauryl, myristyl, cetyl, and stearyl alcohols. They are used as substitutes for the corresponding naturally derived fatty alcohols. Very low toxicity.

FDA (FOOD and DRUG ADMINISTRATION) • The U.S. Food and Drug Administration is part of the Public Health Service of the U.S. Department of Health and Human Services. It is the regulatory agency responsible for ensuring the safety and wholesomeness of all foods sold in interstate commerce except meat, poultry, and eggs, which are under the jurisdiction of the U.S. Department of Agriculture. FDA develops standards for the composition, quality, nutrition, safety, and labeling of foods including food and color additives. It conducts research to improve detection and prevention of contamination. It collects and interprets data on nutrition, food additives, and pesticide residues. The agency also inspects food plants, imported food products, and feed mills that make feeds containing medications or nutritional supplements that are destined for human consumption. And it regulates radiation-emitting products such as microwave ovens. FDA also enforces pesticide tolerances established by the Environmental Protection Agency for all domestically produced and imported foods, except for foods under USDA jurisdiction.

FD and C COLORS • Food, Drug, and Cosmetic Colors. A color additive is a term to describe any dye, pigment, or other substance capable of coloring a food, drug, or cosmetic, on any part of the human body. In 1900, there were more than eighty dyes used to color food. There were no regulations and the same dye used to color clothes could also be used to color candy. In 1906, the first comprehensive legislation for food colors was passed. There were only seven colors, which, when tested, were shown to be composed of known ingredients which demonstrated no harmful effects. Those colors were orange, erythrosine, ponceau 3R, amaranth, indigotin, naphthol yellow, and light green. A voluntary system of certification for batches of color dyes was set up. In 1938, new legislation was passed, superseding the 1906 act. The colors were given numbers instead of chemical names and every batch had to be certified. There were fifteen food colors in use at the time. In 1950, children were made ill by certain coloring used in candy and popcorn. These incidents led to the delisting of FD and C Orange No. 1, Orange No. 2, and FD and C Red No. 32. Since that time, because of experimental evidence of possible harm, Red 1, Yellow 1, 2, 3, and 4 have also been delisted. Violet 1 was removed in 1973. In 1976, one of the most widely used of all colors, FD and C Red No. 2, was removed because it was found to cause tumors in rats. In 1976, Red No. 4 was banned for coloring maraschino cherries (its last use), and carbon black was also banned, because both contain cancer-causing agents.

Earlier, in 1960, scientific investigations were required by law to determine the suitability of all colors in use for permanent listing. Citrus Red No. 2 (limited to 2 ppm) for coloring orange skins has been permanently listed; Blue No. 1, Red No. 3, Yellow No. 5, and Red No. 40 are permanently listed but without any restrictions. In 1959, the Food and Drug Administration approved the use of "lakes," in which the dyes are mixed with alumina hydrate to make them insoluble. *See* FD and C Lakes.

The other food coloring additives remained on the "temporary list." The provisional list permitted colors then in use to continue on a provisional, or interim, basis pending completion of studies to determine whether the colors should be permanently approved or terminated. FD & C Red No. 3 (erythrosin) is permanently listed for use in food and ingested drugs and provisionally listed for cosmetics and externally applied drugs. It is used in foods such as gelatins, cake mixes, ice cream, fruit cocktail cherries, bakery goods, and sausage casings.

The FDA postponed the closing date for the provisionally listed color additives—FD and C Red No. 3, D&C Red No. 33, and D&C Red No. 36—to May 2, 1988, to allow additional time to study "complex scientific and legal questions about the colors before deciding to approve or terminate their use in food, drugs, and cosmetics." The agency asked for sixty days to consider the impact of the October 1987 U.S. Court of Appeals ruling that there is no exception to the Delaney Amendment *(see)*, which says that cancer causing agents may not be added to food. On July 13, 1988, the Public Citizens Health Research Group announced that the FDA agreed to revoke by July 15, 1988, the permanent listing of four color additives used in drugs and cosmetics—D&C Red No. 8, D&C Red No. 9, D&C Red No. 19, and D&C Orange No. 17. In a unanimous decision in October 1987, the U.S. Court of Appeals for the District of Columbia said the FDA lacked legal authority to approve two of the colors, D&C Orange No. 17 and D&C Red No. 19, since they had been found to induce cancer in laboratory animals. The Supreme Court ruled against an appeal on April 18, 1988. Meanwhile, Public Citizen also brought a similar suit, challenging the use of D&C Red No. 8 and D&C Red 9, which was before the U.S. Circuit Court of Appeals in Philadelphia. Under an agreement between FDA and Public Citizen, the case was sent back to the FDA, and the agency delisted these colors as well as D&C Orange No. 17 and D&C Red No. 19. Other countries as well as the World Health Organization maintain there are inconsistencies in safety data and in the banning of some colors, which in turn affects international commerce. As of this writing, there is still a great deal of confusion about the colors, with the FDA maintaining that the cancer risk is minimal—as low as one in a billion—while groups such as Nader's Public Citizen maintain that any cancer risk for a food additive is unacceptable. In 1990, the lakes of Red. No. 3 were removed for all uses from the approved list. The color itself was also removed in 1990 for cosmetic and external drug use. It is still, as of this writing, approved for food and ingested drugs.

FD and C BLUE NO. 1 • Brilliant Blue FD and C. A bright blue, coal-tar derivative, triphenylmethane, it is used as a coloring in bottled soft drinks, gelatin desserts, ice cream, ices, dry drink powders, candy, confections, bakery products, cereals, and puddings. It is also used for hair colorings, face powders, and other cosmetics. May cause allergic reactions. On the FDA permanent list of color additives. Rated 1A—that is, completely acceptable for nonfood use—by the World Health Organization. However, it produces malignant tumors at the site of injection and by ingestion in the rat. Manganese dioxide is now permitted in the manufacturing process. *See* Colors.

FD and C BRILLIANT BLUE NO. 1 ALUMINUM LAKE • Aluminum salt of certified of FD and C Brilliant Blue No. 1 *(see)*. Can be used around the eye in cosmetics. Also permitted for drug use. *See* FD and C Colors, Lakes.

FD and C BLUE NO. 2 • Indigotin. Indigo Carmine. A royal blue powder, a coal-tar derivative, triphenylmethane, almost always contains sodium chloride or sulfate. Easily faded by light. Used in bottled soft drinks, bakery products, cereals, candy, confections, and dry drink powders. Is also in mint-flavored jelly, frozen desserts, candy, confections, and rinses and as a dye in kidney tests and for testing milk. It is a sensitizer in the allergic. Produces malignant tumors at the site of injection when introduced under the skin of rats. The World Health Organization gives it a toxicology rating of B—available data not entirely sufficient to meet requirements acceptable for food use. Permanently listed for foods and drugs in 1987. *See* FD and C Colors.

FD and C CITRUS RED No. 2 • Found in 1960 to damage internal organs and to be a weak cancer-causing agent. Permitted for use only to color orange skins. The World Health Organization said the color has been shown to cause cancer and that toxicological data available were inadequate to allow the determination of a safe limit; they recommended that it not be used as a food color. The FDA ruled on October 28, 1971, that the results of several rodent studies and one dog study using both oral and injected Citrus Red No. 2 showed either no adverse effect or no adverse effect levels. No abnormalities in urinary bladders were reported. The FDA noted that a paper presented in 1965 by the University of Otega Medical School reported a significant level of urinary bladder cancers in rodents fed the dye for up to twenty-four months. The FDA said that since slides of the tissues in photographs were not yet available for examination, and since there has been no confirmation of the studies, the listing of Citrus Red No. 2 should remain unchanged until the Otega results can be confirmed by examination. *See* FD and C Colors.

FD and C GREEN NO. 1 • Guinea Green B. A dull, dark green powder used as a coloring in bottled soft drinks. The certified color industry did not apply for the extension of this color because of the small demand for its use, so it was automatically deleted from the list of color additives in 1966. Rated E by the World Health Organization, meaning it was found to be harmful and not to be used in food. No longer authorized for use by the FDA. *See* FD and C Colors.

FD and C GREEN NO. 2 • Light Green S.F. Yellow. Coloring used in bottled soft drinks. Because of lack of demand for this color, the certified color industry did not petition for extension and it was automatically deleted in 1966. It produces tumors at the site of injection under the skin of rats. No longer authorized for use by the FDA. *See* FD and C Colors.

FD and C GREEN NO. 3 • Fast Green. A sea green color permanently listed for use in food, drugs, and cosmetics, except in the area of the eye, by the FDA in 1983. Used as a coloring in mint-flavored jelly, frozen desserts, gelatin desserts, candy, confections, baking products, and cereals. Has been suspected of being a sensitizer in the allergic. On the FDA permanent list of approved color additives. Produces malignant tumors at the site of injection when introduced under the skin of rats. The World Health Organization gives it a toxicology rating of 1A, meaning that it is completely acceptable. *See* FD and C Colors.

FD and C LAKES • Aluminum or Calcium Lakes. Lakes are pigments prepared by combining FD and C colors with a form of aluminum or calcium, which makes the colors insoluble. Aluminum and calcium lakes are used in confection and candy products and for dyeing eggshells and other products that are adversely affected by water. *See* FD and C Colors for toxicity.

FD and C RED NO. 2 • Amaranth. Formerly one of the most widely used cosmetic and food colorings. A dark, reddish-brown powder that turns bright red when mixed with fluid. A monoazo color, it was used in lipsticks, rouges, and other cosmetics as well as in cereals, maraschino cherries, and desserts. The safety of this dye was questioned by the American scientists for more than twenty years. Two Russian scientists found that FD and C Red No. 2 prevented some pregnancies and caused some stillbirths in rats. The FDA ordered manufacturers using the color to submit data on all food, drug, and cosmetic products containing it. Controversial tests at the FDA's National Center for Toxicological Research in Arkansas showed that in high doses Red No. 2 caused a statistically significant increase in a variety of cancers in female rats. The dye was banned by the FDA in January 1976.

FD and C RED NO. 3 • Erythrosin. Bluish Pink. A cherry red coal-tar derivative, a xanthene color, used in toothpaste, canned fruit cocktail, ice cream, hot dogs, barbecued potato chips, cereals, puddings, fruit salad, sherbets, gelatin desserts, cherry pie mix (up to .01 percent), candy, confections, and mixes as maraschino cherries. Has been determined a carcinogen. It was reported in 1981 by NIH researchers that Red. No. 3 may interfere with transmission of nerve impulses in the brain. It contains iodine and has been shown to affect the thyroid glands of laboratory animals but not of humans. Children who eat large amounts of artificially colored cherries, gelatin desserts, and other FD and C Red No. 3 colored products could be at risk. *See* FD and C Colors. The FDA was supposed to permanently list this color in 1988 but postponed the ruling "to allow the agency additional time to study complex scientific and legal questions about the color before deciding to approve or terminate its use in food." Now permanently listed for food and ingested drugs, its lake use was terminated February 1, 1990. All cosmetic uses were terminated February 1, 1990. In 1996, Red No. 3 was found to be a cancer-causing agent and may contribute to breast cancer. Scientists at Oak Ridge National Laboratory and the Northeastern Illinois University reported Red No. 3 causes breast cancer in the laboratory. When the dye was added to a human cell culture, genetic damage and rapid cell growth occurred even when the concentration of the dye was quite low. The cells responded as if they had been exposed to estrogen, which damaged genetic material and caused rapid reproduction. It is still permitted in food but its lake *(see)* was removed from all uses while Red No. 3 itself was removed from the list for use in cosmetics and external drugs. The FDA has said that it intends "to propose rescinding" its use in food and internal drugs. That was in 1990.

FD and C RED NO. 3 ALUMINUM LAKE • The aluminum salt of certified FD and C Red No. 3 *(see)*. Was terminated February 1, 1990. *See* FD and C Colors, Lakes.

FD and C RED NO. 4 • A monoazo color and coal tar. Used in mouthwashes, bath salts, and hair rinses. The FDA banned it in food in 1964 when it was shown to damage the adrenal glands and bladders of dogs. The agency relented and gave it provisional license for use in maraschino cherries. It was banned in all food in

1976 because it was shown to cause urinary bladder polyps and atrophy of the adrenal glands in animals. It was also banned in orally taken drugs but is still permitted in cosmetics for external use only. *See* also FD and C Colors.

FD and C RED NO. 20 • Permanently listed by the FDA in 1983 for general use in drugs and cosmetics (except in areas around the eyes).

FD and C RED NO. 22 • Permanently listed by the FDA in 1983 for general use in drugs and cosmetics (except in areas around the eyes).

FD and C RED NO. 40 • Allura Red AC. Newest color. Used widely in the cosmetic industry. Approved in 1971, Allied Chemical has an exclusive patent on it. It is substituted for FD and C Red No. 4 in many cosmetics, food, and drug products. Permanently listed because unlike the producers of "temporary" colors, this producer supplied reproductive data. However, many American scientists feel that the safety of Red No. 40 is far from established particularly because all the tests were conducted by the manufacturer. Therefore, the dye should not have received a permanent safety rating. The National Cancer Institute reported that *p*-credine, a chemical used in preparation of Red No. 40 was carcinogenic in animals. In rats, a high (3,800–8,350 mg/kg) oral dose of the coloring caused adverse reproductive effects. The FDA permanently listed Red No. 40 for use in foods and ingested drugs and cosmetics, including use around the eye area. Its lake *(see)* is permitted only for drug and cosmetic use. *See also* Azo Dyes and FD and C Colors.

FD and C VIOLET NO. 1 • Used as a coloring matter in gelatin desserts, ices, carbonated beverages, dry drink powders, candy, confections, bakery products, cereals, puddings, and as the dye used for the Department of Agriculture's meat stamp. A Canadian study in 1962 showed the dye caused cancer in 50 percent of the rats fed the dye in food. The FDA did not consider this valid evidence since the exact nature of the dye used could not be determined and all records and specimens were lost and not available for study. Furthermore, previous and subsequent studies have not confirmed evidence of Violet 1 causing cancer in rats. However, a two-year study with dogs did show noncancerous lesions on the dog's ears after being fed Violet 1. The FDA again felt the study was not adequate but that the ear lesions did appear to be dye-related and that perhaps two years may be too short a period to determine their eventual outcome. The FDA ruled on October 28, 1971, that Violet 1 should remain provisionally listed pending the outcome of a new dog study to be started as soon as possible and to last seven years. The FDA finally banned the use of Violet 1 in 1973. In 1976, however, the U.S. Department of Agriculture found that Violet 1 was still being used as a "denaturant" on carcasses, meats, and food products. The USDA ruled that any such use of mixing Violet 1 with any substance intended for food use would cause the final product to be "adulterated." *See* FD and C Colors.

FD and C YELLOW NO. 5 • Tartrazine. A lemon yellow coal tar derivative, is a pyrazole color used in prepared breakfast cereals, imitation strawberry, jelly, bottled soft drinks, gelatin desserts, ice cream, sherbets, dry drink powders, candy, confections, bakery products, spaghetti, and puddings. Also used as a coloring in hair rinses, hair-waving fluids, and in bath salts. Causes allergic reactions in persons sensitive to aspirin. The certified color industry petitioned for permanent listing of this color in February 1966, with no limitations other than good manufacturing practice. However, in February 1966, the FDA proposed the listing of this color with a maximum rate of use of 300 ppm in food. The color industry had objected to the limitations. Yellow No. 5 was thereafter permanently listed as a color additive without restrictions. Rated 1A by the World Health Organization—acceptable in food. It is estimated that half the aspirin-sensitive people plus 47,000 to 94,000 others in the nation are sensitive to this dye. It is used in about 60 percent of both over-the-counter and prescription drugs. Efforts were made to ban this color in over-the-counter pain relievers, antihistamines, oral decongestants, and prescription anti-inflammatory drugs. Aspirin-sensitive patients have been reported to develop life-threatening asthmatic symptoms when ingesting Yellow No. 5. Since 1981, it is supposed to be listed on the label if it is used. Its lake *(see)* is for drug and cosmetic use only. *See* FD and C Colors. There is reported use of the chemical; it has not yet been assigned for toxicology literature.

FD and C YELLOW NO. 5 ALUMINUM LAKE • For drug and cosmetic use only. *See* FD and C Yellow No. 5, Colors, Lakes.

FD and C YELLOW NO. 6 • Monoazo. Sunset Yellow FCF. A coal-tar, monoazo color, used in carbonated beverages, bakery products, candy, confectionery products, gelatin desserts, and dry drink powders. It is also used in hair rinses as well as other cosmetics. It is not used in products that contain fats and oils. Since there is evidence that this causes allergic reactions, alcoholic beverages that contain it must list it on the label according to the Bureau of Alcohol. Rated 1A by the World Health Organization—acceptable in foods. Permanently listed December 22, 1986. In 1989, a ruling went into effect that it had to be listed on the labels because of its ability to induce allergic reactions. *See* FD and C Colors. There is reported use of the chemical; it has not yet been assigned for toxicology literature.

FD and C YELLOW NO. 6 ALUMINUM LAKE • *See* FD and C Yellow No. 6, Colors, Lakes.

FECULOSE STARCH ACETATE • *See* Modified Starch.

FENAMIPHOS • A wormkiller used in animal feeds, pineapples, and raisins. FDA's residue tolerance is 25 ppm in citrus oil, 0.3 ppm in raisins, 5 ppm in dried apple pomace, 2.5 ppm in citrus molasses, 10 ppm in pineapple bran, and 3 ppm in raisin waste when used for animal feed. EPA considers it extremely hazardous. Poison by ingestion, inhalation, and skin contact.

FENARIMOL • White odorless crystals used as a fungicide in animal feed and apples. Limited to 0.2 ppm in wet and dry apple pomace when used for animal feed. The FDA residue tolerance for meat and meat byproducts of cattle, goats, hogs, or sheep is 0.01 ppm; as a residue in fat, kidney, and livers of cattle, sheep, hogs, goats, and poultry, it is 0.1; in eggs, 0.01; in milk 0.003. Moderately toxic by ingestion. Caused mutations in experimental animals.

FENBENDAZOLE • Panacur. Animal drug used to combat worms in animal feed and in beef and pork. Tolerance of residues in liver of cattle is 0.8 ppm, 5 ppm in swine muscle, and 20 ppm in swine kidney and skin. Can cause mutations.

FENCHOL • *See* Fenchyl Alcohol.

d-**FENCHONE** • A synthetic flavoring occurring naturally in common fennel *(see)*. It is an oily liquid with a camphor smell and practically insoluble in water. Used in berry, liquor, and spice flavorings for beverages, ice cream, ices, candy, baked goods, and liquors. Used medically as a counter irritant.

FENCHYL ALCOHOL • A synthetic berry, lime, and spice flavoring agent for beverages, ice cream, ices, candy, and baked goods. No known toxicity.

FENNEL • Common. Sweet. One of the earliest known herbs from the tall beautiful shrub. The fennel flowers appear in June and are bright yellow, with a characteristic fennel taste. Common fennel is used as a sausage and spice flavoring for beverages, baked goods, meats, and condiments. Sweet fennel has the same function but includes ice cream, ices, and candy. Sweet fennel oil is used in raspberry, fruit, licorice, anise, rye, sausage, root beer, sarsaparilla, spice, wintergreen, and birch beer flavorings for beverages, ice cream, ices, candy, baked goods, gelatin desserts, condiments, meats, and liquors. Organic cosmeticians use compresses of fennel tea to soothe inflamed eyelids and watery eyes. May cause allergic reactions. GRAS.

FENOXAPROP-ETHYL • Acclaim. Furore. Puma. Whip. A selective post-emergent herbicide to control grassy weeds in broad-leaved crops and turf grass. The FDA limits residue to 0.05 ppm on cottonseed, peanuts, peanut hulls, rice grain, and soybeans. The tolerance limits in meat, meat byproducts, and fat of cattle, goats, hogs and sheep is also 0.05 ppm, and in milk, 0.02 ppm.

FENPROSTALENE • Bovilene. An animal drug used to treat beef. FDA residue limits 20 ppb in liver; from 10 to 30 ppm in uncooked edible parts, and 100 ppb at injection site in cattle. A prostaglandin used to induce abortion in feedlot heifers and for estrus control in beef and nonlactating dairy cattle.

FENRIDAZON • A pesticide. The residues allowed by the FDA in fat, meat, and meat byproducts of cattle, goats, hogs, and sheep is 0.5 ppm. Residues in kidney and liver of cattle, goats, hogs, and sheep is 1 ppm. Residues in eggs and milk is 0.05 ppm and in poultry, fat, meat, and meat byproducts, 0.3 ppm.

FENTHION • Mercaptophos. Widely used insecticide in fish, meat, and sauces. FDA limits residues in grass, alfalfa, and rice as well as in fat, meat, and meat byproducts of hogs, poultry, and in milk to 1 ppm. EPA Genetic Toxicology Program *(see)*. A human poison by any route. Caused tumors and birth defects in experimental animals. *See* Organophosphates.

FENUBTATIN OXIDE • A spider and mite-killing compound. The FDA now has a project under way to develop a method to evaluate residues on apples, oranges, and cucumbers to toxicity. At this writing, the agency does not have a method to identify this pesticide.

FENUGREEK SEED • Greek Hay. An annual herb grown in southern Europe, North Africa, and India. The seeds are used in making curry. Fenugreek is a butter, butterscotch maple, black walnut, and spice flavoring for beverages, ice cream, ices, candy, baked goods, syrups, meats, and condiments. The *extract (see)* is a butter, butterscotch, caramel, chocolate, coffee, fruit, maple, meat, black walnut, walnut, root beer, spice, and vanilla flavoring agent for beverages, ice cream, ices, pickles, liquors, and icings. The *oleoresin (see)* is a fruit, maple, and nut flavoring agent for beverages, ice cream, ices, candy, baked goods, puddings, and syrups. It is also used in hair tonic, supposedly to prevent baldness; also added to powders, poultices, and ointments. GRAS.

FENVALERATE • Sumifly. An insecticide used in animal feed, sunflower seeds, and tomatoes. Insecticide residue tolerance of 0.05 ppm on all food items. Limitation of 20 ppm in animal feed. Cyanide and its compounds are on the Community Right-To-Know List. Poison by ingestion. Moderately toxic by skin contact. Highly toxic to fish and bees. Corrosive and causes eye damage. A skin irritant.

FERMENTED AMMONIATED CONDENSED WHEY • *See* Whey.

FERMENTATION DERIVED MILK-CLOTTING ENZYME • Used in the production of cheese as permitted by Standards of Identity *(see)*.

FERRIC AMMONIUM CHLORIDE • A nutrient. GRAS. *See* Ferric Chloride.

FERRIC CHLORIDE • Flavoring agent for various foods. EPA Genetic Toxicology Program *(see)*. Withdrawn as a coloring agent. Moderately toxic by ingestion. Corrosive. Causes adverse reproductive effects in experimental animals. GRAS as a nutrient.

FERRIC CHOLINE CITRATE • *See* Iron Salts.

FERRIC CITRATE • White crystals odorless with a metallic taste. Used as a nutrient supplement in various foods. GRAS. *See* Ferric Chloride.

FERRIC ORTHOPHOSPHATE • *See* Iron Salts.

FERRIC PHOSPHATE • A nutrient supplement. The final report to the FDA of the Select Committee on GRAS Substances stated in 1980 that there is no evidence in the available information that it is a hazard to the public when used as it is now and should continue its GRAS status with limitations on the amounts that can be added to food. *See* Iron Salts.

FERRIC PYROPHOSPHATE and FERRIC SODIUM PYROPHOSPHATE • Nutrients. There is reported use of the chemical; it has not yet been assigned for toxicology literature by the FDA. *See* Iron Salts. GRAS.

FERRIC SULFATE • A flavoring agent. GRAS. There is reported use of the chemical; it has not yet been assigned for toxicology literature. *See* Iron Salts.

FERROCYANIDE SALTS • Salts of ferrocyanic acid obtained by the reaction of cyanide with an iron sulfate. Used as a coloring.

FERROCHOLINATE • Greenish brown solid used as a nutrient supplement. *See* Iron Salts.

FERROUS ASCORBATE • Blue violet solid used as a nutrient supplement. GRAS. *See* Iron Salts.

FERROUS CARBONATE • A nutrient supplement. GRAS. *See* Iron Salts.

FERROUS CITRATE • A nutrient supplement. GRAS. *See* Iron Salts.

FERROUS FUMARATE • Dietary supplement. GRAS. *See* Iron Salts.

FERROUS GLUCONATE • Gluconic Acid. Iron Salt. Iron Gluconate. Ferronicum. Used as a food coloring for ripe olives only, it is a yellowish gray. It is also used to treat iron-deficiency anemia. It may cause gastrointestinal disturbances.

When painted on mouse skin in 2,600 milligram doses per kilogram of body weight, it caused tumors. GRAS. There is reported use of the chemical; it has not yet been assigned for toxicology literature.

FERROUS LACTATE • Lactic Acid. Iron Salt. Iron Lactate. Greenish-white crystals that have a slightly peculiar odor. It is derived from the interaction of calcium lactate with ferrous sulfate or the direct action of the lactic acid on iron fillings. It is used as a food additive and dietary supplement. Causes tumors when injected under the skin of mice. There is no reported use of the chemical and there is no toxicology information available. GRAS.

FERROUS SULFATE • Green or Iron Vitriol. Pale bluish green, odorless crystals, efflorescent in dry air. An astringent and deodorant. Once used in hair dyes. No longer authorized for use. A source of iron used medicinally. *See* Iron Salts. GRAS.

FERROUS SULFATE HEPTAHYDRATE • Pale green crystals or granules used as clarifying agent, dietary supplement, nutrient supplement, processing aid, or stabilizer in baking mixes, cereals, infant foods, pasta products, and wine. Moderately toxic by ingestion. Caused mutations in rats. *See* Iron Salts. Withdrawn by the FDA as a coloring agent for food.

FERULA ASAFOETIDA • *See* Asafoetida Extract.

FIBER • Commonly termed "bulk"—the indigestible carbohydrates, including cellulose, hemicellulose, and gums. Fiber is added to food to reduce calorie content, as a thickening agent, and a stabilizer. If an apple a day keeps the doctor away, it may be because of the fiber content. Scientists have suspected that the high intestinal cancer rate in the United States may be linked to the 80 percent decrease of consumption of fiber in the average diet during the past century. Essentially, there are three classes of fiber found in the fruit, leaves, stems, seeds, flowers, and roots of different plants. The first class is the insoluble cellulose found in the plant-cell wall. Some of the other polysaccharides constitute a second class and are also found in the cell wall (hemicellulose and pectic polyerms), in the endosperm of seeds (mucilages), or in the plant's surface (gums). The third class, the lignins, are noncarbohydrates that infiltrate and contribute to the death of the plant cell, which then becomes part of the woody reinforcing plant structure.

Enzymes from a number of the more than four hundred kinds of bacteria in the human colon are capable of digesting many components of plant fiber. Doctors have found that the water-holding capacity of some fibers may be helpful in treating colon disease. The fiber's bile absorption properties might be used in modifying cholesterol metabolism. Plant fibers are also capable of binding trace metals and bile acids. These properties modify the action of the gut contents. Fibers pass through the gut somewhat like a sponge, probably altering metabolism in the intestine. The fibers appear to protect intestinal cells by removing foreign substances, such as carcinogens produced by charbroiling. Increased fiber consumption has been recommended for relief of some symptoms of diverticular disease, irritable bowel syndrome, and constipation.

FICIN • An enzyme occurring in the latex of tropical trees. A buff-colored powder with an acrid odor. Absorbs water. Concentrated and used as a meat tenderizer. Ten to twenty times more powerful than papain tenderizers. Used to clot milk, as a protein digestant in the brewing industry, and as a chill-proofing agent in beer. Also in cheese as a substitute for rennet in the coagulation of milk, and used for removing casings from sausages. Can cause irritation to the skin, eyes, and mucous membranes, and in large doses can cause purging.

FIELD POPPY EXTRACT • Extract of the petals of *Papaver rhoeas* used in coloring and as an odorant.

FILLED MILK • A combination of skim milk and vegetable oil to replace milk fat. Usually has the same amount of protein and calories as whole milk. Used as a milk substitute. It often contains the high cholesterol fatty acids *(see)* of coconut oil. Nontoxic.

FINOCCHIO • *See* Fennel.

FIR NEEDLE OIL • Fir Oil. Pine. Balsam. An essential oil obtained by the steam distillation of needles and twigs of several varieties of pine trees native to both Canada and Siberia. Used as a scent in perfumes and as a flavoring agent.

FISH GLYCERIDES • *See* Fish Oil and Glycerin.

FISH OIL • A fatty oil from fish or marine mammals used in soap manufacturing. Rich in Omega-3 fatty acids that were reported in the 1980s to reduce fats in the blood and are believed to reduce the risk of coronary artery disease. The final report to the FDA of the Select Committee on GRAS Substances stated in 1980 that it should continue its GRAS status for food packaging with no limitations other than good manufacturing practices. There is reported use of the chemical; it has not yet been assigned for toxicology literature.

FISH PROTEIN CONCENTRATE • Dietary supplement. No known toxicity.

5-A-DAY • Refers to the dietary recommendation to consume five servings of fruits and vegetables every day. The tagline 5-a-day became a promotional message in campaigns to increase fruits and vegetable consumption.

FIXATIVE • A chemical that reduces the tendency of an odor or flavor to vaporize, by making the odor or flavor last longer. An example is musk *(see),* which is used in perfume and undecyl aldehyde as a fixative for citrus flavors.

FLAVONOIDS • A large group of compounds widely distributed throughout nature. They include quercetin, present in onion skins, and anthocyanins, the major commercially used group. *See* Bioflavonoids.

FLAVOR ENHANCERS • *See* Flavor Potentiators.

FLAVOR POTENTIATORS • One of the newest and fastest-growing categories of additives, potentiators enhance the total seasoning effect, generally without contributing any taste or odor of their own. They are effective in minute doses—in parts per million or even less. A potentiator produces no identifiable effect itself but exaggerates one's response. They alter the response of the sensory nerve endings on the tongue and in the nose. The first true potentiators in the United States were the 5′-nucleotides, which are derived from a natural seasoning long in use in Japan: small flakes of dry bonito (a tunalike fish) are often added to modify and improve the flavor of soups, and from bonito a 5'-nucleotide, disodium inosinate *(see)*, has been isolated and identified as a flavor potentiator. Another 5'-nucleotide is disodium guanylate *(see)*, one of the newer additives on the market, which gives one a sensation of "fullness" and "increased viscosity" when eating. The product is advertised as being able to give diners a sense of "full-bodied flavor" when ingesting a food containing it.

FLAVORING COMPOUND • A flavoring composed of two or more substances. The substances may be natural or synthetic, and they are usually closely guarded secrets. Normally, a flavoring compound is complete; that is, it is added to a food without any additional flavorings being necessary. A strawberry flavoring compound, for example, may contain twenty-eight separate ingredients before it is complete.

FLAVORINGS • There are more than two thousand flavorings added to foods, of which approximately five hundred are natural and the rest synthetic. This is the largest category of additive. Lemon and orange are examples of natural flavorings, while benzaldehyde and methyl salicylate *(see both)* are examples from the laboratory.

FLAXSEED • The seed of the flax plant may be "hidden" in cereals and milk of cows fed flaxseed. It is also in flaxseed tea and the laxative Flaxolyn. It is a frequent allergen when ingested, inhaled, or in direct contact. Flaxseeds are the source of linseed oil. Among other hidden sources are: dog food, hair-wave preparations, shampoos, hair tonics, depilatories, patent leather, insulating materials, rugs and some cloths, Roman meal, cough remedies, and muffins.

FLEABANE OIL • Oil of Canada Fleabane. Erigeron Oil. The pale yellow volatile oil from a fresh flowering herb. It takes it name from its supposed ability to drive away fleas. Used in fruit and spice flavorings for beverages, ice cream, ices, candy, baked goods, and sauces. No known toxicity.

FLUAZIFOP-BUTYL • A herbicide used on animal feed. FDA permits a residue of from 0.2 to 1.0 ppm on various feeds.

FLUCYTHRINATE • An herbicide used on animal feed. FDA tolerance is 10 ppm for apple pomace; 0.2 on cottonseed oil; 0.1 ppm in cotton seed, and corn grain, 2.0 on cabbage, 3.0 on corn forage, and 0.2 on sugar bagasse.

FLUORIDE • An acid salt used in toothpaste to prevent tooth decay. *See* Sodium Fluoride.

FLUORIDONE • A herbicide. The FDA residue tolerance in fish and crayfish is 0.05 ppm; as a residue in milk and eggs, 0.05 ppm; as a residue in fat, meat, and meat byproducts of cattle, goats, or hogs, 0.05 ppm. As a residue in kidney and liver of cattle, hogs, or goats, 0.1 ppm, and 0.1 to 1 ppm as a residue on various fruits and vegetables.

FLUORINE COMPOUNDS • Calcium Fluoride. Hydrofluorsillic Acid. Potassium Fluoride. Sodium Fluoride. Sodium Silicofluoride. All have been used in the fluoridation of water. Fluorides cross the placental barrier and the effects on the fetus are unknown. New clinical evidence shows that kidney disturbance sometimes is due to the amount of fluoride it contributes to the blood. Fluorine containing compounds (sodium, potassium, or calcium fluoride) are illegal. A petition for extension in dietary supplements was terminated in 1973. Addition of fluorine compounds to food is limited to that from fluoridation of public water supplies and to that resulting from the fluoridation of bottled water within limits set by the FDA.

4'-FLUORO-4-(4-[2-PYRIDYL]-1*p* IPERAZINYL)BUTYROPHENONE • Azaperone. Suicalm. A sedative and tranquilizer used on animals. Poison by ingestion.

FOAM INHIBITOR • An antifoaming agent such as dimethyl polysiloxane *(see)* used in chewing-gum bases, soft drinks, and fruit juices to keep them from foaming. *See* Defoaming Agent.

FOAM STABILIZERS • Used in soft drinks and brewing. *See* Vegetable Gums.

FOAMING AGENT • Used to help whipped topping peak when it is being whipped with cold milk. A commonly added foaming agent is sodium caseinate *(see)*.

FOLIC ACID • A yellowish orange compound and member of the vitamin B complex, used as a nutrient. Used in cosmetic emollients. Occurs naturally in liver, kidney, mushrooms, and green leaves. Aids in cell formation, especially red blood cells. In 1983, British researchers, in an article published in the prestigious British medical journal *The Lancet,* reported multivitamin supplementation given to pregnant women could prevent the birth of offspring with neural tube defect. In August 1989, the equally prestigious medical publication the *New England Journal of Medicine* carried an article by multiple authors from the National Institute of Child Health and Human Development's Neural Tube Study Group concluding that the use of multivitamins or folate-containing supplements by American women *does not* decrease the risk of having an infant with neural tube defect. Less than three months later, in November 1989, in the respected *Journal of the American Medical Association,* Harvard and Boston University researchers authored an article: "Multivitamin/Folic Acid Supplementation in Early Pregnancy Reduces the Prevalence of Neural Tube Defects." But wait, that's not the end of it. In March of 1993, four years later, The *Journal of the American Medical Association* carried an article by researchers at the Slone Epidemiology Unit, Boston University School of Medicine, concluding that pregnant women's intake of an over-the-counter multivitamin containing folic acid reduces the risk of neural tube defects by 60 percent. In the same issue, an editorial states: "One of the most exciting medical findings of the last part of the 20th century is that folic acid, a simple, widely available, water-soluble vitamin can prevent spina bifida [in which there is incomplete closure of the spine] and anencephaly [in which the brain fails to develop fully] (both are neural tube defects). Not since the rubella vaccine became available 30 years ago have we had a comparable opportunity for primary prevention of such common and serious birth defects."

As of January 1, 1998, manufacturers of enriched breads, flours, corn meals, pastas, rice, and other grain products were required to add the nutrient folic acid to their products—a move to reduce the risk of neural tube birth defects in newborns. Folic acid, when consumed in adequate amounts by women before and during early pregnancy, reduces the risk of such birth defects as spina bifida. It is estimated that folic acid supplementation will reduce by about two thousand per year the number of American babies born with the birth defect. It took ten years for United States government agencies to recommend that *"all women of child-bearing age in the United States who are capable of becoming pregnant should consume 0.4 mg. of folic acid per day for the purpose of reducing their risk of having a pregnancy affected by spina bifida or other neural tube defects.* The FDA denied a claim for folic acid and neural tube birth defects for packaging. However, it was wavering at this writing and may allow such a claim eventually.

FOOD-BORNE DISEASE • Disease, usually gastrointestinal, caused by organisms or their toxins carried in ingested food. Also commonly known as "food poisoning."

FOOD GUIDE PYRAMID • The Food Guide Pyramid is a graphic design used to communicate the recommended daily food choices contained in the 1995 Dietary Guidelines for Americans. The information provided is developed and promoted by the U.S. Department of Agriculture and the U.S. Department of Health and Human Services. The Food Guide Pyramid shows at its wide base what should form the foundation of a healthful diet—six to eleven servings—daily from the bread, cereal, rice, and pasta group. The next level up the tapered pyramid is divided between the vegetable group, three to five servings daily, and the fruit group, two to four servings daily. The next level up the narrowing pyramid is divided between the milk, yogurt, and cheese group, two to three servings daily, and the meat, poultry, fish, dry beans, eggs, and nuts group, two to three servings daily. The smallest part of the pyramid at the top shows the fats, oils, and sweets in the diet that should be used sparingly.

The Food Guide Pyramid's guide to daily food choices are:

- Eat a variety of foods.
- Balance the food you eat with physical activity—maintain or improve your weight.
- Choose a diet with plenty of grain products, vegetables, and fruits.
- Choose a diet low in fat, saturated fat, and cholesterol.
- Choose a diet moderate in sugars.
- Choose a diet moderate in salt and sodium.
- If you drink alcoholic beverages, do so in moderation.

FOOD RED 6 • Formerly Ext. FD and C Red No. 15, FD and C Red No. 1, and Ponceau 3R. One of the first approved certified coal-tar colors. Food Red 6 was delisted as a food additive as possibly harmful. Dark red powder, it changes to cherry red in solution. *See* FD and C Colors.

FOOD STANDARDS • Standards of Identity. The FDA and USDA previously established a "recipe" for about three hundred foods, such as peanut butter and mayonnaise, fixing the ingredients by law. Many of these foods were exempted from the need for ingredient listing. The new labeling law, effective in 1994, requires manufacturers to give full ingredient listings for all foods.

FOOD STARCH ESTERFIED WITH *n*-OCTENYL SUCCINIC ANHYDRIDE TREATED WITH BETA-AMYLASE • Esters *(see)* and enzymes such as beta-amylase change the properties of a compound, often making it more soluble or reducing its allergenic potential. *See* Modified Starch.

FOOD STARCH MODIFIED • Various chemicals are permitted in modifying food starch and are listed under individual chemical names. *See* Modified Starch.

FORMALDEHYDE • Paraformaldehyde. Preservative in defoaming agents and in animal feeds. A colorless gas obtained by the oxidation of methyl alcohol and generally used in watery solution. Formaldehyde generally is known as a disinfectant, germicide, fungicide, defoamer, and preservative, and is used in animal feed, in defoaming agents, and embalming fluid. One ounce taken by mouth causes death within two hours. Skin reaction after exposure. It is a highly reactive chemical that is damaging to the hereditary substances in the cells of several species. It causes lung cancer in rats and has a number of other harmful biological consequences. Researchers from the Division of Cancer Cause and Prevention of the National Cancer Institute recommended in April 1983 that since formaldehyde is involved in DNA damage and inhibits its repair, and potentiates the toxicity of X rays in human lung cells, and since it may act in concert with other chemical agents to produce mutagenic and carcinogenic effects, it should be "further investigated." The question is whether we ingest any formaldehyde when we ingest the animals that ate the feed and the products that had undergone "defoaming" by formaldehyde. The ADI *(see)* set for formaldehyde is 3 mg/kg of body weight. Researchers at Italy's University of Milano studied the health risk from consumption of cheese made using formaldehyde (Grana Padano) and concluded there was no appreciable health risk.

FORMALIN • Fungicide in water of salmon, trout, large mouth bass, catfish, and bluegills. *See* Formaldehyde.

FORMESAFEN SODIUM • A pesticide used on soybeans. FDA tolerance is 0.05 ppm on soybeans.

FORMETANATE HYDROCHLORIDE • A pesticide in citrus molasses resulting from application to growing fruit. The FDA tolerance is 10 ppm in citrus and 8 ppm on growing fruit.

FORMIC ACID • Colorless, pungent, highly corrosive, it occurs naturally in apples and other fruit. Used as a decalcifier and for dehairing hides. Chronic absorption is known to cause albuminuria—protein in the urine. It caused cancer when administered orally in rats, mice, and hamsters in doses from 31 to 49 milligrams per kilogram of body weight. Used as a preservative for silage. Silage is not supposed to be fed to livestock within four weeks of treatment. FDA residue tolerance is 2.25 percent of silage on a dry basis and 0.45 percent when direct cut.

FORMIC ETHER • *See* Ethyl Formate.

FORTIFIED • Fortification of food refers to the addition of nutrients such as vitamin C to breakfast drinks and vitamin D to milk. It actually increases the nutritional values of the original food.

FOS • Abbreviation for Fructooligosaccyarides *(see)*.

FRANKINCENSE • Aromatic gum resin obtained from African and Asian trees and used chiefly as incense. For food use, *see* Olibanum Extract.

FREE • Product contains none or only insignificant amounts of a substance.

FREE RADICALS • Certain oxygen molecules that are underlying factors in aging and degenerative diseases because they damage DNA, the blueprint for life, within the cells. They also adversely affect enzymes, the workhorses of the cells, and damage cell membranes. Free radicals are formed during the course of normal metabolism, as well as from exposure to cigarette smoke and other environmental influences. Fat-soluble antioxidants, beta-carotene and other carotenoids, as well as vitamins C and E and pycnogenol *(see),* are believed to fight the damage from free radicals.

FRESH • A food that has not been heat processed or frozen and supposedly contains no preservatives.

FRUCTOOLIGOSACCHARIDES (FOS) • Sugars that occur naturally in plants such as tomatoes, onions, and bananas. They are not digestible in the stomach and travel unabsorbed to the intestine. In the intestines they promote the growth of beneficial bacteria such as those used to culture yogurt. They are now used in poultry feed to enhance growth and reduce intestinal pathogens. Applications have been made to use them as a food additive for human foods.

FRUCTOSE • A sugar occurring naturally in large numbers of fruits and honey. It is the sweetest of the foodstuffs. It is also used as a medicine, preservative, common sugar, and to prevent sandiness in ice cream. Researchers at the General Clinical Research Center at the University of Colorado School of Medicine in Denver report that fructose is absorbed in the gastrointestinal tract more slowly than sugars like sucrose, which contain glucose. As a result, even though the body converts some fructose to glucose, 80 to 90 percent of the sugar is absorbed intact, and there is only a slight increase in blood glucose levels immediately after consumption. Fructose can be up to two times sweeter than sucrose. Recent advances in enzyme technology have made it possible to produce fructose on a commercial scale. It caused tumors in mice when injected under the skin in 5,000-milligram doses per kilogram of body weight.

FRUIT JUICE • Used to color foods consistent with good manufacturing practices. Permanently listed.

FSIS • Abbreviation for Food Safety and Inspection Service of the United States Department of Agriculture. Personnel are responsible for inspecting meat and poultry facilities.

FULLER'S EARTH • A white or brown naturally occurring earthy substance. A nonplastic variety of kaolin *(see)* containing an aluminum magnesium silicate. Used as an absorbent and to decolorize fats and oils. Used in dry shampoos, hair colorings, beauty masks, and as a dusting powder; also used for lubricants and soaps. No longer permitted in cosmetics.

FUMARIC ACID • White, odorless, derived from many plants and essential to vegetable and animal tissue respiration; prepared industrially. An acidulant used as a leavening agent and a dry acid for dessert powders and confections (up to 3 percent). Also as apple, peach, and vanilla flavoring agent for beverages, baked goods (1,300 ppm), and gelatin desserts (3,600 ppm). Used in baked goods as an antioxidant and as a substitute for tartaric acid *(see).*

FUMARIC ACID FERROUS SALT • A dietary supplement. *See* Ferrous Fumarate.

FUMIGANTS • Chemicals and gases used to kill pests on crops. Among those approved for use by the FDA are carbon tetrachloride with either carbon disulfide or ethylene chloride, with or without pentane; or methyl bromide. Also carbon disulfide, carbon tetrachloride, ethylene dichloride, and ethyl bromide. All are highly toxic and should be applied only by experts in their use.

FUNCTIONAL FOODS • Foods that may provide health benefits beyond basic nutrition.

FUNGAFLOR • Imazalil. Fungicide used in animal feed. Poison by ingestion and causes adverse reproductive effects in experimental animals.

FUNGAL PECTINASE • There is reported use of the chemical; it has not yet been assigned for toxicology literature. *See* Pectins.

FUNGI • A group of simple plantlike organisms that don't have the green coloring known as chlorophyll. Fungi include mushrooms, yeasts, rusts, molds, and smuts.

FURADAN • White crystalline solid widely used as an insecticide in animal feed. Limitation in animal feed is from 2 ppm in grape pomace to 24 ppm in peanut soap-stock fatty acids. Insecticide residue tolerance of 2 ppm in raisins. Extremely hazardous substance, it is on the EPA Genetic Toxicology Program *(see)*. Poisonous by inhalation, ingestion, and skin contact. Causes birth defects in experimental animals.

2-FURALDEHYDE • *See* Furfural.

2-FURAN ACROLEIN • *See* Furyl Acrolein.

FURCELLERAN • Sodium, Calcium, Potassium, and Ammonium. Extracted from red seaweed grown in northern European waters. The processed gum is a white, odorless powder soluble in water as an emulsifier, stabilizer, and thickener in foods. It is a natural colloid and gelling agent. Also used in puddings, ice cream, and jams, in products for diabetics, as a carrier for food preservatives, and in bactericides. It is also used in over-the-counter drugs for weight reducing and toothpastes. On the FDA list of additives to be studied for mutagenic, teratogenic, subacute, and reproductive effects since 1980. It is reportedly more stable than vegetable gums. There is reported use of the chemical; it has not yet been assigned for toxicology literature.

FURFURAL • Artificial Ant Oil. A colorless liquid with a peculiar odor. Occurs naturally in angelica root, apples, coffee, peaches, and skim milk. Used as a solvent, insecticide, fungicide, to decolor resins, and as a synthetic flavoring in butterscotch, butter, caramel, coffee, fruit, brandy, rum, rye, molasses, nut, and cassia flavorings for beverages, ice cream, ices, candy, gelatin, desserts, syrups (the biggest user; up to 30 ppm), and spirits. Darkens when exposed to air. It irritates mucous membranes and acts on the central nervous system. Causes tearing and inflammation of the eyes and throat. Ingestion or absorption of .06 grams produces persistent headache. Used continually, it leads to nervous disturbances and eye disorders (including photosensitivity). The FAO-WHO Expert Committee on Food Additives in June 1998 requested animal studies to investigate whether this additive interacts with DNA in mice and a ninety-day study in rats to identify a no-observed-effect level (NOEL) for liver damage.

FURFURYL ACETATE • Acetic Acid. A synthetic raspberry, fruit, and ginger ale flavoring for beverages, ice cream, ices, candy, baked goods, and chewing gum. No known toxicity.

FURFURYL ALCOHOL • A synthetic flavoring obtained mainly from corncobs and roasted coffee beans. Has a faint burning odor and a bitter taste. Used in butter, butterscotch, caramel, coffee, fruit, and brandy flavorings for beverages, ice cream, ices, candy, baked goods, gelatin desserts, and icings. It is poisonous.

FURFURYL MERCAPTAN • A synthetic fruit, liquor, rum, nut, chocolate, and spice flavoring agent that occurs naturally in coffee and is used for beverages, ice cream, ices, candy, and baked goods. No known toxicity.

2-FURFURYLIDENE BUTYRALDEHYDE • A synthetic fruit, liquor, rum, nut, and spice flavoring agent for beverages, ice cream, ices, candy, and baked goods. No known toxicity.

FURYL ACETONE • *See* (2-Furyl)-2-Propanone.

FURYL ACROLEIN • A synthetic coffee, fruit, cassia, and cinnamon flavoring agent for beverages, ice cream, ices, candy, baked goods, gelatin desserts, and puddings. No known toxicity.

4-(2-FURYL)-3-BUTEN-2-ONE • A synthetic nut, almond, and spice flavoring agent for beverages, ice cream, ices, candy, baked goods, and gelatin desserts. No known toxicity.

(2-FURYL)-2-PROPANONE • A synthetic fruit favoring agent for ice cream, ices, candy, and baked goods. No known toxicity.

FUSEL OIL (REFINED) • A synthetic flavoring that occurs naturally in cognac oil. It is also a product of carbohydrate fermentation to produce ethyl alcohol *(see)* and varies widely in composition. Used in grape, brandy, cordial, rum, rye, scotch, whiskey, and wine flavorings for beverages, ice cream, ices, candy, baked goods, chewing gum, gelatin desserts, puddings, and liquor. Commercial amyl alcohol *(see),* its major ingredient, is more toxic than ethyl alcohol and as little as thirty milligrams has caused death. Smaller amounts cause methemoglobinuria (blood cells in the urine) and kidney damage.

G

g • Abbreviation for *gram (see).*

a-GALACTOSIDASE • Derived from *Mortierella vinaceae,* it is an enzyme used in sugar beet production.

GALANGAL ROOT • East Indian Root. Chinese Ginger. The pungent aromatic *oil* of the galangal root is a bitters, vermouth, spice, and ginger ale flavoring agent for beverages. The *extract* is a bitters, fruit, liquor, spice, and ginger ale flavoring agent for beverages, ice cream, ices, candy, baked goods, and liquors. Related to true ginger, it was formerly used in cooking and in medicine to treat colic. No known toxicity. GRAS. There is reported use of the chemical; it has not yet been assigned for toxicology literature.

GALBANUM OIL • A yellowish to green or brown aromatic bitter gum resin from an Asiatic plant used as incense. The oil is a fruit, nut, and spice flavoring for beverages, ice cream, ices, candy, baked goods, and condiments. Has been used medicinally to break up intestinal gas and as an expectorant. No known toxicity. There is reported use of the chemical; it has not yet been assigned for toxicology literature.

GALLATES (DODECYL, OCTYL, and PROPYL) • These antioxidants are derived from gallic acid, obtained from tannins and molds. The FAO-WHO Expert Committee on Food Additives has held many meetings about these additives. Although the Committee noted there are similarities in the metabolism of the different gallates, it concluded that there was not enough evidence to allocate a group ADI for the gallates. In addition, a 150-day gavage study with dodecyl gallate revealed a no-observed-effect level (NOEL) that was ten-fold lower than the dietary NOEL for propyl gallate. In the ninety-day toxicity study in rats, propyl gallate administered in the diet at 7,450 mg per kg caused changes in blood, spleen, and liver. The Committee allocated an ADI of 0–1.4 mg per kg of body weight for propyl gallate. The Committee concluded that neither octyl or dodecyl gallate were likely to be cancer-causing or gene-toxic. Therefore, the Committee allocated temporary ADIs for these substances. With octyl gallate, a slight anemia was observed at 100 mg per kg of body weight per day in rats when it was administered for two generations. A temporary ADI of 0–01 mg per kg of body weight was allocated for octyl gallate. With dodecyl gallate, reduction in spleen weight and pathological changes in the liver, kidney, and spleen were observed in a 150-day study in rats in which the substance was administered by gavage. A temporary ADI of 0.05 mg per kg of body weight was allocated for dodecyl gallate based on a NOEL of 10 mg per kg of body weight per day in this study and a safety factor of 200. The Committee concluded that additional studies on dodecyl, octyl, and propyl gallate may help to explain the differences in toxicological potency of these compounds. If these studies do not resolve the issue, then the committee said long-term toxicity and cancer studies and gene toxicity studies "might be required."

GALLIC ACID • *See* Propyl Gallate.

GALLOTANNIC ACID • *See* Tannic Acid.

GAMBIR CATECHU • A flavoring. *See* Catechu Extract.

GAMBIR GUM • *See* Catechu Extract.

GARDEN ROSEMARY OIL • *See* Rosemary Extract.

GARDENOL • *See* a-Methylbenzyl Acetate.

GARLIC EXTRACT • An extract from *Allium sativum,* a yellowish liquid with a strong odor used in fruit and garlic flavorings. Garlic is a member of the onion family and was cultivated in Egypt from earliest times and known in China more than two thousand years ago. Garlic contains lots of potassium, fluorine, sulfur, phosphorus, vitamins A and C, as well as seventy-five different sulfur compounds. In addition it contains quercetin, cyanidin, and bioflavonoids *(see all)*. Garlic also contains selenium, which has been found to have anticancer potential. Garlic has been used since ancient times to treat all sorts of ailments, including the Great

Plague in Europe and dysentery during World War I. The herb has recently been found to contain antibiotic, antiviral, and antifungal ingredients. It has also been reported in the scientific literature that garlic may decrease nitrosamines, modulate cancer cell multiplication, increase immunity, and protect the body against ionizing radiation. Three Rutgers University researchers in 1992 reported at the American Chemical Society meeting in Washington, D.C., that chemicals in garlic may protect the liver from damage caused by large doses of the popular nonaspirin painkiller acetaminophen (it's in Tylenol and dozens of other painkillers and cold medications) and may prevent growth of lung tumors associated with tobacco smoke. Garlic also reportedly inhibits the production of prostaglandins *(see),* which may explain why allium oils have antitumor activity. Phytochemicals in garlic are under intensive study for their cholesterol-lowering, immune-enhancing, and cancer-preventive activity, GRAS.

GARLIC OIL • Yellow liquid with a strong odor, obtained from the crushed bulbs or cloves of the plant. Used in fruit and garlic flavorings for beverages, ice cream, ices, candy, baked goods, chewing gum, and condiments. Has been used medicinally to combat intestinal worms. Reevaluated and found to be GRAS by the FDA in 1976. *See* Garlic Extract.

GAS • A product from the controlled combustion in air of butane, propane, or natural gas. It is used for removing or displacing oxygen in the processing, storage, or packaging of citrus products, vegetable fats, vegetable oils, coffee, and wine. No known toxicity when used in packaging.

GASTRONOMY • The study and appreciation of good food and good eating, and a culture's culinary customs, style, and lore. Any interest or study of culinary pursuits relates essentially to the kitchen and cookery, and to the higher levels of education, training, and achievement of the professional chef and the chef apprentice.

GEL • A semisolid, apparently homogenous substance that may be elastic and jellylike (gelatin) or more or less rigid (silica gel) and that is formed in various ways such as by coagulation or evaporation.

GELATINS • Gelatin is a protein obtained by boiling skin, tendons, ligaments, or bones with water. It is colorless or slightly yellow, tasteless, and absorbs five to ten times its weight of cold water. Used as a food thickener and stabilizer and a base for fruit gelatins and puddings. Employed medicinally to treat malnutrition and brittle fingernails. Used in protein shampoos because it sticks to the hair and gives it "more body," peelable face masks, and as a fingernail strengthener. No known toxicity.

GELLAN GUM • Used as a stabilizer and thickener in various foods.

GENE • The smallest genetic unit of a chromosome. It is a piece of DNA which contains the hereditary information for the production of a protein.

GENET, ABSOLUTE • A natural flavoring from flowers used in fruit and honey flavorings for beverages, ice cream, ices, candy, baked goods, and chewing gum. The extract is a raspberry and fruit flavoring for beverages. There is reported use of the chemical; it has not yet been assigned for toxicology literature.

GENETIC TOXICOLOGY PROGRAM • The U.S. Environmental Protection Agency has certain chemicals under study to determine their effects on genes, the parts of the cell that carry inherited characteristics. Damage to the mechanisms of genes can lead to birth defects and cancer, as well as other illnesses.

GENTAMYCIN SULFATE • Garamycin Sulfate. An antibiotic used to treat pork and turkey. FDA residue limitations are 0.1 ppm in turkey and in swine muscle. This drug is also used to treat serious infections in humans and theoretically, resistance to the drug could build up by eating treated pork or turkey. Allergic reactions to the drug in the meat could also occur.

GENTIAN ROOT EXTRACT • The yellow or pale bitter root of central and southern European plants used in angostura, chocolate, cola, fruit, vermouth, maple, root beer, and vanilla flavorings for beverages, ice cream, ices, candy, and liquors. It has been used as a bitter tonic. There is reported use of the chemical; it has not yet been assigned for toxicology literature.

GERANIAL • *See* Citral.

GERANILDEHYDE • *See* Citral.

GERANIOL • Used in perfumery to compound artificial attar of roses and artificial orange blossom oil. Also used in depilatories to mask odors. Oily sweet, with a rose odor, it occurs naturally in apples, bay leaves, cherries, grapefruit, ginger, lavender, and a number of other essential oils. A synthetic flavoring agent that occurs naturally in apples, bay leaves, cherries, coriander, grapefruit, oranges, tea, ginger, mace oil, and the oils of lavender, lavandin, lemon, lime, mandarin, and petitgrain. A berry, lemon, rose, apple, cherry, peach, honey, root beer, cassia, cinnamon, ginger ale, and nutmeg flavoring for beverages, ice cream, ices, candy, baked goods, chewing gum, and toppings. Geraniol is omitted from hypoallergenic cosmetics. Can cause allergic reactions. Whereas no specific toxicity information is available, deaths have been reported from ingestion of unknown amounts of citronella oil *(see)* which is 93 percent geraniol; gastric mucosa was found to be severely damaged. GRAS.

GERANIUM • An essential oil used as flavoring. *See* Geranium Rose Oil. GRAS.

GERANIUM ROSE OIL • A synthetic flavoring agent that occurs naturally in geranium herbs and rose petals. Used in strawberry, lemon, cola, geranium, rose, violet, cherry, honey, rum, brandy, cognac, nut, vanilla, spice, and ginger ale flavorings for beverages, ice cream, ices, candy, baked goods, gelatin desserts, chewing gum, and jelly. A geranium root derivative has been used as an astringent and to treat chronic diarrhea in dogs. A teaspoon may cause illness in an adult and less than an ounce may kill. May affect those allergic to geraniums. There is reported use of the chemical; it has not yet been assigned for toxicology literature.

GERANYL ACETATE • Geraniol Acetate. Clear colorless liquid with the odor of lavender, it is a constituent of several essential oils. Used in berry, lemon, orange, floral, apple, grape, peach, pear, honey, spice, and ginger ale flavorings for beverages, ice cream, ices, candy, baked goods, gelatin desserts, chewing gum, and syrup. It is obtained from geraniol *(see)*. GRAS.

GERANYL ACETOACETATE • A synthetic fruit flavoring agent for beverages, ice cream, ices, candy, and baked goods.

GERANYL BENZOATE • Benzoic Acid. A synthetic flavoring agent, slightly yellowish liquid, with a floral odor. Used in floral and fruit flavorings for beverages, ice cream, ices, candy, baked goods, and candy.

GERANYL BUTYRATE • Geraniol Butyrate. Colorless liquid that occurs in several essential oils, it is used in perfumes. It is used in berry, citrus, fruit, apple, cherry, pear, and pineapple flavorings for beverages, ice cream, ices, candy, baked goods, chewing gum, and gelatin desserts. Used as a synthetic attar of rose. *See* Geraniol.

GERANYL FORMATE • Geraniol Formate. Colorless liquid with a roselike odor, insoluble in alcohol, it occurs in several essential oils. Used in perfumes and soaps as a synthetic neroli bigarade oil *(see)*. A fresh, leafy, rose odor, it is used in berry, citrus, apple, apricot, and peach flavorings for beverages, ice cream, ices, candy, baked goods, gelatins, chewing gum, and puddings. *See* Geraniol.

GERANYL HEXANOATE • Hexanoic Acid. A synthetic citrus and pineapple flavoring agent for beverages, ice cream, ices, candy, and baked goods.

GERANYL ISOBUTYRIC ACID • Isobutyric Acid. A synthetic floral, rose, apple, pear, and pineapple flavoring agent for beverages, ice cream, ices, candy, baked goods, chewing gum, gelatin desserts, and puddings.

GERANYL ISOVALERATE • A synthetic berry, lime, apple, peach, and pineapple flavoring agent for beverages, ice cream, ices, candy, and baked goods.

GERANYL PHENYLACETATE • Phenylacetic Acid. A synthetic flavoring, yellow liquid with a honey-rose odor. Used in fruit flavorings for beverages, ice cream, ices, candy, baked goods, and chewing gum.

GERANYL PROPIONATE • Geraniol Propionate. Colorless liquid with a roselike odor, it is soluble in most oils and is used in perfumery. A synthetic flavoring used in berry, geranium, apple, pear, pineapple, and honey flavorings for beverages, ice cream, ices, candy, baked goods, chewing gum, and gelatin desserts.

GERMANDER • *Teucrium chamaedrys* or *Teucrium scorodonia*. Flavoring in alcoholic beverages only. An American plant. *See* Sage.

GHATTI GUM • Indian Gum. The gummy exudate from the stems of a plant abundant in India and Ceylon. Used as an emulsifier and in butter, butterscotch, and fruit flavorings for beverages. Limited to 0.1 to 0.2 percent of foods in which it is used. Has caused an occasional allergy but when ingested in large amounts has not caused obvious distress. The FDA's reevaluation in 1976 found the gum was GRAS if used at the rate of 0.2 percent for alcoholic beverages and 0.1 percent for all other food categories. In pharmaceutical preparations one part ghatti usually replaces two parts acacia *(see)*. The final report to the FDA of the Select Committee on GRAS Substances stated in 1980 that there is no evidence in the available information that it is a hazard to the public when used as it is now and it should continue its GRAS status with limitations in the amount that can be added to food.

GIBBERELLIC ACID and ITS SALTS • Used for malt beverages and distilled spirits. A plant growth-promoting hormone synthesized in 1978. Mildly toxic by ingestion. It is limited to less than 2 ppm in malt and 0.5 ppm in finished malt beverages. Its tolerance is zero in distilled spirits. Caused tumors in experimental animals.

GIGARTINA EXTRACTS • A stabilizer from red algae of the sea. *See* Algaes. *See* Carrageenan.

GINGER • *Zingiber officinale.* Derived from the rootlike stem of plants culti-vated in all tropical countries, it is used in apple, plum, sausage, eggnog, pump-kin, ginger, ginger ale, and ginger beer flavorings for beverages, ice cream, ices, baked goods (2,500 ppm), and meats. The extract is used for cola, sausage, root beer, ginger, ginger ale, and ginger beer flavorings for beverages, ice cream, ices, candy, baked goods, chewing gum, meats, and condiments. The oleoresin, which is a ginger flavoring, is used in root beer and ginger ale for the same products. Ginger has been used to break up intestinal gas and colic. GRAS.

GINGER OIL • Obtained from the dried rhizomes of *Zingiber officinale,* it is used in flavorings for beverages, ice cream, ices, candy, baked goods, chewing gum, meats, and condiments. It is also used in perfumes. Employed medicinally to break up intestinal gas. A skin irritant. Has been show to be mutagenic in rab-bits. GRAS.

GINSENG • *Panax ginseng* (Asia). *Panax quinquefolia* (North America). *Eleutherococcus senticosus* (Siberian). Root of the ginseng plant, grown in China, Korea, and the United States. The Chinese esteem ginseng as an herb of many uses and have been using it in medicine for more than five thousand years. The Chinese and Koreans also used it in combination with chicken soup. The word *panax* in its botanical name comes from the Greek *panakos,* a panacea. Among its active ingredients are amino acids, essential oils, carbohydrates, peptides, vitamins, min-erals, enzymes, and sterols. In Asia, it is esteemed for its abilities to preserve health, invigorate the system, and prolong life. It is taken in an herbal tea as a daily tonic. North American Indians used ginseng as a love potion. It has been found to normalize high or low blood sugar. It produces a resin, a sugar starch, glue, and volatile oil. Ginseng is used as a flavoring additive in the United States and has a sweetish, licoricelike taste and is widely used in Asian medicines as an aromatic bitter. No known toxicity.

GLUCAMINE • An organic compound that is prepared from glucose *(see).*

GLUCITOL • Sorbitol. Sorbol. White crystalline powder with a sweet taste used as an anticaking agent, curing agent, drying agent, emulsifier, firming agent, fla-voring agent, formulation aid, free-flowing agent, humectant, lubricant, nutritive sweetener, pickling agent, releasing agent, sequestrant, stabilizer, surface-finishing agent, texturizing agent, and thickener. Used in baked goods, baking mixes, low-calorie beverages, hard and soft candy, chewing gum, chocolate, cough drops, frankfurters, frozen dairy desserts, jams, jellies, sausage, and shred-ded coconut. GRAS. Limitation of 99 percent in hard candy and cough drops, 75 percent in chewing gum, 98 percent in soft candy, 30 percent in nonstandardized jams and jellies, 30 percent in baked goods, 17 percent in frozen dairy desserts, 12 percent in all other foods. Mildly toxic by ingestion. Human systemic effects by ingestion include diarrhea. *See also* Sorbitol.

GLUCOAMYLASE • An enzyme used to break down sugars in food processing. No known toxicity.

GLUCODELTA LACTONE • White crystalline powder used as an acidifier, binder, curing agent, leavening agent, pH control agent, pickling agent, and sequestrant *(see)*. Used in meat mixes, dessert mixes, frankfurters, Genoa salami, and sausages. GRAS.

GLUCOMANNAN • A powder extracted from the roots of the konjac plant. The promoters claim that the powder, taken in a capsule before meals, absorbs liquid and swells in the stomach to form a gel and reduces hunger. The FDA was asked to approve it as GRAS but refused to do so unless scientific data were submitted. *See* Konjac Flour.

GLUCONATE • Calcium and Sodium. A sequestrant *(see)* derived from glucose, a sugar. Odorless, tasteless. Used as a buffer for confections and a firming agent for tomatoes and apple slices. Sodium gluconate is also used as a nutrient and dietary supplement. The final report to the FDA of the Select Committee on GRAS Substances stated in 1980 that it should continue its GRAS status with no limitations other than good manufacturing practices.

***d*-GLUCONIC ACID** • A light, amber liquid with the faint odor of vinegar, produced from corn. It is water soluble and is used as a dietary supplement and as a sequestrant *(see)*. The magnesium salt of gluconic acid has been used as an antispasmodic. GRAS.

GLUCONO-DELTA-LACTONE • An acid with a sweet taste; fine, white, odorless. It is used as a leavening agent in jelly powders and soft drink powders where dry food acid is desired. Used in the dairy industry to prevent milk stone, by breweries to prevent beer stone, and is also a component of many cleaning compounds. Also used as a pickling agent. Cleared by the U.S. Department of Agriculture's Meat Inspection Division for use at eight ounces for each one hundred pounds of cured, pulverized meat, or meat food product to speed up the color-fixing process and to reduce the time required for smoking. GRAS.

GLUCOSE • Occurs naturally in blood, grape, and corn sugars. A source of energy for plants and animals. Sweeter than sucrose *(see)*, glucose syrup is used to flavor sausage, hamburger, meat loaf, luncheon meat, chopped or pressed ham. It is also used as an extender in maple syrup. It is used medicinally for nutritional purposes and in the treatment of diabetic coma. Used to soothe the skin and as a filler in cosmetics. No known toxicity in cosmetics, but candy and pastry makers frequently suffer erosions and fissures around their nails, and the nails loosen and sometimes fall off.

***d*-GLUCOSE** • Corn sugar. *See* Glucose.

GLUCOSE GLUTAMATE • Used as a humectant in hand creams and lotions, it occurs naturally in animal blood, grape, and corn sugars, and is a source of energy for plants and animals. It is sweeter than sucrose. Glucose syrup is used to flavor sausage, hamburger, and other processed meats. Also used as an extender in maple syrup and medicinally as a nutrient. Glutamate is the salt of glutamic acid and is used to enhance natural food flavors. The FDA asked for further studies as to its potential mutagenic, teratogenic, subacute, and reproductive effects in 1980. Since then, the FDA has not reported any action.

GLUCURONIC ACID • A carbohydrate that is widely distributed in the animal kingdom.

GLUTAMATE • Ammonium and monopotassium salt of glutamic acid *(see)*. Used to enhance natural flavors and to improve the taste of tobacco. Used to impart meat flavor to foods, to enhance other natural food flavors, and to improve the taste of tobacco. It is used as an antioxidant in cosmetics to prevent spoilage. It is being studied by the FDA for mutagenic, teratogenic, subacute, and reproductive effects. The final report to the FDA of the Select Committee on GRAS Substances stated in 1980 that there is no evidence in the available information that it is a hazard to the public when used as it is now and it should continue its GRAS status with limitations on the amount that can be added to food.

GLUTAMIC ACID • L-Glutamic Acid. A white, practically odorless, free-flowing crystalline powder, a nonessential amino acid *(see)* usually manufactured from vegetable protein. A salt substitute, it has been used to treat epilepsy and to correct stomach acids. It is used to enhance food flavors and to add meat flavor to foods. Glutamic acid with hydrochloride (*see* Hydrochloric Acid) is used to improve the taste of beer. It is also employed as an antioxidant in cosmetics and as a softener in permanent wave solutions to help protect against hair damage. It is being studied by the FDA for mutagenic, teratogenic, subacute, and reproductive effects. The final report to the FDA of the Select Committee on GRAS Substances stated in 1980 that there is no evidence in the available information that it is a hazard to the public when used as it is now and it should continue its GRAS status with limitations on the amount that can be added to food.

GLUTAMINE • A nonessential amino acid *(see)* used as a medicine, dietary supplement, and as a culture medium. Mildly toxic by ingestion. Caused adverse reproductive effects in experimental animals.

GLUTARAL • *See* Glutaraldehyde. *See* Glutaric Acid.

GLUTARALDEHYDE • A food flavoring. An amino acid *(see)* that occurs in green sugar beets. It has a faint agreeable odor and is used as a fixing agent for enzymes added to foods. It is used as a flavor enhancer in foods. Also used as a component of microcapsules. Caused birth defects in experimental animals. A severe human skin irritant. *See* Glutaric Acid.

GLUTARIC ACID • Pentanedioic Acid. A crystalline fatty acid that occurs in green sugar beets, meat, and in crude wood. Very soluble in alcohol and ether. Widely used in Asian medicine as an aromatic bitter. It is used in American cosmetics as a demulcent *(see)*. No known toxicity.

GLUTEN • A mixture of proteins from wheat flour, obtained as an extremely sticky, yellowish gray mass by making a dough and then washing out the starch. It consists almost entirely of two proteins, gliadin and glutelin, the exact proportions of which depend upon the variety of wheat. Contributes to the porous and spongy structure of bread. There is no reported use of the chemical and there is no toxicology information available.

GLY- • The abbreviation for glycine *(see)*.

(MONO)GLYCERIDE CITRATE • Aids the action of and helps dissolve antioxidant formulations for oils and fats, such as shortenings for cooking. No known toxicity.

GLYCERIDES • Monoglycerides, Diglycerides, and Monosodium Glycerides of Edible Fats and Oils. Any of a large class of compounds that are esters *(see)* of the sweet alcohol glycerin. They are also made synthetically. Emulsifying and defoaming agents. Used in bakery products to maintain "softness," in beverages, ice cream, ices, ice milk, milk, chewing-gum base, shortening, lard, oleomargarine, confections, sweet chocolate, chocolate, rendered animal fat, and whipped toppings. The diglycerides are on the FDA list of food additives to be studied for possible mutagenic, teratogenic, subacute, and reproductive effects. The glycerides are also used in cosmetic creams as texturizers, emulsifiers, and emollients. The final report to the FDA of the Select Committee on GRAS Substances stated in 1980 that it should continue its GRAS status with no limitations other than good manufacturing practices.

GLYCERIN • Glycerol. Any byproduct of soap manufacture obtained by adding alkalies *(see)* to fats and fixed oils. A sweet (about 0.6 times as cane sugar), warm-tasting substance. Used as a humectant in tobacco and in marshmallows, pastilles, and jellylike candies; as a solvent for colors and flavors; as a bodying agent in combination with gelatins and edible gums; as a plasticizer in edible coatings for meat and cheese. It is also used in beverages, confectionery, baked goods, chewing gum, gelatin desserts, meat products, soda-fountain fudge. Also used in perfumery. A solvent, humectant, and emollient in many cosmetics, it absorbs moisture from the air and therefore helps keep moisture in creams and other products, even if the consumer leaves the cap off the container. Also helps the products to spread better. Among the many products containing glycerin are cream rouge, face packs and masks, freckle lotions, hand creams and lotions, hair lacquer, liquid face powder, mouthwashes, protective creams, skin fresheners, and toothpastes. In concentrated solutions it is irritating to the mucous membranes, but as used, nontoxic, nonirritating, nonallergenic. Contact with a strong oxidizing agent such as chromium trioxide, potassium chlorate, or potassium permanganate *(see)* may produce an explosion. The final report to the FDA of the Select Committee on GRAS Substances stated in 1980 that it should continue its GRAS status with no limitations other than good manufacturing practices.

GLYCEROL • *See* Glycerin.

GLYCEROL TRIBUTYRATE • A synthetic flavoring. GRAS. There is reported use of the chemical; it has not yet been assigned for toxicology literature. *See* Glyceryl Tributyrate.

GLYCERYL ABIETATE • A density adjuster for citrus oil used in the preparation of alcoholic beverages and still and carbonated fruit drinks. Also cleared as a plasticizing material in chewing-gum base. No known toxicity.

GLYCERYL BEHENATE • Used to form tablets. There is no reported use of the chemical and there is no toxicology information available. GRAS. *See* Behenic Acid.

GLYCERYL CAPRATE • The monoester of glycerin and caprylic acid *(see both)*.

GLYCERYL CAPRYLATE • *See* Glycerin and Caprylic Acid.

GLYCERYL CAPRYLATE/CAPRATE • A mixture of caprylic acid and capric acid *(see both)*.

GLYCERYL COCONATE • *See* Glycerin and Coconut Oil.

GLYCERYL DILAURATE • *See* Glycerin and Lauric Acid.

GLYCERYL DIOLEATE • The diester of glyceric and oleic acid *(see both)*.

GLYCERYL DISTEARATE • The diester of glycerin and stearic acid *(see both)*.

GLYCEROL ESTER OF PARTIALLY DIMERIZED ROSIN • A hard, pale, amber-colored resin produced by combining rosin *(see)* with food-grade glycerin. It is used in chewing-gum bases.

GLYCEROL ESTER OF POLYMERIZED ROSIN • Softener for chewing-gum base.

GLYCEROL ESTER OF WOOD ROSIN • Made from refined, pale yellow-colored wood rosin and food-grade glycerin *(see)*. A hard, pale amber-colored resin, it is used as a chewing-gum base and as a beverage stabilizer. No known toxicity.

GLYCEROL ESTER OF TALL OIL ROSIN • A softener for chewing-gum base.

GLYCERYL HYDROSTEARATE • *See* Glyceryl Monostearate.

GLYCERYL HYDROXYSTEARATE • The monoester of glycerin and hydroxy-stearic acid *(see both)*.

GLYCERYL ISOSTEARATE • *See* Glyceryl Monostearate.

GLYCERYL-LACTO ESTERS OF FATTY ACIDS • Emulsifiers. *See* Glycerol and Fatty Acids.

GLYCERYL LACTOOLEATE and LACTOPALMITATE OF FATTY ACIDS • Food emulsifiers used in shortening where free and combined lactic acid does not exceed 1.75 percent of shortening plus additive. They add calories but are considered nontoxic. The final report to the FDA of the Select Committee on GRAS Substances stated in 1980 that it should continue its GRAS status with no limitations other than good manufacturing practices.

GLYCERYL LANOLATE • The monoester of glycerin and lanolin *(see both)*.

GLYCERYL LINOLEATE • The monoester of glycerin and linoleic acid *(see both)*.

GLYCERYL MONO- and DIESTERS • Manufactured by reacting edible glycerides with ethylene oxide. These are used as defoamers in yeast production. No known toxicity. The final report to the FDA of the Select Committee on GRAS Substances stated in 1980 that it should continue its GRAS status with no limitations other than good manufacturing practices.

GLYCERYL MONOOLEATE • A flavoring agent. GRAS. *See* Glyceryl and Oleic Acid.

GLYCERYL MONOSTEARATE • An emulsifying and dispersing agent used in oleomargarine, shortenings, and other food products including noodles. Restricted to less than 2 percent of macaroni and less than 3 percent of noodle products. It is a mixture of two glyceryls, a white, waxlike solid or beads, and is soluble in hot organic solvents such as alcohol. GRAS.

GLYCERYL MYRISTATE • *See* Glycerin and Myristic Acid.

GLYCERYL OLEATE • *See* Glycerin and Oleic Acid.

GLYCERYL PABA • The ester of glycine and para-aminobenzoic acid *(see both)*.

GLYCERYL PALMITOSTEARATE • A mixture of fatty acid glycerides, it is a fine powder or waxy solid. It is used in food processing. *See* Glycerides and Fatty Acids. GRAS.

GLYCERYL RICINOLEATE • *See* Glycerin.

GLYCERYL SESQUIOLEATE • *See* Glycerin.

GLYCERYL STARCH • *See* Starch and Glycerols.

GLYCERYL STEARATE • An emulsifier. *See* Glycerin.

GLYCERYL TRIACETATE • *See* Triacetin. GRAS.

GLYCERYL TRIBUTYRATE • *See* Tributyrin.

GLYCERYL TRIMYRISTATE • *See* Glycerin and Myristic Acid.

GLYCERYL TRIUNDECANOATE • The triester of glycerin and undecenoic acid *(see both)*.

GLYCINE • An amino acid *(see)* classified as nonessential. Made up of sweet-tasting crystals, it is used as a dietary supplement and as a gastric antacid. Used with saccharin to mask its aftertaste. Mildly toxic by ingestion. Restricted to less than 0.2 percent of the finished beverage or beverage base.

GLYCOCHOLIC ACID • A product of mixing cholic acid and glycine, it is the chief ingredient of bile in vegetarian animals. It is used as an emulsifying agent for dried egg whites up to .1 percent. No known toxicity. The final report to the FDA of the Select Committee on GRAS Substances stated in 1980 that it should continue its GRAS status with no limitations other than good manufacturing practices. There is no reported use of the chemical and there is no toxicology information available.

GLYCOFUROL • The ethoxylated ether of tetrahydrofurfuryl alcohol. *See* Furfurol.

GLYCOGEN • Distributed throughout cell protoplasm, it is an animal starch found especially in liver and muscle. Used as a violet dye and in biochemical research. No known toxicity.

GLYCOLIC ACID • Contained in sugarcane juice, it is an odorless, slightly water-absorbing acid used to control the acid/alkali balance in cosmetics and whenever a cheap organic acid is needed. It is also used in copper brightening, decontamination procedures, and in dyeing. It is a mild irritant to the skin and mucous membranes. The final report to the FDA of the Select Committee on GRAS Substances stated in 1980 that it should continue its GRAS status with no limitations other than good manufacturing practices.

GLYCOL DISTEARATE • Alcohol from glycol. *See* Glycols.

GLYCOLS • Propylene Glycol. Glycerin, Ethylene Glycol, Carbitol. Diethylene Glycol. *Glycol* literally it means "glycerin" plus "alcohol." A group of syrupy alcohols derived from hydrocarbons *(see)* and used in foods as emulsifiers and in chewing-gum bases and in cosmetics as humectants. The FDA cautions manufacturers that glycols may cause adverse reactions in users. Propylene glycol and glycerin *(see both)* are considered safe. Other glycols in low concentrations may be harmless for external application but ethylene glycol, carbitol, and diethylene glycol are hazardous in concentrations exceeding 5 percent even in preparations for use on small areas of the body. Therefore, in sunscreen lotions and protective creams where the area of application is extensive, they should not be used at all. Wetting agents *(see)* increase the absorption of glycols and therefore their toxicity.

GLYCOL STEARATE SE • An emulsifier. *See* Glycols and Stearates.

GLYCOPHEN • Promidione. Rovral. A fungicide used in animal feed, ginseng (dried), grape pomace (dried), raisin waste, raisins, and soap stock. FDA residue tolerance of 300 ppm in raisins, 4 in dried ginseng, and 225 ppm in dried grape pomace and raisin waste for animal feed. Moderately toxic by ingestion.

GLYCOSIDES • Many flowering plants contain cardiac glycosides. The most well known are foxglove, lily of the valley, and squill. The cardiac glycosides have the ability to increase the force and power of the heartbeat without increasing the amount of oxygen needed by the heart muscle. Among the glycosides are cyanogens, goitrogens, estrogens, and saponins. They are found in lima beans, cassava, flax, broccoli and other brassicas, most legumes, and grasses.

GLYCYRRHETINIC ACID • Used as a flavoring, to soothe skin, and as a carrier. Prepared from licorice root, it is soluble in chloroform, alcohol, and acetic acid *(see)*. It has been used medicinally to treat a disease of the adrenal gland. No known toxicity when used in cosmetics.

GLYCYRRHETINYL STEARATE • The stearic acid ester of glycyrrhetinic acid *(see)*.

GLYCYRRHIZA and GLYCYRRHIZA EXTRACT • GRAS. *See* Glycyrrhizin, Ammoniated.

GLYCYRRHIZIC ACID • Used as a flavoring, coloring, and to soothe the skin in cosmetics. Extracted from licorice, the crystalline material is soluble in hot water and alcohol. *See* Glycyrrhetinic Acid.

GLYCYRRHIZIN, AMMONIATED • Licorice. Product of dried root from the Mediterranean region used in licorice, anise, root beer, wintergreen, and birch beer flavorings for beverages, ice cream, ices, candy, and baked goods. It is used as a sugar substitute. It is one hundred times as sweet as sugar. It is also used to flavor tobacco and pharmaceuticals, as a demulcent and expectorant, and as a drug vehicle. It doesn't have calories. The final report to the FDA of the Select Committee on GRAS Substances stated in 1980 that it should continue its GRAS status with limitations on amounts that can be added to food. Cases have been reported of avid licorice eaters who develop high blood pressure. *See* Licorice.

GLYOXYLIC ACID • Used as a coloring. Syrup or crystals that occur in unripe fruit, young leaves, and baby sugar beets. Malodorous and strongly corrosive. Forms a thick syrup, very soluble in water, sparingly soluble in alcohol. It absorbs water from the air and condenses with urea to form allantoin *(see)* and gives a nice blue color with sulfuric acid. It is a skin irritant and corrosive.

GLYPHOSATE • A broad spectrum, postemergent herbicide used in animal feed. FDA residues allowed are 0.4 ppm in dried citrus pulp, 20 ppm in soybean hulls, and 30 ppm in sugarcane molasses.

GONADORELIN • A hormone used as an injection for cattle to increase growth. In humans it can cause such side effects as nausea, headache, and flushing.

GONADOTROPIN (SERUM) • A hormone capable of promoting growth and function of testes and ovaries when injected into cattle. It is also used in human medicine.

GRADE • Grading and inspection assure purity, wholesomeness, and appearance. The USDA has established grades for more than three hundred food products. Grading for most products is done voluntarily at the manufacturers' request (and expense) by a USDA inspector, and a USDA grade symbol may then appear on the package; lack of a symbol does not mean substandard product. Unfortunately, these grades lack continuity among product categories (Grade AA is the highest grade for eggs; Grade A is the highest for milk). Meat and poultry, however, whether fresh or processed and packaged must be inspected and carry an inspection stamp.

GRAINS OF PARADISE • Pungent aromatic seeds of a tropical African plant of the ginger family. It is a natural flavoring used in fruit, ginger, ginger ale, and pepper flavorings for beverages, ice cream, ices, and candy. No known toxicity. GRAS.

GRAM (g) • A metric unit of weight. There are about twenty-eight grams in one ounce. Food labels list fat, protein, carbohydrate, and fiber in grams (g) per serving.

GRAMINIS • *See* Dog Grass Extract.

GRAM-NEGATIVE, -POSITIVE • Classification of bacteria according to whether or not they accept a stain named after Hans Gram, a Danish bacteriologist. Different life processes and vulnerabilities of germs are reflected by their gram-positive or gram-negative characteristics. An antibiotic may be effective against certain gram-positive germs and have no effect on gram-negative ones and vice versa.

GRAPE COLOR EXTRACT • The extract of the pulp of *Vitis vinifera* used as a coloring for nonbeverage food. Permanently listed since 1981, although it is exempt from certification.

GRAPE JUICE • The liquid expressed from fresh grapes used as a coloring.

GRAPE POMACE • Source of natural red and blue colorings. Also used as an animal feed. *See* Anthocyanins.

GRAPE SKIN EXTRACT • Enocianina. Used in still and carbonated drinks and ades, beverage bases, and alcoholic beverages. Permanently listed since 1966. Does not require certification. No known toxicity.

GRAPEFRUIT OIL • The yellow, sometimes reddish liquid is an ingredient in fragrances obtained by expression from the fresh peel of the grapefruit, lemon, lime, orange, and peach flavorings for beverages, ice cream, ices, candy, baked goods, gelatin desserts, chewing gum (1,500 ppm), and toppings. An experimental tumor-causing agent. A skin irritant. GRAS.

GRAPE-SEED OIL • An ingredient in fragrances obtained by expression from the fresh peel of the grapefruit. The yellow, sometimes reddish liquid is also used in fruit flavorings. No known toxicity.

GRAPE SKIN EXTRACT • Enocianina. A purple-red liquid extracted from the residue of grapes pressed for use in grape juice and wine. Used for coloring in still and carbonated drinks and ales, beverage bases, and alcoholic beverages. Regarding the spraying of grapes, specifications by the FDA restrict pesticide residues to not more than 10 ppm lead and not more than 1 ppm arsenic.

GRAS • The Generally Recognized As Safe List was established in 1958 by Congress. Those substances that were being added to food over a long time, which under conditions of their intended use were generally recognized as safe by qualified scientists, would be exempt from premarket clearance. Congress had acted on a very marginal response—on the basis of returns from those scientists sent questionnaires. Approximately 355 out of 900 responded, and only about 100 of those responses had substantive comments. Three items were removed from the originally published list. Since then, developments in the scientific fields and in consumer awareness have brought to light the inadequacies of the testing of food additives and, ironically, the complete lack of testing of the Generally Recognized as Safe List. President Nixon directed the FDA to reevaluate items on the GRAS list. The reevaluation was completed and a number of items were moved from the list. Although there were a number of others on the list, some of them top priority, to be studied in 1980, nothing has been reported by the FDA on their status since then.

GREEN • *See* FD and C Greens (Nos. 1, 2, 3).

GREEN BEAN EXTRACT • The extract of the unripe beans of domesticated species of *Phaseolus.*

GREEN TEA EXTRACT • A number of studies in the 1990s have suggested green tea may help prevent certain human illnesses. An ingredient, epigallocatechin gallate (EGCG), reported carries twice the antioxidant power of red wine and vitamins C and E. *See* Antioxidants.

GROUND LIMESTONE • Used as a flavoring. GRAS.

GROUNDSEL EXTRACT • Extract of *Senecio vulgaris,* a North American maritime shrub or tree.

GUAIAC • A resin from Mexican and West Indian trees, especially *Guaiacum santum* and *Guaiacum officinale.* Brownish lumps that are insoluble in water but soluble in alcohol. Used as a flavoring in alcoholic beverages only. *See* Guaiac Wood Oil. There is reported use of the chemical; it has not yet been assigned for toxicology literature.

GUAIAC WOOD OIL • Yellow to amber, semisolid mass with a floral odor. Soluble in alcohol. Derived from steam distillation of guaiac *(see)* wood. A gum resin used in fruit and rum flavorings for beverages, ice cream, ices, candy, and baked goods. The oil is a raspberry, strawberry, rose, fruit, honey, ginger, and ginger ale flavoring for beverages, ice cream, candy, baked goods, gelatin desserts, and chewing gum. Formerly used to treat rheumatism. Used as a perfume fixative and modifier, soap odorant, and in fragrances. *See* Guaiac.

GUAIACYL ACETATE • A synthetic berry flavoring for beverages, ice cream, ices, candy, gelatin, chewing gum, and baked goods.

GUAIACYL PHENYLACETATE • A synthetic berry, coffee, honey, tobacco, and smoke flavoring agent flavoring for beverages, ice cream, ices, candy, baked goods, and toppings.

GUAIOL • *Michelia champaca,* an alcohol from guaiac *(see)* wood.

GUANIDOETHYL CELLULOSE • *See* Guaiac Wood Oil.

GUANYLIC ACID SODIUM SALT • Disodium Guanylate. A flavor enhancer used in canned foods, poultry, sauces, snack items, and soups. Mildly toxic by ingestion. Has caused mutations in experimental animals.

GUAR GUM • Guar Flour. From ground nutritive seed tissue of plants cultivated in India, it has five to eight times the thickening power of starch. A free-flowing powder, it is used as a stabilizer for frozen fruit, icings, glazes, and fruit drinks, and as a thickener for hot and cold drinks. Also a binder for meats, confections, baked goods, cheese spreads, cream cheese, ice cream, ices, French dressing, and salad dressing. Keeps tablet formulations from disintegrating, and is used in cosmetic emulsions, toothpastes, lotions, and creams. Employed also as a bulk laxative, appetite suppressant, and to treat peptic ulcers. The FDA's reevaluation in 1976 found guar gum to be GRAS if used as a stabilizer, thickener, and firming agent at .35 percent in baked goods, 1.2 percent in breakfast cereals, 2 percent in fats and oils, 1.2 percent in gravies, 1 percent in sweet sauces, toppings, and syrups, and 2 percent in processed vegetables and vegetable juices. In large amounts, it may cause nausea, flatulence, or abdominal cramps. The final report to the FDA of the Select Committee on GRAS Substances stated in 1980 that there is no evidence in the available information that it is a hazard to the public when used as it is now and it should continue its GRAS status with limitations on amounts that can be added to food. In 1997, however, the FDA banned it from use as an active ingredient in drugs because it swells when wet and had been used in weight-loss products to produce a feeling of fullness. One brand resulted in hospitalization of at least ten patients and one death from a blood clot after surgery to remove a throat blockage.

GUARANA GUM • The dried paste consisting mainly of crushed seed from a plant grown in Brazil. Contains about 4 percent caffeine. Used in cola flavorings for beverages and candy. *See* Caffeine for toxicity. There is reported use of the chemical; it has not yet been assigned for toxicology literature.

GUARANINE • *See* Caffeine.

GUAVA • Extracted from the fruit of a small shrubby American tree widely cultivated in warm regions. The fruit is sweet, sometimes acid, globular, and yellow. It is used to flavor jelly. GRAS.

GUINEA GREEN B • *See* FD and C Green No. 1.

GUM • True plant gums are the dried exudates from various plants obtained when the bark is cut or other injury is suffered. Gums are soluble in hot or cold water and sticky. Today the term gum, both for natural and synthetic sources, usually refers to resins. Gums are also used as emulsifiers, stabilizers, and suspending agents. No known toxicity.

GUM ACACIA • *See* Gum Arabic.

GUM ARABIC • Acacia Gum. The exudate from acacia trees grown in the Sudan. Used in face masks, hairsprays, setting lotions, rouge, and powders for compacts. Serves as an emulsifier, stabilizer, and gelling agent. Used in ice cream and vanilla powder. It may cause allergic reactions such as hay fever, dermatitis, gastrointestinal distress, and asthma. GRAS.

GUM BENJAMIN • *See* Benzoin.

GUM BENZOIN • Used as a preservative in creams and ointments and as a skin protective. It is the balsamic resin from benzoin grown in Thailand, Cambodia, Sumatra, and Vietnam. Also used to glaze the polish confections. No known toxicity.

GUM DAMMAR • *See* Dammar.

GUM GHATTI • *See* Ghatti Gum.

GUM GLUTEN • Used as a stabilizer in macaroni products. *See* Gluten.

GUM GUAIAC • Resin from the wood of the guaiacum used widely as an antioxidant in edible fats or oils, beverages, rendered animal fat, or a combination of such fats and vegetable fats. It is also used in cosmetic creams and lotions. Brown or greenish brown. Formerly used in treatment of rheumatism. No known toxicity. The final report to the FDA of the Select Committee on GRAS Substances stated in 1980 that it should continue its GRAS status with no limitations other than good manufacturing practices.

GUM KARAYA • Sterculia Gum. It is the dried exudate of a tree native to India. Karaya came into wide use during World War I as a cheaper substitute for gum tragacanth *(see)*. Karaya swells in water and alcohol but does not dissolve. It is used as a stabilizer in cheese, dressings for foods, ice cream, and fruit jelly and jam. Because of its high viscosity at low concentrations, its ability to produce highly stable emulsions, and its resistance to acids, it is widely used in frozen food products. In 1971, however, the FDA put this additive on the list of chemicals to be studied for teratogenic, mutagenic, subacute, and reproductive effects. It can cause allergic reactions such as hay fever, dermatitis, gastrointestinal diseases, and asthma. GRAS.

GUM ROSIN • *See* Rosins.

GUM SUMATRA • *See* Gum Benzoin.

GUM TRAGACANTH • The dried gummy exudate from plants found in Iran, Asia Minor, and Syria. A thickener and stabilizer, odorless, and with a gluelike taste. Used in fruit jelly, ornamental icings, fruit, sherbets, water ices, salad dressing, French dressing, confections, and candy. An emulsifier used in brilliantine, shaving cream, toothpaste, face packs, foundation cream, hairspray, mascara, depilatories, compact powder, rouge, dentifrice, setting lotion, eye makeup, and hand lotion. Also employed in compounding drugs and pastes. One of the oldest known natural emulsifiers, its history predates the Christian era by hundreds of years; it has been recognized in the U.S. Pharmacopoeia since 1829. It has a long shelf life and is resistant to acids. Aside from occasional allergic reactions, it can be ingested in large amounts with little harm except for diarrhea, gas, or constipation. When reevaluated it was found to be GRAS in the following percentages: 0.2 for baked goods; 0.7 percent in condiments and relishes; 1.3 percent in fats and oils; 0.8 percent in gravies and sauces; 0.2 percent in meat products; 0.2 percent in processed fruits; and 0.1 percent in all other categories.

GUTA HANG KANG • A chewing-gum base.

GUTHION • Azinphos-methyl. A pesticide used to combat mites. It inhibits nerve transmission. *See* Organophosphates.

H

HALOFUGINONE HYDROBROMIDE • An animal antibiotic used in broiler chicken feed. The FDA's residue limitation is 0.3 ppm in uncooked chicken liver and 0.1 in uncooked edible tissue of chicken.

HALOXON • Galloxon. An antiworm medicine for animals. FDA residue tolerance is 0.1 ppm in edible tissues of cattle, sheep, and goats.

HALSOSALT • Made from cornstarch that is fermented to produce lysine, a salty amino acid, it is being proposed as a salt substitute.

HAW BARK • Black Extract. Extract of the fruit of a hawthorn shrub or tree. Used in butter, caramel, cola, maple, and walnut flavorings for beverages, ice cream, ices, candy, and baked goods. Has been used as a uterine antispasmodic.

HAZELNUT OIL • The oil obtained from the various species of the hazelnut tree, genus *Corylus*.

HCL • The abbreviation for Hydrochloride.

HEATHER EXTRACT • An extract of *Calluna vulgaris,* also called ling extract.

HECTORITE • An emulsifier and extender. A clay consisting of silicate of magnesium and lithium, it is used in the chill-proofing of beer. The dust can be irritating to the lungs. No known toxicity of the skin.

HEDEOMA OIL • *See* Pennyroyal Oil.

HELIOTROPIN • Piperonal. Used in cherry and vanilla flavors. A purple diazo dye used in perfumery and soaps. Consists of colorless, lustrous crystals that have a heliotrope odor. Usually made from oxidation of piperic acid. Ingestion of large amounts may cause central nervous system depression. Applications to the skin may cause allergic reactions and skin irritations. Not recommended for use in cosmetics or perfumes.

HELIOTROPINE • *See* Heliotropin.

HELIOTROPYL ACETATE • *See* Piperonyl Acetate.

HELIUM • This colorless, odorless, tasteless gas is used as propellant for foods packed in pressurized containers. No known toxicity. The final report to the FDA of the Select Committee on GRAS Substances stated in 1980 that it should continue its GRAS status with no limitations other than good manufacturing practices. There is no reported use of the chemical and there is no toxicology information available.

HEMICELLULOSE EXTRACT • Used in feed as a source of metabolizable energy. It is in the cell walls of all plants and of some seaweeds and contains a variety of sugars. Nontoxic.

HEMLOCK OIL • Spruce Oil. A natural flavoring extract from North American or Asian nonpoisonous hemlock. Used in fruit, root beer, and spice flavorings for beverages, ice cream, ices, candy, baked goods, gelatin desserts, puddings, and chewing gum. There is no reported use of the chemical and there is no toxicology information available.

HENDECANAL • *See* Undecanal.

HENDECEN-9-OL • *See* 9-Undecanal.

10-HENDECENYL ACETATE • *See* 10-Undecen-1-yl Acetate.

2,4-HEPTADIENAL • Slightly yellow liquid used as a flavoring agent in various foods. Poisonous by skin contact. Moderately toxic by ingestion. Severe skin irritant.

γ-HEPTALACTONE • A synthetic coconut, nut, and vanilla flavoring for beverages, ice cream, ices, candy, and baked goods.

HEPTALDEHYDE • *See* Heptanal.

HEPTANAL • Heptaldehyde. Oily, colorless liquid with a penetrating fruit odor made from castor oil. A synthetic flavoring agent used in citrus, apple, melon, cognac, rum, and almond flavorings for beverages, ice cream, ices, candy, baked goods, and liqueurs. Used in perfumery. Mildly toxic by ingestion.

HEPTANAL DIMETHYL ACETAL • A synthetic fruit, melon, and mushroom flavoring agent for beverages, ice cream, ices, candy, baked goods, chewing gum, and condiments.

HEPTANAL GLYCERYL ACETAL • A synthetic mushroom flavoring for beverages, ice cream, ices, candy, and baked goods.

2,3-HEPTANEDIONE • A synthetic raspberry, strawberry, butter, fruit, rum, nut, and cheese flavoring agent for beverages, ice cream, ices, candy, baked goods, and chewing gum.

HEPTANOIC ACID • Enanthic Acid. Found in various fusel oils and in rancid oils, it has the faint odor of tallow. It is made from grapes and is a fatty acid used chiefly in making esters *(see)* for flavoring materials.

2-HEPTANOL • A synthetic flavoring agent, liquid, and miscible with alcohol and ether. *See* Heptyl Alcohol for use.

2-HEPTANONE • A synthetic flavoring agent, liquid, with a penetrating odor, used to give a "peppery" smell to such cheeses as Roquefort. Found in oil of cloves and in cinnamon bark oil. Used in berry, butter, fruit, and cheese flavorings for beverages, ice cream, ices, candy, baked goods, chewing gum, and condiments (25 ppm). Used also in perfumery as a constituent of artificial carnation oils. Found naturally in oil of cloves and in cinnamon bark oil. The lethal concentration in air for rats is 4,000 ppm. In high doses it is narcotic, and a suspected irritant to human mucous membranes.

3-HEPTANONE • A synthetic melon flavoring agent for beverages, ice cream, ices, candy, and baked goods. *See* 2-Heptanone, which is a similar compound.

4-HEPTANONE • A synthetic strawberry and fruit flavoring agent for beverages, ice cream, ices, candy, baked goods, and gelatin desserts. *See* 2-Heptanone, which is a similar compound.

HEPTYL ACETATE • A synthetic berry, banana, melon, pear, and pineapple flavoring agent for beverages, ice cream, ices, candy, and baked goods. No known toxicity. *See* 2-Heptanone.

HEPTYL ALCOHOL • 1-Heptanol. Colorless, fragrant liquid miscible with alcohol. A synthetic flavoring agent with a fatty, citrus odor, used in fruit flavorings for beverages, ice cream, ices, candy, and baked goods. Moderately toxic by ingestion and skin contact. Used in perfumery. *See* 2-Heptanone.

HEPTYL ALDEHYDE • *See* Heptanal.

HEPTYL BUTYRATE • Butyric Acid. A synthetic raspberry, floral, violet, apricot, melon, and plum flavoring agent for beverages, ice cream, ices, candy, baked goods.

γ-HEPTYL BUTYROLACTONE • *See γ-*Undecalactone.

HEPTYL CINNAMATE • A synthetic cinnamon flavoring.

HEPTYL FORMATE • Used in artificial fruit essences. A skin irritant. *See* 2-Heptanone.

HEPTYL HEPTANOATE • Colorless liquid with fruity odor used in artificial fruit essences. *See* 2-Heptanone.

HEPTYL ISOBUTYRATE • A synthetic coconut, apricot, peach, pineapple, and plum flavoring agent for beverages, ice cream, ices, candy, and baked goods. No known toxicity.

HEPTYL PELARGONATE • Liquid with pleasant odor used in flavors and perfumes. *See* 2-Heptanone.

n-HEPTYLIC ACID • *See* Heptanoic Acid.

HEPTYLPARABEN • A preservative used in fermented malt beverages to inhibit microbiological spoilage. It is also used in noncarbonated soft drinks and fruit based beverages when allowed by established standards of identity. The FDA tolerance is 12 ppm. *See* Parabens.

HERB ROBERT EXTRACT • Extract of the entire plant, *Geranium robertianum*. *See* Geranium Oil.

HESPERIDIN • A natural bioflavonoid *(see)*. Fine needles from citrus fruit peel. Used as a synthetic sweetener.

HEXACHLOROPHENE • An antibacterial used in animal products, but the FDA restricts its use. In 1969 scientists reported microscopically visible brain damage in rats from small concentrations of this chemical. The company that had the patent on hexachlorophane, the Swiss-based Givaudan Corporation, sold the chemical only to those companies that could demonstrate a safe and effective use for it. However, when the patent ran out, it was sold for many purposes. It is still used in small amounts in some cosmetic products for humans.

1-HEXADECANOIC ACID • *See* Palmitic Acid.

1-HEXADECANOL • Cetyl Alcohol. A synthetic chocolate flavoring agent for ice cream, ices, and candy. Moderately toxic by ingestion. An eye and human skin irritant.

ω-6-HEXADECENLACTONE • Ambrettolide. 6-Hexadecenolide. A synthetic fruit flavoring agent for beverages, ice cream, ices, candy, baked goods, gelatin desserts, and chewing gum.

6-HEXADECENOLIDE • *See* ω-6-Hexadecenlactone.

HEXADECYLIC ACID • *See* Palmitic Acid.

2,4-HEXADIENOATE • *See* Allyl Sorbate.

HEXAHYDROPYRIDENE • *See* Piperidine.

HEXAHYDROTHYMOL • *See* Menthol.

HEXAKIS • A pesticide to kill mites in animal feeds. The residue tolerance set by the FDA range from 20 ppm in raisin waste to 100 ppm in dried grape pomace. A corrosive skin and eye irritant.

γ-**HEXALACTONE** • A synthetic butter, fruit, honey, and vanilla flavoring for beverages, ice cream, ices, candy, baked goods, chewing gum, and gelatin desserts.

HEXALDEHYDE • *See* Hexanal.

HEXAMETHYLENETETRAMINE (HMT) • Methenamine. Odorless powder or crystals used in adhesives, coatings, as a stabilizers for lubricating and insulating oils, as a urinary antibacterial and as a urinary antiseptic for animals. It is used in production of Provolone cheese. Studies at Italy's University of Milano concluded there was no appreciable health risk from ingestion of cheese made with this additive.

HEXANAL • Hexaldehyde. Hexoic Aldehyde. A synthetic flavoring agent occurring naturally in apples, coffee, cooked chicken, strawberries, tea, and tobacco leaves (oils). Used in butter, fruit, honey, and rum flavorings for beverages, ice cream, ices, candy, baked goods, chewing gum, and gelatin desserts.

1-HEXANAL • *See* Hexyl Alcohol.

2,3-HEXANDIONE • A synthetic strawberry, butter, citrus, banana, pineapple, rum, and cheese flavoring agent for beverages, ice cream, ices, candy, and baked goods. No known toxicity.

HEXANE • A colorless volatile liquid derived from distillation of petroleum and used as a solvent for spice oleoresins *(see)*. Also used in low-temperature thermometers instead of mercury, usually with a blue or red dye. The FDA residue tolerance is 25 ppm in spices; 2.2 percent by weight in hops extract added before or during cooking of beer; 25 ppm in modified hop extract for beer; 5 ppm as residue in fish protein isolate. It is a mild central nervous system depressant that may be irritating to the respiratory tract.

HEXANEDIOIC ACID • *See* Adipic Acid.

1,2,6-HEXANETRIOL • An alcohol used as a solvent. No known skin toxicity.

HEXANOIC ACID • A synthetic flavoring agent that occurs naturally in apples, butter acids, cocoa, grapes, oil of lavender, oil of lavandin, raspberries, strawberries, and tea. Used in butter, butterscotch, chocolate, berries, strawberries, and tea. Used in butter, butterscotch, chocolate, berries, fruit, rum, pecan, and cheese flavorings for beverages, ice cream, ices, candy, baked goods, chewing gum, and condiments. Moderately toxic by ingestion and skin contact. Severe eye irritant. Has caused mutations in laboratory animals.

HEXANOL • Hexyl Alcohol. Used as an antiseptic and preservative in cosmetics, it occurs as the acetate *(see)* in seeds and fruits of *Heracleum sphondylium* and *Umbelliferae*. Colorless liquid slightly soluble in water, it is miscible with alcohol.

HEXAZINONE • A weed killer used in various plant products. Moderately toxic by ingestion and mildly toxic by skin contact. Has caused adverse reproductive effects in laboratory animals.

2-HEXEN-1-OL • A synthetic flavoring that is a colorless liquid with a fruity odor. It occurs naturally in grapes; similar in compound to 3-Hexen-1-ol *(see)*. Used in fruit and mint flavorings for beverages, ice cream, ices, candy, and baked goods. Moderately toxic by ingestion and mildly toxic by skin contact.

3-HEXEN-1-OL • Leaf Alcohol. Blatteralkohol. A synthetic flavoring that occurs naturally in leaves of odoriferous plants and grapefruit, raspberries, and tea. Strong odor. Used in fruit and mint flavorings for beverages, ice cream, ices, candy, and baked goods.

2-HEXEN-1-YL ACETATE • A synthetic fruit flavoring agent for beverages, ice cream, ices, candy, and baked goods.

2-HEXENAL • A synthetic berry and fruit flavoring agent that occurs naturally in apples and strawberries and is used for beverages, ice cream, ices, candy, and baked goods. No known toxicity.

cis-3-HEXENAL • A synthetic fruit flavoring agent for beverages, ice cream, ices, and candy. No known toxicity.

2-HEXENOIC ACID • *See* Methyl Hexenoate.

cis-3-HEXENYL 2-METHYL BUTYRATE • Colorless liquid with a strong fruity odor used as a flavoring in various foods.

HEXITOL OLEATE • An emulsifier that was used in ice cream but has been banned by the FDA.

HEXOIC ACID • *See* Caproic Acid.

HEXOIC ALDEHYDE • A synthetic berry, apple, pear, and pineapple flavoring agent for beverages, ice cream, ices, candy, baked goods, and chewing gum.

HEXONE • Colorless liquid with a fruity odor used as a flavoring agent in various foods. Moderately toxic by ingestion. Mildly toxic by inhalation. Very irritating to the skin, eyes, and mucous membranes. A human systemic irritant by inhalation. Narcotic in high concentration.

HEXYL ACETATE • Acetic Acid, Hexyl Ester. A synthetic berry, apple, pear, and pineapple flavoring agent for beverages, ice cream, ices, candy, baked goods, and chewing gum. Mildly toxic by ingestion.

2-HEXYL-4-ACETOXYTETRAHYDROFURAN • A synthetic fruit flavoring agent for beverages, ice cream, ices, candy, and baked goods. Although allowed as a food additive, there is no current reported use of the chemical, and therefore, although toxicology information may be available, it is not being updated, according to the FDA.

HEXYL ALCOHOL • 1-Hexanol. A synthetic flavoring agent that occurs naturally in apples, oil of lavender, strawberries, and tea. Used in berry, coconut, and fruit flavorings for beverages, ice cream, ices, candy, baked goods, chewing gum, and gelatin desserts. Also used in antiseptics and in perfumery. *See* Hexanol and also Fatty Alcohols.

HEXYL-2-BUTENOATE • Colorless liquid with a fruity odor used as a flavoring in various foods. GRAS.

HEXYL CINNAMALDEHYDE • Yellow liquid with a jasmine odor used as a flavoring agent in various foods. Moderately toxic by ingestion. A skin irritant.

a-HEXYL CINNAMALDEHYDE • A synthetic flavoring, pale yellow liquid with a jasminelike odor. Used in berry, fruit, and honey flavorings for beverages, ice cream, ices, candy, baked goods, and gelatin desserts.

HEXYL ESTER • *See* Hexyl Acetate.

HEXYL FORMATE • Formic Acid. A synthetic raspberry and fruit flavoring agent for beverages, ice cream, ices, candy, and baked goods.

HEXYL 2-FUROATE • A synthetic coffee, maple, and mushroom flavoring agent for candy and condiments.

HEXYL HEXANOATE • Hexanoic Acid. A synthetic fruit flavoring agent for beverages, ice cream, ices, candy, and baked goods.

HEXYL ISOVALERATE • A colorless liquid with a fruity odor used as a flavoring in various foods.

2-HEXYL-5 (or 6)-KETO-1,4-DIOXANE • A synthetic cream flavoring agent for beverages, ice cream, ices, candy, and baked goods. No known toxicity.

HEXYL LAURATE • *See* Lauric Acid.

HEXYL 2-METHYL BUTYRATE • Colorless liquid; strong, fresh, green fruity odor used as a flavoring agent.

HEXYL OCTANOATE • Octanoic Acid. A synthetic fruit flavoring agent for beverages and puddings.

HEXYL PROPIONATE • Propionic Acid. A synthetic fruit flavoring agent for beverages, ice cream, ices, candy, and baked goods.

HEXYLENE GLYCOL DIACETATE • *See* 1,3-Nonanediol Acetate.

2-HEXYLIDENE CYCLOPENTANONE • A synthetic fruit flavoring agent for beverages, ice cream, ices, candy, and baked goods. No known toxicity.

4-HEXYLRESORCINOL • A pale yellow, heavy liquid that becomes solid upon standing at room temperature. It has a pungent odor and a sharp astringent taste and has been used medicinally as an antiworm medicine and antiseptic. In foods, it is used as a color stabilizer, enzyme browning inhibitor, and a processing aid. It can cause severe gastrointestinal irritation; bowel, liver, and heart damage has been reported. Concentrated solutions can cause burns of the skin and mucous membranes.

HEXYTHIAZOX • A white, odorless, crystalline pesticide used to kill mites on pears. FDA residue tolerance is 0.3 ppm.

HICKORY BARK EXTRACT • A natural flavoring extract from the hickory nut tree and used in butter, caramel, rum, maple, nut, spice, tobacco, and smoke flavorings for beverages, ice cream, ices, candy, baked goods, condiments, and liquors. There is no reported use of the chemical and there is no toxicology information available. GRAS.

HICKORY SMOKE CONDENSATE (HSC) • A food flavoring popular in the United States. Available data have suggested that this additive has tumor initiating and promoting potential. Researchers at Japan's Nagoya City University Medical School gave rats a diet containing 5 percent HSC and the animals did develop precancerous lesions. No effect was observed at lower doses.

HIGH AMYLOSE CORNSTARCH • Cornstarch that has been treated with enzymes to make it sweeter.

HIGH FRUCTOSE CORN SYRUP • Corn syrup *(see)* that has been treated with enzymes to make it sweeter. It is about one and a half times sweeter than sugar. It does have calories. Used in beverages, candy, frozen desserts, dairy drinks, canned fruits, processed ham, hamburger, ice cream, luncheon meat, meat loaf, poultry, and sausage. A combination of fructose and dextrose *(see both)* is a low-cost addition to pickles, ketchup, and syrups. There is reported use of the chemical; it has not yet been assigned for toxicology literature.

HIGH POTENCY • A nutrient in a food that is 100 percent or more of the RDI *(see)* established for that product. The term may also be used with multi-ingredient products if two-thirds of the nutrients are present at 100 percent of the RDI.

HINOKITIOL • The organic compound distilled from the leaves of arborvitae, it is a pale yellow oil with a camphor smell and is used in perfumery and flavoring. Low toxicity.

HIP BERRY EXTRACT • *See* Rose Hips Extract.

HISTAMINE • A chemical released by mast cells and considered responsible for much of the swelling and itching characteristics of hay fever and other allergies.

HISTIDINE • L forms only (L-Histidine is the natural form). A basic essential amino acid *(see)* used as a nutrient. It is a building block of protein, used as a nutrient. Soluble in water. It is used in cosmetic creams. Histidine has been on the FDA list of additives that need further study since 1980. GRAS.

HOMOCYSTEINE • An amino acid found in high concentrations in blood when there is a risk of a heart attack in young women. Women who have high homocysteine levels tend to have low folate levels.

HONEY • Used as a coloring, flavoring, and emollient in cosmetics. Formerly used in hair bleaches. The common, sweet, viscous material taken from the nectar of flowers and manufactured in the sacs of various kinds of bees. The flavor and color depend upon the plants from which it was taken. Honey has been used to cure meat for thousands of years. Recently, researchers at Clemson University in South Carolina rediscovered that this natural preservative confers excellent protection against oxidation and boosts shelf life in popular processed meats.

HONEYDEW MELON JUICE • Liquid expressed from fresh honeydew.

HONEYSUCKLE • The common fragrant tubular flowers filled with honey, which are used in perfumes. No known toxicity.

HOPS • *Humulus lupulus.* Used in beer brewing and in fruit and root beer flavorings for beverages. Derived from the carefully dried pineconelike fruit of the hop plant grown in Europe, Asia, and North America. Light yellow or greenish, it is an oily liquid with a bitter taste and aromatic odor. A solid extract is used in bitters, fruit, and root beer flavorings for beverages, ice cream, ices, candy, and baked goods. Hops oil is used in raspberry, grape, whiskey, and spice flavorings for beverages, ice cream, ices, candy, baked goods, chewing gum, and condiments. Hops at one time were thought to be a sedative. GRAS.

HOPS OIL • *See* Hops.

HOREHOUND EXTRACT • Hoarhound. A flavoring extracted from a mintlike plant cultivated in Europe, Asia, and the United States, *Marrubium vulgare.* It has a very bitter taste and is used in maple, nut, and root beer flavorings for beverages, ice cream, ices, candy, and baked goods. It is also a bitter tonic and expectorant. GRAS.

HORMONES • A hormone is a chemical produced by a gland and secreted into the blood stream, affecting the function of distant cells or organs. United States beef producers have been using growth hormones, a very powerful chemical from the pituitary gland at the base of the brain, to increase the cattle's weight from 10 to 20 percent for the same amount of feed. Diethylstilbestrol, another hormone, an estrogen, was used by beef and poultry producers to increase the weight of meat for which they are paid by the pound. The FDA has tried to ban diethylstilbestrol for that purpose because it has been shown to be carcinogenic, but spot checks have shown that it is still present in some meat and poultry products. In 1988, the twelve-nation European Community put a ban on American beef because of the use of growth hormones in raising cattle for meat. The American position is that the growth hormones approved for cattle by the Department of Agriculture are not harmful to humans. Environmentalists who testified in favor of the European legislators have maintained that such hormones create tumors and genetic deformities in children. Hormones are still being used in feed and by implantation in cattle, chickens, and turkeys, as you can determine by checking listings, including those for estradiol, mibolerone, testosterone propionate, and trenbolone.

HORSE CHESTNUT • The seeds of *Aeschylus hippocastanum.* A tonic, natural astringent for skin, and fever-reducing substance that contains tannic acid *(see).* No known toxicity.

HORSEMINT LEAVES EXTRACT • *Monarda* spp. A flavoring extract from any of several coarse, aromatic plants, grown from New York to Florida and from Texas to Wisconsin. Used in fruit flavorings for beverages (600 ppm). Formerly used as an aromatic stimulant and to break up intestinal gas. GRAS.

HORSE NETTLE • Solanum. Bull Nettle. Radical Weed. Air-dried ripe fruit of *Solanum carolinense,* a South American nightshade plant. It is also grown in Florida. It is used as a sedative and anticonvulsant.

HORSERADISH EXTRACT • Scurvy Grass. *Armoracia lapathifolia.* A condiment ingredient utilizing the grated root from the tall, coarse, white-flowered herb native to Europe. Often combined with vinegar or other ingredients. Contains ascorbic acid *(see)* and acts as an antiseptic in cosmetics. It contains vitamin C and is used by herbalists to treat arthritis pain by stimulating blood flow to inflamed joints. Potential adverse reactions include diarrhea and sweating if taken internally in large amounts. GRAS.

HOUSELEEK EXTRACT • Extract of the common houseleek *Sempervivum tectorium* native to the mountains of Europe and to the Greek Islands. Its longevity led to its being named sempervivum, which means "ever alive." It has been used to treat shingles, gout, and to get rid of bugs. Its pulp was applied to the skin for rashes and inflammation, and to remove warts and calluses. The juice was used to reduce fever and to treat insect stings. Houseleek juice mixed with honey was prescribed for thrush, and an ointment made from the plant was used to treat ulcers, burns, scalds, and inflammation.

HPP • Hydrolyzed Plant Protein. *See* Hydrolyzed Vegetable Protein.

HUMECTANT • A substance used to preserve the moisture content of materials, used to preserve moisture in confections and tobacco. Glycerin, propylene, glycol, and sorbitol *(see all)* are widely used humectants. *See* individual substances for toxicity.

HUMULUS • A hop plant, a herbaceous vine with palmate leaves and pistillate flowers. No known toxicity. *See* Hops.

HVP • *See* Hydrolyzed Vegetable Protein.

HYACINTH, ABSOLUTE • *Hyacynthus Orientalis.* The extract of the common fragrant flower. Once used as a flavoring for chewing gum and in perfumes and soaps, it is now permitted only for alcoholic beverage flavoring. Dark green liquid with a penetrating odor, the juice of hyacinth is very irritating to the skin and can cause allergic reactions. The bulb can cause severe gastrointestinal symptoms. There is reported use of the chemical; it has not yet been assigned for toxicology literature.

HYACINTHIN • *See* Phenylacetaldehyde.

HYBRID SAFFLOWER OIL • The oil derived from the seeds of a genetic strain that contains mostly oleic acid triglyceride, as distinct from safflower oil.

HYDRATED • Combined with water.

HYDRATED ALUMINA • *See* Aluminum Hydroxide.

HYDRATED SILICA • An anticaking agent used to keep loose powders free-flowing. *See* Silica and Hydrated.

HYDRATROPALDEHYDE • *See* 2-Phenylpropionaldehyde.

HYDRATROPALDEHYDE DIMETHYL ACETAL • *See* 2-Phenylpropionaldehyde Dimethyl Acetal.

HYDRAZINE • Colorless fuming liquid used as a solvent and catalyst for inorganic materials. Used in steam in contact with food. FDA allows zero residue. A reducing agent *(see)* and chlorine scavenger, it is a highly toxic chemical. It is a cancer-causing agent and direct liquid contact with skin or eyes may produce severe burns. Vapors are highly irritating to the nose and throat and may cause injury to the lungs, liver, and kidneys. The FDA has zero tolerance for residue on food.

a-HYDRO-OMEGA-HYDROXY-POLY(OXYETHYLENE)POLY(OXYPROPY-LENE)(51-57 MOLES)POLY (OXYETHYLENE)BLOCK COPOLYMERS, (MOL WT. 14,000) • Dough conditioner. FDA tolerance, 0.5 percent of flour used. *See* Copolymer Condensates of Ethylene Oxide and Propylene Oxide.

a-HYDRO-OMEGA-HYDROXY-POLY(OXYETHYLENE)POLY(OXYPRO-PYLENE)(55-61 MOLES)POLY(OXYETHYLENE)BLOCK COPOLYMERS, (MOL WT. 9,760–13,200) • Solubilizer and stabilizer in flavor concentrations. FDA permits use according to general manufacturing principles. *See* Copolymer Condensates of Ethylene Oxide and Propylene Oxide.

a-HYDRO-OMEGA-HYDROXY-POLY(OXYETHYLENE)POLY(OXYPRO-PYLENE)(53-59 MOLES)POLY(OXYETHYLENE)(14-16 MOLES)BLOCK CO-POLYMER, (MOL WT. 3,500–4,125) • A solubilizing and dispersing agent in combination with dioctyl sodium sulfosuccinate *(see)*. FDA tolerance is 10 ppm total in finished beverage or fruit drink. *See* Copolymer Condensates of Ethylene Oxide and Propylene Oxide.

HYDROBIOTIC FEED • *See* Verxite Granule and Flakes.

HYDROCARBONS • A large class of organic compounds containing only carbon and hydrogen. Petroleum, natural gas, coal, and bitumens are common hydrocarbon products. Hydrocarbons also include mineral oils, paraffin wax, and ozokerite. *See all.*

HYDROCHLORIC ACID • An acid used as a modifier for food starch, in the manufacture of sodium glutamate *(see),* and gelatin, for the conversion of cornstarch to syrup (0.012 percent), and to adjust the pH (acid-alkalinity balance) in the brewing industry (0.02 percent). Also used as a solvent. A clear, colorless, or slightly yellowish corrosive liquid, it is a water solution of hydrogen chloride of varying concentrations. Used in hair bleaches to speed up oxidation in rinses and to remove color. Inhalation of the fumes causes choking and inflammation of the respiratory tract. Ingestion may corrode the mucous membranes, esophagus, and stomach, and cause diarrhea. Circulatory collapse and death can occur. GRAS.

HYDROCHLOROFLUORCARBON, 22, 142b, 152a • Propellants and refrigerants derived from chlorofluorocarbon, any of several compounds comprised of carbon, fluorine, chlorine, and hydrogen. Though safer than many propellant gases, their use has diminished because of suspected effects on stratospheric ozone.

HYDROCINNAMALDEHYDE • Colorless to slightly yellow liquid with a strong hyacinth odor used as a flavoring agent in various foods. A human skin irritant.

HYDROCINNAMIC ALCOHOL • Colorless, thick liquid with a sweet hyacinth odor used as a flavoring agent in various foods. Moderately toxic by ingestion. Mildly toxic by skin contact.

HYDROCINNAMYL ACETATE • Colorless liquid with a spicy, floral odor used as a flavoring agent in various foods. Mildly toxic by ingestion.

HYDROCORTISONE SODIUM SUCCINATE • A-Hydrocort. Solu-Cortef. An adrenal gland hormone used to decrease severe inflammation. Used to treat cows, and the FDA permits up to 10 ppb in milk. The drug also suppresses the immune response. Has caused adverse reproductive effects in laboratory animals.

HYDROGEN CYANIDE • A colorless gas or liquid with a characteristic odor. In veterinary preparations used to treat mastitis, inflammation of the udders. As a fumigant, the FDA tolerances are 200 ppm in cocoa, 125 ppm in cereal flours, 90 ppm in cereals cooked before eaten, and 50 ppm in uncooked ham, bacon, and sausage. In humans, high concentrations may cause shortness of breath, paralysis, unconsciousness, convulsions, and respiratory arrest. Chronic exposure over long periods may cause fatigue and weakness. Exposure to 150 ppm from thirty minutes to an hour may endanger life. Death may result from a few minutes exposure to 300 ppm. Average fatal dose is 50 to 60 mg. The compressed gas is used for exterminating rodents and insects. Must be handled by specially trained experts.

HYDROGEN PEROXIDE • A bleaching and oxidizing agent, a detergent, and antiseptic. An unstable compound readily broken down into water and oxygen. It is made from barium peroxide and diluted phosphoric acid. Generally recognized as safe as a preservative and germ killer in milk and cheese as well as in cosmetics. Bleaches tripe and butter; used in the treatment of eggs before drying and in cheddar and Swiss cheeses. A 3 percent solution is used medicinally as an antiseptic and germicide. A strong oxidizer, undiluted it can cause burns of the skin and mucous membranes. In 1980, the Japanese notified the World Health

Organization that hydrogen peroxide was a suspect as a cancer-causing agent. It was widely used in Japanese fish cakes. The noodles were dipped in dilute hydrogen peroxide for disinfections. The fish meat and raw flour were also mixed with hydrogen peroxide. In laboratory rats, it was discovered that in the sixty-fifth week, the lining of the duodenum was thickened but no cancers occurred. The Japanese Welfare Ministry decided that hydrogen peroxide is safe for food when it is entirely decomposed and that the food should not contain any residual. GRAS.

HYDROGEN SULFIDE • Colorless gas with a terrible odor. It is derived from sulfuric acid and as a byproduct of petroleum refining. Highly flammable. Toxic by inhalation. Strong irritant to the eyes. Used as a source of sulfur and hydrogen in the manufacture of food additives.

HYDROGENATED CORN SYRUP • Used in cat and dog food as a humectant *(see). See also* Corn Syrup.

HYDROGENATED HONEY • Controlled hydrogenation *(see)* of honey.

HYDROGENATED MENHADEN OIL • Obtained along the West coast of North America from the menhaden fish, somewhat larger than herring. The oil contains myristic acid, palmitic acid, and linoleic acid *(see all)*. Used as a substitute for linseed oil. Hydrogenated menhaden oil is used as a substitute for tallow. GRAS.

HYDROGENATED OIL • Oil that is partially converted from naturally polyunsaturated fats to saturated. Makes liquid oils partially solid. May adversely affect the levels of fat in the blood and has been linked to colon cancer in some reports. *See* Hydrogenation.

HYDROGENATED PEANUT OIL • *See* Hydrogenation and Peanut Oil.

HYDROGENATED SOYBEAN OIL • *See* Soybean Oil and Hydrogenation.

HYDROGENATED SOY GLYCERIDE • *See* Soybean Oil and Hydrogenation.

HYDROGENATED SPERM OIL • Used to coat bakery pans so the products will not stick.

HYDROGENATED STARCH HYDROLYSATE • The end product of the hydrogenation of corn syrup. *See* Hydrogenation and Corn Syrup.

HYDROGENATED TALLOW • A component used in the production of beet sugar and yeast in amounts to inhibit foaming. *See* Hydrogenation. No known toxicity. The final report to the FDA of the Select Committee on GRAS Substances stated in 1980 that it should continue its GRAS status with no limitations other than good manufacturing practices.

HYDROGENATED TALLOW ACID • *See* Hydrogenated Tallow.

HYDROGENATED TALLOW ALCOHOL • *See* Hydrogenated Tallow, which has the same uses. The final report to the FDA of the Select Committee on GRAS Substances stated in 1980 that it should continue its GRAS status with no limitations other than good manufacturing practices.

HYDROGENATED TALLOW BETAINE • *See* Hydrogenated Tallow and Betaine.

HYDROGENATED TALLOW GLYCERIDE • *See* Hydrogenated Tallow and Glycerides.

HYDROGENATED TALLOWTRIMONIUM CHLORIDE • *See* Quaternary Ammonium Compounds.

HYDROGENATED VEGETABLE GLYCERIDE • An emollient to prevent the skin from losing moisture. *See* Vegetable Oils and Hydrogenation.

HYDROGENATION • The process of adding hydrogen gas under high pressure to liquid oils. It is the most widely used chemical process in the edible fat industry. Used in the manufacture of petrol from coal and in the manufacture of margarine and shortening. Used primarily in the cosmetic and food industries to covert liquid oils to semisolid fats, Crisco, for example, at room temperature. Reduces the amount of acid in the compound and improves color. Usually the higher the amount of hydrogenation the lower the unsaturation in the fat and the less possibility of flavor degradation or spoilage due to oxidation. Hydrogenated oils still contain some unsaturated components that are susceptible to rancidity. Therefore, the addition of antioxidants is still necessary.

HYDROLYSIS • Decomposition that changes a compound into other compounds by taking up the elements of water. For example, hydrolysis of salt into an acid and a base or hydrolysis of an ester into an alcohol and an acid. *See* Hydrolyzed.

HYDROLYZED • Subject to hydrolysis or turned partly into water. *Hydrolysis* is derived from the Greek *hydro,* meaning "water," and *lysis,* meaning "a setting free." It occurs as a chemical process in which the decomposition of a compound is brought about by water, resolving into a simpler compound. Hydrolysis also occurs in the digestion of foods. The proteins in the stomach react with water in an enzyme reaction to form peptones and amino acids *(see).*

HYDROLYZED ANIMAL PROTEIN • Protein from animals that has been split into smaller units by acids, alkalis, or enzymes.

HYDROLYZED CASEIN • *See* Casein and Hydrolyzed.

HYDROLYZED KERATIN • The widely used hydrolysate of keratin, a protein obtained from hair, wool, horn, nails, claws, beaks, membranes of eggshells, and nerve tissues. Acid, enzyme, or other forms of hydrolysis derive the hydrolysate. The word *animal* was removed from this ingredient name. Used in dietary protein supplements.

HYDROLYZED LEATHER MEAL • Used in swine feed up to 1 percent of weight.

HYDROLYZED MILK PROTEIN • *See* Acid Hydrolyzed Proteins.

HYDROLYZED PLANT PROTEIN • A protein obtained from various foods such as soybeans, corn, or wheat and then broken down into amino acids by a chemical process, acid hydrolysis. Hydrolyzed plant or vegetable protein is used as a flavor enhancer in numerous processed foods like soups, chillies, sauces, and some meat products like frankfurters. *See* Hydrolyzed Vegetable Protein.

HYDROLYZED PROTEIN • Used as a flavoring and flavor enhancer. The word *animal* was removed from this ingredient's name. Also used in gels and in animal feed. *See* Acid Hydrolysates of Protein and Hydrolyzed.

HYDROLYZED (SOURCE) PROTEIN EXTRACT • *See* Acid Hydrolysates of Proteins.

HYDROLYZED SOY PROTEIN • *See* Soybean and Hydrolyzed.

HYDROLYZED VEGETABLE PROTEIN (HPP, HVP) • The hydrolysate (liquefaction) of vegetable protein derived by acid, enzyme, or other method of hydrolysis. A flavor enhancer used in soup, beef, and stew. High salt and gluta-mate content with low quality protein. On the GRAS list, but the Select Committee of the Federation of American Societies for Experimental Biology (FASEB) advised the FDA that hydrolyzed vegetable protein contains dicar-boxylic amino acid (a building block of the protein that affects growth) when used at present levels in strained and junior baby foods. They said that the effects of this substance on children should be studied further. The effects on adults of veg-etable and animal protein hydroxylates demonstrate "no current hazard," but the FASEB voiced uncertainties about future consumption levels for those products and recommended further studies. The source of HVP must now be listed on the label. *See* Acid Hydrolysates of Protein.

HYDROLYZED YEAST • The hydrolysate of yeast (liquefaction) derived from acid, enzyme, or other method of hydrolysis.

HYDROLYZED YEAST PROTEIN • *See* Hydrolyzed Yeast.

HYDROQUINONE • Used in bleach, freckle creams, and in suntan lotions. A white crystalline phenol *(see)* that occurs naturally but is usually manufactured in the laboratory. Hydroquinone combines with oxygen very rapidly and becomes brown when exposed to air. Death has occurred from the ingestion of as little as 5 grams. Ingestion of as little as one gram (one-thirtieth of an ounce) has caused nausea, vomiting, ringing in the ears, delirium, a sense of suffoca-tion, and collapse. Industrial workers exposed to the chemical have suffered clouding of the eye lens. Application to the skin may cause allergic reactions. It can cause depigmentation in a 2 percent solution. When injected into the abdomen of mice in 28 milligram doses per kilogram of body weight, it caused bladder cancers, but other studies in which animals were fed the chemical did not show it to induce cancer. However, it did cause atrophy of the liver and aplastic anemia.

HYDROQUINONE DIMETHYL ETHER • White flakes with sweet clover odor used as a fixative in foods, perfumes, dyes, cosmetics, and especially in suntan preparations. *See* Hydroquinone.

1-HYDROXY-2-BUTANONE • *See* Acetoin.

2-HYDROXY-*p*-CYMENE • *See* Carvacrol.

5-HYDROXY-4-OCTANONE • A synthetic butter, butterscotch, fruit, cheese, and nut flavoring agent for beverages, ice cream, ices, candy, and baked goods. No known toxicity.

HYDROXY PROPYLMETHYL CELLULOSE CARBONATE • Prepared from wood pulp or cotton by treatment with methyl chloride. Used as a substitute for water-soluble gums, to render paper greaseproof, and as a thickener. The final report to the FDA of the Select Committee on GRAS Substances stated in 1980 that it should continue its GRAS status with limitations on amounts that can be added to food.

***p*-HYDROXYANISOLE** • *See* Guaiacol.

***o*-HYDROXYBENZALDEHYDE** • *See* Benzyl Acetate.

***p*-HYDROXYBENZOATE** • *See* Propylparaben.

o-**HYDROXYBENZOIC ACID** • *See* Salicylic Acid.

p-**HYDROXYBENZOIC ACID** • Prepared from *p*-bromophenol. Used as a preservative and fungicide. *See* Benzoic Acid for toxicity.

p-**HYDROXYBENZYL ISOTHIOCYANATE** • A derivative of mustard oil used in flavoring. The final report to the FDA of the Select Committee on GRAS Substances stated in 1980 that it should continue its GRAS status with no limitations other than good manufacturing practices.

2-**HYDROXYCAMPHANE** • *See* Borneol.

HYDROXYCITRONELLAL • Colorless liquid obtained by the addition of citronellol. Used as a fixative and a fragrance in perfumery for its sweet lilylike odor. It can cause allergic reactions.

HYDROXYCITRONELLAL DIETHYL ACETAL • A synthetic citrus and fruit flavoring agent for beverages, ice cream, ices, candy, and baked goods.

HYDROXYCITRONELLAL DIMETHYL ACETAL • A synthetic flavoring agent, colorless liquid, with a light floral odor. Used in fruit and cherry flavorings for beverages, ice cream, ices, candy, and baked goods.

HYDROXYCITRONELLOL • A synthetic lemon, floral, and cherry flavoring agent for beverages, ice cream, ices, candy, baked goods, gelatin desserts, and chewing gum.

(Z)-4-**HYDROXY-6-DODECENOIC ACID LACTONE** • One of the newer synthetic flavorings.

HYDROXYLAMINE HCL • An antioxidant for fatty acids and soaps, sodium nitrite *(see)*. May be slightly irritating to skin, eyes, and mucous membranes, and may cause a depletion of oxygen in the blood when ingested. In the body it is reportedly decomposed to sodium nitrite.

HYDROXYLATE • The process in which an atom of hydrogen and an atom of oxygen are introduced into a compound to make the compound more soluble.

HYDROXYLATED LECITHIN • An emulsifier and antioxidant used in baked goods, ice cream, and margarine. It is also used as a defoaming agent for processing beet sugar and yeast. According to the FAO-WHO Expert Committee on Food Additives, the safety of hydroxylated lecithin (*see* Lecithin) has not been adequately established. It has been cleared by the FDA for use as a food emulsifier.

HYDROXYLATION • The process in which an atom of hydrogen and an atom of oxygen are introduced into a compound to make that compound more soluble.

HYDROXYMETHYLCELLULOSE • Thickener and bodying agent derived from plants. Used to thicken cosmetics and as a setting aid in hair products. *See* Carboxymethyl Cellulose.

HYDROXYOCTACOSANYL HYDROXYSTEARATE • *See* Stearic Acid and Hydroxylation.

4-(*p*-**HYDROXY PHENYL)-2-BUTANONE** • A synthetic fruit flavoring for beverages, ice cream, ices, candy, baked goods, gelatin desserts, and chewing gum.

HYDROXYPHENYL GLYCINEAMIDE • Derived from the nonessential amino acid glycine *(see)* used as a buffering agent and as a violet scent.

HYDROXYPROLINE • L-Proline. The hydroxylated *(see)* amino acid used to add "protein" to a compound. There is no reported use of the chemical and there is no toxicology information available.

HYDROXYPROPYLAMINE NITRITE • *See* Isopropanolamine Nitrite.

HYDROXYPROPYL CELLULOSE • A thickener. *See* Hydroxymethylcellulose.

HYDROXYPROPYL GUAR • Guar Gum. 2-Hydroxypropyl Ether. *See* Guar Gum.

HYDROXYPROPYL METHYLCELLULOSE • An emulsifier used in food except standard foods which do not provide for such use. *See* Cellulose Gums.

HYDROXYPROPYL STARCH, HYDROXYPROPYL STARCH OXIDIZED, and HYDROXYPROPYL DISTARCHPHOSPHATE • These are all modified starches. The final report to the FDA of the Select Committee on GRAS Substances stated in 1980 that while no evidence in the available information on these starches demonstrates a hazard to the public when they are used at levels that are now current and in the manner now practiced, uncertainties exist requiring that additional studies should be conducted. In 1980, the FDA said GRAS status would continue while tests were being completed and evaluated. The FDA has reported nothing new since then.

HYDROXYQUINOLINE SULFATE • Was used as a component of a cottage cheese coagulant but has been banned by the FDA.

HYDROXYSTEARIC ACID • *See* Stearic Acid.

HYDROXYSTEARMIDE MEA • A mixture of ethanolamide of hydroxystearic acid. *See* Stearic Acid.

HYDROXYSTEARYL METHYLGLUCAMINE • An amino sugar. *See* Glucose.

HYGROMYCIN • A broad spectrum antibiotic from *Streptomyces hygroscopicus* used in animal feed. The FDA allows zero residue in eggs of poultry and in uncooked edible tissues and byproducts of swine and poultry.

HYPERACTIVITY • See Attention Deficit Hyperactivity Disorder (ADHD).

HYPERICUM • Hypericin. Blue black needles obtained from pyridine *(see)*. The solutions are red or green with a red cast. Small amounts seem to be a tranquilizer and have been used as an antidepressant in medicine. It can produce a sensitivity to light.

HYPERSENSITIVITY • The condition in persons previously exposed to an antigen in which tissue damage results from an immune reaction to a further dose of the antigen. Classically, four types of hypersensitivity are recognized, but the term is often used to mean the type of allergy associated with hay fever and asthma.

HYPERTENSION • High Blood Pressure. Hypertension is the persistently elevated arterial blood pressure. It is the most common public health problem in developed countries. Emphasis on lifestyle modifications has given diet a prominent role for both the primary prevention and management of hypertension.

HYPNONE • *See* Acetophenone.

HYPO • Prefix from the Greek, meaning "under" or "below," as in hypoacidity—acidity in a lesser degree than is usual or normal.

HYPOGLYCEMIA • Low blood sugar—the opposite of diabetes.

HYPOPHOSPHORIC ACID • Crystals used in baking powder, sodium salt. No known toxicity.

HYPOTHALAMUS • Brain control area involved in emotion, movement, and eating. Less than the size of a peanut and weighing a quarter of an ounce, this small area deep within the brain also oversees appetite, blood pressure, sexual behavior, sleep, and emotions, and sends orders to the pituitary gland.

HYSSOP EXTRACT • Extract of *Hyssopus officinalis*. A synthetic flavoring from the aromatic herb. Used in bitters. The *extract* is liquor flavoring for beverages, ice cream, and ice. Native to southern Europe. It was used to calm the nerves. The *oil* is a liquor and spice flavoring. GRAS. There is reported use of the chemical; it has not yet been assigned for toxicology literature.

I

ICELAND MOSS EXTRACT • The extract of *Lichen islandicus*. A water-soluble gum that gels on cooling. Used to flavor alcoholic beverages only.

IgE • Antibodies that are responsible for the majority of allergic reactions. Medical scientists feel that if their efforts succeed in suppressing IgE formation they will have a method of not only more effectively treating allergies but also of preventing many of them from occurring. *See also* Antibody.

IGF-I • Abbreviation for insulinlike growth factor. A natural protein required for normal growth, it is associated with the use of recombinant bovine somatotropin *(see)*. Allegations have been made that milk from treated cows may cause breast cancer. The consumption of dietary IGF-I in milk, the FDA maintains, plays no role in inducing or promoting any human disease, including breast cancer.

IMAZALIL • An antifungal used on dried citrus pulp for animal feed. FDA residue tolerance is 25 ppm in the pulp and 0.01 to 0.50 ppm in cattle fats, swine, sheep, and milk.

IMAZETHAPYR • An herbicide used on soybeans. FDA residue tolerance is 0.1 ppm.

IMIDAZOLE • Glyoxaline. White crystalline base made by the action of ammonia and formaldehyde on glyoxal. It is used as a biological control of pests and as an antihistamine.

IMIDAZOLIDINYL UREA • A bactericidal preservative with a low toxicity in animals. Sensitivity reactions have been reported in humans.

IMIDAZOLINE • A derivative of imidazole *(see)* also called *glyoxalidine*.

IMITATION • A flavor containing any portion of nonnatural materials. For instance, unless a strawberry flavoring is made entirely from strawberries, it must be called imitation. When a processor fails to use all the standard ingredients in mayonnaise, he must call it salad dressing. Imitation means that the product contains fewer vitamins, minerals, or other nutrients than the food it resembles. With reference to a fragrance, it means containing all or some portion of nonnatural materials. For instance, unless a strawberry flavoring used in lipstick is made entirely from strawberries, it must be called imitation.

IMITATION MILK • Contains no milk derivative. Usually contains water, sugar, and vegetable fat. A source of protein (such as soybean) with various additive flavorings. Imitation milk contains 1 percent protein compared to 3.5 percent in whole cow's milk.

IMMORTELLE EXTRACT • *Erytherina micopteryx.* A natural flavoring extract from a red flowered tropical tree. The name derives from the French *immortel,* "immortal" or "everlasting." Used in raspberry, fruit, and liquor flavoring for beverages, ice cream, ices, baked goods, candy, gelatin desserts, and chewing gum. GRAS.

IMPERATORIA • *Peucedanum ostruthium.* A flavoring from a tropical grass used in malt beer. Used in alcoholic beverages only.

INDIAN GUM • *See* Ghatti Gum.

INDIAN TRAGACANTH • *See* Karaya Gum.

INDIGO • Probably the oldest known dye. Prepared from various *Indigofera* plants native to Bengal, Java, and Guatemala. Dark blue powder with a coppery luster. No known skin irritation.

INDIGO CARMINE • *See* FD and C Blue No. 2.

INDOLE • A white, lustrous, flaky substance with an unpleasant odor, occurring naturally in jasmine oil and orange flowers and used as a synthetic flavoring agent in raspberry, strawberry, bitters, chocolate, orange, coffee, violet, fruit, nut, and cheese flavorings for beverages, ice cream, ices, candy, baked goods, and gelatin desserts. Also used in perfumes. It can be extracted from coal tar and feces; in highly diluted solutions, the odor is pleasant. The lethal dose in dogs is 60 milligrams per kilogram of body weight. Moderately toxic by ingestion and skin contact. Has caused tumors and cancer in laboratory animals.

INORGANIC BROMIDES PRESENT AS A RESULT OF FUMIGATION OF PROCESSED FOODS WITH ORGANIC BROMIDES and/or FROM USE ON RAW PRODUCTS • The FDA's residue tolerances are: less than 25 ppm in malt beverages; 125 ppm on all processed food; less than 125 ppm in animal feed grain milled fractions; less than 250 ppm in concentrated tomato products and dried figs; less than 325 ppm in Parmesan or Roquefort cheeses; less than 400 ppm in dried egg, or processed herbs, spices, and dog food; less than 90 in dried citrus pulp for use as cattle feed. *See* Bromides.

INOSINATE • A salt of inosinic acid used to intensify flavor, as with sodium glutamate *(see).* Inosinic acid is prepared from meat extract; also from dried sardines. No known toxicity.

INOSITOL • A dietary supplement of the vitamin B family used in emollients. Found in plant and animal tissues. Isolated commercially from corn. A fine, white crystalline powder, it is odorless with a sweet taste. Stable in air. No known toxicity. The final report to the FDA of the Select Committee on GRAS Substances stated in 1980 that it should continue its GRAS status with no limitations other than good manufacturing practices.

INSECTICIDE • A class of crop protection and specialty chemicals used to control insects on farms and forests, as well as nonagricultural applications such as residential lawns, golf courses, and public tracts of land.

INSOL. FIBER • Label listing for insoluble fiber *(see both)*.

INSOLUBLE • A substance that cannot be dissolved.

INSOLUBLE GLUCOSE ISAMASE ENZYME PREPARATIONS • GRAS. *See* Enzymes.

INTENSE SWEETENERS • Intense sweeteners are nonnutritive sweeteners, also referred to as low-calorie sweeteners. Intense sweeteners can replace nutritive sweeteners in most foods at a caloric saving of approximately 16 calories per teaspoon. Thus, caloric reduction may be achieved when low-calorie sweetened foods and beverages are substituted for their full-calorie counterparts. Examples of intense sweeteners in use in the U.S. food supply are saccharin, aspartame, and acesulfame K.

INTERMEDIATE • A chemical substance found as part of a necessary step between one organic compound and another, as in the production of dyes, pharmaceuticals, or other artificial products that develop properties only upon oxidation. Used frequently for artificial colors.

INTERNATIONAL AGENCY FOR RESEARCH ON CANCER (IARC) • A United Nations organization that gathers information on suspected environmental carcinogens and summarizes available data with appropriate references. Included in these reviews are synonyms, physical and chemical properties, uses and occurrence, and biological data relevant to the evaluation of the risk of cancer to humans. The more than forty monographs in the series contain an evaluation of about nine hundred materials.

INTRINSIC FACTOR COMPLEX • A dietary supplement of liver-stomach concentration. FDA has deemed it illegal.

INVERT SUGAR • Inversol. Colorose. A mixture of 50 percent glucose and 50 percent fructose. It is sweeter than sucrose. Commercially produced by "inversion" of sucrose. Honey is mostly invert sugar. Invert sugar is used in confectionery and in brewing. Like glycerin *(see)* it holds in moisture and prevents drying out. Used medicinally in intravenous solutions. No known toxicity. The final report to the FDA of the Select Committee on GRAS Substances stated in 1980 that there is no evidence in the available information that it is a hazard to the public when used as it is now and it should continue its GRAS status with limitations on amounts that can be added to food.

INVERTASE FROM SACCHAROMYCES CEREVISIAE • An enzyme used in processing.

IODINE SOURCES • Calcium Iodate, Cuprous Iodide, Potassium Iodate, and Potassium Iodide. Discovered in 1811 and classed among the rarer earth elements, it is found in the earth's crust as bluish black scales. Nearly two hundred products contain this chemical. They are prescription and over-the-counter medications. Iodine is an integral part of the thyroid hormones, which have important metabolic roles, and is an essential nutrient for humans. Iodine deficiency leads to thyroid enlargement or goiter. Nutritionists have found that the most efficient way to add iodine to the diet is through the use of iodized salt. The FDA has ordered all table salts to specify whether the product contains iodide. However, many commercially prepared food items do not contain iodized salt. Iodized salt contains up to .01 percent; dietary supplements contain .16 percent. Cuprous and potassium iodides are used in table salts; potassium iodide is in some drinking water; and potassium iodate is used in animal feeds. Dietary iodine is absorbed from the intestinal tract, and the main human sources are from food and water. Seafoods are good sources, and dairy products may be good sources if the cows eat enriched grain. Adult daily iodine requirement is believed to be 110 to 150 milligrams. Growing children and pregnant or lactating women may need more. Iodine compounds are used in expectorants and thinners, particularly in the treatment of asthma and in contrast media for X rays and fluoroscopy. They can produce a diffuse red pimply rash, hives, asthma, and sometimes, anaphylactic shock. Iodine is also used as an antiseptic and germicide in cosmetics.

IONONE • Used as a scent in perfumery and as a flavoring agent in foods. It occurs naturally in *Boronia,* an Australian shrub. Colorless to pale yellow with an odor reminiscent of cedar wood or violets. It may cause allergic reactions.

IPRODIONE • Glycophene. A fungicide used on various commodities including cattle, goats, hogs, chickens, sheep, and eggs. FDA residue tolerance on animal feed ranges from 10 to 300 ppm.

IPRONIDAZOLE • A feed additive withdrawn for animal use January 17, 1989.

IRIS FLORENTINA • *See* Orris.

IRISH MOSS • Emulsifier for frozen desserts, dressings, fruits, jelly, and preserves. *See* Carrageenan.

***a*-IRISONE** • *See* Ionone, *a*-Ionone.

***b*-IRISONE** • *See* Ionone, *b*-Ionone.

IRON • An essential mineral element that occurs widely in foods, especially organ meats such as liver, red meats, poultry, and leafy vegetables. The principal foods to which iron or iron salts are added are enriched cereals and some beverages, including milk, poultry stuffing, cornmeal, corn grits, and bread. *Iron ammonium citrate* is an anticaking agent in salt. *Iron-choline citrate* is cleared for use as a source of iron in foods for special dietary use. *Iron peptonate,* a combination of oxide and peptone, is made soluble by the presence of sodium citrate and is used in the treatment of iron-deficiency anemia. The recommended daily allowances for children and adults is from 0.2 milligram to 1 milligram and 18 milligrams per day for pregnant women. Iron ascorbate, carbonate, chloride, citrate, fumarate, gluconate, lactate, oxide, phosphate, pyrophospate, sulfate, and reduced iron are dietary supplements. GRAS. Iron is potentially toxic in all forms.

IRON AMMONIUM CITRATE • A salt for human or animal consumption. An anticaking agent that the FDA says should be less than 25 ppm. *See* Iron Salts.

IRON CAPRYLATE, IRON LINOLEATE, IRON NAPHTHENATE, and IRON TALLATE • All are used in packaging. Iron naphthenate was said by the Select Committee on GRAS Substances to have so little known about it that there was nothing upon which to base an evaluation of it when it is used as a food ingredient. As for the others, the final report to the FDA of the Select Committee on GRAS

Substances stated in 1980 that they should continue GRAS status with no limitations other than good manufacturing practices. There is no reported use of iron caprylate, iron naphthenate, or iron linoleate and there is no toxicology information available.

IRON-CHOLINE CITRATE COMPLEX • Used in animal feed. *See* Iron and Citrate Salts.

IRON (HARMLESS SALTS OF) • Used as nutrients in flour, macaroni, and noodles and bakery products. *See* Iron Salts.

IRON OXIDE • Any of several natural or synthetic oxides of iron (iron combined with oxygen) varying in color from red-brown or black-orange to yellow. Used for dyeing eggshells and for pet food. There is no reported use of the chemical and there is no toxicology information available. *See* Iron for toxicity.

IRON, REDUCED • Elemental iron obtained by a chemical process. It is a grayish black powder used as a nutrient and dietary supplement.

IRON SALTS • Iron Sources. Ferric, Choline Citrate, Ferric Orthophosphate, Ferric Phosphate, Ferric Sodium Pyrophosphate, Ferrous Fumarate, Ferrous Gluconate, Ferrous Lactate, and Ferrous Sulfate. Widely used as enrichment for foods, *ferric phosphate* is used as a food supplement, particularly in bread enrichment. *Ferric pyrophosphate* is a grayish blue powder used in ceramics. *Ferric sodium pyrophosphate* is used in prepared breakfast cereals, poultry stuffing, enriched flours, self-rising flours, farina, cornmeal, corn grits, bread, and rolls. The final report to the FDA of the Select Committee on GRAS Substances stated in 1980 that there is no evidence in the available information that it is a hazard to the public when used as it is now and should continue as GRAS with limitations on amounts that can be added to food. It may cause gastrointestinal disturbances. *Ferrous lactate* is greenish white with a sweet iron taste. Air and light affect it. It is also used to treat anemia. The final report to the FDA of the Select Committee on GRAS Substances stated in 1980 that there is no evidence that ferrous lactate is hazardous and therefore it should continue as GRAS with limitations. *Ferrous sulfate* is blue-green and odorless and oxidized in air and is used as a wood preservative, weed killer, and to treat anemia. Large quantities can cause gastrointestinal disturbances. For ferric choline citrate, *see* Choline Chloride. Among other irons used are ferrous gluconate, ferrous fumarate, sodium ferric EDTA, sodium ferricitropyrophosphate, ferrous citrate, and ferrous ascorbate. Iron salts are used in cosmetics mainly for coloring and as astringents.

a-IRONE • A synthetic flavoring derived from the violet family and usually isolated from irises and orris oil. A light yellow, viscous liquid, it gives off the delicate fragrance of violets when put in alcohol. It is also used to flavor dentifrices and in perfumery. *See* Orris for toxicity.

IRRADIATED ENZYMES • Used to control insects. FDA requires that the dose does not exceed 10 kilograys.

IRRADIATED ERGOSTEROL • *See* Vitamin D_2.

IRRADIATED FOOD • To control pests in any food or to inhibit maturation of fresh food. FDA regulations say the dose cannot exceed 1 kilogray.

IRRADIATED MEATS • Minimum dose 44 kilograms for sterilization of frozen packaged meats.

IRRADIATED PORK • Control of *Trichinella spiralis*. FDA says minimum dose is 0.3 kilograys. Maximum dose 1 kilograys.

IRRADIATED POULTRY • To control pathogens in fresh or frozen uncooked poultry. FDA says dose must not exceed 30 kilograys.

IRRADIATED POULTRY FEED • Dose ranges from 2 to 25 kilogray gamma radiation from cobalt-60 to render poultry feed salmonella *(see)* negative.

IRRADIATED SPICES, HERBS, and SEASONINGS • To control insects and/or microorganisms. FDA says dose is not to exceed 30 kilograys.

IRRADIATED YEAST • A nutrient in enriched farina, a source of vitamin D.

ISO • Greek for "equal." In chemistry, it is a prefix added to the name of one compound to denote another composed of the same kinds and numbers of atoms but different from each other in structural arrangement.

ISOAMYL ACETATE • A synthetic flavoring agent that occurs naturally in bananas and pears. Colorless, pearlike odor and taste, it is used in raspberry, strawberry, butter, caramel, coconut, cola, apple, banana, cherry, grape, peach, pea, pineapple, rum, cream soda, and vanilla flavorings for beverages, ice cream, ices, candy, baked goods, chewing gum (2,700 ppm), and gelatin desserts. Also used in perfuming shoe polish among other industrial uses. Exposure to 950 ppm for one hour has caused headache, fatigue, shoulder pain, and irritation of the mucous membranes.

ISOAMYL ACETOACETATE • A synthetic fruit and apple flavorings for beverages, ice cream, ices, candy, and baked goods.

ISOAMYL ALCOHOL • A synthetic flavoring agent that occurs naturally in apples, cognac, lemons, peppermint, raspberry, strawberry, and tea. Used in chocolate, apple, banana, brandy, and rum flavorings for beverages, ice cream, ices, candy, baked goods, gelatin desserts, chewing gum, and brandy. A central nervous system depressant. Vapor exposures have caused marked irritation of the eyes, nose, and throat, and headache. Amyl alcohols are highly toxic, and ingestion has caused human deaths from respiratory failure. Isoamyl alcohol may cause heart, lung, and kidney damage.

ISOAMYL BENZOATE • A synthetic berry, apple, cherry, plum, prune, liquor, rum, and maple flavoring agent for beverages, ice cream, ices, candy, gelatin desserts, baked goods, and chewing gum. Also used in perfumery and cosmetics.

ISOAMYL CINNAMATE • A synthetic strawberry, butter, caramel, chocolate, cocoa, fruit, peach, pineapple, and honey flavoring agent for beverages, ice cream, candy, and baked goods.

ISOAMYL FORMATE • Formic Acid. A synthetic flavoring agent, colorless, liquid, with a fruity smell. Used in strawberry, apple, apricot, banana, peach, and pineapple flavorings for beverages, ice cream, candy, baked goods, gelatin desserts, and chewing gum. *See* Formic Acid for toxicity.

ISOAMYL 2-FURANBUTYRATE • A synthetic chocolate, coffee, fruit, and whiskey flavoring agent for beverages, ices, candy, baked goods, and gelatin.

ISOAMYL 2-FURANPROPIONATE • A synthetic chocolate, coffee, fruit, and whiskey flavoring agent for beverages, ice cream, ices, candy, and baked goods.

a-**ISOAMYL FURFURYLACETATE** • *See* Isoamyl 2-Furanpropionate.

a-**ISOAMYL FURFURYLPROPIONATE** • *See* Isoamyl 2-Furanbutyrate.

ISOAMYL ISOBUTYRATE • A synthetic fruit and banana flavoring agent for beverages, ice cream, ices, candy, baked goods, gelatin desserts, puddings, and chewing gum (2,000 ppm). Used in manufacture of artificial rum and fruit essences.

ISOAMYL ISOVALERATE • A synthetic flavoring agent, clear, colorless, liquid, with an apple odor. Occurs naturally in bananas and peaches. Used in raspberry, strawberry, apple, apricot, banana, cherry, peach, pineapple, honey, rum, walnut, vanilla, and cream soda flavoring for beverages, ice cream, ices, candy, baked goods, gelatin desserts, puddings, jellies, liqueurs, and chewing gum. No known toxicity.

ISOAMYL LAURATE • The ester of isoamyl alcohol and lauric acid *(see both)* used as a synthetic fruit flavoring for beverages, ice cream, ices, candy, and baked goods.

ISOAMYL NONANOATE • A synthetic chocolate, fruit, and liquor flavoring agent for beverages, ice cream, ices, candy, baked goods, and gelatin desserts.

ISOAMYL OCTANOATE • A synthetic chocolate, fruit, and liquor flavoring agent for beverages, ice cream, ices, candy, baked goods, and gelatin desserts.

ISOAMYL PHENYLACETATE • A synthetic butter, chocolate, cocoa, peach, honey, licorice, and anise flavoring agent for beverages, ice cream, ices, candy, baked goods, toppings, and gelatin desserts.

ISOAMYL PYRUVATE • A synthetic flavoring agent, colorless, liquid, with a pleasant odor. Used in root beer and fruit flavorings for beverages, ice cream, ices, candy, and baked goods. Also used in perfumery and soaps. *See* Salicylic Acid for toxicity.

ISOASCORBIC ACID • Preservative. GRAS. *See* Erythorbic Acid.

ISOBORNEOL • A synthetic fruit and spice flavoring agent for beverages, ice cream, ices, candy, baked goods, and chewing gum. *See* Borneol for toxicity.

ISOBORNYL ACETATE • A synthetic pine odor in bath preparations. Also used as a synthetic fruit flavoring for beverages, ice cream, ices, candy, baked goods, and gelatin.

ISOBUTANE • A propellant. There is no reported use of the chemical and there is no toxicology information available. GRAS. *See* Butanes.

ISOBUTRYALDEHYDE • A synthetic flavoring agent that occurs naturally in soy sauce, tea, tobacco, and coffee. It has a pungent odor. Used in berry, butter, caramel, fruit, liquor, and wine flavorings for beverages, ice cream, ices, candy, baked goods, and liquor.

ISOBUTYL ACETATE • The ester of isobutyl alcohol and acetic acid used as a synthetic flavoring agent. A clear, colorless liquid with a fruity odor. Used in raspberry, strawberry, butter, banana, and grape flavorings for beverages, ice cream, ices, candy, baked goods, gelatin desserts, chewing gum, and icings. It may be mildly irritating to mucous membranes, and in high concentrations it is narcotic.

ISOBUTYL ACETOACETATE • A synthetic berry and fruit flavoring agent for beverages, ice cream, ices, candy, and baked goods. *See* Isobutyl Acetate for toxicity.

ISOBUTYL ALCOHOL • Present in fusel oil; also produced by fermentation of carbohydrates. Colorless liquid with an odor of amyl alcohol, it is used in the manufacture of synthetic fruit flavorings and as a solvent. It is mildly irritating to skin and mucous membranes and, in high concentrations, narcotic.

ISOBUTYL ANTHRANILATE • A synthetic mandarin orange, cherry, and grape flavoring agent for beverages, ice cream, ices, candy, baked goods, and chewing gum (1,700 ppm).

ISOBUTYL BENZOATE • A synthetic berry, cherry, plum, and pineapple flavoring agent for beverages, ice cream, ices, candy, and baked goods.

ISOBUTYL BUTYRATE • A synthetic berry, apple, banana, pineapple, liquor, and rum flavoring agent for beverages, ice cream, ices, candy, puddings, liquors, and baked goods.

2(4)-ISOBUTYL-4(2),DIMETHYLDIHYDRO-4H-1,3,5-DIMETHYLDIHYDRO-4H-1,3,5-DITHIAZINE • A newer synthetic flavoring.

ISOBUTYL 2-FURANPROPIONATE • A synthetic berry and pineapple flavoring agent for beverages, ice cream, ices, gelatin desserts, chewing gum, and ices.

ISOBUTYL HEXANOATE • A synthetic apple and pineapple flavoring agent for beverages, ice cream, ices, chewing gums, and baked goods.

ISOBUTYL ISOBUTYRATE • A synthetic strawberry, butter, fruit, banana, and liquor flavoring agent for beverages, ice cream, ices, candy, gelatin desserts, puddings, liquors, and baked goods.

ISOBUTYL PABA • *See* Propylparaben.

ISOBUTYL PALMITATE • *See* Palmitate.

ISOBUTYL PARABEN • *See* Parabens.

ISOBUTYL PELARGONATE • The ester of isobutyl alcohol and pelargonic acid *(see both)*.

ISOBUTYL PHENYLACETATE • A synthetic butter, caramel, chocolate, fruit, honey, and nut flavoring agent for beverages, ice cream, ices, candy, puddings, maraschino cherries, and baked goods.

ISOBUTYL PROPIONATE • A synthetic strawberry, butter, peach, and rum flavoring agent for beverages, ice cream, candy, and baked goods. Used in the manufacture of fruit essences.

ISOBUTYL SALICYLATE • A synthetic flavoring agent; colorless liquid with an orchid odor. Used in fruit and root beer flavorings for beverages, ice cream, ices, candy, and baked goods. *See* Salicylic Acid for toxicity.

ISOBUTYL STEARATE • The ester of isobutyl alcohol and stearic acid. *See* Fatty Alcohols. Used in waterproof coatings, polishes, face creams, rouges, ointments, soaps, dyes, and lubricants. No known toxicity.

ISOBUTYLENE/ISOPYRENE COPOLYMER • A copolymer of isobutylene and isoprene monomers derived from petroleum and used as resins. A chewing-gum base. Isobutylene is used to produce antioxidants for foods, food supplements, and packaging. Vapors may cause asphyxiation.

ISOBUTYLENE/MALEIC ANHYDRIDE COPOLYMER • A copolymer of isobutylene and maleic anhydride monomers derived from petroleum and used as a resin. Strong irritant.

ISOBUTYLENE RESIN, POLYISOBUTYLENE • A component of chewing-gum base.

a-ISOBUTYLPHENETHYL ALCOHOL • A synthetic butter, caramel, chocolate, fruit, and spice flavoring agent for beverages, ice cream, ices, candy, baked goods, liqueurs, and chocolate. See Isoamyl Alcohol for toxicity.

ISOBUTYRIC ACID • A synthetic flavoring agent that occurs naturally in bay, bay leaves, parsley, and strawberries. It has a pungent odor. Used in butter, butterscotch, fruit, liquor, rum, cheese, nut, vanilla, and cream soda flavorings for beverages, ice cream, ices, candy, baked goods, chewing gum, and margarine. It is a mild irritant. A pungent liquid that smells like butyric acid *(see)*.

ISOCETYL ALCOHOL • *See* Cetyl Alcohol.

ISOCETYL ISODECANOATE • *See* Cetyl Alcohol.

ISOCETYL PALMITATE • *See* Cetyl Alcohol and Palmitate.

ISOCETYL STEARATE • *See* Cetyl Alcohol and Stearic Acid.

ISOCETYL STEAROYL STEARATE • The ester of isocetyl alcohol, stearic alcohol, and stearic acid. *See* Fatty Acids.

ISOEUGENOL • An aromatic liquid phenol oil obtained from eugenol *(see)* by mixing with an alkali. A synthetic flavoring agent, pale yellow, viscous, with a floral odor. Occurs naturally in mace oil. Used in mint, fruit, spice, cinnamon, and clove flavorings for beverages, ice cream, ices, baked goods, chewing gum (1,000 ppm), and condiments. Used in the manufacture of vanillin *(see)*. Moderately toxic by ingestion. Has caused mutations in experimental animals.

ISOEUGENYL ACETATE • A synthetic berry, fruit, and spice flavoring agent for beverages, ice cream, ices, candy, baked goods, and chewing gum.

ISOEUGENOL ACETATE • *See* Acetylisoeugenol.

ISOEUGENYL ETHYL ETHER • A synthetic flavoring agent, white, crystalline, with a spicy, clovelike odor. Used in fruit and vanilla flavorings for beverages, ice cream, ices, candy, and baked goods.

ISOEUGENYL FORMATE • A synthetic spice flavoring agent used in condiments. *See* Formic Acid for toxicity.

ISOEUGENYL METHYL ETHER • A synthetic raspberry, strawberry, cherry, and clove flavoring agent for beverages, ices, ice cream, candy, baked goods, gelatin desserts, and chewing gum.

ISOEUGENYL PHENYLACETATE • A synthetic fruit, honey, and spice flavoring agent for beverages, ice cream, ices, candy, and baked goods.

ISOJASMONE • *See* Jasmone.

ISOLATE • A substance that is freed from chemical contaminants.

ISOLEUCINE • L Form. An essential amino acid not synthesized within the human body. Isolated commercially from beet sugar, it is a building block of protein. Used as a nutrient and dietary supplement. The FDA asked for further study of this nutrient in 1980. GRAS.

ISOMALT • A candidate for an artificial sweetener, it has 45 to 65 percent the sweetness of sugar. A component of bread obtained by the action of enzymes on starch. It contains calories and is physically similar to sugar. It is a free-flowing, white crystalline. It has a sweet taste reportedly without any aftertaste. While it is not as sweet as sugar, it may be enhanced with an intense sweetener such as acesulfame K *(see)*. It is used in fifteen countries in candies, gums, ice cream, jams, and baked goods.

ISONONYL ISONONANOATE • The ester *(see)* produced by the reaction of nonyl alcohol with nonanoic acid. Used in fruit flavorings for lipsticks and mouthwashes. Occurs in cocoa, oil of lavender. No known toxicity.

ISOPARAFFINIC PETROLEUM HYDROCARBONS, SYNTHETIC • Coating agent, insecticide formulations, used on eggs, fruits, pickles, vegetables, wine, and vinegar. *See* Paraffin.

ISOPHORONE • White, watery liquid that is irritating to skin and eyes. It is used in solvents for polyvinyl and nitrocellulose resins, and pesticides.

ISOPROPANOL • *See* Isopropyl Alcohol.

ISOPROPANOLAMINE • An emulsifying agent with a light ammonia odor that is soluble in water. It is used as a plasticizer and in insecticides as well as in cosmetic creams. No known toxicity.

ISOPROPYL ALCOHOL • Isopropanol. An antibacterial, solvent, and denaturant *(see)*. Solvent for the spice oleoresins. The FDA permits residues of 250 ppm or less in modified hop extract; 50 ppm in spice oleoresins; 6 ppm in manufacture of lemon oil; 2 percent by weight in hop extract as residue from extraction of hops in manufacture of beer. It is also used in defoaming agents for processing beet sugar and yeast, on food-processing equipment and on food-contact sufraces as well as on glass containers for holding milk. It is prepared from propylene, which is obtained in the cracking of petroleum. Also used in antifreeze compositions and as a solvent for gums, shellac, and essential oils. Ingestion or inhalation of large quantities of the vapor may cause flushing, headache, dizziness, mental depression, nausea, vomiting, narcosis, anesthesia, and coma. The fatal ingested dose is around a fluid ounce.

ISOPROPYL CITRATE • A sequestrant and antioxidant agent used in oleomargarine and salad oils. The final report to the FDA of the Select Committee on GRAS Substances stated in 1980 that it should continue its GRAS status with no limitations other than good manufacturing practices. When heated to decomposition it emits acrid smoke and irritating fumes.

ISOPROPYL FORMATE • Formic Acid. A synthetic berry and melon flavoring agent for beverages, ice cream, candy, and baked goods.

ISOPROPYL HEXANOATE • A synthetic pineapple flavoring agent for beverages, ice cream, ices, candy, and baked goods.

ISOPROPYL ISOBUTYRATE • A synthetic pineapple flavoring agent for beverages, ice cream, ices, candy, and baked goods.

ISOPROPYL ISOSTEARATE • *See* Stearic Acid and Propylene Glycol.

ISOPROPYL ISOVALERATE • A synthetic pineapple and nut flavoring agent for beverages, ice cream, ices, candy, and baked goods.

ISOPROPYL PHENYLACETATE • A synthetic butter, caramel, and honey flavoring agent for beverages, ice cream, ices, candy, and baked goods.

ISOSAFROEUGENOL • White crystalline powder with a vanilla odor used as a flavoring agent in various foods. Moderately toxic by ingestion.

ISOSTEARIC ACID • A saturated fatty acid that has the same uses as stearic acid and oleic acids *(see both)*.

ISOTHIOCYANATES • Found in mustard, horseradish, radishes, they seem to induce protective enzymes.

ISOTHIOUREA • Antifungal agent used on citrus fruit. Prohibited from direct addition or use in human food.

ISOVALERIC ACID • Occurs in valerian, hop oil, tobacco, and other plants. Colorless liquid with a disagreeable taste and odor used in flavors and perfumes. A poison by skin contact. Moderately toxic by ingestion. A corrosive skin and eye irritant. *See* Valeric Acid.

ISOVALERIC ACID, ALLYL ESTER, BENZYL ESTER, BUTYL ESTER, ETHYL ESTER • Flavoring agents in various foods. The allyl ester is under IARC review. The allyl form is poisonous by ingestion. The others are mildly toxic by ingestion. Moderately toxic by skin contact. Skin irritants.

ISOVINYL FORMATE • Formic Acid. A synthetic fruit flavoring agent for beverages, ices cream, ices, candy, and baked goods. *See* Formic Acid for toxicity.

ISOVINYL PROPIONATE • *See* Isovinyl Formate.

I.U. • International Unit. A term for measurement of vitamins that are fat soluble (do not mix with water and need fat for proper absorption). Vitamins A, E, D, and K are usually measured in I.U.'s.

IVA • *Achillea moschata jacq.* A flavoring for alcoholic beverages only from a small American ground pine that smells like skin. There is no reported use of the chemical and there is no toxicology information available.

IVERMECTIN • Mectizan. Hyvermectin. A drug used to treat river blindness in humans, it is used to treat worms in animals, especially beef, pork, and reindeer. FDA limits residues to 15 ppb in cattle and reindeer liver, and 20 ppb in swine liver. Poison by injection under the skin. Potential adverse human effects include dizziness, fever, headache, tender swollen glands, rash, and fatigue.

J

JAGUAR GUM • *See* Guar Gum.

JAMBUL OLEORESIN • Java Plum. *Syzygium jambolanum.* Used medically as an antidiarrheal medication. Used as a flavoring in foods.

JAPAN WAX • Japan Tallow. Sumac Wax. Vegetable Wax. Japan Tallow. A fat squeezed from the fruit of a tree grown in Japan and China. Pale yellow, flat cakes, disks or squares, with a fatlike rancid odor and taste. Used as a substitute for beeswax in cosmetic and in food packaging, also floor waxes and polishes. It is related to poison ivy and may cause allergic contact dermatitis. The final report to the FDA of the Select Committee on GRAS Substances stated in 1980 that there were insufficient relevant biological and other studies upon which to base an evaluation of it when it is used as a food ingredient. It remains GRAS for packaging.

JASMINE • Oil and Spiritus (alcoholic solution). The oil is extracted from a tropical shrub with extremely fragrant white flowers and is used in raspberry, strawberry, floral, and cherry flavorings for ice cream, ices, candy, baked goods, gelatin desserts, chewing gum, and jelly. The spiritus is used in blackberry, strawberry, and fruit flavoring for beverages, ice cream, ices, candy, baked goods, gelatin, and cherries. Used in perfumes. May cause allergic reactions. GRAS. There is reported use of the chemical; it has not yet been assigned for toxicology literature.

JASMINE ABSOLUTE • Oil of jasmine obtained by extraction with volatile or nonvolatile solvents. Sometimes called the "natural perfume" because the oil is not subjected to heat and distilled oils. *See* Absolute. May cause allergic reactions. There is reported use of the chemical; it has not yet been assigned for toxicology literature.

JASMONATES • Derived from fragrant compounds with the odor of jasmine flowers (*see* Jasmine Absolute), these have been found to keep stored potatoes from sprouting.

JASMONE • Derived from the oil of jasmine flowers, it is used in flavorings and perfumery.

JASMONYL • *See* 1,3-Nonanediol Acetate.

JELUTONG • *Dyer costulata hook.* Any of several trees with a milky white exudate. Resembles chicle and is used chiefly in waterproofing and in chewing gum.

JOJOBA OIL • The oil extracted from the beanlike seeds of the desert shrub, *Simondsia chinensis.* A liquid wax used as a lubricant and as a substitute for sperm oil, carnauba wax, and beeswax. Mexicans and Indians have long used the bean's oily wax as a hair conditioner and skin lubricant. United States companies are now promoting the ingredient in shampoos, moisturizers, sunscreens, and conditions as a treatment for crow's feet, wrinkles, stretch marks, and dry skin. May cause allergic reactions.

JUNIPER • Extract, Oil, and Berries. A flavoring from the dried ripe fruit of trees grown in northern Europe, Asia, and North America. The greenish yellow extract is used in liquor, root beer, sarsaparilla, wintergreen, and birch beer flavorings for beverages, ice cream, ices, candy, and baked goods. The *oil* is used in berry, cola, pineapple, gin, rum, whiskey, root beer, ginger, and meat flavorings for beverages, ice cream, ices, candy, baked goods, gelatin desserts, chewing gum, meats, and liquors. The *berries* are used in gin flavoring for condiments and liquors. Juniper is used also in fumigating and was formerly a diuretic for reducing body water. The oil is mildly toxic by ingestion, a human skin irritant and allergen, and if taken internally, a severe kidney irritation similar to that caused by turpentine may result. GRAS. There is reported use of the chemical; it has not yet been assigned for toxicology literature.

K

KABAT • Altosid. Methoprene. Amber liquid used as an insect growth regulator in animal feed, dried apples, apricots, barley cereal, beef, corn cereal, corn meal, grits, hominy, macaroni, oat cereal, dried peaches, potable water, dried prunes, raisins, rice cereal, rye cereal, spices, wheat cereal, and wheat flour. FDA's insect growth regulator residue tolerance is 10 ppm in the grains, rice, and dried fruits. Exempt from the tolerance is potable water. Moderately toxic by skin contact. Mildly toxic by ingestion. Has caused mutations in laboratory animals.

KADAYA • *See* Karaya Gum.

KAOLIN • China Clay. Used as an anticaking agent in food. Aids in the covering ability of face powder and in absorbing oil secreted by the skin. Used in baby powder, bath powder, face masks, foundation cake makeup, liquid powder, face powder, dry rouge, and emollients. Originally obtained from Kaoling Hill in Kiangsi Province in southeast China. Essentially a hydrated aluminum silicate *(see)*. It is a white or yellowish white mass or powder, insoluble in water and absorbent. Used medicinally to treat intestinal disorders, but in large doses it may cause obstructions, perforations, or granuloma (tumor) formation. It is also used in the manufacture of porcelain, pottery, bricks, and color lakes *(see)*. No known toxicity for the skin. The final report to the FDA of the Select Committee on GRAS Substances stated in 1980 that it should continue its GRAS status with no limitations other than good manufacturing practices. *See* also Clays.

KARAYA GUM • Kaday. Katilo. Kullo. Kuterra. Sterculia. Indian Tragacanth. Mucara. The exudate of a tree found in India. The finely ground white powder is used as a stabilizer in gelatins, gumdrops, prepared ices, and ice cream, and as a filler for lemon custard. Also a citrus and spice flavoring agent for beverages, ice cream, ices (1,300 ppm), candy, meats, baked goods, toppings (3,500 ppm), and emulsions (18,000 ppm). Used instead of the more expensive gum tragacanth *(see)* and in bulk laxatives. Reevaluated by the FDA in 1976 and found to be GRAS in the following percentages: 0.3 for frozen dairy desserts and mixes; 0.02 percent for milk products; 0.9 percent for soft candy; and 0.002 for all other food categories. GRAS.

KATILO • *See* Karaya Gum.

KAUTSCHIN • *See* d-Limonene.

KELP • Recovered from the giant Pacific marine plant *Macrocystis pyriferae.* Used as seasonings or flavoring and to provide iodine when used in dietary foods. It has many minerals that are associated with seawater and, as a result, is very high in sodium. The FDA residue tolerance is less than 0.225 mg per day without reference to age or physical state; 0.045 mg per day for infants; 0.105 mg per day for those under 4 years; 0.225 per day for adults and children. For pregnant or lactating women, 0.20 mg per day. It is a source of iodine in foods for special dietary use. The Japanese report that kelp reduced normal thyroid function, probably because of its iodine content. The FDA has also reported that high levels of arsenic have been found in people who eat a lot of kelp as a vegetable. The final report to the FDA of the Select Committee on GRAS Substances stated in 1980 that it should continue its GRAS status with no limitations other than good manufacturing practices. There is reported use of the chemical; it has not yet been assigned for toxicology literature search. *See* Algae, Brown.

KETONAROME • *See* Methylcyclopentenolone.

KETONE C-7 • *See* 2-Heptanone.

2-KETOPROPIONALDEHYDE • *See* Pyruvaldehyde.

a-KETOPROPIONALDEHYDE • *See* Pyruvic Acid.

KG • Abbreviation for *kilogram,* which is equal to about 2.205 pounds.

KIDNEY BEAN EXTRACT • Extract of *Phaseolus vulgaris,* the beans were used as a nutrient and a laxative by the American Indians. No known toxicity.

KILOGRAM (kg) • Equal to about 2.205 pounds.

KOLA NUT EXTRACT • Guru Nut. A natural extract from the brownish seed, about the size of a chestnut, produced by trees in Africa, West Indies, and Brazil. Contains caffeine *(see)*. Used in butter, caramel, chocolate, cocoa, coffee, cola, walnut, and root beer flavorings for beverages, ice cream, ices, candy, and baked goods. Has been used to treat epilepsy. GRAS.

KONJAC FLOUR • Konjac Mannan. Konnyaku. Yam Flour. It is derived from the tubers of *Amorphophallus konjac,* a large plant grown in Japan for its flour. A food additive that is expected to increase in use as a gelling agent, thickener, emulsifier, and stabilizer in such foods as soup, gravy, mayonnaise, and jam. There is a long history of use in traditional Japanese and Chinese goods; the average consumption of konjac flour from these uses is estimated to be between two and three grams per person per day and sometimes as high as four grams. The anticipated maximum consumption of konjac flour from food additive uses is about three grams per person per day. Human studies conducted for up to sixty-five days at dose levels of up to 8.6 grams of konjac flour per person per day. Volunteers consuming approximately 5.2 g or more reported loose stools, flatulence, diarrhea, and abdominal pain or distension. Studies with normal and diabetic volunteers demonstrated that consumption of 7.2 to 8.6 grams of konjac flour per day for 17 days significantly decreased mean fasting blood sugar levels; in addition, a dose of 3.9 to 5 grams consumed in a single meal or administered with glucose was reported to delay the increase in blood sugar and insulin levels for several hours following the meal, also delaying their return to baseline levels. The test meal also appeared to impair vitamin E absorption (up to 30 percent decrease) and influenced the absorption of co-administered drug glibenclamide (a diabetes medication). On the basis of the available toxicological data and the long history of use of konjac in food, the Committee allocated temporary ADI *(see)* "not specified" for konjac flour and said a review should be done of konjac's affect on vitamin E and other fat-soluble vitamins. Also, it was noted that consumption of dry konjac has been associated with obstruction of the esophagus and that it should be consumed only in hydrated form.

KONNYAKU • *See* Konjac Flour.

KOSHER • Parv. U. Hebrew word meaning "proper" or "fit," used especially for food prepared according to Orthodox dietary and religious laws. Forbidden are pork, horseflesh, shellfish, and parts of beef and lamb. All meat and poultry must be killed by a Jew trained in the prescribed ritual, then soaked or salted to remove all blood. Milk and its products must not be eaten with meat. The notifications on packages meaning the product has been prepared under dietary laws are *U* or *Parv.*

KRAMERIA EXTRACT • Rhatany Extract. A synthetic flavoring derived from the dried root of either of two American shrubs. Used in raspberry, bitters, fruit, and rum flavorings. Used in cosmetics as an astringent. Low oral toxicity. Large doses may produce gastric distress. Can cause tumors and death after injection, but not after ingestion.

KULLO • *See* Karaya Gum.

KUTEERA • *See* Karaya Gum.

L

LABDANUM • Absolute, Oil, and Oleoresin. A synthetic musk flavoring agent. It is a volatile oil obtained by steam distillation from gum extracted from various rockrose shrubs. Golden yellow, viscous, with a strong balsamic odor and a bitter taste. The absolute is used in raspberry, fruit, and vanilla flavorings for beverages, ice cream, ices, candy, baked goods, gelatin desserts, and chewing gum. The oil is used in fruit and spice flavorings for beverages, ice cream, ices, candy, and baked goods. The oleoresin *(see)* is used in fruit and vanilla flavorings for beverages, ice cream, ices, candy, and baked goods. Also used in perfumes, especially as a fixative. Mildly toxic by ingestion. A skin irritant. There is reported use of the chemical; it has not yet been assigned for toxicology literature.

LABRADOR TEA EXTRACT • Hudson Bay Tea. Marsh Tea. The extract of the dried flowering plant or young shoots of *Ledum palustre* or *Ledum groelandicum,* a tall, resinous evergreen shrub found in bogs, swamps, and moist meadows. Brewed like tea, it has a pleasing odor and is stimulating. It was used by the Indians and settlers as a tonic supposed to purify blood. It was also employed to treat wounds. The *Ledum palustre* contains, among other things, tannin and valeric acid *(see both)*. No known toxicity.

LACTASE ENZYME PREPARATION FROM *SACCHAROMYCES FRAGILIS* or *KLUVEROMYCES LACTIS* • An enzyme that breaks down lactose *(see)*. There is no reported use of the chemical and there is no toxicology information available. GRAS.

LACTIC ACID • Butyl Lactate. Ethyl Lactate. Odorless, colorless, usually a syrupy product normally present in blood and muscle tissue as a product of the metabolism of glucose and glycogen. Present in sour milk, beer, sauerkraut, pickles, and other food products made by bacterial fermentation. It is produced commercially by fermentation of whey, cornstarch, potatoes, and molasses. Used as an acidulant in beverages, candy, olives, dried egg whites, cottage cheese, confections, bread, rolls, buns, cheese products, frozen desserts, sherbets, ices, fruit jelly, butter, preserves, jams (sufficient amounts may be added to compensate for the deficiency of fruit acidity), and in the brewing industry. Also used in infant-feeding formulas. Used in blackberry, butter, butterscotch, lime, chocolate, fruit, walnut, spice, and cheese flavorings for beverages, ice cream, ices, candy, baked goods, gelatins, puddings, chewing gum, toppings, pickles, and olives (24,000 ppm). Also used in skin fresheners. It is caustic in concentrated solutions when taken internally or applied to the skin. In cosmetic products, it may cause stinging in sensitive people, particularly in fair-skinned women. The final report to the FDA of the Select Committee on GRAS Substances stated in 1980 that it should continue its GRAS status with no limitations other than good manufacturing practices.

LACTIC YEASTS • Obtained from milk. *See* Lactic Acid.

LACTOFEN • A pesticide used on soybeans. FDA tolerance is 0.05 ppm.

LACTOFLAVIN • *See* Riboflavin.

LACTOSE • Milk Sugar. Saccharum Lactin. D-Lactose. A slightly sweet-tasting, colorless sugar present in the milk of mammals (humans have 6.7 percent and cows 4.3 percent). Occurs as a white powder or crystalline mass as a byproduct of the cheese industry. Produced from whey *(see)*. It is inexpensive and is widely used in the food industry as a culture medium, such as in souring milk, and as a humectant *(see)* and nutrient in infant or debilitated patient formula. Also used as a medical diuretic and laxative. Used widely as a base in eye lotions. Stable in air but readily absorbs odors. It is generally nontoxic. However, it was found to cause tumors when injected under the skin of mice in 50-milligram doses per kilogram of body weight.

LACTITOL • A candidate for approval as an artificial sweetener. It has 30 to 40 percent the sweetness of sugar and does contain calories. It has potential for baked goods, chewing gum. *See* Lactose.

LACTOSE HYDROLYZED • A nutritive sweetener used in cheeses. *See* Lactose.

LACTYLIC ESTERS OF FATTY ACIDS • Emulsifiers used in food products. *See* Esters and Fatty Acids.

LACTYLIC STEARATE • Salt of stearic acid *(see)* used as a dough conditioner to add volume and to keep baked products soft; it makes bread less sticky. *See* Stearic Acid for toxicity.

LADY'S-MANTLE EXTRACT • From the dried leaves and flowering shoots of *Achemilla vulgaris.* A common European herb covered with spreading hairs, it has been used for centuries by herbalists to concoct love potions.

LAKES, COLOR • A lake is an organic pigment prepared by precipitating a soluble color with a form of aluminum, calcium, barium potassium, strontium, or zirconium, which then makes the colors insoluble. Not all colors are suitable for making lakes.

LAMINARIA • Seaweed from which algin is extracted. *See* Alginates. GRAS.

LANALOOL • Synthetic flavoring. GRAS.

LANOLIN • Wool Fat. Wool Wax. A product of the oil glands of sheep. Used as a chewing-gum base component. Used in lipstick, liquid powder, mascara, nail polish remover, protective oil, rouge, eye shadow, foundation creams, foundation cake makeup, hair conditioners, eye creams, cold creams, brilliantine hairdressings, ointment bases, and emollients. A water-absorbing base material and a natural emulsifier, it absorbs and holds water to the skin. Chemically a wax instead of a fat. Contains about 25 to 30 percent water. Advertisers have found that the words "contains lanolin" help to sell a product and have promoted it as being able to "penetrate the skin better than other oils," although there is little scientific proof of this. Lanolin has been found to be a common skin sensitizer causing allergic contact skin rashes. It will not prevent or cure wrinkles and will not stop hair loss. It is not used in pure form today because of its allergy-causing potential. Products derived from it are less likely to cause allergic reactions.

LANOLIN ALCOHOLS • Sterols, triterpene, alcohols. Aliphatic Alcohols. Derived from lanolin *(see),* lanolin alcohols are available commercially as solid waxy materials that are yellow to amber in color or as pale to golden-yellow liquids. They are widely used as emulsifiers and emollients in hand creams and lotions, and while less likely to cause an allergic reaction than lanolin, still may do so in the sensitive.

LANTANA • *See* Oregano.

LARCH GUM • Larch Turpentine. Venice Turpentine. Oleoresin *(see)* from *Larix decidua,* grown in middle and southern Europe. A yellow, sometimes greenish, tenacious, thick liquid with a pleasant aromatic odor, it has a hot, somewhat bitter taste. It becomes hard and brittle on prolonged exposure. It is used as a stabilizer, thickener, and texturizer. No known toxicity.

LARD and LARD OILS • Pork Fat and Oils. It is the purified internal fat from the abdomen of the hog. It is a soft white unctuous mass, with a slight characteristic odor and a bland taste. It is used in packaging and in chewing-gum bases. Easily absorbed by the skin, it is used as a lubricant, emollient, and base in shaving creams, soaps, and various cosmetic creams. Insoluble in water. When lard was fed to laboratory animals in doses of from 2 to 25 percent of the diet, the male mice had a shortened life span and increased osteoarthritis. This was thought to be due to the large amounts of fat and not specifically to lard. The final report to the FDA of the Select Committee on GRAS Substances stated in 1980 that it should continue its GRAS status with no limitations other than good manufacturing practices. There is no reported use of the chemical and there is no toxicology information available.

LARD GLYCERIDE • *See* Lard.

LARIXINIC ACID • *See* Maltol.

LASALOCID • An antibiotic used in beef, chicken, and lamb. Tolerance residue of 10.3 ppm in chicken skin, 0.7 ppm, in cattle liver, and 1.2 ppm in sheep muscle. Poison by ingestion and injection. An eye and skin irritant.

LASOLOCID SODIUM • An antibiotic feed additive. The tolerated residue in edible tissues of chicken is 0.05 ppm; 4.8 ppm in cattle liver.

LASSO • *See* Alachlor.

LATEX • Synthetic Rubber. Component of chewing-gum base. The milky, usually white juice or exudate of plants obtained by tapping. Used in beauty masks for its coating ability and in balloons, condoms, and gloves. Any of various gums, resins, fats, or waxes in an emulsion of water and synthetic rubber of plastic are now considered latex. Ingredients of latex compounds can be poisonous, depending upon which plant products are used. Can cause skin rash. In May 1991, the FDA cautioned doctors and manufacturers about potential allergic reactions to latex products. Allergic reactions caused the death of four patients undergoing medical procedures involving an inflatable latex cuff. The FDA also reported fifty cases of life-threatening allergic reactions involving latex gloves and, in other instances, contact with rubber dental devices, balloons, and racquetball handles.

LAUREL BERRIES • *Laurus nobilis.* The fresh berries and leaf extract of the laurel tree. The berries are used as a flavoring for beverages and the leaf extract is a spice flavoring for vegetables. There is no reported use of the chemical and there is no toxicology information available. *See* Laurel Leaf Oil. GRAS.

LAUREL GALLATE • An antioxidant, the laurel ester gallic acid. *See* Propyl Gallate.

LAUREL LEAF OIL • Derived from steam distillation of the leaves of *Laurus nobilis,* it is a yellow liquid with a spicy odor used as a flavoring agent. Moderately toxic by ingestion. A skin irritant. GRAS.

LAURIC ACID • Dodecanoic Acid. A common constituent of vegetable fats, especially coconut oil and laurel oil. A white, glossy powder, insoluble in water, and used in the manufacture of miscellaneous flavors for beverages, ice cream, candy, baked goods, gelatins, and puddings. Its derivatives are widely used as a base in the manufacture of soaps, detergents, and lauryl alcohol (*see* Fatty Alcohols) because of their foaming properties. Has a slight odor of bay and makes large copious bubbles when in soap. A mild irritant but not a sensitizer.

LAURIC ALDEHYDE • *See* Lauric Acid.

LAUROAMPHOACETATE • A preservative. *See* Imidazole.

LAUROAMPHODIACETATE • A preservative. *See* Imidazole.

LAUROAMPHODIPROPIONATE • *See* Propionic Acid and Lauric Acid.

LAUROAMPHODIPROPIONIC ACID • A preservative. *See* Lauric Acid and Propionic Acid.

LAUROAMPHOHDROXYPROPYLSULFONATE • *See* Imidazolin.

LAUROAMPHOPROPINOATE • *See* Lauric Acid and Propionic Acid.

LAUROSTEARIC ACID • *See* Lauric Acid.

LAURYL ACETATE • Dodecyl Acetate. Colorless liquid with fruity odor used in flavoring.

LAURYL ALCOHOL, SYNTHETIC • *See* Fatty Alcohols.

a-LAURYL-OMEGA-HYDROXYPOLY(OXYETHYLENE) • Sanitation compound. May be used on beverage containers including milk containers and equipment.

LAVANDIN OIL • A flavoring from a hybrid related to the lavender plant, pale yellow liquid with a camphor-lavender smell. Used in berry and citrus flavorings for beverages, ice cream, ices, candy, baked goods, and chewing gum. Used in soaps and perfumes. A skin irritant. GRAS. There is reported use of the chemical; it has not yet been assigned for toxicology literature.

LAVENDER OIL • *Lavandul officinalis*. The colorless liquid extracted from the fresh, flowery tops of the plant. Smells like lavender and is used in ginger ale flavoring for beverages. *Lavender absolute* is a fruit flavoring for beverages, ice cream, ices, candy, and baked goods. *Lavender concrete* is a fruit flavoring for beverages, ice cream, ices, candy, and baked goods. Lavender was once used to break up stomach gas. Used in skin fresheners, powders, shaving preparations, mouthwashes, dentifrices, and perfumes. It can cause allergic reactions and has been found to cause adverse skin reactions when the skin is exposed to sunlight. GRAS.

LEAD • This metal can enter the body in two ways—by ingestion and inhalation. Lead can build up in the body even if you are exposed to small amounts for a long time. In general, the more lead in your body, the more likely harm will occur. It is one of the most hazardous of toxic metals because its poison is cumulative and its toxic effects are many and severe. Among these are leg cramps, muscle weakness, numbness, depression, brain damage, coma, and death. Obvious symptoms of lead toxicity may occur in some people with levels as low as 40 micrograms of lead per deciliter of blood. The good news is that the almost complete elimination of lead-soldered side seams in canned foods in a number of countries has contributed to a reduction in lead exposure. The FDA reports that the mean level in canned foods in the U.S. has decreased from 0.20 mg/kg in 1982–83 to 0.01 mg/kg since 1988–89. Most relevant to the concern about infant exposure to lead is that the concentration of lead in canned evaporated milk has decreased from 0.11 mg/kg in 1982–83 to undetectable levels (less than 0.01 mg/kg) since 1985–86. The lead content of drinking water may be greater than 100 micrograms per liter where lead pipes or lead solder are used in plumbing. The lead content of drinking water in Canada and the U.S. is generally below 5 micrograms per liter and averages 1 or 2 micrograms per liter. The World Health Organization recommends lead content of drinking water should not exceed 10 micrograms per liter. The FAO-WHO Expert Committee on Food Additives recommends PTWI *(see)* of 25 micrograms per kg of body weight for all age groups. The experts also said there is a need for continued epidemiological studies on the effects of lead on intellectual development in children. In particular, information is needed on whether a reduction in blood lead concentrations leads to reversal of lead-related intellectual deficits.

LEAF ALCOHOL • *See* 3-Hexen-1-ol.

LEATHER MEAL, HYDROLYZED • Used in feed. FDA tolerance, 1 percent by weight of feed.

LEAVENING • From the Latin *levare*, "to raise." It is a substance, such as yeast, acting to produce fermentation in dough or liquid. Leavening serves to lighten or enliven, such as baking soda when it produces a gas that lightens dough or batter.

LECHEA CASPI or DE VACA • A genus of herbs that have branched stems and have minute purplish flowers.

LECITHIN • From the Greek, meaning "egg yolk." A natural antioxidant and emollient composed of units of choline, phosphoric acid, fatty acids, and glycerin *(see all)*. Commercially isolated from eggs, soybeans, corn, and egg yolk and used as an antioxidant in prepared breakfast cereal, candy, sweet chocolate, bread, rolls, buns, and oleomargarine. Egg yolk is 8 to 9 percent lecithin. Hydroxylated lecithin is a defoaming component in yeast and beet sugar production. Lecithin with or without phosphatides (components of fat) is an emulsifier for sweet chocolate, milk chocolate, bakery products, frozen desserts, oleomargarine, rendered animal fat, or a combination of vegetable-animal fats. Also used in eye creams, lipsticks, liquid powders, hand creams and lotions, soaps, and many other cosmetics. Also a natural emulsifier and spreading agent. Nontoxic. The final report to the FDA of the Select Committee on GRAS Substances stated in 1980 that it should continue its GRAS status with no limitations other than good manufacturing practices.

LECITIHIN, HYDROXYLATED LECITHIN • *See* Lecithin and Hydroxylated.

LEEK OIL • *Sempervivum tectorium.* Native to the mountains of Europe and to the Greek Islands, its longevity led to its being named *sempervivum,* which translated means "ever alive." It is used as flavoring. It has been used to treat shingles, gout, and to get rid of bugs. Its pulp was applied to the skin for rashes and inflammation, and to remove warts and calluses. The juice was used to reduce fever and to treat insect stings. The juice mixed with honey was prescribed for thrush, a fungal infection of the mouth, and an ointment made from the plant was used to treat ulcers, burns, scalds, and inflammation. There is reported use of the chemical; it has not yet been assigned for toxicology literature search.

LEGUMES • Plants that include seeds in a pod, such as beans and peas. The Leguminosae family includes over eighteen thousand species and is one of the most economically important plant families in the world. They include the phytochemicals being studied as health factors. Phytochemicals from legumes are utilized as food additives, fungicides, and anticancer agents.

LEMON • Extract and Oil. The common fresh fruit. The *lemon extract* is used in flavorings for beverages, ice cream, ices, candy, baked goods, and icings. *Lemon oil* is a blueberry, loganberry, strawberry, butter, grapefruit, lemon, lime, orange, cola, coconut, honey, wine, rum, root beer, and ginger ale flavoring for beverages, ice cream, ices, candy, baked goods, gelatin desserts, chewing gum

(1,900 ppm), condiments, meats, syrups, icings, and cereals. Lemon oil is suspected of being a cancer-causing agent. GRAS.

LEMON BALM • Sweet Balm. Garden Balm. Used in perfumes and as a soothing facial treatment. An Old World mint cultivated for its lemon-flavored fragrant leaves. Often considered a weed, it has been used by herbalists as a medicine and to flavor foods and medicines. It reputedly imparts long life. Also used to treat earache and toothache. Nontoxic.

LEMON EXTRACT • *See* Lemon Oil.

LEMON JUICE • *See* Lemon.

LEMON OIL • Cedro Oil. Used in perfumes and food flavorings, it is the volatile oil expressed from the fresh peel. A pale yellow to deep yellow, it has a characteristic odor and taste of the outer part of fresh lemon peel. It can cause an allergic reaction and has been suspected of being a co-agent cause of cancer.

LEMON OIL, TERPENELESS • A lemon fruit, ginger, and ginger ale flavoring agent for beverages, ice cream, ices, candy, baked goods, gelatin desserts, chewing gum, and toppings. Terpene, which is removed to improve flavor, is a class of unsaturated hydrocarbons. *See* Lemon for toxicity.

LEMON PEEL • From the outer rind, the extract is used as a flavor in medicines and in beverages, confectionery, and cooking. *See* Lemon for toxicity.

LEMON VERBENA EXTRACT • Extract of *Lippia citriodoral*. Flavoring in alcoholic beverages only. *See* Lemongrass Oil.

LEMONGRASS OIL • Indian Oil of Verbena. Used in perfumes, especially those added to soap. It is the volatile oil distilled from the leaves of lemon grasses. A yellowish or reddish brown liquid, it has a strong odor of verbena. Also used in insect repellent. Used in lemon and fruit flavorings for beverages, ice cream, ices, candy, baked goods, gelatin desserts, and chewing gum. Death reported when taken internally; an autopsy showed lining of the intestines was severely damaged.

LEUCINE • L and DL forms. An essential amino acid *(see)* for human nutrition not manufactured in the body. It is isolated commercially from gluten, casein, and keratin *(see all)*. The L form is a food additive that the FDA says can be 3.5 percent of table weight. Used in aspartame *(see)* tabs as a lubricant. It has a sweet taste. It has caused birth defects in experimental animals.

L-LEUCINE • *See* Leucine.

LEVAMISOLE • Ergamisol. A drug that appears to restore depressed immune function. Used as an animal drug and in animal feed to fight parasites. It is employed in treatment of beef, lamb, and pork. FDA limitations are 0.1 ppm in cattle, sheep, and swine. Poisonous by ingestion and other routes. Human systemic effects by ingestion include coma, skin rash, and irritation, and fever. There was a great deal of controversy over the pricing of this drug in 1992, when it was revealed that while the veterinary drug cost $14, for a human cancer patient the cost was up to $1,500. The company that produces the drug explained that it backed fourteen hundred studies involving forty thousand patients, and that this was factored into the cost of the drug for humans.

LEVULINIC ACID • Crystals used as intermediate for plasticizers, solvents, resins, flavors, and pharmaceuticals.

LEVULOSE • *See* Fructose.

L-GLUTAMIC ACID • *See* Glutamic Acid.

LICORICE • Liquorice. Glycyrrhizin. Monoammonium Glycrrhizinate. Ammoniated Glycyrrhizin. Extract, extract powder, and root. A black substance derived from a plant, *Glycyrrhiza glabra,* "sweet root," belonging to the Leguminosae and cultured from southern Europe to Central Asia. It is used in fruit, licorice, anise, maple, and root beer flavorings for beverages, ice cream, ices, candy (29,000 ppm), baked goods, gelatin, chewing gum, and syrups. *Licorice root* is used in licorice and root beer flavorings for beverages, candy, baked goods, chewing gum (3,200 ppm), tobacco, and medicines. Some people known to have eaten licorice candy regularly and generously had raised blood pressure, headaches, and muscle weakness. It can cause asthma, intestinal upsets, and contact dermatitis. No known skin toxicity. Tentatively affirmed as GRAS in 1983.

LIGHT GREEN • *See* FD and C Green No. 2.

LIGNIN • Sulfate. Ammonium. Calcium. Magnesium. Sodium and lignin from Abaca. Binding agent in animal feed from plant fibers. The FDA says it can be up to 4 percent of finished pellets in animal feed. It is also used on flakes and as a surfactant in molasses used in feeds.

LIME OIL • A natural flavoring extracted from the fruit of a tropical tree. Colorless to greenish. Used in grapefruit, lemon, lemon-lime, lime, orange, cola, fruit, rum, nut, and ginger flavorings for beverages, ice cream, ices, candy, baked goods, gelatin desserts, chewing gum (3,100 ppm), and condiments. Terpeneless (*see* Lemon Oil) lime oil is used in lemon, lime, lemon-lime, cola, pineapple, ginger, and ginger ale flavorings for beverages, ice cream, ices, candy, baked goods, gelatin desserts, chewing gum, and syrups. Also used in perfumery and as an antiseptic. A source of vitamin C. Can cause an adverse reaction when skin is exposed to sunlight. GRAS. There is reported use of the chemical, it has not yet been assigned for toxicology literature.

LIME WATER • Calcium Hydroxide *(see)* solution. Clear, colorless, and odorless, it is strongly alkaline. Used to prepare many food additives such as emulsifiers and waterproofing compounds. *See* Calcium Stearate, for example.

LIMESTONE, GROUND • Flavoring agent. GRAS.

LIMINOIDS • Found in citrus fruits, they seem to induce protective enzymes.

LIMONENE • D, L, and DL forms. A synthetic flavoring agent that occurs naturally in star anise, buchu leaves, caraway, celery, oranges, coriander, cumin, cardamom, sweet fennel, common fennel, mace, marigold, oil of lavandin, oil of lemon, oil of mandarin, peppermint, petitgrain oil, pimento oil, orange leaf (absolute), orange peel (sweet oil), origanum oil, black pepper, peels of citrus, macrocarpa bunge, and hops oil. Used in lime, fruit, and spice flavorings for beverages, ice cream, ices, candy, baked goods, gelatin desserts, and chewing gum. A skin irritant and sensitizer. GRAS. It caused loss of weight and tumors in some experimental animals and therefore, the FAO-WHO Expert Committee on Food Additives recommended its used be reduced and restricted to 75 nanograms per kilogram of body weight per day. For D and L limonene, the Committee the principal toxicological finding was that *d*-limonene worsens spontaneously occurring nerve damage in mature male rats with subsequent occurrence of kidney tumors. The Committee concluded that "the postulated mechanism for *d*-limonene-induced neuropathy and renal tumors in the male rat was probably not relevant to humans." The ADI *(see)* was established based upon the significant decreases in the body weight gain associated with the administration of *d*-limonene to male and female rats and mice and female rabbits. It was based on the lowest NOEL *(see)* for this effect, which was 150 mg per kg of body weight per day administered by gavage in a two-year study of male rats. At its latest meeting, the Committee concluded that the ADI should not be set on the basis of the highest dose level in the long-term rat study, where kidney damage in male rats precluded testing at higher doses. The Committee noted that no toxicity, other than decreased weight gain, had been observed at nonfatal doses in female rats or in other species, and that current patterns of use indicate that most *d*-limonene consumption would be associated with natural sources. The Committee therefore withdrew the previous ADI for *d*-limonene and allocated an ADI "not specified."

LINALOE WOOD OIL • Bois de Rose Oil. A natural flavoring agent that is a colorless to yellow volatile essential oil distilled from a Mexican tree. It has a pleasant flowery scent and is soluble in most fixed oils. Used in berry citrus, fruit, liquor, and ginger flavorings for beverages, ice cream, ices, candy, baked goods, and liquors. Also used in perfumes. May cause allergic reactions. There is reported use of the chemical; it has not yet been assigned for toxicology literature.

LINALOOL • A synthetic flavoring that occurs naturally in basil, bois de rose oil, cassia, coriander, cocoa, grapefruit, grapefruit oil, oranges, peaches, tea, bay and bay-leaf extract, ginger, lavender, laurel leaves, and other oils. Used in flavorings such as blueberry, chocolate, and lemon. Used in perfumes and soaps instead of bergamot or French lavender. It is a fragrant, colorless liquid. May cause allergic reactions and is mildly toxic by ingestion.

LINALYL ACETATE • A colorless, fragrant liquid, slightly soluble in water, it is the most valuable constituent of bergamot and lavender oils, which are used in perfumery. It occurs naturally in basil, jasmine oil, lavandin oil, lavender oil, and lemon oil. It has a strong floral scent. Colorless, it is used in berry, citrus, peach, pear, and ginger flavorings for beverages, ice cream, ices, candy, baked goods, gelatin desserts, and chewing gum. GRAS.

LINALYL ANTHRANILATE • A synthetic berry, citrus, fruit, and grape flavoring agent for beverages, ice cream, ices, candy, and baked goods.

LINALYL BENZOATE • A synthetic flavoring, brownish yellow, with a roselike odor. Used in berry, citrus, fruit, and peach flavorings agent for beverages, ice cream, ices, candy, gelatin desserts, and baked goods.

LINALYL CINNAMATE • A synthetic loganberry, floral, rose, fruit, grape, and honey flavoring agent for beverages, ice cream, ices, candy, and baked goods.

LINALYL FORMATE • Formic Acid. A synthetic flavoring agent that occurs naturally in oil of lavandin. Used in berry, apple, apricot, peach, and pineapple flavorings for beverages, ice cream, ices, candy, and baked goods. *See* Formic Acid for toxicity.

LINALYL HEXANOATE • A synthetic fruit flavoring agent for beverages, ice cream, ices, candy, and baked goods.

LINALYL ISOBUTYRATE • A synthetic flavoring, colorless to slightly yellow, with a fruity odor. Used in berry, citrus, fruit, banana, black currant, cherry, pear, pineapple, plum, nut and spice flavorings for beverages, ice cream, ices, candy, and baked goods.

LINALYL ISOVALERATE • A synthetic flavoring, colorless to slightly yellow, with a fruity odor. Used in loganberry, apple, apricot, peach, pear, and plum flavorings for beverages, ice cream, ices, candy, gelatin desserts, and baked goods.

LINALYL OCTANOATE • A synthetic citrus, rose, apple, pineapple, and honey flavoring agent for beverages, ice cream, ices, candy, gelatin desserts, and baked goods.

LINALYL PROPIONATE • A synthetic currant, orange, banana, pear, and pineapple flavoring agent for beverages, ice cream, ices, candy, and baked goods.

LINCOMYCIN • Lincocin. An antibacterial introduced in 1965, it is used to treat respiratory tract, skin, soft tissue, gynecologic, and urinary tract infections; osteomyelitis, blood poisoning caused by streptococci, pneumococci, and staphylococci. FDA tolerance for residues are 0.1 ppm for edible tissues of chickens and swine 0.1 ppm in milk. Potential adverse reactions may include blood problems, dizziness, headache, low blood pressure, sore tongue, ringing in the ears, nausea, vomiting, severe colitis, persistent diarrhea, abdominal cramps, itching around the anus, vaginitis, jaundice, rashes, hives, pain at injection site, and serious allergic reactions. Antidiarrheal medicines reduce oral absorption of lincomycin. Lincomycin may reduce the effectiveness of drugs to treat myasthenia gravis.

LINDEN FLOWERS • *Tilia Glabra vent.* A natural flavoring extract from the flowers of the tree grown in Europe and the United States. Used in raspberry and vermouth flavorings for beverages (2,000 ppm). Also used in fragrances. GRAS. There is reported use of the chemical, it has not yet been assigned for toxicology literature.

LINOLEAMIDE • A releasing agent that prevents food from sticking to containers. *See* Linoleic Acid.

LINOLEIC ACID • An essential fatty acid *(see)* prepared from edible fats and oils. Component of vitamin F and a major constituent of many vegetable oils, for example, cottonseed and soybean. Used in emulsifiers and vitamins. Large doses can cause nausea and vomiting. When given in large doses to rats, weight loss and progressive secondary anemia developed. No known skin toxicity and, in fact, may have emollient properties. The final report to the FDA of the Select Committee on GRAS Substances stated in 1980 that it should continue its GRAS status with no limitations other than good manufacturing practices.

LINOLENIC ACID • Polyunsaturated acid produced in the body as a metabolite of linoleic acid. A nutrient used in the treatment of eczema. In the diet of Mediterranean people alpha-linolenic acid is believed to be important in the prevention of heart disease.

LINSEED OIL • Golden amber or brown oil with a peculiar odor and bland taste. Used in paints, varnishes, as a film, in printing inks, and for its protein. *See* flaxseed.

LIPASE • Any class of enzymes that break down fat to glycerol and fatty acids *(see both)*. It is used in the manufacture of cheeses.

LIVER-STOMACH CONCENTRATE WITH INTRINSIC FACTOR COMPLEX • A dietary supplement illegal in foods.

LOAEL • Lowest Observable Adverse Effect Level. Used to signify the lowest dose of a substance that causes an adverse effect in an experimental animal. *See also* NOEL.

LOCUST BEAN GUM • St. John's Bread. Carob Bean Gum. A thickener and stabilizer in cosmetics and foods. Also used in depilatories. A natural flavor extract from the seed of the carob tree cultivated in the Mediterranean area. The history of the carob tree dates back more than two thousand years when the ancient Egyptians used locust bean gum as an adhesive in mummy binding. It is alleged that the "locust" (through confusion of the locusts with carob) and wild honey, which sustained John the Baptist in the wilderness, was from this plant, thus the name St. John's Bread. The carob pods are used as feed for stock today because of their high protein content. Some health food enthusiasts also eat them for the same purpose. They are also used as a thickener and stabilizer (*see* Gum, Carob Bean). Carob bean extract is used in raspberry, bitters, butter, butterscotch, caramel, chocolate, cherry, brandy, wine, maple, root beer, spice, vanilla, cream soda, and grape flavorings for beverages, ice cream, ices, candy, baked goods, gelatin desserts (600 ppm), icings and toppings (1,000 ppm). A University of Minnesota pediatric cardiologist reported in 1981 that locust bean may lower blood cholesterol levels. Dr. James Zavoral and associates found that twenty-eight adults and children with histories of familial hypercholesterolemia were fed food products rich in locust bean gum. Some of those included breads, cookies, crackers, and Tater Tots. After four weeks on the special diets their cholesterol dropped 10 percent, and after six weeks, 20 percent. The final report to the FDA of the Select Committee on GRAS Substances stated in 1980 that it should continue its GRAS status with limitations on amounts that can be added to food.

LOVAGE • Smallage. *Levisticum officinale.* Flavoring obtained from the root of an aromatic herb native to southern Europe and grown in monastery gardens centuries ago for medicine and food flavoring. It has a hot, sharp, biting taste. The yellow brown oil is extracted from the root or other parts of the herb. It has a reputation for improving health and inciting love; Czechoslovakian girls reportedly wear it in a bag around their necks when dating boys. It supposedly has deodorant properties when added to bathwater. Used in bitters, maple, and walnut flavorings for beverages, ice cream, ices, candy, baked goods, chewing gum, and table syrups. The *extract* is used in berry, butter, butterscotch, caramel, maple, meat, black walnut, and spice flavorings for the same foods as above, plus condiments and icings. The *oil,* yellow-brown and aromatic, is used in butter, butterscotch, caramel, coffee, fruit, licorice, liquor, maple, nut, walnut, and spice flavorings for the same food as is the extract. There is reported use of the chemical; it has not yet been assigned for toxicology literature.

LOW CALORIE • Fewer than forty calories per serving.

LOW CHOLESTEROL • Twenty milligrams or less per serving.

LOW FAT • Three grams or less per serving.

LOW-FAT MILK • *See* Milk.

LOW SATURATED FAT • 1 gram or less per serving.

LOW SODIUM • 140 milligrams or less per serving.

LPE • Lysophosphatidylethanolamine. A compound found in many plants and animal tissues, it is purified from egg yolks and soybeans. When applied before harvest, this compound accelerates the development of fruit flavor and color. It is also believed to make fruit last longer on grocers' shelves and in refrigerators. At this writing, it was being tested on cranberries, peaches, tomatoes, grapes, and cut flowers.

LUNGMOSS • Lungwort. *Sticta pulmonacea ach.* Any of several plants once thought helpful in pulmonary diseases. Used as a flavoring in foods. There is no reported use of the chemical and there is no toxicology information available.

LUPULIN EXTRACT • Lupine. Hops. Extract of *Lupinus alba.* The seed has been used as a food since earliest times. A natural flavoring agent from a plant *(Humulus lupulis)* grown in Europe, Asia, and North America. Used in beer brewing. Formerly used as aromatic bitters and as a sedative. At one time veterinary usage was recommended for treatment of nymphomania. It contains lupulone, which is active against fungus and bacteria, and humulone, which is an antibiotic. It produces a light blue dye. GRAS. There is reported use of the chemical; it has not yet been assigned for toxicology literature.

LUTEIN • *See* Xanthophyll.

LYCOPENE • Red crystals, insoluble in water. The main pigment of tomato, paprika, grapefruit, and rose hips. Being studied as a compound to prevent heart disease and cancer. No known toxicity.

LYSINE • L form. An essential amino acid *(see)* isolated from casein, fibrin, or blood. It is used for food enrichment for wheat-based foods. Lysine improves their protein quality and results in improved growth and tissue synthesis. Employed in the fortification of specialty bread and cereal mixes up to .25 percent to .5 percent of the weight of flour. On the FDA list for further study since 1980. GRAS.

L-LYSINE • *See* Lysine.

LYSOPHOSPHOPHATIDYLETHANOLAMINE • *See* LPE.

LYSOZYME • Found in animal tissue and used in cheese production to inhibit the growth of *Clostridium tyrobutyricum.* The use level is less than 40 mg of lysozyme per liter of cheese milk, resulting in a concentration of less than 400 mg of lysozyme per kg of cheese. In studies related to allergenic effects, the reactions produced by egg-white lysozyme in humans were less severe than those seen with other proteins such as albumin, which have a long history of use as food components. On the basis of available data, the FAO-WHO Expert Committee on Food Additives concluded that the low additional intake of lysozyme via cheese was not a hazard to the consumer health, provided that the enzyme complied with the specifications.

M

MACE • Oil and Oleoresin. Obtained by team distillation from the ripe, dried seed of the nutmeg. Colorless to pale yellow, with the taste and odor of nutmeg. Used in bitters, meat, and spice flavorings for beverages, ice cream, ices, baked goods, condiments, and meats (2,000 ppm). The oil is used in chocolate, cocoa, coconut, cola, fruit, nut, spice, and ginger ale flavorings for beverages, ice cream, ices, candy, baked goods, chewing gum, condiments, and meats. The oleoresin *(see)* is used in sausage and spice flavorings for baked goods, condiments, meats, and pickles. *See* Nutmeg for toxicity. The final report to the FDA of the Select Committee on GRAS Substances stated in 1980 that while no evidence in the available information on it demonstrates a hazard to the public at current use levels, uncertainties exist, requiring that additional studies be conducted. The FDA continued the GRAS status while tests were being completed and evaluated in 1980.

MADURAMICIN AMMONIUM • Cygro. An antiparasite medication used in chicken feed to prevent infection. FDA residue tolerances are: 0.24 ppm in muscle, 0.72 ppm in liver, and 0.48 ppm in fat. When used as a medication to treat infection, the residue tolerances are the same as in uncooked chicken, except for 0.48 ppm in uncooked chicken fat.

MAGNESIA • Slightly alkaline white powder taken from any one of several ores such as periclase. Named after Magnesia, an ancient city in Asia Minor. An antacid. No known toxicity.

MAGNESIUM • Magnesium Acetate, Magnesium Phosphate, Magnesium Sulfate, Magnesium Oxide, Magnesium Silicate, Magnesium Chloride, Magnesium Carbonate, Magnesium Cyclamate, Magnesium Stearate, and Magnesium Hydroxide. A silver-white, light, malleable metal that occurs abundantly in nature and is widely used in combination with various chemicals as a powder. *Magnesium acetate* is used as a buffer and neutralizer in nonalcoholic beverages. GRAS. *Magnesium phosphate,* a white, odorless powder, and *magnesium sulfate* are used as mineral supplements for food, leavening agents, and pH control agents. Recommended daily allowances, according to the National Academy of Sciences, are 40 milligrams for infants, 100 to 300 milligrams for children, 350 milligrams for adult males and females. *Magnesium sulfate* is used also as a corrective in the brewing industry and for fertilizers. *Magnesium silicate,* a fine, white, odorless and tasteless power, is used in table salt and vanilla powder as an anticaking agent. In table salt it is limited to 2 percent. *Magnesium chloride* is used for color retention and as a firming agent in canned peas. *Magnesium carbonate* is used as an alkali for sour cream, butter, ice cream, cacao products, and canned peas. It is also used as a drying agent and an anticaking agent. Magnesium carbonate is also used as a perfume carrier and coloring agent. Used in baby powder, bath powder, tooth powders, face masks, liquid powders, face powders, dry rouge. It is a silver white, crystalline salt that occurs in nature as magnetite or dolomite. Can be prepared artificially and is also used in paint, printing ink, table salt, and as an antacid. Nontoxic to the intact skin but may cause irritation when applied to abraded skin. *Magnesium chloride* is used as a buffer and neutralizer in nonalcoholic beverages and is used for color retention and as a firming agent. GRAS. *Magnesium citrate* is a buffer and neutralizer in nonalcoholic beverages. *Magnesium cyclamate* was banned in 1969 as an artificial sweetener. *Magnesium hydroxide* is used as an alkali in dentifrices and skin creams, in canned peas, and as a drying agent and color retention agent for improved gelling in the manufacture of cheese, and GRAS. Slightly alkaline, crystalline compound obtained by hydration of magnesia *(see)* or precipitation of seawater by lime. Toxic when inhaled. Harmless to skin and in fact soothes it. *Magnesium oxide* is used in canned peas, frozen desserts, and as a dietary supplement, and is considered GRAS. *Magnesium phosphate* is a nutrient supplement considered GRAS. *Magnesium phosphide* is a fungicide in animal feeds. *Magnesium silicate* is used in vanilla powder and is considered GRAS. *Magnesium stearate,* a soft, white powder, tasteless, odorless, and insoluble in water, is used as a dietary supplement, in food packaging, and as an emulsifying agent in cosmetics. Magnesium was reevaluated by the FDA in 1976 as not harmful in presently used current levels. However the FAO-WHO Expert Committee on Food Additives recommends further study of magnesium silicate because kidney damage in dogs has been reported upon ingestion. Magnesium carbonate, chloride, sulfate, stearate, phosphate, and silicate are all GRAS according to the final report to the FDA of the Select Committee on GRAS Substances and they should continue their GRAS status with no limitations other than good manufacturing practices.

MAGNESIUM CAPRATE • There is no reported use of the chemical and there is no toxicology information available.

MAGNESIUM CAPRYLATE • There is no reported use of the chemical and there is no toxicology information available.

MAGNESIUM CARBONATE • GRAS. *See* Magnesium.

MAGNESIUM CHLORIDE • GRAS. *See* Magnesium.

MAGNESIUM CYCLAMATE • Nonnutritive sweetener removed from the market September 1, 1969. Legal only in products complying with drug provision of the law.

MAGNESIUM GLUCONATE • A buffering agent in soda water. *See* Magnesium.

MAGNESIUM GLYCEROPHOSPHATE • There is no reported use of the chemical and there is no toxicology information available.

MAGNESIUM HYDROXIDE • Permitted as an optional ingredient in standardized food. Does not have to be listed. GRAS. *See* Magnesium.

MAGNESIUM LACTATE • Buffering and neutralizing agent in cacao products and in canned peas. *See* Magnesium.

MAGNESIUM LAURATE • There is no reported use of the chemical and there is no toxicology information available.

MAGNESIUM MYRISTATE • There is no reported use of the chemical and there is no toxicology information available.

MAGNESIUM OLEATE • There is no reported use of the chemical and there is no toxicology information available.

MAGNESIUM OXIDE • Magnesia. White, odorless powder used as an alkali, anticaking agent, firming agent, free-flow agent, lubricant, neutralizing agent, nutrient, pH control agent, and releasing agent. It is used as a neutralizer in frozen dairy products, butter, cacao products, and canned peas. Inhalation can cause fever in humans. Also used as a dietary supplement. Has caused tumors in hamsters. GRAS. *See* Magnesium.

MAGNESIUM PHOSPHATE • Di-, Tri-, Basic. A dietary supplement. GRAS. *See* Magnesium.

MAGNESIUM PHOSPHIDE • A fumigant used in animal feed and on processed foods. FDA residue tolerance is 0.01 ppm in processed foods and 0.1 ppm in animal feeds. A poison. Moderately toxic by inhalation. *See* Magnesium.

MAGNESIUM SALTS of FATTY ACIDS • *See* Magnesium and Fatty Acids.

MAGNESIUM SILICATE • An anticaking agent. GRAS. *See* Magnesium.

MAGNESIUM STEARATE • Miscellaneous uses as a migratory substance from packaging materials, stabilizer, defoaming agent, anticaking agent. *See* Magnesium.

MAGNESIUM SULFATE • Nutrient supplement. GRAS. *See* Magnesium.

MAIDENHAIR FERN • Venus Hair. Extract of the leaves of the fern, *Adiantum capillus-veneris*. Used as a flavoring in alcoholic beverages only and to soothe irritated skin in herbal creams.

MALATHION • Yellow liquid derived from diethyl maleate and dimethyldithiophosphoric acid, it is an insecticide against such pests as aphids, the leaf-cutter bee, and the Mediterranean fruit fly. Toxic when absorbed through the skin and can damage transmission of nerve signals. In dehydrated citrus pulp for animal feed, the FDA allows a tolerance of 50 ppm; in nonmedicated cattle feed concentrate blocks from application of pesticide to paper used in packaging, the residue tolerance allowed in the blocks is 10 ppm.

MALEIC HYDRAZIDE • Regulates the growth of unwanted "suckers" on about 90 percent of the United States tobacco crop. It is also applied to 10 to 15 percent of domestic potatoes and onions to prevent sprouting after harvest. It is highly toxic to humans and has produced central nervous system disturbances and liver damage in experimental animals. It has led to liver and other tumors in some mice. However, other studies, including one done for the National Cancer Institute and published in 1969, report no carcinogenic effects. It has produced genetic damage in plant and animal systems, a fact that often signals a cancer-causing effect. The FDA residue tolerance for potato chips is 160 ppm from use as a preharvest pesticide.

MALIC ACID • A colorless, crystalline compound with a strong acid taste that occurs naturally in a wide variety of fruits, including apples and cherries. A flavoring agent and aid in aging wine. It has a strong acid taste. Used as an alkali in frozen dairy products, beverages, baked goods, confections, fruit, butter, and jelly and jam preserves "in amount sufficient to compensate for the deficiency of fruit in artificially sweetened fruit." An alkali and antioxidant in cosmetics and ingredient of hair lacquer. Irritating to the skin and can cause allergic reaction when used in hair lacquers. The final report to the FDA of the Select Committee on

GRAS Substances stated in 1980 that it should continue its GRAS status with no limitations other than good manufacturing practices.

MALLOW EXTRACT • From the herb family. A moderate purplish red that is paler than magenta rose. Used in coloring and also as a source of pectin *(see)*. No known toxicity.

MALT EXTRACT • Extracted from barley that has been allowed to germinate, then heated to destroy vitality, and dried. It contains sugars, proteins, and salts from barley. The extract is mixed with water and allowed to solidify. It is used as a nutrient and as a texturizer in cured meat and poultry. FDA limitations are 2.5 percent in cured meat. It is also widely used in the brewing industry. GRAS.

MALT SYRUP • Component of caramel coloring. *See* Malt Extract.

MALTITOL and MALTITOL SYRUP • Obtained by the hydrogenate from maltose *(see)*. A candidate for a sugar substitute, it has 90 percent the sweetness of sugar and does contain calories. It has the potential for use in confections and candy coatings. In a cancer study in rats, changes were observed in the adrenal gland, which included increased incidence of both benign and malignant tumors of the adrenal glands in both sexes and a "slight increase" in breast cancer in female rats. The FAO-WHO Expert Committee on Food Additives did not consider these cancers to be related to treatment. The Committee, however, recommended that the information database on adrenal overgrowth and tumors associated with polyols and other poorly absorbed carbohydrates *(see both)* be reviewed that the mechanisms of appearance of these lesions and their toxicological significance be assessed at a future meeting.

MALTODEXTRIN • The sugar obtained by hydrolysis of starch. A combination of maltol *(see)* and dextrin *(see)* used as a texturizer and flavor enhancer in candies, particularly chocolate. No known toxicity. The final report to the FDA of the Select Committee on GRAS Substances stated in 1980 that it should continue its GRAS status with no limitations other than good manufacturing practices.

MALTOL • A white, crystalline powder with a butterscotch odor, found in the bark of young larch trees, pine seeds, chicory, wood tars, and in roasted malt. It imparts a "freshly baked" odor and flavor to bread and cakes. Used as a synthetic chocolate, coffee, fruit, maple, nut, and vanilla flavoring agent for beverages, ice cream, ices, candy, baked goods, gelatin desserts, chewing gum, and jelly.

MALTOSE • Malt Sugar. Colorless crystals derived from malt extract and used as a nutrient, sweetener, culture medium, and stabilizer. It is soluble in water and used as a supplement of sugar for diabetics. It is also used in brewing and as a stabilizer. It is nontoxic but it has been reported to cause tumors when injected under the skin of mice in doses of five hundred milligrams per kilogram of body weight. There is no reported use of the chemical and there is no toxicology information available.

MANDARIN OIL • Obtained by expression of the peel of a ripe mandarin orange, *Citrus reticulata blanco*. Clear dark orange to reddish yellow, with a pleasant orangelike odor. It is an orange, tangerine, cherry, and grape flavoring for beverages, ice cream, ices, candy, baked goods, chewing gum, and gelatin desserts. GRAS. There is reported use of the chemical; it has not yet been assigned for toxicology literature.

MANEB • A pesticide used on growing grapes. The residue tolerances are 28 ppm in raisins, 20 ppm in brain of barley, oats, rye, and wheat, and 1 ppm in flours of barley, oats, rye, and wheat. *See* Zinc.

MANGANESE BACITRACIN • An antibiotic in animal feed. *See* Bacitracin and Manganese Sources.

MANGANESE CHLORIDE • Dietary supplement. GRAS. *See* Manganese Sources.

MANGANESE CITRATE • A light, pink-white fine, granular solid. It is used as a nutrient. GRAS. *See* Manganese Sources.

MANGANESE GLUOCONATE • Dietary supplement. GRAS. There is reported use of the chemical; it has not yet been assigned for toxicology literature. *See* Manganese Sources.

MANGANESE GLYCEROPHOSPHATE • Dietary supplement. GRAS. *See* Manganese Sources.

MANGANESE HYPOPHOSPHITE • Dietary supplement. GRAS. *See* Manganese Sources.

MANGANESE SOURCES • Manganese Acetate, Manganese Carbonate, Manganese Chloride, Manganese Citrate, Manganese Sulfate, Manganese Glycerophosphate, Manganese Hypophosphite, and Manganese Oxide. A mineral supplement first isolated in 1774, manganese occurs in minerals and in minute quantities in animals, plants, and in water. The chloride, citrate, gluconate, glycerate, hypophosphite, and sulfate are all used as dietary supplements and nutrients and are considered GRAS. Many forms are used in dyeing. Manganous salts are activators of enzymes and are necessary to the development of strong bones. They are used as nutrients and as dairy substitutes. Toxicity occurs by inhalation. Symptoms include languor, sleepiness, wakefulness, emotional disturbances, and Parkinson-like symptoms. *Manganese chloride, citrate, glycerophosphate,* and *hypophosphite* are all considered GRAS according to the final report of the Select Committee on GRAS Substances and should continue their GRAS status as nutrients with no limitations other than good manufacturing practices. However, *manganese oxide,* according to the Committee, does not have enough known about it upon which to base an evaluation when it is used as a food ingredient.

MANGANESE SULFATE • Dietary Supplement. GRAS. There is reported use of the chemical; it has not yet been assigned for toxicology literature. *See* Magnesia.

MANGANOUS OXIDE • A dietary supplement derived by reduction of the dioxide in hydrogen or by heating the carbonate without air. It is also used in ceramics, paints, bleaching tallow, animal feeds, and fertilizers. GRAS.

MANNITOL • Widespread in plants but mostly prepared from seaweed. It is about 70 percent as sweet as sugar and it does contain calories. White, crystalline solid, odorless, and sweet tasting. Used as a texturizer in chewing gum, up to 31 percent, hard candy up to 5 percent, and pressed mints, 98 percent. It is also used in soft candy at 40 percent, frostings at 8 percent, jams and jellies at 15 percent.

It has been used as a sweetener in "sugar-free" products but has calories and carbohydrates. The FDA says that "excess consumption may have a laxative effect: if ingested daily, it must carry that warning on the label." In 1982, the FDA reported that it does not cause cancer in rats. GRAS on an interim basis.

MANNOSE • A carbohydrate occurring in some plants. It has a sweet taste.

MAO INHIBITORS • *See* Monoamine Oxidase Inhibitors.

MAPLE, MOUNTAIN • Flavoring. No known toxicity.

MARGARINE • Oleomargarine. A butter substitute made from animal or vegetable fats or oils. If oils are used they are "hardened" into fats by the process of hydrogenation *(see)*. Skimmed milk, water, salt, coloring matter *(see* Carotene), artificial flavors, lecithin *(see)*, and small amounts of vitamins are usually added. By federal regulations, margarine contains at least 80 percent fat. No known toxicity.

MARIGOLD, POT • A natural plant extract. The oil is used in various flavorings for beverages, ice cream, ices, candy, and baked goods. There is reported use of the chemical; it has not yet been assigned for toxicology literature. *See* Tagetes. GRAS.

MARJORAM, POT • Sweet Marjoram. *Marjorana onites*. The natural extract of the flowers and leaves of two varieties of the fragrant marjoram plant. The oleoresin *(see)* is used in sausage and spice flavorings for condiments and meats. The seed is used in sausage and spice flavorings for meats (3,500 ppm) and condiments. Sweet marjoram is used in sausage and spice flavorings for beverages, baked goods (2,000 ppm), condiments, meats, and soups. The sweet oil is used in vermouth, wine, and spice flavorings for beverages, ice creams, ices, candy, baked goods, and condiments. Also used in hair preparations, perfumes, and soaps. Can irritate the skin. The redness, itching, and warmth experienced when applied to the skin are carried by local dilation of the blood vessels or by local reflex. May produce allergic reactions. Essential oils such as marjoram are believed to penetrate the skin easily and produce systemic effects. GRAS.

MARSHMALLOW ROOT • *See* Althea Root.

MASSARANDUBA CHOCOLATE • *Manilkara solimoesensis gilly*. Used in chewing-gum base.

MATÉ EXTRACT • Paraguay Tea Extract. St. Bartholomew's Tea. Jesuits' Tea. A natural flavoring extract from small gourds grown in South America where maté is a stimulant beverage. Among its constituents are caffeine, purines, and tannins. *See* Caffeine and Tannic Acid for toxicity. GRAS.

MATRICARIA EXTRACT • Wild Chamomile Extract. Extract of the flower heads of *Matricaria chamomilla*. Used as a soothing tea and tonic internally and externally as a soothing medication for contusions and other inflammation. *See* Tannic Acid. GRAS.

MATRICARIA OIL • Camomile Oil. Wild Chamomile Extract. The volatile oil distilled from the dried flower heads of *Matricaria chamomilla*. Used internally as a tonic and soothing tea and externally as a soothing medication for contusions and other inflammation. *See* Matricaria Extract.

MATURING AGENTS • *See* Bleaching Agents.

MAYONNAISE • The common salad dressing. Semisolid, made with eggs, vegetable oil, and vinegar or lemon juice.

MCG • Abbreviation for microgram, a metric measurement that is $\frac{1}{1000}$ of one milligram.

MELAMINE • Cyanuramide. Used in the manufacture of paper and paperboard for packaging materials. An experimental cancer-causing and tumor-causing agent. Moderately toxic by ingestion. An eye, skin, and mucous membrane irritant. Causes skin rash in humans.

MELENGESTROL ACETATE • A progesterone used to treat animals and to suppress ovulation when added to animal feed. Residue limitation is zero according to the FDA.

MELISSA • Essential oil. *See* Balm Oil. GRAS.

MELONAL • *See* 2,6-Dimethyl-5-Heptenal.

MENADIONE • Vitamin K_3. Dietary Supplement. Extension of a petition has been filed to permit a limit of 1 mg per day. Its use was revoked March 22, 1963. No food additive regulation authorizing use of menadione in prenatal supplements or any other food products has been issued. However, menadione is permitted as a nutritional supplement in chicken and turkey feed for prevention of vitamin K-deficiency and in swine feed. Used as a preservative in emollients. A synthetic with properties of vitamin K. Bright yellow crystals that are insoluble in water are used medically to prevent blood clotting and in food to prevent souring of milk products. Can be irritating to mucous membranes, respiratory passages, and the skin.

MENHADEN OIL • Hydrogenated and Partially Hydrogenated *(see)*. Pogy Oil. Moss Bunker Oil. Obtained along the coast of Africa from the menhaden fish, which are a little larger than herrings. The fish glycerides of menhaden are reddish and have strong fishy odor. Used as a nutrient. Also used in soaps and creams.

MENTHA ARVENSIS OIL • From *Mentha arvensis,* it is a colorless to yellow liquid with a minty odor used as a flavoring agent. GRAS. Has caused reproductive problems in experimental animals.

p-**MENTHA-1,8-DIEN-7-OL** • A synthetic citrus, fruit, mint, and vanilla flavoring agent for beverages, ice cream, ices, candy, and baked goods. It is found naturally in caraway. Can cause skin irritation.

MENTHADIENOL • Although allowed as a food additive, there is no current reported use of the chemical, and therefore, although toxicology information may be available, it is not being updated, according to the FDA.

MENTHOL • A flavoring agent that can be obtained naturally from peppermint or other mint oils and can be made synthetically by hydrogenation *(see)* of thymol *(see)*. Used in butter, caramel, fruit, peppermint, and spearmint flavorings for beverages, ice cream, ices, candy, baked goods, chewing gum (1,100 ppm), and liquor. Also used in perfumes, emollient creams, hair tonics, mouthwashes, shaving creams, preshave lotions, aftershave lotions, body rubs, liniments, and skin fresheners. It gives that "cool" feeling to the skin after use. It is a local anesthetic. It is nontoxic in low doses, but in concentrations of 3 percent or more it exerts an irritant action that can, if continued too long, induce changes in all layers of the mucous membranes. It can also cause severe abdominal pain, nausea, vomiting, vertigo, and coma when ingested in its concentrated form. The lethal dose in rats is 2.0 grams per kilogram of body weight. GRAS.

MENTHONE • A synthetic flavoring agent that occurs naturally in raspberries and peppermint oil. Bitter, with a slight peppermint taste. Used in fruit and mint flavorings for beverages, ice cream, ices, candy, baked goods, and chewing gum. May cause gastric distress. There is reported use of the chemical; it has not yet been assigned for toxicology literature.

MENTHYL ACETATE • A natural flavoring agent that occurs naturally in peppermint oil. Colorless, with a mint odor. Used in fruit, mint, and spice flavorings for beverages, ice cream, ices, candy, baked goods, and chewing gum; also in perfumes and toilet waters. Mildly toxic by ingestion. A skin irritant. GRAS.

N-MERCAPTO METHYL PHTALIMIDE • Phosphamidon. An organophosphate insecticide limited to 0.2 ppm tolerance by the FDA as a residue in meat by products of cattle. *See* Organophosphates for toxicity.

METALAXYL • A fungicide used in animal feed, dried hops, potato chips, processed potatoes, soybean meal, sugar beet molasses, processed tomatoes, and wheat-milling fractions. FDA limits residues to 7 ppm in citrus oil, 4 ppm in processed potatoes including potato chips, and 3 ppm in processed tomatoes.

METALDEHYDE • A polymer of acetaldehyde *(see)* used as a slug and snail poison on strawberries at the time of harvest. FDA residue tolerance is zero. Ingestion may cause severe abdominal pain, nausea, vomiting, diarrhea, fever, convulsions, and coma.

METHACRYCLIC ACID-DIVINDYL BENZENE COPOLYMER • Used as a carrier for vitamin B_{12} in nutritional supplements.

METHANEARSONIC ACID • Used in or on cottonseed hulls used for animal feed. *See* Arsenic.

METHANE DICHLORIDE • Colorless, volatile liquid with the odor of chloroform used to dilute color and extract chemicals. It is used to decaffeinate coffee, fruits, hops, spices, and vegetables. FDA permits residues of 30 ppm in spice oleoresins, 2.2 percent in hops extract, and 10 ppm in decaffeinated coffee. Moderately toxic by ingestion. An experimental cancer-causing and tumor-causing agent. Human systemic effects by ingestion and inhalation include numbness, altered sleep, convulsions, euphoria, and changes in cardiac rate. It causes birth defects in experimental animals and may be mutagenic in humans. It is an eye and severe skin irritant.

METHANETHIOL • Methyl Mercaptan. A pesticide and fungicide isolated from the roots of a plant. Occurs in the "sour" gas of West Texas, in coal tar, and in petroleum. Produced in the intestinal tract by action of bacteria. Found in urine after ingestion of asparagus. Its odor may cause nausea and it may be narcotic in high concentrations.

METHANOL • Methyl Alcohol. Wood Alcohol. Wood Spirit. A solvent and denaturant obtained by the destructive distillation of wood. Flammable, poisonous liquid with a nauseating odor. Better solvent than ethyl alcohol. It is used primarily in antifreeze compounds, paints, cements, inks, varnishes, shellacs, wood strippers, windshield wiper solvents, gasoline antifreeze, automotive radiators, and as a solvent for dyes. It is also used in the fuel Sterno, in home heating oil extenders, as an octane booster in gasoline, and as a fuel for soldering torches. It is a softening agent for plastics. It is the raw material for making formaldehyde. In the food industry, it is used to extract hops and spices. It is on the Community-Right-To-Know List *(see)*. Methanol is highly toxic and readily absorbed from all routes of exposure. It possesses narcotic properties. Toxic effects are primarily on the nervous system. Symptoms include headache, dizziness, confusion, abdominal pain, lung problems, weakness, and coma. Ingestion can cause blindness and death. Lesser exposure causes blurring of vision, headache, and GI disturbances. It is also a dangerous fire hazard. If you must use a product containing methanol, make sure you do so either outdoors or in a well-ventilated area. Use gloves.

METHDIATHION • Insecticide. The residue tolerances are 0.03 ppm in milk, 0.05 ppm residue in fat, meat, and meat byproducts of cattle, goats, hogs, poultry, and sheep.

METHILANIN • *See* Acimeton.

METHIONINE • D and DL Forms. An essential amino acid *(see)* that occurs in protein. Used as a dietary substance. It is attracted to fat and Rutgers University researchers patented a process to impregnate a carrier material with methionine for use in deep-frying cooking oil to impart a "fresh" potato or potato chip flavor to snack foods, soups, or salad dressings. Not to be used in baby foods. Used as a texturizer in cosmetic creams. Methionine is mildly toxic by injection and has caused birth defects in experimental animals. On the FDA list of additives requiring further study since 1980.

METHOPRENE • A growth inhibitor that mimics juvenile hormone in insects. It is used in animal feed or mineral blocks for cattle. The FDA residue tolerances are: 22.7 to 45.4 mg per 100 pounds body weight; 0.05 ppm as residues in eggs and milk; 0.1 ppm as residues in meat and meat byproducts of cattle, goats, hogs, and sheep; 0.3 ppm as residues in fat of cattle, goats, hogs, and sheep; 0.05 ppm as residues in fat and meat of poultry.

2-METHOXY-3,6-DICHLOROBENZOIC ACID • Banex. A herbicide used in animal feed and on sugarcane. The FDA residue tolerance is 2 ppm on sugarcane molasses and 2 ppm in sugarcane molasses when used for animal feed. In the EPA Genetic Toxicology Program *(see)*. Moderately toxic by ingestion.

4-METHOXY-2-METHYL-2-BUTANETHIOL • The FDA has not yet done a search of the toxicology literature concerning this additive.

***p*-METHOXY A-METHYLCINNAMALDEHYDE** • A flavoring.

2-METHOXY-4-METHYLPHENOL • Creosol. A synthetic flavoring that occurs naturally in cassia and is used in fruit, rum, nut, and clove flavorings for beverages, ice cream, ices, candy, baked goods, and liqueurs. About the same toxicity as phenol, a highly caustic, poisonous compound derived from benzene.

2-METHOXY-3 (5)-METHYLPYRAZINE • A colorless liquid with the odor of roasted hazelnuts used as a flavoring agent in various foods. GRAS.

3-L-METHOXYPROPANE-1,2-DIOL • A synthetic flavoring.

1-METHOXY-4-PROPENYL BENZENE • *See* Anethole.

2-METHOXY-4-PROPENYL PHENOL • *See* Isoeugenol.

***p*-METHOXYACETOPHENONE** • *p*-Acetanisole. Crystalline solid with a pleasant odor. Soluble in alcohol and fixed oils and derived from the interaction of anisole and acetyl chloride with aluminum chloride and carbon disulfide. Used in perfumery as a synthetic floral odor and in flavoring.

4-METHOXYACETOPHENONE • Colorless to pale yellow solid with a hawthorn odor used as a flavoring agent in various foods. Moderately toxic by ingestion. Human systemic effect by inhalation was increased pulse rate. A skin irritant.

0-METHOXY BENZALDEHYDE • A synthetic flavoring agent that occurs naturally in cassia oil and used in spice and cinnamon flavorings for beverages, baked goods, and chewing gum. *See* Benzyl Acetate.

***p*-METHOXYBENZALDEHYDE** • Anisaldehyde. A synthetic flavoring agent that occurs naturally in hawthorn, fennel, oil of anise, star, anise, and Tahiti vanilla beans. Used in raspberry, strawberry, butter, caramel, chocolate, apricot, cherry, peach, licorice, anise, nut, black, walnut, walnut, spice, and vanilla flavorings for beverages, ice cream, ices, candy, baked goods, gelatin desserts, and chewing gum. *See* Benzyl Acetate.

METHOXYBENZENE • *See* Anisole.

***p*-METHOXY BENZYL ACETATE** • *See* Anisyl Acetate.

***p*-METHOXY BENZYL ALCOHOL** • *See* Anisyl Alcohol.

***p*-METHOXYBENZYL FORMATE** • *See* Anisyl Formate.

1-METHOXYCARBONYL-1-PROPEN-2-YL DIMETHYL PHOSPHATE • Mevinphos. An organophosphate pesticide in dehydrated parsley as a result of application to the growing crop. FDA residue tolerance is 4 ppm. *See* Organophosphates for toxicity.

***p*-METHOXYCINNAMALDEHYDE** • A flavoring.

METHOXYETHANOL • *See* Ethanol.

4*p*-METHOXYPHENYL-2-BUTANONE • A synthetic fruit, licorice, and anise flavoring agent for beverages, ice cream, ices, candy, baked goods, chewing gum, and gelatin desserts. A flavoring agent used in foods, it has a pale yellow color and a sweet floral odor. No known toxicity.

1-(*p*-METHOXYPHENYL)-1-PENTEN-3-ONE • A synthetic butter, cream, fruit, maple, nut, and vanilla flavoring agent for beverages, ice cream ices, candy, and baked goods. No known toxicity.

1-(*p*-METHOXYPHENYL)-2-PROPANONE • A synthetic flavoring agent that occurs naturally in star anise. Used in fruit and vanilla flavorings for beverages, ice cream, ices, candy, and baked goods. No known toxicity.

2-METHOXYPYRAZINE • A colorless to yellow liquid with a nutty, cocoalike odor used as a flavoring in a variety of foods. Skin and eye irritant. GRAS.

***p*-METHOXYTOLUENE** • *See* *p*-Methyl Anisole.

4-METHOXYTOLUENE-2,5-DIAMINE HCL • A colorless liquid used in perfumery and flavorings. *See* Toluene.

METHIONINE HYDROXY ANALOG and ITS CALCIUM SALTS • A nutrient for animal feeds. GRAS.

METHYL ABIETATE • *See* Abietic Acid.

METHYL ACETAMIDE • *See* Methyl Acetate.

METHYL ACETATE • Acetic Acid. Colorless liquid that occurs naturally in coffee, with a pleasant apple odor. Used in perfume to emphasize floral odors, especially that of rose, and in toilet waters having a lavender odor. Also naturally occurs in peppermint oil. A flavoring used in fruit, rum, and nut flavorings for beverages, ice cream, ices, candy, baked goods, gelatin desserts, puddings, and liquor. Used as a solvent for many resins and oils. May be irritating to the respiratory tract and, in high concentrations, may be narcotic. Since it has an effective fat-solvent drying effect on skin, it may cause skin problems such as chafing and cracking.

4-METHYL ACETOPHENONE • Colorless liquid with a fruit odor, it is used as a flavoring agent in various foods. Moderately toxic by ingestion. A human skin irritant.

METHYLACETOPYRONONE • White crystalline powder used as a preservative in various foods. Poison by ingestion. Causes tumors in experimental animals. GRAS.

METHYL 1-ACETOXYCYCLOHEXYL KETONE • A flavoring agent. The FAO-WHO Expert Committee on Food Additives determined this substance needs further study.

2-METHYLALLYL BUTYRATE • *See* Butyric Acid.

METHYL ACRYLATE • 2-Propanoic Acid, Methyl Ester. Derived from Ethylene Chlorohydrin, it is transparent and elastic. Used to coat paper and plastic film. Can be highly irritating to the eyes, skin, and mucous membranes. Convulsions occur if vapors are inhaled in high concentrations. GRAS for packaging. The final report to the FDA of the Select Committee on GRAS Substances stated in 1980 that there were insufficient relevant biological and other studies upon which to base an evaluation of it when used as a food ingredient. There is no reported use of the chemical and there is no toxicology information available.

METHYL ALCOHOL • Solvent for spice oleoresins and in hops extract for beer. Clear, colorless liquid derived from carbon monoxide and hydrogen under pressure. Toxic by ingestion. Can cause blindness. Used in the manufacture of formaldehyde, acetic acid and other compounds. Used to denature (*see* Denaturant) alcohol. FDA tolerance for residues on spices is less than 50 ppm or less than 2.2 percent by weight.

METHYL AMYL KETONE • *See* 2-Heptanone.

METHYL ANISATE • Anisic Acid. A synthetic fruit, melon, liquor, root beer, and spice flavoring agent for beverages, ice cream, ices, candy, and baked goods.

***p*-METHYL ANISOLE** • *See* Ylang-Ylang Oil.

METHYL ANTHRANILATE • Occurs naturally in neroli, ylang-ylang, bergamot, jasmine, and other essential oils. Colorless to pale yellow liquid with a bluish fluorescence and a grapelike odor. It is made synthetically from coal tar *(see)*. Used in loganberry, strawberry, orange, floral, rose, violet, cherry, grape, melon, liquor, wine, and honey flavorings for beverages, ice cream, ices, candy, baked goods, chewing gum (2,200 ppm), and liquors. Used as an "orange" scent for ointments, in the manufacture of synthetic perfumes, and in suntan lotions. Can irritate the skin. GRAS.

N-METHYL ANTHRANILIC ACID, METHYL ESTER • *See* Methyl Anthranilate.

METHYL BENZENE ACETATE • A colorless liquid with a honey or jasmine odor, it is used a flavoring agent in a variety of foods. Moderately toxic by ingestion and skin contact.

METHYL BENZOATE • Essence of oil of Niobe. Made from methanol and benzoic acid *(see both)*. Colorless, transparent liquid with a pleasant fruity odor. Used in fruit rum, liquor, nut, spice, and vanilla flavorings for beverages, ice cream, ices, candy, and baked goods. Also used in perfumes.

METHYL BENZO CARBOXYLATE • Colorless liquid with a fragrant odor used as a flavoring agent in various foods. Moderately toxic by ingestion. Mildly toxic by skin contact.

METHYL-5-BENZOYL BENZIMIDAZOLE-2-CARBAMATE • Vermirax. Telmin. Mebendazole. An antiworm medicine for animals. In the EPA Genetic Toxicology Program. Poison by ingestion. Causes mutations in animals.

METHYL BROMIDE • Prepared from the action of hydrobromic acid on methanol *(see)* it is used as a fumigant in warehouses and for extracting oils from nuts, seeds, and flours. Inhalation causes dizziness, headache, vomiting, abdominal pain, mental confusion, convulsions, pulmonary edema, coma, and death. Chronic exposure can cause central nervous system depression or kidney injury. FDA tolerance for various crops is from 5 to 200 ppm.

METHYL-1-(BUTYL CARBAMOYL) 2-BENZIMIDAZOLYLCARBAMATE • BBC. Benylate. Benomyl. A fungicide used on apples, apricots, bananas, cherries, mangoes, nectarines, peaches, pears, pineapples, plums, raisins, and tomato products (concentrated). FDA residue tolerances are: 50 ppm in raisins and concentrated tomato products; 125 ppm in dried grape pomace and raisin waste; 70 ppm in dried apple pomace; 50 ppm in dried citrus pulp; 20 ppm in rice hulls. In EPA Genetic Toxicology Program *(see)*. Poison by ingestion. A human skin irritant. May cause birth defects.

METHYL *p*-tert-BUTYPHENYLACETATE • A synthetic chocolate, fruit, and honey flavorings for beverages, ice cream, ices, candy, and baked goods.

METHYL BUTYRATE • A synthetic flavoring agent that occurs naturally in apples. Colorless, used in fruit and rum flavorings for beverages, ice cream, candy, and baked goods.

METHYL CHLORIDE • Chloromethane. Colorless gas or colorless liquid with a sweet taste, it is used as a spray for pesticides in food storage and processing areas. It is not supposed to contact fatty foods. The FDA tolerance for modified hop extract for beer is up to 250 ppm. Poisonous, it can cause severe injury to liver and kidney.

METHYL CINNAMATE • White crystals, strawberrylike odor, and soluble in alcohol. Derived by heating methanol, cinnamic acid, and sulfuric acid. A synthetic strawberry, butter, cream, cherry, grape, peach, plum, and vanilla flavoring agent for beverages, ice cream, ices, candy, baked goods, chewing gum, and condiments. Used also in perfumes. *See* Cinnamic Acid.

METHYL DISULFIDE • A synthetic onion flavoring agent for baked goods, condiments, and pickle products. No known toxicity.

METHYL ESTER OF FATTY ACIDS • Produced from edible fats and oils. Used in dehydrating grapes to produce raisins. *See* Esters and Fatty Acids.

METHYL ESTER OF HIGHER FATTY ACIDS • Used in animal feed. *See* Fatty Acids.

METHYL ESTER OF ROSIN PARTIALLY HYDROGENATED • Used as a constituent of chewing-gum base. *See* Rosin and Hydrogenated.

METHYL ESTERS OF FATTY ACIDS PRODUCED FROM EDIBLE FATS and OILS • Used in dehydrating grapes to produce raisins. FDA tolerance is less than 3 percent of weight or less than 200 ppm in raisins.

METHYL ESTERS OF HIGHER FATTY ACIDS • Used in animal feed. No known toxicity.

METHYL ETHYL CELLULOSE • A foaming, aerating, and emulsifying agent prepared from wood pulp or chemical cotton. Used in vegetable-fat whipped topping and emulsifying agent. Used as a bulk laxative but absorbed from the bowel. *See* Sodium Carboxymethyl Cellulose for toxicity.

METHYL FORMATE • Colorless liquid with a sweet odor used as a fumigant in raisins and dried currants. FDA residue tolerance of 250 ppm as formic acid *(see)* in raisins and dried currants.

METHYL GLUCOSIDE OF FATTY ACIDS OF EDIBLE COCONUT OIL • Used in the manufacture of beet sugar and as an aid in crystallization of sucrose and dextrose. Used as a surfactant in molasses meant for animal feed. No known toxicity except that coconut is thought to contribute to cholesterol clogging of the arteries.

METHYL HEPTANOATE • A synthetic berry, grape, peach, and pineapple flavoring agent for beverages, ice cream, ices, candy, and baked goods.

METHYL HEPTENONE • *See* 6-Methyl-5-Hepten-2-One.

6-METHYL-5-HEPTEN-2-ONE • Methyl Heptenone. A synthetic flavoring agent that occurs naturally in oil of lavender and oil of lemon. Used in berry, citrus, banana, melon, pear, peach, and pineapple flavorings for beverages, ice cream, ices, candy, baked goods, and gelatin desserts. Moderately toxic by ingestion. A skin irritant.

METHYL HEXENOATE • A synthetic pineapple flavoring agent for beverages, ice cream, ices, candy, and baked goods.

METHYL-*p*-HYDROXYBENZOATE • Methylparaben. A preservative in beverages, baked goods, candy, and artificially sweetened jellies and preserves. Methylparaben may cause allergic skin reaction. On the FDA list of additives requiring further study. GRAS.

METHYL ISOBUTYL KETONE • A synthetic fruit flavoring agent for beverages, ice cream, ices, candy, and baked goods. Used as solvent for cellulose and lacquer. Similar in toxicity to methyl ethyl ketone, which is irritating to the eyes and mucous membranes, but likely more toxic. Causes intestinal upsets and central nervous system depression.

METHYL ISOBUTYRATE • A synthetic fruit flavoring agent for beverages, ice cream, ices, candy, and baked goods.

1-METHYL-4-ISOPROPYLCYCLOHEXADIENE-1,3 • A colorless liquid with a lemony odor, it is used as a flavoring agent in various foods. Moderately toxic by ingestion.

METHYL LAURATE • The ester of methyl alcohol and lauric acid. Derived from coconut oil. A synthetic flavoring agent for beverages, ice cream, ices, candy, and baked goods. It is also used in detergents, emulsifiers, wetting agents, stabilizers, resins, lubricants, and plasticizers.

METHYL LINOLEATE • The ester of methyl alcohol and linoleic acid, it is a colorless oil derived from safflower oil and used in detergents, emulsifiers, wetting agents, stabilizers, resins, lubricants, and plasticizers.

METHYL MERCAPTAN • A synthetic flavoring agent that occurs naturally in caseinate, cheese skim milk, coffee, and cooked beef. Used in coffee flavorings for beverages, ice cream, ices, candy, and baked goods. *See* Methanethiol for toxicity.

METHYL-2-METHYL BUTYRATE • Colorless liquid with a sweet, applelike odor used as a flavoring agent in various foods. No known toxicity.

METHYL MYRISTATE • *See* Myristic Acid.

METHYL b-NAPHTHYL KETONE • Orange Crystals. 2′ Acetonaphthone. A synthetic flavoring agent used in berry, strawberry, citrus, fruit, grape, and vanilla flavorings for beverages, ice cream, ices, candy, baked goods, gelatin desserts, and chewing gum. *See* Methyl Isobutyl Ketone for toxicity.

METHYL NONANOATE • A synthetic berry, citrus, pineapple, honey, and cognac flavoring agent for beverages, ice cream, ices, candy, and baked goods.

METHYL 2-NONENOATE • A synthetic berry and melon flavoring agent for beverages, ice cream, ices, candy, and baked goods.

METHYL 2-NONYNOATE • A synthetic berry, floral, violet, fruit, and banana flavoring agent for beverages, ice cream, ices, candy, and gelatin desserts, baked goods, and condiments. No known toxicity.

METHYL OCTANOATE • A synthetic flavoring agent that occurs naturally in pineapple. Used in pineapple and berry flavorings for beverages, ice cream, ices, candy, and baked goods.

METHYL 2-OCTYNOATE • A synthetic flavoring agent used in berry, raspberry, strawberry, floral, violet, fruit, peach, liquor, and muscatel flavorings for beverages, ice cream, ices, candy, baked goods, gelatin desserts, chewing gum, and jellies.

METHYLPARABEN • Methyl-*p*-hydroxybenzoate. Preservative. Used in jellies and preserves. The FDA allows zero residue in milk from dairy cows treated with mastitis formulations. GRAS.

METHYL PELARGONATE • Nonanoic Acid. Methyl Ester. The ester of ethyl alcohol and pelargonic acid used in perfume and flavorings. No known toxicity.

4-METHYL-2-PENTANONE • A synthetic fruit flavoring for beverages, ice cream, ices, candy, and baked goods.

2-METHYL-4-PHENYL-2-BUTYL ACETATE • A synthetic fruit and tea flavoring agent for beverages, ice cream, ices, candy, and baked goods. No known toxicity.

METHYLBENZYL ACETATE • Colorless liquid with a sweet, nutty odor. Used as a flavoring agent in various foods.

α-METHYLBENZYL ALCOHOL • A flavoring agent in foods and beverages derived from alcohol and benzoic acid *(see both)* and also appears naturally in a variety of foods. The FAO-WHO Expert Committee on Food Additives found that in short-term toxicity studies, high rates of mortality were associated with dose levels of 1,000 mg and 2,000 mg per kg of body weight per day in mice and 2,000 mg per day in rats. It also adversely affected body weight, long-term survival rates and caused birth defects. The Committee said the intake of this compound from all sources is extremely low. On the basis of the evidence available, the Committee concluded that the higher incidence of benign tumors in the kidneys of male rats was not relevant to humans. In view of the "limited database," the Committee concluded that the available data could be used to set an ADI by application of a safety factor of 1,000 to the minimal-effect level of 93 mg per kg of body weight per day. Accordingly, an ADI of 0–0.1 mg per kg of body weight per day was allocated for this additive.

1-(3-METHYL)BUTYL BENZOATE • Amyl Benzoate. Isopentyl Benzoate. Used as a flavoring agent in various foods. Mildly toxic by ingestion. A skin irritant.

2-METHYLBUTYL ISOVALERATE • *See* Valeric Acid.

METHYLCELLULOSE • A white fibrous powder prepared from wood pulp used as a binder, bodying agent, bulking agent, emulsifiers, film former, stabilizer, thickener, in baked goods, fruit pie fillings, meat patties, and vegetable patties. It is used as a laxative because it swells with water and increases the bulk and moisture content of the stool, which encourages bowel movements. GRAS.

METHYLCHLOROPINDOL • Coccidiostat. An antibiotic drug for animals used on beef and in feed as well as cereal grains, chicken, fruits, goat, lamb, milk, pork, turkey, and vegetables. FDA limits it to 0.2 ppm in cereal grains, vegetables, and fruits; 15 ppm in uncooked liver and kidney; 5 ppm in uncooked muscle of chickens and turkeys; and 3 ppm in uncooked kidney.

METHYLCINNAMATE • *See* Cinnamic Acid.

6-METHYLCOUMARIN • A white needlelike substance from benzene with a coconut odor, it is used as a flavoring agent in various foods. Moderately toxic by ingestion.

METHYLENE CHLORIDE • Dichloromethane. Methane Dichloride. Methylene Dichloride. Aerothene NM. Solaestine. Freon 30 Somethine. F-30. A colorless gas that compresses into colorless liquid of pleasant odor and sweet taste. It is widely used as a degreaser; solvent for spices, waxes, oils, paint, and varnish thinner; as cleansers in many industries and work settings; in aerosols, including pesticides; in refrigeration, and air-conditioning equipment; in coffee decaffeination and spice extraction processes. Methylene chloride is nonflammable and a good grease remover and therefore products may contain very high percentages of the chemical. For instance, paint strippers are usually 40 to 80 percent methylene chloride. Some which may be labeled "nonflammable" are almost 100 percent. Spray paints may contain up to 33 percent of the chemical. High concentrations are narcotic. Methylene chloride enters your body when you breathe it in the air. Once it enters the body, methylene chloride generates carbon monoxide, which interferes with the blood's ability to pick up and deliver oxygen. The body responds to lack of oxygen by driving the heart to work harder. People with angina (chest pains) from coronary artery disease are extremely sensitive to carbon monoxide and may have increased chest pains from exposure to methylene chloride, even below the legal exposure limit (100 parts per million over an eight-hour workshift). There is no one watching how consumers use the products. The use of a paint remover in a poorly ventilated setting has been implicated in fatalities, according to a report in the November 8, 1990 issue of the *American Journal of Emergency Medicine.* Since smoking increases the carbon monoxide level in the blood, smokers are doubly affected. Small amounts can also be absorbed through the skin. Damage to the liver, kidney, and central nervous system can occur, and persistent postrecovery symptoms after inhalation include headache, nervousness, insomnia, and tremor. It is also a skin irritant. Methylene chloride is considered to have "poor warning properties" since most people cannot smell it until it reaches a hazardous level (100–500 ppm). If you can smell it, you may be overexposed. Methylene chloride causes cancer in animals and is considered a potential cancer-causing agent in humans. The FAO-WHO Expert Committee on Food Additives said that epidemiological studies have not shown any carcinogenic effect of dichloromethane after occupational exposure. However, the Committee noted that the power to detect excess risk in these studies was limited. On the basis of the available data, the Committee concluded that the use of dichloromethane as an extraction solvent in food processing should be limited to use for spice oleoresins and the decaffeination of tea and coffee and for food additives that included residues of dichloromethane. FDA residue tolerances are: 30 ppm in spice oleoresins, less than 10 ppm in decaffeinated roasted coffee and decaffeinated instant coffee, and 2.2 percent as a residue in hops extract added before or during cooking of beer.

METHYL ESTER OF ROSIN, PARTIALLY HYDROGENATED • Used as a chewing-gum base.

3-METHYL-3-PHENYL GLYCIDIC ACID, ETHYL ESTER • A synthetic strawberry flavoring. GRAS.

METHYL PHENYLACETATE • Colorless liquid with a honeylike odor used in strawberry, chocolate, peach, and honey flavorings for beverages, ice cream, ices, baked goods, candy, gelatin desserts, chewing gum, and syrup. Also used in perfumery. Moderately toxic by ingestion and skin contact. *See* Phenyl Acetate.

2-METHYL-4-PHENYLBUTYRALDEHYDE • A synthetic nut flavoring agent for beverages, ice cream, ices, candy, and baked goods.

3-METHYL-2-PHENYL BUTYRATE • A synthetic fruit flavoring for beverages, ice cream, ices, and candy.

METHYL 4-PHENYLBUTYRATE • A synthetic strawberry, fruit, and honey flavoring agent for beverages, ice cream, ices, candy, and baked goods.

METHYL PIPERAZINE • Colorless liquid that absorbs water. Used as a surfactant *(see)*.

METHYL PREDNISOLONE • Medrol. Meprolone. A-MethaPred. Solu-Medrol. A hormone secreted by the adrenal gland that affects carbohydrate and protein metabolism. It was introduced as a medication in 1957 to treat severe inflammation or for immunosuppression or to decrease residual damage following spinal cord trauma. Used to treat cows. FDA limits residue to 10 ppb in milk. Most adverse reactions are the result of dose- or length-of-time of administration. Should be taken with food or milk to reduce GI irritation. Potential adverse reactions include euphoria, insomnia, psychotic behavior, high blood pressure, swelling, cataracts, glaucoma, peptic ulcer, GI irritation, increased appetite, high blood sugar, growth suppression in children, delayed wound healing, acne, skin eruptions, muscle weakness, pancreatitis, hairiness, decreased immunity, and acute adrenal gland insufficiency. When withdrawn, there may be rebound inflammation, fatigue, weakness, joint pain, fever, dizziness, lethargy, depression, fainting, a drop in blood pressure upon arising from a seated or prone position, shortness of breath, loss of appetite, and high blood sugar. Sudden withdrawal may be fatal. Contraindicated in systemic fungal infections. Should be used cautiously in patients with GI ulceration or kidney disease, high blood pressure, diabetes, chickenpox, osteoporosis, Cushing's syndrome, blood clotting disorders, seizures, myasthenia gravis, congestive heart failure, tuberculosis, herpes, and emotional instability. FDA tolerance in milk from treated cows is 10 ppb.

METHYL SALICYLATE • Salicylic Acid. Oil of Wintergreen. Found naturally in sweet birch, cassia, and wintergreen. Used in strawberry, grape, mint, walnut, root beer, sarsaparilla, spice, wintergreen, birch beer, and vanilla flavorings for beverages, ice cream, ices, candy, baked goods, chewing gum (8,400 ppm), and syrup. The volatile oil obtained by maceration. Used in perfumery and as a counterirritant, local anesthetic, and disinfectant in cosmetics and in sunburn lotions as a ultraviolet absorber. Toxic by ingestion. Use in foods restricted by the FDA. Lethal dose 30 cc in adults, 10 milliliters in children. The FDA proposed that liniments and other liquid preparations containing more than 5 percent methyl salicylate be marketed in special child-resistant containers.

METHYL SILICONE • Prepared by hydrolyzing *(see)* dimethyldichlorosilane or its esters, it is used to help compounds resist oxidation. No known toxicity. *See* Silicones.

METHYL SULFIDE • A synthetic flavoring agent that occurs naturally in caseinate, cheese, coffee, coffee extract, and skim milk. Disagreeable odor. Used in chocolate, cocoa, fruit, and molasses flavorings for beverages, ice cream, ices, candy, baked goods, gelatin desserts, and syrups. Used also as a solvent for minerals. No known toxicity.

METHYL 9-UNDECENOATE • A synthetic citrus and honey flavoring agent for beverages, ice cream, ices, candy, and baked goods.

2-METHYLUNDECANAL • Colorless to slightly yellow liquid with a fatty odor; used as a flavoring agent.

METHYL 2-UNDECYNOATE • A synthetic floral and violet flavoring agent for beverages, ice cream, ices, candy, and baked goods.

METHYL VALERATE • A synthetic flavoring agent that occurs naturally in pineapple. Used in fruit flavorings for beverages, ice cream, ices, candy, and baked goods.

2-METHYL VALERIC ACID • A synthetic chocolate flavoring agent for candy.

METHYLACETALDEHYDE • *See* Propionaldehyde.

METHYLACETIC ACID • *See* Propionic Acid.

2-METHYLALLYL BUTYRATE • A synthetic pineapple flavoring for beverages, ice cream, ices, candy, and baked goods. No known toxicity.

o-METHYLANISOLE • A synthetic fruit and nut flavoring for beverages, ice cream, ices, candy, and baked goods.

p-METHYLANISOLE • A synthetic berry, maple, black walnut, walnut, and spice flavoring agent for beverages, ice cream, ices, candy, baked goods, gelatin desserts, puddings, condiments, and syrups.

METHYLBENZYL ACETATE • A synthetic flavoring agent, colorless, with a gardenia odor. Used in cherry and fruit flavoring agent, colorless with a gardenia odor. Used in cherry and fruit flavorings for beverages, ice cream, ices, candy, baked goods, gelatin desserts, and chewing gum.

a-METHYLBENZYL ACETATE • Acetic Acid. A synthetic berry and fruit flavoring agent for beverages, ice cream, ices, candy, baked goods, chewing gum, and toppings.

a-METHYLBENZYL ALCOHOL • A synthetic flavoring agent, colorless, with a hyacinth odor. Used in strawberry, rose, fruit, and honey flavorings for beverages, ice cream, ices, candy, baked goods, gelatin desserts, and chewing gum. Methyl alcohol is wood alcohol, a widely used solvent in paints, varnishes, and paint removers. Readily absorbed from the gastrointestinal tract; as little as two teaspoonfuls is considered toxic if ingested. The fatal dose lies between 2 and 8 ounces.

a-METHYLBENZYL BUTYRATE • A synthetic berry and fruit flavoring agent for beverages, ice cream, ices, candy, and baked goods.

a-METHYLBENZYL ISOBUTRYATE • A synthetic fruit flavoring agent for beverages, ice cream, ices, candy, and baked goods. No known toxicity.

a-METHYLBENZYL FORMATE • Formic Acid. A synthetic fruit and berry flavoring agent for beverages, ice cream, ices, candy, and baked goods. *See* Formic Acid for toxicity.

2-METHYLBUTYALDEHYDE • A synthetic flavoring agent that occurs naturally in coffee and tea. Used in chocolate and fruit flavoring for beverages, ice cream, ices, candy, and baked goods. No known toxicity.

3-METHYLBUTYRALDEHYDE • A synthetic flavoring agent that occurs naturally in coffee extract, oil of lavender, and peppermint oil. Used in butter, chocolate, cocoa, fruit, and nut flavorings for beverages, ice cream, ices, candy, baked goods, and gelatin desserts.

2-METHYLBUTYRIC ACID • A synthetic fruit flavoring agent for beverages, ice cream, ices, and candy.

METHYLCELLULOSE • Cellulose, Methyl Ether. A binder, thickener, dispersing, and emulsifying agent, it is prepared from wood pulp or chemical cotton by treatment with alcohol. Swells in water. Soluble in cold water and insoluble in hot. The commercial product has a methoxyl content of 29 percent. It is used as a bodying agent for beverages and canned fruits sweetened with artificial sweeteners; a thickener for kosher food products; a bulking agent for low-calorie crackers; a binder in nonwheat baked goods for nonallergic diets; a beer foam stabilizer; a condiment carrier; in food products for diabetics and low-calorie dietetic products; an edible film for food products; a leavening agent for prepared mixes; a clarifier for vinegar and beverages; and in imitation jellies and jams, processed cheese, confectionery, and toppings. It is also used in wave-setting lotions, foam stabilizers, bath oils, and other cosmetic products. It is a bulk laxative. Ingestion of large doses may cause flatulence, distension of the abdomen or intestinal obstruction, and may also affect the absorption of minerals or other drugs. A dose injected into the abdomen of rats causes cancer. Nontoxic on the skin. The final report to the FDA of the Select Committee on GRAS Substances stated in 1980 that there is no evidence in the available information that it is a hazard to the public when used as it is now and it should continue its GRAS status with limitations in the amounts that can be added to foods. *See also* Carboxymethyl Cellulose. GRAS.

6-METHYLCOUMARIN • A synthetic flavoring agent used in butter, caramel, coconut, fruit, nut, root beer, and vanilla flavorings for beverages, ice cream, ices, candy, baked goods, gelatin desserts, puddings, and chewing gum. Unlike methyl-coumarin, which is listed as GRAS by the Flavor Extract Manufacturers Association, coumarin, once widely used in foods, is banned. Prolonged feeding of coumarin causes liver injury.

METHYLCYCLOPENTENOLONE • A synthetic flavoring agent used in berry, butter, butterscotch, caramel, maple, hazelnut, pecan, walnut, fruit, and vanilla flavorings for beverages, ice cream, ices, candy, baked goods, chewing gum, gelatin desserts, and syrups. No known toxicity.

METHYLENE CHLORIDE • A colorless gas that compresses into colorless liquid of pleasant odor and sweet taste. A solvent in the microencapsulation of thiamin hydrochloride *(see)* intended for use in both dry beverages and dry gelatin mixes. One of the most commonly used solvents, it is used to remove caffeine from coffee and tea. The FDA estimates, based on coffee industry tests, that about 0.1 ppm remain in most brands decaffeinating this way. Once absorbed into the body, methylene chloride generates carbon monoxide, affecting the blood's ability to pick up oxygen. Because of public concern about methylene chloride, some brands are now using other methods of decaffeinating. Methylene chloride is also used as a solvent for nail enamels and for cleansing creams. Used as an anesthetic in medicine. High concentrations are narcotic. Damage to the liver, kidney, and central nervous system can occur, and persistent postrecovery symptoms after inhalation include headache, nervousness, insomnia, and tremor. Can be absorbed through the skin and is then converted to carbon monoxide which, in turn, can cause stress in the cardiovascular system. It is also a skin irritant.

5-METHYLFURFURAL • A synthetic honey, maple, and meat flavoring for beverages, ice cream, ices, candy, and baked goods.

2-METHYLOCTANAL • A synthetic citrus flavoring agent for beverages, ice cream, ices, candy, and baked goods.

METHYLPARABEN • Methyl *p*-Hydroxybenzoate. Preservative in jelly and preserves. Used in bubble baths, cold creams, eyeliners, and liquid makeup. It is an antimicrobial and preservative made of small, odorless, colorless crystals that have a burning taste. FDA residue tolerance in milk from cows treated with mastitis formulations is zero. Nontoxic in small amounts but can cause allergic skin reactions. *See* Methyl-*p*-Hydroxybenzoate. GRAS.

2-METHYLPENTANOIC ACID • *See* 2-Methyl Valeric Acid.

***b*-METHYLPHENETHYL ALCOHOL** • A synthetic berry, rose, melon, and honey flavoring agent for beverages, ice cream, ices, and candy, baked goods.

METHYLPHENYL ETHER • *See* Anisole.

METHYLPROTOCATECHUIC ALDEHYDE • *See* Vanillin.

4-METHYLQUINOLINE • A synthetic butter, honey, and nut flavoring agent for beverages, ice cream, ices, candy, and baked goods. No known toxicity.

METHYLTHEOBROMINE • *See* Caffeine.

2-METHYLUNDECANAL • A synthetic flavoring agent, colorless, with a fatty odor. Used in a variety of foods.

2-METHYLRESORCINOL • Orcin. An aromatic compound with white crystalline prisms derived from lichen; used in medicine and as a reagent for sugars and starches. *See* Resorcinol.

METOLACHLOR • An odorless, preemergent herbicide. FDA residue tolerances are: 0.02 ppm in cattle, goats, sheep, hog fat, meat byproducts, and in eggs; 0.05 ppm as residue in cattle, goat, hog, sheep liver; 0.1 ppm as residues in corn grain and cottonseed; 0.3 ppm as residues in sorghum grain; 0.2 ppm as residues in soybean; 2 ppm as residues in or on sorghum forage, fodder; and 8 ppm as residue in or on corn forage or fodder.

METOSERPATE HYDROCHLORIDE • An animal drug used in chicken. FDA limits residue to 0.02 ppm in chicken. Crystals from benzene and cyclohexane. Used as a sedative. Poisonous by ingestion.

METSULFURON METHYL • A pre- and postemergent herbicide. FDA tolerances for residues in or on grain, green forage, hay, straw of barley and wheat, 0.05 to 20 ppm; 0.1 ppm as a residue in meat and meat byproducts of cattle, hogs, and sheep; and 0.05 ppm as a residue in milk.

MEXICAN SAGE • *See* Oregano.

mg • Abbreviation for a milligram, a metric measurement that is $\frac{1}{1000}$ of a gram.

MIBOLERONE • Crystalline solid used as an animal feed drug. A male hormone, it used in dog food to increase growth. Caused adverse reproductive effects and birth defects in experimental animals.

MICROCAPSULES • Used for flavoring oils, these tiny vessels contain succinylated gelatin, arabinogalactan, silicon dioxide, glutaraldehyde, and octanal *(see all)*.

MICROCRYSTALLINE CELLULOSE • Used in frozen desserts. No longer listed as GRAS. Limited in standardized products. *See* Cellulose.

MICROPARTICULATED PROTEIN PRODUCT • Thickener and texturizer in frozen dessert products. May not be used to replace milk fat in standardized frozen desserts. GRAS.

MIEHEI, or *MUCOR PUSILLUS* • Enzyme used to clot milk for making cheese.

MILFOIL • *See* Yarrow.

MILK • Milk may be a hidden ingredient in cream of rice, macaroni, filled candy bars, Ovaltine, Junket, prepared flours, frankfurters, and other sausages. Some people are allergic to milk. *See also* Nonfat Dry Milk. The Food and Drug Administration ruled, starting January 1, 1998, lower-fat milk products must follow the same criteria as most other foods labeled "low fat." This means that such products as 2 percent milk, which contains about 5 grams of fat per serving, cannot be labeled "low fat" because the fat content is more than 3 grams per serving, which is the upper limit permitted in food products labeled "low fat." Actually, 2 percent milk has two-thirds the fat of whole milk. Milk with zero fat will be called "fat free" or "nonfat" instead of "skim" and 1 percent milk will be "low fat." "Milk is so important to good nutrition, and now consumers can fit it into low-fat diets as well," said Donna E. Shalala, Secretary of Health and Services. "And folic acid fortification of bakery products is one of the safest scientific approaches we know to protect the future of our children."

Whole milk normally contains 3.25 percent milkfat or 8 grams of fat per serving (a serving is defined as 1 cup). Milk labeled 1 percent milk fat contains 2.5 grams of fat per serving, and thus qualifies for the "low fat" claim, but 2-percent does not.

Standards of identity for lower-fat dairy products were adopted some time before the Nutrition Labeling and Education Act of 1990 (NLEA). In 1993, when regulations for NLEA went into effect, nutrient content claims, including "low fat," were defined. However, since standards of identity for lower-fat milk products were already in place using the same terms, milk products with standards were exempted from the new labeling rules. The rule revokes the old standards of identity for lower-fat milk products. Now, fat claims on milk products will mean the same as they do for other foods. Although 2 percent milk, with its 5 grams of fat, may not be called "low fat," the product does qualify for a "reduced fat" claim. "Reduced fat" means that the fat content of the food has been reduced by at least 25 percent per serving compared to the full-fat food. Because whole milk contains 8 grams of fat, 2 percent milk with its 5 grams of fat has more than a 25 percent reduction in fat. "Light" may be used on milk whose fat has been reduced by 50 percent or more per serving; for example, 4 grams of fat or about 1.5 percent milk fat. "Nonfat" and "fat-free" are defined as less than 0.5 grams of fat per serving. These terms and "skim" may be used on milk products that qualify. Lower-fat dairy products may continue to show the percent of milk fat as long as the declaration is not false or misleading. For example, the percent–milk fat declaration cannot be more than twice the size of the name of the food. Lower-fat milk must also show a "Nutrition Facts" panel, as do most packaged food. The renaming of lower-fat dairy products applies to twelve products. They are low-fat milk, skim milk, low-fat cottage cheese, sweetened condensed skimmed milk, low-fat dry milk, evaporated skimmed milk, acidified low fat milk, cultured low-fat milk, acidified skim milk, cultured skim milk, sour half-and-half, and acidified sour half-and-half. FDA has decided to defer action on claims for yogurt to allow the industry time to resolve nutritional and technical problems in the manufacture of low-fat products. The new rules giving consistency to claims for milk fat with other food products are based on petitions from the Center for Science in the Public Interest, the Milk Industry Foundation, and the American Dairy Products Institute.

MILK-CLOTTING ENZYME FROM *BACILLUS CEREUS* • Derived from *Bacillus cereus*, used to clot milk in cheese making. There is no reported use of the chemical and no toxicology information available.

MILK-CLOTTING ENZYME FROM *ENTOTHIA PARASITICA, MUCOR PUSILLUS* • Used to clot milk for cheese making. The FDA has not done a search of the toxicology literature concerning this additive.

MILLET EXTRACT • An extract of the seeds of *Panicum miliaceum*.

MILLIGRAM (mg) • A metric unit of weight equal to one-thousandth of a gram. Food labels list cholesterol and sodium in milligrams (mg) per serving.

MILO STARCH • *See* Modified Starch. The final report to the FDA of the Select Committee on GRAS Substances stated in 1980 that it should continue its GRAS status with no limitations other than good manufacturing practices.

MIMOSA, ABSOLUTE • *Acacia decurrens*. Black Wattle Flowers. Reddish yellow solid with a long-lasting, pleasant odor resembling ylang-ylang, used in perfumes. Derived from trees, shrubs, and herbs native to tropical and warm regions. Mimosa droops and closes its leaves when touched. A natural flavoring agent used in raspberry and fruit flavorings for beverages, ice cream, ices, candy, and baked goods. Also used in tanning. May produce allergic skin reactions.

MINERAL OIL • White Oil. It is a mixture of refined liquid hydrocarbons *(see)* derived from petroleum. Colorless, transparent, odorless, and tasteless. It is used as a defoaming component in the processing of beet sugar and yeast; as a coating for fresh fruits and vegetables; a lubricant and binder for capsules and tablets, supplying small amounts of flavor in spice condiments and vitamins. Also employed as a lubricant in food-processing equipment; a dough-divider oil; pan oil; and a lubricant in meat-packing plants. It is also used in confectionery as a sealant. It is also employed in baby creams, baby lotions, bay oil, brilliantine hairdressings, cleansing creams, cold creams, emollients, moisturizing creams, eye creams, foundation creams and makeup, hair conditioners, hand lotions, lipsticks, mascaras, rouge, shaving creams, compact facial powders, makeup removers, suntan creams, oils, and ointments. Also a cosmetic lubricant, protective agent, and binder. When heated, it smells like petroleum. It stays on top of the skin and leaves a shiny protective surface. May inhibit absorption of digestive fats and it has a mild laxative effect. A human cancer-causing agent by inhalation. Causes birth defects if inhaled by humans and also causes testicular tumors in the fetus. An eye irritant. FDA tolerances include: 200 ppm in dried fruits and vegetables from use as a releasing agent in drying pans; less than 0.095 percent in meat from use as hot melt coating; less than 0.10 percent in egg white solids; and less than 0.06 percent as a releasing agent, binder, and/or lubricant in or on capsules or tablets containing concentrates of flavors, spices, condiments, and nutrients intended for addition to food. The FAO-WHO Expert Committee on Food Additives requested in June 1998 that studies of the compositional factors in mineral oils that influence their absorption and toxicity be done in rats for at least one year. In addition, a one-year study of the potential effects on the immune system was requested. The results of the study will be evaluated in 2002.

MIXED CARBOHYDRASE and PROTEASE ENZYME PRODUCTS • Enzymes. GRAS. *See* Enzymes.

MOCA • Bis Amine. Curalin M. Packaging adhesive prohibited from indirect addition to human food from food contact surface. IARC review *(see)*. EPA Genetic Toxicology Program and Community Right-To-Know List *(see both)*. Moderately toxic by ingestion. Caused cancer and tumors in experimental animals.

MODIFIED CELLULOSE • *See* Cellulose Gums.

MODIFIED SEA SALT • Salts derived from seawater with a reduced sodium chloride content.

MODIFIED STARCH • Ordinary starch that has been altered chemically to modify such properties as thickening or jelling. Babies have difficulty in digesting starch in its original form. Modified starch is used in baby food on the theory that it is easier to digest. Questions about safety have arisen because babies do not have the resistance of adults to chemicals. Among chemicals used to modify starch are propylene oxide, succinic anhydride, 1-octenyl succinic anhydride, aluminum sulfate, and sodium hydroxide *(see all)*. On the FDA top priority list for reevaluation since 1980. Nothing new reported by the FDA since.

MOENOMYCIN • Bambermycin. Menomycin. An antibiotic produced by *Streptomyces roseoflavus* used as an animal feed drug for poultry, calves, and swine. An eye and skin irritant. Poison by ingestion. Moderately toxic by ingestion.

MOLASSES EXTRACT • Extract of sugarcane, a thick, brown, viscid syrup. Separated from raw sugar in the successive processes of sugar manufacture and graded according to its quality. It is a natural flavoring agent for candy, baked goods, ice cream, and medicines. GRAS.

MOLYBDATE ORANGE • A solution of lead chromate, lead molybdate, and lead sulfate. Used in printing inks. Toxic by ingestion.

MOLYBDENUM • A dietary supplement. The dark gray, powdered mineral is a trace element in animal and plant metabolism. Resembles chromium and tungsten in many of its properties. Low order of toxicity.

MONAMINE OXIDASE INHIBITOR (MAO) • An enzyme that acts in the nervous system to break down certain types of neurotransmitters (chemical messengers sent between nerve cells) such as dopamine, norepinephrine, and serotonin *(see all)*.

MONARDA SPECIES • *See* Horsemint Leaves Extract.

MONESIN • Antibiotic isolated from *Streptocyces cinnamonensis*. Used in feed to combat parasites and fungus infections. It is also used to increase weight gain in cattle. FDA residue limits are: 0.05 ppm in edible tissues of cattle; 1.5 ppm in muscle tissue of chicken and turkey; 3 ppm as residue in skin with fat of chicken and turkey; and 4.5 ppm as residue in liver of chicken. Used as a medicated block for cattle; in liquid feed for cattle; in goat feed.

MONOAMINE • Containing one amine group.

MONOAMINE OXIDASE INHIBITOR MEDICATIONS (MAOIs) • A class of antidepressant medications usually prescribed for people who have certain forms of depression with symptoms including an increase in weight, appetite, or sleep. MAOIs may also be used for cases of mixed anxiety and depression, depression accompanied by pain, panic disorder, post-traumatic stress disorder, and bipolar depression. The drug works by raising the level of neurotransmitters by preventing their destruction by enzymes. People taking MAOIs must adhere to a special diet because of the interaction of the medications with certain foods. Foods that contain tyramine such as cheeses, yogurt, sour cream, beef or chicken livers, and red wines should be avoided. The combination of MAOIs and tyramine can shoot up blood pressure to dangerous levels. Symptoms include headache, increased or decreased heart rate, nausea and vomiting, sweating, fever or cold clammy skin, and chest pain.

4-MONOAMINOPHOSPHATIDE • *See* Lecithin.

MONOAMMONIUM GLUTAMATE • Miscellaneous uses. GRAS. *See* Glutamate, Ammonium.

MONOAZO COLOR • A dye made from diazonium and phenol, both coal tar derivatives. *See* Coal Tar.

MONOCALCIUM PHOSPHATE • Calcium Phosphate, Monobasic. Buffer and neutralizing agent in self-rising cereal flours or meals. The FDA allows residues of up to 0.75 parts per 100 parts of flour; 4.5 parts including sodium bicarbonate per 100 parts of cereal product; 75 percent in phosphated flour, in self-rising cereal flours or meals; in fruit butters, jellies, and preserves; 0.1 percent in finished product of canned vegetables. GRAS. *See* Calcium Phosphate.

MONOCHLORACETIC ACID • A banned preservative. Any amount in beverages and other food will be considered adulterated by the FDA.

MONO- and DI-GLYCERIDES of FATS or OILS • Mono- and di-glycerides of edible fat-forming acids used as emulsifiers in oleomargarine. GRAS. *See* Glycerides.

MONOETHANOLAMINE • Used in flume water for washing sugar beets prior to slicing. See ethanolamine.

MONOGLYCERIDE CITRATE • Aids the action of and helps dissolve antioxidant formulations that retard rancidity in oils and fats. *See* Citrate Salts for toxicity. The final report to the FDA of the Select Committee on GRAS Substances stated in 1980 that there were insufficient relevant biological and other studies upon which to base an evaluation of it when it is used as a food ingredient.

MONOGLYCERIDES DISTILLED • Used to treat mastitis in dairy animals.

MONOGLYCERIDES OF FATTY ACIDS • Stabilizers in shortenings. *See* Fatty Acids. No known toxicity.

MONOGLYCEROL CITRATE • A preservative. *See* Glycerols.

MONOISOPROPYL CITRATE • A sequestrant and plasticizer and antioxidant aid used in fats, lard, meat, oleomargarine, packaging materials, sausage, and shortening. GRAS. *See* Isopropyl Citrate.

MONOMER • A molecule that by repetition in a long chain builds up a large structure or polymer *(see)*. Ethylene, the gas, for instance, is the monomer of polyethylene *(see)*.

MONOPOTASSIUM GLUTAMATE • Flavor enhancer and salt substitute used on meat. EPA Genetic Toxicology Program *(see)*. Mildly toxic by ingestion. Human systemic effects by ingestion: headache. GRAS. *See* Glutamate.

MONOPOTASSIUM PHOSPHATE • A derivative of edible fat. Used as an emulsifying agent in food products and as a buffer in prepared cereal. Cleared by the USDA's Meat Inspection Department to decrease the amounts of cooked-out juices in canned hams, pork shoulders, pork loins, chopped hams, and bacon. Monosodium phosphate is a urinary acidifier but has no known toxicity. The final report to the FDA of the Select Committee on GRAS Substances stated in 1980 that it should continue its GRAS status with no limitations other than good manufacturing practices.

MONOSACCHARIDE LACTATE CONDENSATE • The condensation product of sodium lactate and the sugars, glucose, fructose, ribose, glucosamine, and deoxyribose.

MONOSODIUM GLUTAMATE (MSG) • Accent. Zest. The monosodium salt of glutamic acid *(see),* one of the amino acids. Occurs naturally in seaweed, sea tangles, soybeans, and sugar beets. Used to intensify meat and spice flavorings in meats, condiments, pickles, soups, candy, and baked goods. Believed responsible for the so-called Chinese Restaurant Syndrome in which diners suffer from chest pain, headache, and numbness after eating a Chinese meal. Causes brain damage in young rodents and brain damage effects in rats, rabbits, chicks, and monkeys. Baby-food processors removed MSG from baby-food products. Depression, irritability, and other mood changes have been reported. On the FDA list of additives needing further study for mutagenic, teratogenic, subacute, and reproductive effects. Studies have shown that MSG administered to animals during the neonatal period resulted in reproductive dysfunction when both males and females became adults. Females treated with MSG had fewer pregnancies and smaller litters, while males showed reduced fertility. The final report to the FDA of the Select Committee on GRAS Substances stated in 1980 that while no evidence in the available information on it demonstrates a hazard to the public at current use levels, uncertainties exist requiring that additional studies be conducted. In 1995, a report from the Federation of American Societies for Experimental Biology (FASEB), an independent body of scientists that advises the FDA, identified two groups of people who may develop a condition: "MSG symptom complex." One group is those who may be intolerant to MSG when eaten in large quantities. The second is a group of people with severe, poorly controlled asthma. In addition to being prone to MSG symptoms these people may suffer temporary worsening of asthmatic symptoms after consuming MSG. The MSG dosage that produced reactions ranged from 0.5 grams to 2.5 grams. This report made the FDA propose that foods containing significant amounts of free glutamate (not bound in protein along with other amino acids) declare glutamate on the label. GRAS status has continued since 1980 while tests were being completed and evaluated.

MONOSODIUM METHYLARSONATE • Arsonate Liquid. Weed-E-Rad. An herbicide used on animal feed and cottonseed hulls. FDA residue limit is 0.9 ppm in cottonseed hulls when used for animal feed. Arsenic and its compounds are on the Community Right-To-Know List and in the EPA Genetic Toxicology Program *(see both)*. Moderately toxic by ingestion. A skin and eye irritant.

MONOSODIUM PHOSPHATE • Used as an emulsifier for cheeses, frozen eggs, and jellies. The FDA's tolerance is set at less than 5 percent. In medicine it is used as a laxative. GRAS.

MONOSODIUM PHOSPHATE DERIVATIVES OF DIGLYCERIDES • Derived from edible fats or oils or edible fat-forming fatty acids and used as emulsifiers. GRAS.

MONOSTARCH PHOSPHATE • A modified starch *(see)*. The final report to the FDA of the Select Committee on GRAS Substances stated in 1980 that there is no evidence in the available information that it is a hazard to the public when used as it is now and it should continue its GRAS status with limitations on amounts that can be added to food.

MONOTERPENES • Found in parsley, carrots, broccoli, cabbage, cucumbers, squash, yams, tomatoes, eggplant, peppers, mint, basil, citrus fruits, they have some antioxidant properties. Have been found to inhibit cholesterol production and aid protective enzyme activity.

MONOUNSAT FAT • The listing on food labels for monounsaturated fat *(see)*.

MONOUNSATURATED FATS • The saturation of fat refers to the chemical structure of its fatty acids. Saturated fats, which are hard at room temperature—lard, suet, and butter fat are examples—consist primarily of fatty acids that contain a full load of hydrogen atoms. Monounsaturated fatty acids, however, can accept two additional hydrogen atoms. Fats that contain primarily monounsaturated fatty acids are liquid at room temperature but may become thickened when refrigerated. Polyunsaturated fats, which are liquid at room temperature, remain so even in the refrigerator and consist mainly of fatty acids that can hold four or more additional hydrogen atoms. Examples of polyunsaturated fats are safflower and corn oil. Examples of monounsaturated fats are olive oil, rapeseed oil, cashews, and avocados. Once thought to be neutral, monounsaturated fats may be beneficial for blood cholesterol levels. This concept evolved from epidemiological studies of populations who have a diet high in monounsaturated and a lower artery disease rate than populations eating a high saturated fat diet. Some even suggest that monounsaturated fats may be even better than polyunsaturates in preventing heart disease. Monounsaturated fats are manufactured normally by the body and are believed to be less likely to have some of the side effects thought to occur with polyunsaturates.

MORANTEL • Paratect. Suiminth. A worm medicine used to treat cattle that leaves residues in beef and milk. FDA limits residues to from 1.2 ppm to 4.8 ppm in cattle and to 0.4 ppm in milk.

MORELLONE • *See* 3-Benzyl-4-Heptanone.

MORPHOLINE • Salt Fatty Acid. Coating on fresh fruits and vegetables. Broad industrial uses. Used as a surfactant *(see)* and an emulsifier in cosmetics. Prepared by taking the water out of diethanolamine *(see)*. A mobile, water-absorbing liquid that mixes with water, it has a strong ammonia odor. A cheap solvent for resins, waxes, and dyes. Also used as a corrosion inhibitor, antioxidant, plasticizer, viscosity improver, insecticide, fungicide, local anesthetic, and antiseptic. Irritating to the eyes, skin, and mucous membranes. It may cause kidney and liver injury and can produce sloughing of the skin. A strong alkali, corrosive to the skin, irritating to the eyes and mucous membranes. May cause liver and kidney injury. *See* diethanolamine for potential cancer hazard.

MORPHOLINE STEARATE • A coating and preservative. *See* Morpholine.

MOSCHUS MOSCHIFERUS • *See* Musk Tonquin.

MOUNTAIN ASH EXTRACT • The extract from the berries of a European tree or shrub, *Sorbus aucuparia.* High in vitamin C, it has been used by herbalists to cure and prevent scurvy and to treat nausea. Used in cosmetics as an antioxidant. No known toxicity.

MOUNTAIN MAPLE EXTRACT • Extract from a tall shrub or bushy tree found in the eastern United States. Used in chocolate, malt, and maple flavoring for beverages, ice cream, ices, candy, and baked goods.

MOXIDECTIN • Cydectin. Antibacterial used for treatment and control of infections and infestations of certain internal and external parasites. The FDA allows a 0.5 percent solution as a pour-on for beef and nonlactating dairy cattle at 500 micrograms per kilogram of body weight. The ADI *(see)* is 4 mg/kg/day and residue tolerance in cattle is 50 ppb in muscle and 200 ppb in liver.

MSG • *See* Monosodium Glutamate.

MUCILAGE • A solution in water of the sticky principles of vegetable substances. Used as a soothing application to the mucous membranes.

MUCOSA • Mucous membrane lining the digestive tract.

MUCOUS MEMBRANES • The thin layers of tissues that line the respiratory and intestinal tracts and are kept moist by a sticky substance called mucus. These membranes line the nose and other parts of the respiratory tract, and are found in other parts of the body that have communication with air.

MUGWORT • The extract of the flowering herb, *Artemisia absinthium. See* Wormwood and Sesquiterpene Lactones.

MUIRA PUAMA EXTRACT • A wood extract used as an aromatic resin and fat. No known toxicity.

MULBERRY EXTRACT • An extract of the dried leaves of various species of *Morus,* which produces a purplish black dye.

MULLEIN FLOWERS • The flowers from common mullein, *Verbascum thapsis.* Used as a flavoring in alcoholic beverages only and in henna hair coloring. There is no reported use of the chemical and there is no toxicology information available.

MUSHROOM EXTRACT • The extract of various species of mushrooms used as an oil and plasticizer.

MUSK • The dried secretion from preputial follicles of the northern-Asian small hornless deer, which has musk in its glands. Musk is a brown, unctuous, smelly substance associated with attracting the opposite sex and is promoted by stores for such purposes. As *musk ambrette* it is used in fruit, cherry, maple, mint, nut, black walnut, pecan, spice, and vanilla flavorings for beverages, ice cream, ices, candy, baked goods, gelatin desserts, pudding, and chewing gum. Musk ambrette, as a synthetic fixative, is widely used as a fragrance agent in perfumes, soaps, detergents, creams, lotions, and dentifrices in the United States at an estimated 100,000 pounds per year. It reportedly damages the myelin, the covering of nerve fibers. It can cause photosensitivity *(see)* and contact dermatitis. The problem is mostly with aftershave lotions. *(Musk tetralin,* in use for twenty years as a fragrance ingredient, was identified as a neurotoxin and removed from the market in 1978.) Musk ambrette has been generally recognized as safe as a food additive by the FDA. As *musk tonquin* it is used in fruit, maple, and molasses flavorings for beverages, ice cream, ices, candy, baked goods, and syrups. As *musk ketone* it is used in chewing gum and candy. Musk, of course, is also used in perfumery. At one time it was a stimulant and nerve sedative in medicine. Can cause allergic reactions. GRAS.

MUSTARD • Black, Brown, and Red. Pulverized dried, ripe seeds of the mustard plant *(Brassica nigra)* grown in Europe and Asia and naturalized in the U.S. Used in mustard and spice flavorings for condiments (5,200 ppm) and meats (2,300 ppm). Used as an emetic. Has been used as a counterirritant on the skin. Used in soaps, liniments, and lubricants. It has an intensely pungent odor that can be irritating. It is a strong skin blisterer and is used diluted as a counterirritant *(see)* and rubefacient *(see).* Can cause allergic reactions. May cause a sensitivity to light. On the FDA list of products to be studied for possible mutagenic, teratogenic, subacute, and reproductive effects. The final report to the FDA of the Select Committee on GRAS Substances stated in 1980 that it should continue its GRAS status with no limitations other than good manufacturing practices.

MUSTARD • Yellow and White. The pulverized dried, ripe seeds of the mustard plant *(Brassica alba)* grown in Europe and Asia and naturalized in the U.S. Used in sausage and spice flavoring for beverages, baked goods, condiments (8,200 ppm), meats, and pickles (3,800 ppm). Used as an emetic. The final report to the FDA of the Select Committee on GRAS Substances stated in 1980 that it should continue its GRAS status with no limitations other than good manufacturing practices. *See* Mustard, Black, for toxicity.

MUSTARD OIL • *See* Allyl Isothiocyanate.

MUTAGEN • A substance that induces mutation *(see)*.

MUTAGENIC • Having the power to cause mutations. A mutation is a sudden change in the character of a gene that is perpetuated in subsequent divisions of the cells in which it occurs. It can be induced by the application of such stimuli as radiation, certain food chemicals, or pesticides. Certain food additives such as caffeine have been found to "break" chromosomes.

MUTATION • A change in the genetic material of the cell.

MYCLOBUTANIL • A systemic fungicide used on fruits. FDA limits residue to 5 ppm in apple or grape pomace for feed; 10 ppm in grapes and raisins; 25 ppm in raisin waste; 0.05 ppm residue in meat, fat, and meat byproducts of cattle, goats, hogs, poultry, and sheep; 0.3 ppm residue in liver of cattle, goats, hogs, poultry, and sheep; 0.02 ppm in eggs.

MYCOBUTANOL • A fungicide. The FDA allows 5 ppm residue in apples; 10 ppm residues in grapes; 10 ppm residue in raisins; 25 ppm in raisin waste; 0.05 ppm in meat, fat, and meat byproducts of cattle, goats, hogs, poultry, and sheep; and 0.3 ppm residue in liver of cattle, goats, and hogs.

MYRCENE • A synthetic flavoring agent that occurs naturally in galbanum oil, pimenta oil, orange peel, palma rosa oil, and hop oil. Pleasant aroma. Used in fruit, root beer, and coriander flavorings for beverages, ice cream, ices, candy, and baked goods. A moderate skin and eye irritant. Found to cause birth defects in experimental animals.

MYRISTALDEHYDE • A synthetic citrus and fruit flavoring agent for beverages, ice cream, ices, candy, baked goods, and gelatin desserts.

MYRISTIC ACID • Used in shampoos, shaving soaps, and creams. A solid organic acid that occurs naturally in butter acids (such as nutmeg butter to the extent of 80 percent), oil of lovage, coconut oil, mace oil, cire d'abeille in palm seed fats, and in most animal and vegetable fats. Used in butter, butterscotch, chocolate, cocoa, and fruit flavorings for beverages, ice cream, ices, candy, baked goods, and gelatin desserts. A human skin irritant. Causes mutations in laboratory animals.

MYRISTIC FRAGRANS HOUTT • *See* Mace, also Nutmeg.

MYRISTYL ALCOHOL • *See* Fatty Alcohols.

MYRJ 45 (POLYOXYETHYLENE 8-STEARATE) • An emulsifier the use of which is unauthorized in food.

MYROXYLON • *See* Balsam Peru.

MYRRH • Used in perfumes, dentifrices, and skin topics. One of the gifts of the Magi, it is a yellowish to reddish brown, aromatic bitter gum resin that is obtained from various trees, especially from East Africa and Arabia. Used by the ancients as an ingredient of incense and perfumes and as a remedy for localized skin problems. The gum is used in fruit, liquor, tobacco, and smoke flavorings for beverages, baked goods, ice cream, ices, candy, chewing gum, and soups. The oil is used in honey and liquor flavorings for beverages, ice cream, ices, candy, and baked goods. The gum resin has been used to break up intestinal gas and as a topical stimulant.

MYRTLE LEAVES • The extract of the leaves of *Myrtus communis,* a European shrub used in alcoholic beverages only. There is no reported use of the chemical and there is no toxicology information available.

MYRTRIMONIUM BROMIDE • *See* Quaternary Ammonium Compounds.

N

NAPHTHA • Obtained from the distillation of petroleum, coal tar, and shale oil. It is a common diluent *(see)* found in nail lacquer. Naphtha is an imprecise term because various fractions of petroleum may be called that. Among the common naphthas that are used as solvents are coal tar/naphtha and petroleum/naphtha. Naphthas are used as solvents for asphalts, road tars, pitches, paints, dry-cleaning fluids, in cleansing compounds, engraving and lithography, rubber cements, and naphtha soaps. Causes upper respiratory tract irritation. Although allowed as a food additive, there is no current reported use of the chemical, and, therefore, although toxicology information may be available, it is not being updated, according to the FDA.

NAPHTHALENE • A coal tar *(see)* derivative. Used to manufacture dyes, solvents, fungicides, smokeless powder, lubricants, as a moth repellent, and a topical and internal antiseptic. It has been used as a dusting powder to combat insects on animals. Naphthalene can enter your body through inhalation, skin absorption, ingestion, and eye and skin contact. It may produce damage to the eyes, liver, kidneys, skin, red blood cells, and the central nervous system. Has reportedly caused anemia in infants exposed to clothing and blankets stored in naphthalene mothballs. Can cause allergic contact dermatitis in adults and children.

2-NAPHTHALENTHIOL • Derived from naphthalene *(see),* it has a disagreeable odor. It is used in the manufacture of food additives.

NAPHTHYL ANTHRANILATE • A synthetic fruit and grape flavoring agent for beverages, ice cream, ices, baked goods, and candy.

***b*-NAPHTHYL ETHYL ETHER** • White crystals with an orange-blossom odor. Used in perfumes, soaps, and flavoring.

***b*-NAPHTHYL METHYL ETHER** • White crystals with a menthol odor. Used to perfume soaps. A synthetic berry, fruit, honey, and nut flavoring agent for beverages, ice cream, ices, chewing gum, candy, and baked goods.

NARASIN • An antibiotic in broiler chicken feed that is used to combat parasites and as a growth stimulant. It is derived from *Streptomyces aureofaciens. See* Antibiotics.

NARINGIN EXTRACT • Naringin is in the flowers, fruit, and rind of the grapefruit tree. Most abundant in immature fruit. Extracted from grapefruit peel. Used in bitters, grapefruit, and pineapple flavorings for beverages, ice cream, ices, and liquors. GRAS.

NASTURTIUM EXTRACT • The extract of the leaves and stems of *Tropaaeolum majus.* A member of the mustard family, it has pungent and tasty leaves. It is very rich in vitamin A and C as well as containing vitamins B and B_2. It is soothing to the skin and supposedly has blood-thinning factors and increases the flow of urine. No known toxicity.

NATAMYCIN • Pimaricin. Natacyn. Myprozine. A fungicide produced from *Streptomyces natalensis* from soil near Pietermaritzburg, South Africa. It is applied to surface cuts and slices of cheese where standards permit to inhibit mold. FDA residue tolerance is 200 to 300 ppm. A drug used to treat fungal infections of the eye or eyelid in humans. Potential adverse reactions include swelling around the eyes and "black eyes" from blood gathering there. *See* Antibiotics.

NATIONAL HEALTH and NUTRITION EXAMINATION SURVEY (NHANES) • A series of surveys that include information from medical history, physical measurements, biochemical evaluation, physical examination, and dietary intake of population groups within the United States. The U.S. Department of Health and Human Services conducts the NHANES approximately every five years.

NATIONAL TOXICOLOGY PROGRAM (NTP) • Under the aegis of the National Institute of Environmental Health Sciences, the NTP tests chemicals for all federal agencies upon request. The program's staff also tests for cancer-causing agents.

NATURAL • The Federal Trade Commission requires that food advertised as "natural" may not contain synthetic or artificial ingredients and may not be more than minimally processed. For example, minimal processing includes such actions as washing or peeling fruits or vegetables; homogenizing milk; canning, bottling, and freezing food; baking bread; aging and roasting meats; and grinding nuts. It does not include processes that, in general, cannot be done in a home kitchen and involve certain types of chemicals or sophisticated technology; for example, chemically bleached foods will not qualify as minimally processed.

N-BUTANE • *See* Butane.

NDGA • Illegal antioxidant. *See* Nordihydroguaiaretic Acid.

NEO-DHC • *See* Dihydrochalcones.

NEOFOLINONE • Occurs naturally in oil of lavender, orange leaf (absolute), palma rosa oil, rose, neroli, and oil of petitgrain. Used in citrus, honey, and neroli flavorings for beverages, ice cream, ices, candy, baked goods, chewing gum, gelatin desserts, and puddings. No known toxicity.

NEOHESPERIDINE DIHYDROCHALCONE • *See* Dihydrochalcones.

(d)-NEOMENTHOL • A flavoring agent that occurs naturally in Japanese mint oil. Used in mint flavorings for beverages, ice cream, candy, and baked goods. *See* Menthol for toxicity.

NEOMYCIN SULFATE • Biosol Veterinary. Otobiotic. Neomix. Sulfate. Bactine First Aid Antibiotic. Campho-Phenique Triple Antibiotic Ointment. Mycitracin Plus Pain Reliever. Mycifradin. Myciguent. Neosporin Ointment. Neosulf. Introduced in 1951, it is one of the most widely used antibiotics for humans. The oral form is used to treat infectious diarrhea caused by *Escherichia coli (see)*. Among potential adverse reactions: headache, lethargy, ear problems, nausea, vomiting, kidney dysfunction, skin rashes, and hypersensitivity reactions. Interacts with Cephalothin, dimenhydrinate, oral anticoagulants (decreases vitamin K), IV loop diuretics, Cisplatin, methoxyflurane, and other aminoglycoside antibiotics. In animals it is used as an animal drug to treat cattle. FDA residue limitations are 0.25 ppm in calves and 0.15 ppm in milk.

NEQUINATE • An animal drug used to treat chicken. FDA residue limitation is 0.1 ppm in chickens. A coccidiostat *(see)* is added to chicken feed to inhibit or delay the onset of coccidiosis, a common and serious disease of many species that involves intestines and lungs. It has been reported in individuals with AIDS.

NEROL • A primary alcohol used in perfumes, especially in rose and orange blossom scents. Occurs naturally in oil of lavender, orange leaf, palma rosa oil, rose, neroli, and oil of petitgrain. It is colorless, with the odor of rose. Used in citrus, neroli, and honey flavorings for beverages, ice cream, ices, candy, baked goods, gelatin desserts, puddings, and chewing gum. Similar to turpentine in toxicity.

NEROLI BIGARADE OIL • Used chiefly in cologne and in perfumes. Named for the putative discoverer, Anna Mariade la Tremoille, prince of Nerole (1670). A fragrant, pale yellow essential oil obtained from the flowers of the sour orange tree, Citrus aurantium. It darkens upon standing. Used in berry, orange, cola, cherry, spice, and ginger ale flavorings for beverages, ice cream, ices, candy, baked goods, and chewing gum. GRAS.

NEROLIDOL • A sesquiterpene alcohol. A straw-colored liquid with an odor similar to rose and apple. Occurs naturally in balsam Peru and oils of orange flower, neroli, sweet orange, and ylang-ylang. Also made synthetically. Used in perfumery and flavoring. *See* Nerol.

NEROSOL • *See* Nerol.

NERYL ACETATE • A synthetic citrus, fruit, and neroli flavoring for beverages, ice cream, ices, candy, and baked goods.

NERYL BUTYRATE • A synthetic berry, chocolate, cocoa, citrus, and fruit flavoring agent for beverages, ice cream, ices, candy, and baked goods.

NERYL FORMATE • Formic Acid. A synthetic berry, citrus, apple, peach, and pineapple flavoring agent for beverages, ice cream, ices, candy, and baked goods. *See* Formic Acid for toxicity.

NERYL ISOBUTYRATE • A synthetic citrus and fruit flavoring agent for beverages, ice cream, ices, candy, and baked goods.

NERYL ISOVALERATE • A synthetic berry, rose, and nuts flavoring agent for beverages, ice cream, ices, candy, and baked goods.

NERYL PROPIONATE • A synthetic berry and fruit flavoring agent for beverages, ice cream, ices, candy, and baked goods.

NETSON • *See* Acimeton.

NETTLES • A troublesome weed, with stingers, it has a long history and was used in folk medicine. Its flesh is rich is minerals and plant hormones, and it supposedly stimulates hair growth and shines and softens hair. Also used to make tomatoes resistant to spoilage, to encourage the growth of strawberries, and to stimulate the fermentation of humus. Hemp belongs to the nettle family.

NEURAL TUBE DEFECT • In simple terms, a neural tube defect (NTD) is a malformation of the brain or spinal cord (neurological system) during embryonic development. Infants born with spina bifida, where the spinal cord is exposed, can grow to adulthood but usually suffer from paralysis or other disabilities. Babies born with anencephaly, where most or all of the brain is missing, usually die shortly after birth. These NTDs make up about 5 percent of all U.S. birth defects each year. If all women of childbearing age consumed sufficient folic acid (either through diet or supplements), 50 percent to 70 percent of birth defects of the brain and spinal cord could be prevented, according to the U.S. Centers for Disease Control and Prevention. Folic acid is critical in the first four to six weeks of pregnancy when the neural tube is formed. This means adequate diet or supplement use should begin before pregnancy occurs. A leading CDC authority refers to folic acid as "the sleeping giant of preventive medicine" for its potential to eliminate much of the risk of NTDs—if only it were consumed in the right quantities by the right people at the right time.

NEURON • The basic nerve cell of the central nervous system containing a nucleus within the cell body, an axon (a trunklike projection containing neurotransmitters), and dendrites (spiderlike projections that send and receive messages).

NEUROTENSIN • A peptide of thirteen amino acid derivatives that helps to regulate blood sugar by its effects on a number of hormones, including insulin and glucagon. It is also thought to play a part in pain suppression.

NEUROTRANSMITTERS • Molecules that carry chemical messages between nerve cells. Neurotransmitters are released from a nerve cell, diffuse across the minute distance between two nerve cells (synaptic cleft) and bind to a receptor at another nerve site.

NEUTRALIZING AGENT • A substance, such as ammonium bicarbonate or tartaric acid *(see both),* used to adjust the acidity or alkalinity of certain foods. *See* pH.

NHANES • Abbreviation for National Health and Nutrition Examination Survey *(see).*

NIACIN • Nutrient. Nicotinic Acid. Nicotinamide. White or yellow crystalline powder, it is an essential nutrient that participates in many energy-yielding reactions and aids in the maintenance of a normal nervous system. It is a component of the vitamin B complex. Added to prepared breakfast cereals, peanut butter, baby cereals, enriched flours, macaroni, noodles, breads, rolls, cornmeal, corn grits, and farina. Niacin is distributed in significant amounts in liver, yeast, meat, legumes, and whole cereals. Recommended daily intake is 18 to 19 milligrams for men and 13 to 15 milligrams for women. *Nicotinic acid* is a component of the vitamin B complex. The final report to the FDA of the Select Committee on GRAS Substances stated in 1980 that it should continue its GRAS status with no limitations other than good manufacturing practices.

NIACINAMIDE • Nicotinamide. Vitamin B. A dietary supplement. Also used as a skin stimulant. A white or yellow, crystalline, odorless powder used to treat pellagra, a vitamin-deficiency disease, and in the assay of enzymes for substrates. No known skin toxicity. The final report to the FDA of the Select Committee on

GRAS Substances stated in 1980 that it should continue its GRAS status with no limitations other than good manufacturing practices.

NIACINAMIDE ASCORBATE • A complex of ascorbic acid *(see)* and niacinamide *(see)*. Occurs as a yellow powder that is practically odorless but which may gradually darken on exposure to air. Used as a dietary supplement. *See* Niacin.

NICARBAZIN • Nicoxin. Nicrazin. An animal drug used in chicken feed to inhibit or delay coccidiosis *(see)*. FDA residue limitations are 4 ppm in uncooked muscle, liver, skin, and neck of chickens.

NICKEL • Metal that occurs in the earth. Lustrous, white, hard metal that is used as a catalyst for the hydrogenation *(see)* of fat. Nickel may cause dermatitis in sensitive individuals and ingestion of large amounts of the soluble salts may cause nausea, vomiting, and diarrhea. The final report to the FDA of the Select Committee on GRAS Substances stated in 1980 that it should continue its GRAS status with no limitations other than good manufacturing practices.

NICKEL SULFATE • Occurs in the earth's crust as a salt of nickel. Obtained as green or blue crystals and is used chiefly in nickel plating. Used in hair dyes and astringents. It has a sweet astringent taste. Used as a mineral supplement up to 1 milligram per day. It acts as an irritant and causes vomiting when swallowed. Its systemic effects include blood vessel, brain, and kidney damage, and nervous depression. Frequently causes skin rash when used in cosmetics. The lethal dose varies widely. The dose in guinea pigs is 62 milligrams per kilogram.

NICOTINAMIDE • *See* Niacin.

NICOTINAMIDE–ASCORBIC ACID COMPLEX • A dietary supplement in multivitamin preparations.

NICOTINIC ACID • *See* Niacin.

NIGER GUTTA • *Ficus platyphylla del.* The coagulated latex from a tree that is mixed with chicle *(see)* to make chewing gum.

NIOSH • Abbreviation for National Institute of Occupational Safety and Health. Congress set up this institute in 1970 to play a key role in helping to protect workers and their health on the job. The agency was to conduct occupational-health research; to inspect manufacturers' plants at employers' and workers' requests, and for its own studies; and to recommend standards for safe exposure to hazardous substances. NIOSH is supposed to work closely with OSHA *(see)*, the organization responsible for setting the legally permitted exposures to hazards in the workplace. NIOSH, through its investigations into plant conditions and studies of already available data, provides OSHA with the scientific background needed to determine these rules. When a workplace crisis arises, the two agencies often work in tandem to find out how the workers were harmed and to help the industry correct the problem. Under the law, NIOSH documents summarizing its findings about a hazard should be used by OSHA to help in setting health and safety regulations for the industry.

NISIN PREPARATION • Crystals from *Streptococcus lactis* used as a preservative and antimicrobial agent in cheese spreads. FDA limits residue to 250 ppm in the finished product. It is also used in canned vegetables and fruit. GRAS.

NITAPYRIN • An insecticide. The FDA limits residues in cottonseed to 1.0 ppm; in the fat, meat, and meat byproducts of cattle, goats, hogs, poultry, and sheep to 0.05 ppm.

NITARSONE • A feed additive of which 0.5 ppm is arsenic *(see)* as a residue in muscle meat and eggs of chicken.

NITER • *See* Nitrate.

NITRATE • Potassium and Sodium. *Potassium nitrate,* also known as saltpeter and niter, is used as a color fixative in cured meats. *Sodium nitrate,* also called Chile saltpeter, is used as a color fixative in cured meats. Both nitrates are used in matches and to improve the burning properties of tobacco. They combine with natural stomach saliva and food substances (secondary amines) to create nitrosamines, powerful cancer-causing agents. Nitrosamines have also been found in fish treated with nitrates. Researchers at Michael Reese Medical Center's Department of Pathology in Chicago induced cancer in mice by giving single doses of one three-thousandth (0.3 microgram) of a gram of nitrosamine for each gram of the animal's weight. This is in contrast to the way other researchers have induced cancer in laboratory animals with nitrosamines by using repeated small doses or single large doses. The tumors that developed were analogous to human liver tumors. Nitrosamines caused pancreatic cancer in hamsters, similar to human pancreatic cancers. Nitrates have caused deaths from methemoglobinemia (it cuts off oxygen to the brain). Because nitrates are difficult to control in processing, they are being used less often. However, they are still employed in long curing processes, such as for country hams, as well as dried, cured, and fermented sausages. In the early seventies, baby-food manufacturers voluntarily removed nitrates from their products. The U.S. Department of Agriculture, which has jurisdiction over meats, and the FDA, which has jurisdiction over processed poultry, has asked manufacturers to show that the use of nitrates is safe. Efforts to ban nitrates have failed because manufacturers claim there is no good substitute for them.

Nitrates change into nitrites on exposure to air. Our major intake of nitrates in foodstuffs comes primarily from vegetables or water supplies that are high in nitrate content, or from nitrates used as additives in meat curing. Nitrates are natural constituents of plants. They occur in very small amounts in fruits but are high in certain vegetables—spinach, beets, radishes, eggplant, celery, lettuce, collards, and turnip greens—as high as more than 3,000 ppm. The two most important factors responsible for large accumulations of nitrates in vegetables are the high levels of fertilization with nitrate fertilizers and the tendency of the species to accumulate nitrate.

NITRITE • Potassium and Sodium. *Potassium nitrite* is used as a color fixative in the more than $125 billion a year cured-meat business. *Sodium nitrite* has the peculiar ability to react chemically with the myoglobin molecule and impart red-bloodedness to processed meats, to convey tanginess to the palate, and to resist the growth of *Clostridium botulinum* spores. It is used as a color fixative in cured meats, bacon, bologna, frankfurters, deviled ham, meat spread, potted meats, spiced ham, Vienna sausages, smoke-cured tuna fish products, and in smoke-cured shad and salmon. Nitrite combines with natural stomach and food chemicals (secondary amines) to create nitrosamines, powerful cancer-causing agents. The U.S. Department of Agriculture, which has jurisdiction over processed meats, and the FDA, which has jurisdiction over processed poultry, asked manufacturers to show that the use of nitrites was safe and that nitrosamines were not formed in the products as preliminary tests showed in bacon. Processors claimed there was no alternate chemical substitute for nitrite. They said alternate processing methods could be used, but the products would not look or taste the same. Baby-food manufacturers voluntarily removed nitrites from baby foods in the early seventies. The FDA found that adding vitamin C to processed meats prevents or at least retards the formation of nitrosamines. In May 1978, the USDA announced plants to require bacon manufacturers to reduce their use of nitrite from 150 to 120 ppm and to use preservatives that retard nitrosamine formation. Processors would have been required to keep nitrosamine levels to 10 ppm under the interim plan.

But in August 1978 a new concern about nitrite was raised. The USDA and the FDA issued a joint announcement that the substance has been directly linked to cancer by a Massachusetts Institute of Technology study. That work was later disputed. In 1982, amyl and butyl nitrites used by homosexual men were linked to Kaposi's sarcoma and other abnormalities of the immune system.

Researchers at Michael Reese Medical Center linked infinitesimal amounts of nitrite to cancer in young laboratory mice, especially in the liver and lungs. Dr. Koshlya Rijhsinghani and her colleagues gave single doses of one three-thousandth (0.3 microgram) of a gram of nitrosamine for each gram of the animal's weight. This method differs from the way other researchers have induced cancer in mice with nitrosamines by repeated small doses of single large doses. Nitrosamines also produce cancer in hamsters similar to pancreatic cancers in humans.

In 1980, the FDA revoked its proposed phase-out because manufacturers said there was no adequate substitute for nitrites. In 1977 Germany banned nitrites and nitrates except in certain species of fish. However, a Committee on Nitrite and Alternative Curing Agents in Food, formed by the National Research Council in the United States, concluded that there was no single agent or process that could replace nitrite completely: "Several chemical and physical treatments appear to be comparable in inhibiting outgrowth of *Clostridium botulinum* spores in types of meat products but none confers the color and flavor that consumers have come to expect in nitrite-cured meats." Until the all-purpose agent comes along or until consumer preference changes, the best compromise probably will be continued use of nitrite in conventional amounts with vitamins C and E added to block formation of nitrosamines, or the use of smaller amounts of nitrite in combination with biological acidification, irradiation, or the chemicals potassium sorbate, sodium hypophosphite, or fumarate esters, the Committee said.

To reduce nitrosamines in bacon, the U.S. Department of Agriculture requires meat packers to add sodium ascorbate or sodium erythorbate (vitamin C) to the curing brine. This offers only a partial barrier because ascorbate is soluble in water and its activity in fat is limited. Vitamin E, however, inhibits nitrosation in fatty tissues. The Committee suggested that both C and E be added to provide more complete protection. If you must eat nitrite-laced meats, include a food or drink high in Vitamin C at the same time—for example, orange juice, grapefruit juice, cranberry juice or lettuce.

NITRO • A prefix denoting one atom of nitrogen and two of oxygen. *Nitro* also denotes a class of dyes derived from coal tars. Nitro dyes can be absorbed through the skin. When absorbed or ingested they can cause a lack of oxygen in the blood. Chronic exposure may cause liver damage. *See* FD and C Colors.

NITROCELLULOSE • Any of several esters *(see)* obtained as white fibrous flammable solids by adding nitrate to cellulose, the cell walls of plants. Used in food processing and in skin protective creams, nail enamels, and lacquers. No known toxicity.

NITROFURAZONE • Aldomycin. Furacillin. Coxistat. Nitrofurazone. A once widely used antibiotic in animal feed for pigs and poultry. FDA withdrew permission for its use in 1991. A human sensitizer. IARC review and EPA Genetic Toxicology Program *(see both)*. Potential adverse reactions include kidney toxicity, redness, itching, burning, water retention, severe blistering, and allergic skin rash.

3-([5-NITROFURFURYLIDENE] AMINO)2-OXAZOLIDONE • Bifuron. Corizium. Diafuron. Enterotoxon. Furazone. Furazolidone. Furoxone. A widely used antiprotozoal *(see)* drug in animals, particularly for pigs. It is also a human medication for diarrhea and enteritis caused by *Giardia lamblia* and *Vibrio cholerae.* Taken by mouth, it works inside the intestines to counteract cholera, colitis, and/or diarrhea caused by the bacteria. Potential adverse reactions include joint pain, fever, itching, skin rash or redness, nausea, vomiting, diarrhea, stomach pain, headache, and sore throat. Severe high blood pressure and other side effects may occur if combined with MAO inhibitors *(see),* ephedrine, and tricyclic antidepressants with this drug. Severe high blood pressure and other undesirable side effects may occur if the following are eaten or drunk while taking this drug: aged cheese, caviar, yeast or protein extracts, fava or broad beans; smoked or pickled meat, poultry, or fish; fermented sausages (bologna, pepperoni, salami, summer sausage) or other fermented meat; or any overripe fruit. You should not drink dark beer, red wine, sherry, or liqueurs. If the human medication is taken, the above foods and drinks are to be avoided for at least two weeks after stopping furazolidone. The FDA says that residues must be zero in meat sent to market, but who can do adequate testing for its presence all the time?

NITROGEN • A gas that is 78 percent by volume of the atmosphere and essential to all living things. Odorless. Used as a preservative for cosmetics, in which it is nontoxic. In high concentrations, it can asphyxiate. Toxic concentration in humans is 90 ppm; in mice, 250 ppm. GRAS.

NITROGEN OXIDES • Nitrous Oxide *(see),* Nitric Oxide, Nitrogen Dioxide, Nitrogen Trioxide, Nitrogen Pentoxide. Bleaching agent for cereal flour, *nitrogen dioxide* is a deadly poison gas. Short exposure may cause little pain or discomfort but several days later, fluid retention and inflammation of the lungs can cause death. About 200 ppm can be fatal. There is no reported use of the chemical and there is not toxicology information available, according to the FDA.

3-NITRO-4-HYDROXYPHENYLARSONIC ACID • Roxarsone. Tufts of pale yellow needles used to control intestinal infections and to improve growth and feed efficiency. FDA limits are 0.5 ppm as arsenic in muscle meat and eggs of chickens as residue; 2 ppm as arsenic in edible byproducts, turkey, and swine; 0.5 ppm as arsenic in muscle tissue and byproducts other than liver and kidney. *See* Arsenic.

NITROMIDE with SULFANITRAN • A feed additive used in chicken feed. Both ingredients are antibacterials. FDA tolerance is zero residue for nitromide in uncooked edible chicken.

4-NITROPHENYLARSONIC ACID • Nitarsone. An animal feed drug used to combat intestinal parasites chiefly affecting turkeys, chickens, and other birds. FDA says the feed additive is not to be used as level in excess of the amount reasonably required to accomplish the intended effect. An arsenic compound, it is on the Community Right-To-Know List *(see)*. Poison by ingestion.

NITROSYL CHLORIDE • Nonexplosive, very corrosive, reddish yellow gas, intensely irritating to the eyes, skin, and mucosa. Used as a bleaching agent for cereal flour. Inhalation may cause pulmonary edema and hemorrhage.

NITROUS OXIDE • Laughing Gas. A whipping agent for whipped cosmetic creams and a propellant in pressurized cosmetic containers. Slightly sweetish odor and taste. Colorless. Used in rocket fuel. Less irritating than other nitrogen oxides but narcotic in high concentrations and it can asphyxiate. GRAS.

NOAEL • No Observed Adverse Effect Level. *See* NOEL.

NOBELITIN • A substance found in citrus fruit that has been found to have anti-cancer properties in laboratory studies.

NOEL • Test results that show a given dose of a substance has a No Observed Effect Level or sometimes called a No Observed Adverse Effect Level. The safety factor usually has a value of one hundred in the case of a NOEL derived from long-term animal study, on the assumption that humans are ten times as sensitive as the test animal used and that there is a ten-fold range of sensitivity within the human population.

NONADIENAL • Cucumber Aldehyde or Alcohol. A flavoring agent used in various foods. A moderate skin irritant.

***g*-NONALACTONE** • Aldehyde C-18. Prunolide. Coconut Aldehyde. A synthetic berry, coconut, fruit, and nut flavoring agent for beverages, ice cream, ices, candy, baked goods, gelatin desserts, chewing gum, and icings.

NONALOL • *See* Nonyl Alcohol.

NONANAL • Pelargonic Aldehyde. Colorless liquid with an orange-rose odor. A synthetic flavoring that occurs naturally in lemon oil, rose, sweet orange oil, mandarin, lime, orris, and ginger. Used in lemon and fruit flavorings for beverages, ice cream, ices, candy, baked goods, chewing gum, and gelatin desserts. Used also in perfumery. A severe skin irritant. *See* Aldehyde.

1,3-NONANEDIOL ACETATE • Colorless to slightly yellow mixture of isomers used in synthetic berry and fruit flavoring for beverages, ice cream, ices, candy, and baked goods. No known toxicity. *See* Nonanoic Acid and Acetic Acid.

NONANNOYL 4-HYDROXY-3-METHOXY BENZYLAMIDE • Perlargonyl Vanillylamide. A synthetic spice flavoring agent for candy, baked goods, and condiments.

NONANOIC ACID • Pelargonic Acid. Nonoic acid. Nonglic Acid. A colorless, oily liquid that is insoluble in water, it occurs in the oil of pelargonium plants such as the geranium. Used in berry, fruit, nut, and spice flavorings for beverages, ice cream, ices, candy, baked goods, and shortenings. It is practically insoluble in water and is used in producing salts and in the manufacture of lacquers. Can be very irritating to the skin.

2-NONANOL • *See* Nonyl Alcohol.

3-NONANON-1-YL-ACETATE • A synthetic berry, rose, fruit, and cheese flavoring agent for beverages, ice cream, ices, candy, and baked goods. Although allowed as a food additive, there is no current reported use of the chemical, and, therefore, although toxicology information may be available, the FDA is not updating it.

2-NONENAL • *See* Isoamyl Nonanoate.

NONFAT DRY MILK • The solid residue produced by removing the water from defatted cow's milk. Comparisons between whole and dry milk: 100 grams fluid whole milk contains 68 calories; 87 grams of water; 3.5 grams of protein; 3.9 grams of fat; 0.7 gram of ash; 4.9 grams of carbohydrates; 118 milligrams of calcium; 93 milligrams of phosphorus; 0.1 milligram of iron; 50 milligrams of sodium; 140 milligrams of potassium; 160 international units of vitamin A; 0.04 milligram of vitamin B_1; 0.17 milligram of B_2; 0.1 milligram of nicotinic acid; and 1 milligram of vitamin C. Total calories for one cup of milk is 166. Nonfat dry milk has 362 calories per 100 grams; 3.5 grams of water; 35.6 grams of protein; 1 gram of fat; 7.9 grams of ash; 52 grams of total carbohydrates; 1,300 milligrams of calcium; 1,030 milligrams of phosphorus; 0.6 milligrams of iron; 77 milligrams of sodium; 1,130 milligrams of potassium; 40 international units of vitamin A; 0.35 milligrams of vitamin B_1; 196 milligrams of vitamin B_2; 1.1 milligrams of nicotinic acid; and 7 milligrams of vitamin C. The total calories for a tablespoon of dry nonfat milk is 28. *See* Milk.

NONNUTRITIVE SWEETENERS • Sugar substitutes that contain no calories. Saccharin and cyclamates *(see both)* are examples.

NONYL ACETATE • An ester produced by the reaction of nonyl alcohol and acetic acid *(see)*. Pungent odor suggestive of mushrooms but when diluted it resembles the odor of gardenias. Insoluble in water. Used for beverages, ice cream, ices, candy, and baked goods.

NONYL ALCOHOL • Nonalol. A synthetic flavoring, colorless to yellow with a citronella oil odor. Occurs in oil of orange. Used in butter, citrus, peach, and pineapple flavorings for beverages, ice cream, ices, candy, and chewing gum. Also used in the manufacture of artificial lemon oil. In experimental animals it has caused central nervous system and liver damage.

NONYL CARBINOL • *See* 1-Decanol.

NONYL ISOVALERATE • A synthetic fruit and hazel nut flavoring agent for beverages, ice cream, ices, candy, and baked goods.

γ-NONYL LACTONE • Yellowish to almost colorless liquid with a coconutlike odor. Used in perfumery and flavors. *See* Nonyl Alcohol.

NONYL NONANOATE • Nonyl Pelargonate. Liquid with a floral odor used in flavors, perfumes, and organic synthesis. *See* Nonyl Alcohol.

NOOTKATONE • From a cypress tree grown in northwest Washington State and British Columbia. It is named after the Nootka people who populated the area. It smells like cedar. It is used in flavorings and perfumes.

NOPINENE • *See b*-Pinene.

NORBIXIN • From the seeds of Bixa zorellana used in a suspension of vegetable oil for coloring in food. *See* Annatto.

NORDIHYDROGUAIARETIC ACID (NDGA) • An antioxidant used in brilliantines and other fat-based cosmetics. Occurs in resinous exudates of many plants. White or grayish white crystals. Lard containing 0.01 percent NGDA stored at room temperature for nineteen months in diffuse daylight showed no appreciable rancidity or color change. It was used as an antioxidant in prepared pie-crust mix, candy, lard, butter, ice cream, and pressure-dispensed whipped cream. Canada banned the additive in food in 1967 after it was shown to cause cysts and kidney damage in a large percentage of rats tested. The FDA removed it from the GRAS list in 1968 and prohibited its use in products over which it has control. The U.S. Department of Agriculture, which controls antioxidants in lard and animal shortenings, banned it in 1971.

NOREPINEPHRINE • Noradrenaline. A hormone released by the adrenal gland, it possesses the ability to stimulate that epinephrine but has minimal inhibitory effects. It has little effect on the lungs' smooth muscles and metabolic processes and differs from epinephrine in its effect on the heart and blood vessels.

NORFLURAZON • A herbicide used in feed and hops used for animal feed. FDA tolerance limits are 1 ppm in dried citrus molasses, 3 ppm in citrus pulp, and 0.1 ppm in milk, fat, meat, and meat byproducts of cattle, goats, hogs, poultry, and sheep.

NORVALINE • A protein amino acid *(see)* soluble in hot water and insoluble in alcohol. *See* Valeric Acid.

NOTE • A distinct odor or flavor. *Top* note is the first note normally perceived when a flavor is smelled or tasted; usually volatile and gives "identity." *Middle* or *main* note is the substance of the flavor, the main characteristic. *Bottom* note is what is left when top and middle notes disappear. It is the residue when the aroma or flavoring evaporates.

NOVATONE • *See* Acetanisole.

NOVOBIOCIN • Albamycin. An antibiotic from *Streptomyces niveus,* it is used in animal feed for beef, chicken, duck, and turkey. FDA residue limitations are 0.1 in milk, 1 ppm in cattle, chickens, turkeys, and ducks. Moderately toxic by ingestion.

NTP • Abbreviation for National Toxicology Program *(see)*.

NUCLEIC ACIDS • Originally isolated from the cell nuclei, they are carriers and mediators of genetic information. There are two types, DNA (deoxyribonucleic acid) and RNA (ribonucleic acid). DNA has one less oxygen molecule in its component sugar ribose and is double-stranded. The messages carried by DNA are carried out by RNA. The two types are components of all cells so that any food in which cells are concentrated are rich sources of nucleic acids. Organ meats, poultry, and fish are examples. Butter, fat, fruits, milk, nuts, vegetables, and carbohydrates are low in nucleic acids. *See* Purines, disodium guanylate, and disodium inosinate.

NUTMEG • A natural flavoring extracted from the dried ripe seed of *Myristica fragrans houtt.* Used in cola, vermouth, sausage, eggnog, and nutmeg flavorings for beverages, ice cream, ices, baked goods (2,000 ppm), condiments, meats, and pickles. The oil is used in loganberry, chocolate, lemon, cola, apple, grape, muscatel, rum, sausage, eggnog, pistachio, root beer, cinnamon, dill, ginger, mace, nutmeg, and vanilla flavorings for beverages, ice cream, ices, candy, baked goods, chewing gum, condiments, meats, syrups, and icings. In common household use since the Middle Ages, nutmeg is still a potentially toxic substance. Ingestion of as little as 3 whole seeds or 5 to 15 grams of grated spice can cause flushing of the skin, irregular heart rhythm, absence of salivation, and central nervous system excitation, including euphoria and hallucinations. GRAS.

NUTRACEUTICALS • One term used to describe substances in or parts of a food that may be considered to provide medical or health benefits beyond basic nutrition, including disease prevention. *See also* Functional Foods.

NUTRASWEET • *See* Aspartame.

NUTRIENT CONTENT CLAIM • Descriptor. A claim on a food product that directly or by implication characterizes the level of a nutrient in the food such as "low fat" or "high in oat bran." Nutrient content claims are also known as descriptors.

NYSTATIN • Mycostatin. Nadostine. Nilstat. Nystex. O-V Statin. Yellow to light tan powder with a cereal-like odor, it is used in animal feed for poultry and pigs. FDA requires zero residue in eggs, swine, and poultry. Antifungal medication introduced in 1954. It is used in human medicine to treat oral, vaginal, and intestinal infections caused by *Candida albicans* (Moniliales) and other *Candida* species. In cream or ointment it is used to treat infant eczema, itching around the anus or vagina, and localized forms of candidiasis. Potential adverse reactions include nausea, vomiting, and diarrhea. Skin applications may cause occasional contact dermatitis from preservatives in some formulations. Nystatin is in the EPA Genetic Toxicology Program. Moderately toxic by ingestion. Causes birth defects in experimental animals.

O

OAK BARK EXTRACT • Oak Chip Extract. The extract from the white oak used in bitters and whiskey flavorings for beverages, ice cream, ices, candy, whiskey (1,000 ppm), and baked goods. Contains tannic acid *(see)* and is exceedingly astringent. The Indians used it in a wash for sore eyes and as a tonic. Used in astringents in herbal cosmetics.

OAKMOSS, ABSOLUTE • Any one of several lichens, *Evernia* spp., that grow on oak trees and yield a resin for use as a fixative *(see)* in perfumery. Stable green liquid with a long-lasting characteristic odor. Soluble in alcohol. Used in fruit, honey, and spice flavorings for beverages, ice cream, ices, candy, baked goods, gelatin desserts, condiments, and soups. A common allergen in aftershave lotions.

OAK WHITE, CHIPS EXTRACT • *See* Oak Bark Extract.

OAK WOOD, ENGLISH • *Quercus robur.* Used as a coloring in alcoholic beverages only.

OATS • Whole grain oats contain more soluble fiber than other whole grains such as wheat, corn, or rye. They contain more protein and lipids than other grains. Oats contain naturally occurring phytochemicals that have been associated with protection from a variety of chronic diseases. Whole grains contain naturally occurring phytoestrogens, which have been linked to decreased risk of hormone-related diseases such as breast cancer. Oats were discovered to lower cholesterol in 1963. They are also a good source of selenium, iron, calcium, manganese, magnesium, zinc, and copper. Cheerios, a breakfast cereal, has been permitted to make the claim that they help to reduce cholesterol by the American Heart Association and the FDA. Presumably, other oat cereals will also be able to make the claim.

OAT BRAN • The broken coat of oats, *Avena sativa. See* Oats and Oat Flour.

OAT EXTRACT • The extract of the seeds of oats, *Avena sativa. See* Oat Flour.

OAT FLOUR • Flour from the cereal grain that is an important crop grown in the temperate regions. Light yellowish or brown to weak greenish or yellow powder. Slight odor; starchy taste. Makes a bland ointment for cosmetic treatments, including soothing baths. No known toxicity.

OAT GUM • A plant extract used as a thickener and stabilizer in foods and cosmetics. Also an antioxidant in butter, creams, and candy up to 1.5 percent. It is used as a thickener and stabilizer in pasteurized cheese spread and cream cheese. In foods, it can cause an allergic reaction including diarrhea and intestinal gas.

OATMEAL • Meal obtained by grinding of oats from which the husks have been removed.

OBESITY or OVERWEIGHT • Although precise definitions vary among experts, overweight has been traditionally defined as 10 to 20 percent above an optimal weight for height, derived from statistics. Some scientists argue that the amount and distribution of an individual's body fat is a significant indicator of health risk and therefore should be considered in defining overweight. Abdominal fat has been linked to more adverse health consequences than fat in the hips or thighs. Thus, calculations of waist-to-hip ratio are preferred by some health experts to help determine if an individual is overweight.

OCIMENE • A terpene obtained from sweet basil oil. Used in flavors and perfumes.

OCIMUM BASILICUM • *See* Basil Extract.

OCOTEA CYMBA RUM OIL • An oil obtained by steam distillation from the wood of a Brazilian tree. Used chiefly as a source of safrole *(see),* a natural oil, and as a substitute for sassafras *(see).* No known toxicity.

OCTADECANOIC ACID • Abracol S.L.G. Dermagine. Distearin. Orbon. Stearic

Acid, Monoester with Glycerol. Pure white or cream-colored, waxlike solid used as a coating agent, emulsifier, lubricant, solvent, and texturizer in baked goods, shortening, fruits, ice cream, nuts, peanut butter, puddings, and whipped toppings. *See* Stearic Acid.

9-OCTADECENOIC ACID • *See* Oleic Acid.

1-OCTADECANOL • *See* Stearic Acid.

OCTAFLUOROCYCLOBUTANE • A nonflammable gas. A refrigerant, propellant, and aerating agent in foamed or sprayed food products. Used alone or in combination with carbon dioxide or nitrous oxide *(see both)*. Nontoxic when used alone.

OCTAHYDROCOUMARIN • One of the newer flavoring agents. *See* Coumarin.

OCTALACTONE • D and G. *See* Lactic Acid.

OCTANAL • Octanaldehyde. Found in many essential oils *(see)* including a number of citrus oils, it is a colorless to light yellow liquid with an orange odor. It is used as a flavoring agent in many foods. Mildly toxic by ingestion.

OCTANOIC ACID • Colorless, oily liquid with a bad odor derived from coconut, it is used as an antimicrobial agent in other food additives and as a defoaming agent, flavoring agent, and lubricant. It is used in baked goods, soft candies, cheese, fats, frozen dairy desserts, gelatins, meat products, oils, packaging materials, puddings, and snack foods. Mildly toxic by ingestion and a skin irritant, it has caused mutations in experimental animals. FDA residue limits are 0.0013 percent in baked goods; 0.04 percent in frozen dairy desserts; 0.005 percent in meat products; 0.005 percent in soft candies; 0.016 percent in snack foods; and 0.001 percent in other food categories when used in accordance with good manufacturing practices. GRAS as an indirect additive.

N-OCTANOIC (CAPRYLIC) ACID • Preservative and other miscellaneous uses. Can be up to 0.013 percent baked products; 0.04 percent cheeses; 0.005 percent fats and oils; 0.016 percent snack foods; 0.001 percent all other food categories. Used in a lye peeling solution for fruits and vegetables and is a component of sanitizing solution. GRAS in cheese wraps. *See* Caprylic Acid.

1-OCTANOL • Caprylic Alcohol. Used in the manufacture of flavorings and perfumes. Colorless, viscous liquid, soluble in water, insoluble in oil. Occurs naturally in oil of lavender, oil of lemon, oil of lime, oil of lovage, orange peel, and coconut oil. It has a penetrating, aromatic scent. May cause skin rash.

3-OCTANOL • Colorless liquid with a strong nutty odor; used as a flavoring agent in various foods. It is a moderate skin and eye irritant.

2-OCTANONE • A synthetic fruit and cheese flavoring agent for beverages, ice cream, ices, candy, and baked goods.

3-OCTANONE • A synthetic flavoring that occurs naturally in oil of lavender. Used in citrus, coffee, peach, cheese, and spice flavorings for beverages, ice cream, ices, candy, and baked goods. No known toxicity.

1-OCTEN-3-OL • A synthetic fruit and spice flavoring agent for beverages, ice cream, ices, candy, baked goods, condiments, and soups.

1-OCTENYL SUCCINIC ANHYDRIDE • A starch modifier incorporating up to

3 percent of the weight of the product. Limited to 2 percent in combination with aluminum sulfate *(see)*.

OCTODECANOIC ACID • *See* Stearic Acid.

OCTOXYNOL • Waxlike emulsifiers, dispersing agents, and detergents derived from phenol *(see)* and used as a surfactant. The numbers from −1 to −70 after the additive signify the viscosity.

OCTYL ACETATE • Acetic Acid. Octyl Ester. A colorless liquid with an orange-jasmine scent, it is used as a flavoring agent in various foods. Moderately toxic by ingestion.

OCTYL ALCOHOL, SYNTHETIC • Caprylic Alcohol. Colorless, viscous liquid soluble in water and insoluble in oil. Used as a solvent in the manufacture of perfumes and of food additives. Occurs naturally in the oils of lavender, lemon, lime, lovage, orange peel, and coconut. It has a penetrating aromatic scent. Moderately toxic by ingestion. A skin irritant. Has caused mutations in experimental animals.

***n*-OCTYL BICYCLOHEPTENE DI CARBOXIMIDE** • Dimethyl Carbate. Pyrodone. Octacide 264. A widely used insecticide in various foods. FDA residue tolerance is 10 ppm. Moderately toxic by ingestion and skin contact. Has caused adverse reproductive effects in experimental animals. Large doses can cause central nervous system stimulation followed by depression.

OCTYL BUTYRATE • Butyric Acid. A synthetic strawberry, butter, citrus, fruit, cherry, melon, peach, pineapple, pumpkin, and liquor flavoring agent for beverages, ice cream, ices, candy, and baked goods.

OCTYL FORMATE • Formic Acid. A synthetic flavoring, colorless with a fruity odor. Used in citrus and fruit flavorings for beverages, ice cream, ices, candy, and baked goods. *See* Formic Acid for toxicity.

OCTYL GALLATE • A salt of gallic acid made from the tannins of nutgalls or from the *Penicilliun glaucum* or *Aspergillus niger,* it is used as an antioxidant in margarine with a limit of 0.02 percent set by the FDA. Mildly toxic by ingestion. When heated to decomposition emits acrid smoke and irritating fumes. *See* Gallates.

OCTYL HEPTANOATE • A synthetic citrus, coconut, and fruit flavoring for beverages, ice cream, ices, candy, and baked goods.

OCTYL ISOBUTYRATE • Isobutyric Acid. A synthetic citrus, fruit, melon peach, liquor, and wine flavoring agent for beverages, ice cream, ices, candy, and baked goods.

OCTYL ISOVALERATE • Isovaleric Acid. A synthetic berry, butter, citrus, apple, cherry, grape, honey, and nut flavoring agent for beverages, ice cream, ices, candy, and baked goods.

OCTYL OCTANOATE • Octanoic Acid. A synthetic citrus, grape, and pineapple flavoring agent for beverages, ice cream, ices, candy, and baked goods.

OCTYL PHENYLACETATE • Phenylacetic Acid. A synthetic berry, apple, banana, grape, peach, pear, and honey flavoring agent for beverages, ice cream, ices, candy, and baked goods.

OCTYL PROPIONATE • Propionic Acid. A synthetic berry, citrus, and melon flavoring agent for beverages, ice cream, ices, candy, and baked goods.

1-OCTYL SUCCINIC ANHYDRIDE • Modifier for food starch. *See* Modified Starch.

ODORLESS LIGHT PETROLEUM HYDROCARBONS • Liquids with a faint odor used as coating agents, defoamers, and in insecticide formulations for beet sugar, eggs, fruits, pickles, vegetables, vinegar, and wine. *See* Petroleum.

OIL OF NIOBE • *See* Methyl Benzoate.

OIL OF SASSAFRAS • Used in dentifrices, perfumes, and soaps to correct disagreeable odors. It is 80 percent safrole. May produce allergic reactions in sensitive persons. It is illegal for use in foods.

OIL OF SASSAFRAS, SAFROLE FREE • This flavoring agent without the safrole is permitted in foods.

OLEAMIDE • An agent that prevents sticking to pans. *See* Oleic Acid.

OLEANDOMYCIN HYDROCHLORIDE • An antibiotic produced by *Streptomyces antibioticus* used in animal feed for chickens, swine, and turkeys. Moderately toxic by ingestion. FDA requires zero residue in chickens, turkeys, and swine for market.

OLEIC ACID • Obtained from various animal and vegetable fats and oils. Colorless. On exposure to air, it turns a yellow to brown color and develops a rancid odor. Used as a defoaming agent; as a synthetic butter, cheese, and spice flavoring agent for beverages, ice cream, ices, candy, and baked goods, and condiments; as a lubricant and binder in various foods; and as a component in the manufacture of food additives. Used in preparations of soft soap, permanent wave solutions, vanishing creams, brushless shave creams, cold creams, brilliantines, nail polish, toilet soaps, and lipsticks. Possesses better skin-penetrating properties than vegetable oils. Also employed in liquid makeup, liquid lip rouge, shampoos, and preshave lotions. Low oral toxicity but is mildly irritating to the skin. It caused tumors when injected under the skin of rabbits in 3,120-milligram doses per kilogram of body weight and when painted on the skin of mice in 62-milligram doses per kilogram of body weight. The final report to the FDA of the Select Committee on GRAS Substances stated in 1980 that it should continue its GRAS status with no limitations other than good manufacturing practices. The final report of the Committee also said that oleic acid should continue its GRAS status for packaging with no limitations other than good manufacturing practices.

OLEIC ACID DERIVED FROM TALL OIL FATTY ACIDS • Used as a component in the manufacture of food-grade additives on fresh citrus fruit and in processing beet sugar and yeast. *See* Oleic Acid and Tall Oil.

OLEINIC ACID • *See* Oleic Acid.

OLEORESIN • A natural plant product consisting of essential oil and resin extracted from a substance, such as ginger, by means of alcohol, ether, or acetone. The solvent alcohol, for example, is percolated through the ginger. Although the oleoresin is very similar to the spice from which it is derived, it is not identical because not all the substances in the spice are extracted. Oleoresins are usually more uniform and more potent than the original product. The normal use range of an oleoresin is from one-fifth to one-twentieth the corresponding amount for the crude spice. Certain spices are extracted as oleoresins for color rather than for flavor. Examples of color-intensifying oleoresins are those from paprika and turmeric *(see both)*.

OLESTRA • Sucrose Polyester. Olean. A fat substitute developed by Procter and Gamble that cannot be digested. It has no calories. It is aimed at replacing conventional fats in french fries and baked desserts. It is a mixture of esters *(see)* of sucrose *(see)* prepared by the reaction of sucrose with edible fatty acids *(see)*. It occurs as a solid, soft gel or liquid at room temperature depending on the fatty acids used. It looks, cooks, and tastes like ordinary fat, but adds no fat or calories to foods with which it is cooked. Potato chips made with Olean, for example, contain no fat and only 75 calories vs. 10 grams of fat and 150 calories in regular chips. Use of Olestra in foods requires addition of specific amounts of vitamins A, D, E, and K to these foods. Olestra may cause abdominal cramping and loose stools in some individuals and the FDA requires this observation to be on the labels of all foods made with olestra.

Henry Blackburn, MD, of the University of Minnesota, writing an editorial in the April 11, 1996, issue of the *New England Journal of Medicine* wrote he was concerned that Olestra would be used for a long time by millions of people without good direct evidence that its use "would benefit them, reduce weight among the obese, prevent weight gain among those at risk for conditions associated with obesity, or reduce caloric intake substantially in representative population—all purported reasons for adding Olestra to the food supply." He said there is no regulatory requirement as there is for drugs that the petitioner demonstrate a benefit. He said members of the committee that approved Olestra expressed the view that the gastrointestinal symptoms associated with it were at most an "annoyance," not a serious health problem, and required only a warning label on the product. He wrote that this shifts the responsibility to the public when experts knowingly approved a "gastrointestinal hazard." The American Medical Association, on the other hand, noted that approximately 150 studies, including 43 clinical trials, have been conducted with Olestra in advance of FDA approval, making it "one of the most thoroughly tested foodstuffs to come to market in America."

OLIBANUM EXTRACT • Frankincense Extract. The extract of *Boswellia carteri* of various species. The volatile, distilled oil from the gum resin of a plant found in Ethiopia, Egypt, and Arabia. It was one of the gifts of the Magi. It is used in cola, fruit, and spice flavorings for beverages, ice cream, ices, candy, and baked goods.

OLIVE OIL • A monounsaturated fat *(see)*. Superior to mineral oils in penetrating power. Used in brilliantine hairdressings, emollients, eyelash oils, lipstick, nail polish removers, shampoos, soaps, face powders, hair colorings, antiwrinkle and massage oils. It is a pale yellow or greenish fixed oil obtained from ripe olives grown around the Mediterranean Sea. May cause allergic reactions. Has been reported to be beneficial to blood cholesterol.

OMEGA-3 FATTY ACIDS • Found in fish oils, reported to lower fats in the blood and thus reduce the risk of coronary artery disease. The FDA denied a claim for omega-3 fatty acids in reducing the risk of coronary heart disease because studies relating fish intake and risk of coronary heart disease were "conflicting and inconsistent." The FDA said the most compelling evidence was a well-controlled study that showed fish consumption may reduce the chance of death from a second heart attack. However, these studies did not establish that the effects were due specifically to omega-3 fatty acids. Data revealed that omega-3 may raise blood LDL (the bad kind of cholesterol) of people with high blood fats and may interfere with blood glucose control in diabetics. *See* Fish Oil.

ONION EXTRACT • Extract of the bulbs of onion, *Allium cepa,* discovered in Asia. Used in meat, onion, and spice flavorings for beverages, ice cream, ices, baked goods, condiments, meats, and pickles. Skin irritant. When heated to decomposition it emits acrid smoke and irritating fumes. GRAS.

OPOPANAX • Bisabol. An odorous, myrrh-type gum resin from a southern European or African herbs. Once used in medicine. Now used as a flavoring.

ORANGE B • Dull orange crystals derived from coal tar. Coloring for casing of frankfurters and sausages. The color additive was limited to not more than 150 ppm by weight of finished food. In 1978, the FDA said use could result in exposure of consumers to beta-naphthylamine, a known cancer-causing agent. Although it was permanently listed by the FDA, the only manufacturer of it stopped making it. *See* FD & C Colors.

ORANGE BITTER, FLOWERS and PEEL • The essential oil is used as a flavoring. GRAS.

ORANGE BLOSSOMS • Orange blossoms, absolute, is a natural flavoring derived from the fruit of the bitter plant species. Used in citrus and fruit flavorings for beverages, ice cream ices, candy, baked goods, and chewing gum. The flowers provide a natural flavoring extract for citrus and cola flavorings for beverages (2,000 ppm). The orange leaf extract is used as a natural fruit flavoring for beverages, ice cream, ices, and baked goods. Orange peel bitter oil is expressed from the fresh fruit and is used in orange and fruit flavorings for beverages, ice cream, ices, candy, gelatin desserts, chewing gum, and liquors. GRAS.

ORANGE CRYSTALS • *See* Methyl *b*-Naphthyl Ketone.

ORANGE FLOWER, BITTER OIL • *See* Nerol.

ORANGE LEAF • *See* Orange Blossoms.

ORANGE OIL • Sweet Orange Oil. Yellow to deep orange, highly volatile, unstable liquid with a characteristic orange taste and odor expressed from the fresh peel of the ripe fruit of the sweet orange plant species. Once used as an expectorant, it is now employed in perfumery, soaps, and flavorings. Used in orange and fruit flavorings for beverages, ice cream, ices, candy, baked goods, gelatin desserts, and chewing gum. Inhalation or frequent contact with oil of orange may cause severe symptoms such as headache, dizziness, and shortness of breath. Perfumes, colognes, and toilet water containing oil of orange may cause allergic reaction in the hypersensitive. Omitted from hypoallergenic cosmetics.

ORANGE PEEL, BITTER OIL • *See* Orange Blossoms.

ORANGE PEEL, SWEET EXTRACT • From the fresh rind of the fruit. Sweetish, fragrant odor; slightly bitter taste. Used in orange and ginger ale flavorings for beverages, ice cream, ices, candy, and baked goods. GRAS.

ORANGE PEEL, SWEET OIL (TERPENELESS) • From the fresh rind of the fruit. Sweetish, fragrant odor; slightly bitter taste. Used in orange and fruit flavoring for beverages, ice cream, ices, candy, baked goods, gelatin desserts, and puddings.

ORANGE-SWEET and LEAF, FLOWER, PEEL • Used as a flavoring. *See* Orange Blossoms and Orange Oil.

OREGANO • Mexican Oregano. Mexican Sage. Origanum. The wild marjoram *(see)* plant, but spicier, ordinarily found in Eurasia. Used in loganberry, cherry, sausage, root beer, and spice flavorings for beverages, baked goods, condiments (2,800 ppm), and meats. *See* Origanum Oil for toxicity. GRAS.

ORGANIC • The term usually means produce grown without pesticides, herbicides, or synthetic fertilizers on land that has been free of such chemicals for one to seven years. The U.S. Department of Agriculture proposed regulations in 1997 that raw products be 100 percent organic and that processed foods contain 95 percent organic ingredients. Processed foods with 50 percent to 95 percent organic content could be labeled as "made with certain organic ingredients," while those with less than 50 percent organic content must specify the organic ingredients. Those selling or labeling products that do not meet the standards could be fined up to $10,000. About half the states now have their own organic food regulations, and they would be permitted to issue stricter standards than the ones enforced by the USDA subject to approval by the agriculture secretary. The Organic Trade Association estimates there are up to 12,000 organic farmers in the United States, out of roughly 2 million farms nationwide. They tend to be smaller operations, usually selling vegetable and other specialty crops at local farmer's markets and to small groceries through cooperatives. Organic farmers face higher costs because their natural fertilizers and pest-control efforts tend to be more expensive and they must hire more workers to replace the mechanization common in conventional farming.

ORGANOPHOSPHATES • Compounds containing phosphorus that belong to several groups including:

- Phospholipids or phosphatides, which are widely distributed in plants and animals. Lecithin is an example.

- Esters of phosphinic and phosphonic acids, which are used as plasticizers, insecticides, resin modifiers, and flame retardants.

- Pyrophosphates, which are the basis for many insecticides that inhibit cholinesterase, an enzyme necessary for nerve transmission. Tetraethyl pyrophosphate (TEPP), which is highly toxic, was developed during World War II.

- The phosphoric esters of glycerol, glycol, and other fatty alcohols that are used in fertilizers.

Organophosphates, pesticides, and insecticides can be extremely toxic. They can kill quickly or slowly depending on the amount of exposure. Most are easily absorbed through the skin, eyes, stomach, and lungs. Among the organophosphate pesticides in use are azinphosmethyl, carbophenothion, demeton, diazinon, dichlorvos, dicrotophos, dimethoate, endothion, EPN, fensulfothion, fenthion, Hinosan, methyl demeton, methyl parathion, mevinphos, mipafox, monocrotophos, naled, parathion, phorate, phosphamidon, Phostex, tetraethyl pyrophosphate (TEPP), thiometon, and trichlorfon.

Organophosphorous compounds are now being studied for delayed neurotoxicity. It can occur in factory workers exposed during the production of organophosphorous chemicals, which are used as plasticizers, lubricants, fire retardants, and pesticides.

ORIGAN • *See* Oregano.

ORIGANOL • *See* 4-Carvomenthenol.

ORIGANUM OIL • The volatile oil is obtained by steam distillation from a flowering herb. Yellowish red to dark brown, with a pungent odor. Used in vermouth, sausage, root beer, and spice flavorings for beverages, ice cream, ices, candy, baked goods, condiments, and meats. A teaspoonful can cause illness and less than an ounce has killed adults. GRAS.

ORIZANOL • The ester of ferulic acid and terpene alcohol widely found in plants used in flavorings and perfumes. *See* Cinnamate.

ORMETOPRIM • A feed additive. The FDA tolerance for residue in edible tissues of chickens, ducks, turkeys, salmoids, and catfish is 0.1 ppm.

ORRIS • Orris Root Oil. White Flag. Love Root. Made from the roots of the plant. Yellowish, semisolid, and fragrant oil. Distilled for use in raspberry, blackberry, strawberry, violet, cherry, nut, and spice flavorings for beverages, ice cream, ices, candy, baked goods, gelatin desserts, chewing gum, and icings. It is also used in dusting powders, perfumes, dry shampoos, toothpaste, and sachets. Discontinued in the United States because of the frequent allergic reactions to orris, including infantile eczema, hay fever, stuffy nose, red eyes, and asthma. *See* Orris Root Extract.

ORRIS ROOT EXTRACT • Obtained from dried orris root. Has an intense odor and is used in perfumery. Used in chocolate, fruit, nut, vanilla, and cream soda flavorings for beverages, ice cream, ices, candy, baked goods, gelatin desserts, and chewing gum. Causes frequent allergic reactions.

ORYZALIN • Surflan. Dirimal. A herbicide used in peppermint and spearmint. FDA limits it to 0.1 ppm in peppermint and spearmint oil.

OSMANTHUS, ABSOLUTE • A widely distributed genus of evergreen shrubs or trees, family Oleaceae, with inconspicuous bisexual flowers, and sometimes foliage resembling holly. Used in flavoring and perfumery.

OSTEOPOROSIS • A skeletal disease, in which the bones lose mass and density, the pores in bones enlarge, and the bones generally become fragile. Osteoporosis often is not diagnosed until a fracture occurs, most commonly in the spine, hip, or wrist. The National Osteoporosis Foundation says about 1.5 million such fractures occur each year in the United States.

OTHER CARB • The listing for Other Carbohydrates on food labels. *See* Carbohydrates.

OURICURY WAX • The wax exuded from the leaves of the Brazilian palm tree. The hard brown wax has the same properties and uses as carnauba wax *(see)*.

OXALIC ACID • Occurs naturally in many plants and vegetables, particularly in the Oxalis family; also in many molds. Some plants such as rhubarb, spinach, and amaranthus are high in it. Oxalic acid has the ability to bind some metals such as calcium and magnesium and has therefore been suspected of interfering with the metabolism of these minerals.

OXAMYL • A pesticide. The FDA residue tolerance in pineapple bran is 6 ppm.

OXAZOLINE • A series of synthetic waxes that are versatile and miscible with most natural waxes and can be applied to the same uses.

OX BILE • Oxgall. Emulsifier from the fresh bile of male castrated bovines. Brownish green or dark green; viscous. Characteristic odor. Bitter, disagreeable taste. Used in dried egg whites up to 0.1 percent. No known toxicity. The final report to the FDA of the Select Committee on GRAS Substances stated in 1980 that it should continue its GRAS status with no limitations other than good manufacturing practices.

OXFENDAZOL • Crystals from chloroform and methanol, it is used in a suspension to kill worms in cattle. FDA tolerance is 0.8 ppm in cattle liver.

OXIDIZED POLYETHYLENE • The resin produced by exposing polyethylene *(see)* to air. It is used as a protective coating or component of protective coatings for fresh avocados, bananas, beets, coconuts, eggplant, garlic, grapefruit, lemons, limes, mangos, muskmelons, onions, oranges, papaya, peas (in pods), pineapple, plantain, pumpkin, rutabaga, squash (acorn), sweet potatoes, tangerines, turnips, watermelon, Brazil nuts, chestnuts, filberts, hazelnuts, pecans, and walnuts (all nuts in shells).

OXIDIZED TALLOW • A defoaming component used in yeast and beet sugar production in reasonable amounts required to inhibit foaming. *See* Tallow Flakes.

OXIDIZER • A substance that causes oxygen to combine with another substance. Oxygen and Hydrogen Peroxide are examples of oxidizers.

OXIDES OF NITROGEN • Used as a bleaching agent in flour. *See* Nitrogen.

OXYFLUORFEN • Orange solid used as an herbicide in cottonseed oil, mint oil, and soybean oil. Limitation of 0.25 ppm in the oils.

OXYSTEARIN • A mixture of the glycerides *(see)* of partially oxidized stearic acids *(see)* and other fatty acids *(see)*. Occurs in animal fat and used chiefly in manufacture of soaps, candles, cosmetics, suppositories, pill coatings. Tan, waxy. Used as a crystallization inhibitor in cottonseed and soybean cooking. In salad oils up to 0.125 percent. Also used as a defoamer in the production of beet sugar and yeast. The Select Committee of the Federation of American Societies for Experimental Biology advising on food additives recommended further study of this additive. The final report to the FDA of the Select Committee on GRAS

Substances stated in 1980 that while no evidence in the available information on it demonstrates a hazard to the public at current use levels, uncertainties exist, requiring that additional studies be conduced. GRAS status has continued since 1980 while tests were being completed and evaluated.

OXYTETRACYCLINE • An antibiotic substance used in feed to increase growth and found in edible tissue of chickens and turkeys. FDA permits a residue in the birds of up to 3 ppm in liver and 1 ppm in uncooked muscle, fat, and skin of chickens and turkeys. It is used in combination with carbomycin *(see)* in the drinking water of chickens. It is used in tablet form for cattle. Because it is an antimicrobial, it may cause sensitivity to light, nausea, inflammation of the mucous membranes of the mouth, and diarrhea. *See* Antibiotics.

OZOKERITE • Ceresin. A naturally occurring waxlike mineral; a mixture of hydrocarbons. Colorless or white when pure; horrid odor. Upon refining, it yields a hard white microcrystalline wax known as ceresin *(see)*. An emulsifier and thickening agent used in lipstick and cream rouge. No known toxicity.

OZONE • A colorless gas or dark blue liquid used as an antimicrobial agent in bottle water. Under the EPA Genetic Toxicology Program *(see)*. Toxic effects are from inhalation.

P

PABA • *See* para-Aminobenzoic acid.

PALATONE • *See* Maltol.

PALE CATECHU • *See* Catechu Extract.

PALM KERNEL OIL • The oil from the fruit of the oil palm *Elaeisis guineensis*. A fatty solid with a sweet, nutty flavor. Used as a coating agent, emulsifying agent, and texturizer in confectionery products and margarine. GRAS.

PALM OIL • Palm Butter. Palm Tallow. Yellow-brown, buttery, edible solid at room temperature. Oil palms are native to Central Africa and Malaysia. A reddish yellow to dark dirty red. A fatty mass with a faint violet odor. Used as a shortening, as a substitute for tallow, and in making soaps and ointment. No known toxicity.

PALM OIL GLYCERIDE • *See* Palm Oil.

PALMA ROSA OIL • Geranium Oil. The volatile oil obtained by steam distillation from a variety of partially dried grass grown in East India and Java. Used in rose, fruit, and spice flavorings for ice cream, ices, candy, and baked goods. Believed as toxic as other essential oils, causing illness, ingestion of a teaspoonful and death after ingestion of an ounce. A skin irritant. GRAS.

PALMAMIDE MEA • A mixture of ethanolamides of the fatty acids derived from palm oil *(see)*.

PALMITAMIDE • A substance that keeps food from sticking to a container. Used in packaging material. *See* Palmitic Acid.

PALMITIC ACID • A mixture of solid organic acids obtained from fats consisting chiefly of palmitic acid with varying amounts of stearic acid *(see)*. It is white or faintly yellow and has a fatty odor and taste. Palmitic acid occurs naturally in allspice, anise, calamus oil, cascarilla bark, celery seed, butter acids, coffee, tea, and many animal fats and plant oils. It forms about 21 percent of cow's milk. Obtained from palm oil, Japan wax, or Chinese vegetable tallow. No known toxicity to skin and hair provided no salts of oleic or lauric acids *(see)* are present. Used in butter and cheese flavorings for seasoning preparations. Used as a texturizer in shampoos, shaving creams, and soaps.

PALMITOYL HYDROLYZED ANIMAL PROTEIN • *See* Hydrolyzed Protein.

PALMITOYL HYDROLYZED MILK PROTEIN • The condensation product of palmitic acid chloride and hydrolyzed milk protein. *See* Hydrolyzed and Milk.

PANCREATIC EXTRACT • Hi-Vegi-Lip. A preparation of pancreatic hormones used in disorders of the pancreas to aid digestion of starches, fats, and proteins. Potential adverse reactions include nausea and diarrhea. Should be used cautiously in persons allergic to pork.

PANSY EXTRACT • The extract obtained from *Viola tricolor*. Flavoring in alcoholic beverages only. Also used as a coloring in cosmetics.

PANTHENOL • Dexpanthenol. Vitamin B Complex Factor. A viscous, slightly bitter liquid used as a medicinal supplement in foods to aid digestion and in liquid vitamins. Used in hair products and in emollients. It is good for human tissues. No known toxicity.

***d*-PANTOTHENAMIDE** • Vitamin B Complex. Vitamin B_5. Made synthetically from the jelly of the queen bee, yeast, and molasses. Cleared as a source of pantothenic acid in foods for special dietary use. Pantothenic acid (common sources are liver, rice bran, and molasses) is essential for metabolism of carbohydrates, fats, and other important substances. Nerve damage has been observed in patients with low pantothenic acid. It helps release energy from carbohydrates in the breakdown of fats. Children and adults need from five to ten milligrams per day. *See* Calcium Pantothenate.

PANTOTHENIC ACID • Vitamin B_5. A necessity in human diets. It helps metabolize fats and proteins. Nontoxic.

***d*-PANTOTHENYL ALCOHOL** • The final report to the FDA of the Select Committee on GRAS Substances stated in 1980 that it should continue its GRAS status with no limitations other than good manufacturing practices. *See* Calcium Pantothenate.

PANTOTHENYL ETHYL ETHER • The ethyl ether of the B vitamin panthenol *(see)*.

PANTOTHENYL ETHYL ETHER ACETATE • The ester of acetic acid and the ethyl ether of the B vitamin panthenol *(see)*.

PAPAIN • A proteinase enzyme for meat tenderizing. Prepared from papaya, a fruit, and *Carica papaya,* grown in tropical countries. Used for clearing beverages. Added to enriched farina to reduce cooking time. Used medically to prevent adhesions. It is deactivated by cooking, but because of its protein digesting ability it can dissolve necrotic material with disastrous results. The usual grade used in food digests about thirty-five times its weight of lean meat. It may cause allergic reactions. Has caused birth defects in experimental animals. The final report to the FDA of the Select Committee on GRAS Substances stated in 1980 that it should continue its GRAS status with no limitations other than good manufacturing practices.

PAPAYA • A fruit grown in tropical countries. It contains an enzyme, papain, used as a meat tenderizer and, medicinally, to prevent adhesions. It is deactivated by cooking. Because of its protein-digesting ability, it can dissolve necrotic (dead) material. It may cause allergic reactions. *See* Papain.

PAPRIKA • The finely ground pods of dried, ripe, sweet pepper, *Capsicum annuum*. The strong, reddish orange powder is used in sausage and spice flavorings for baked goods (1,900 ppm), condiments, meats (7,400 ppm), and soups (7,500 ppm). The oleoresin *(see)* is used in fruit, meat, and spice flavorings for beverages, ice cream, ices, candy, baked goods, condiments, and meats. Both paprika and paprika oleoresins are used as red coloring. Permanently listed since 1966 for use in foods consistent with good manufacturing practices. They do not require certification. GRAS.

PAPRIKA OLEORESIN • Essential oil used as a color additive. GRAS. *See* Paprika.

PARA-AMINOBENZOIC ACID • The colorless or yellowish acid found in vitamin B complex. In an alcohol and water solution plus a little light perfume, it is sold under a wide variety of names as a sunscreen lotion to prevent skin damage from the sun. It is also used as a local anesthetic in sunburn products. It is used medicinally to treat arthritis. However, it can cause allergic eczema *(see)* and sensitivity to light in susceptible people, whose skin may react to sunlight by erupting with a rash, sloughing, and/or swelling.

PARABENS • Butylparaben. Heptylparaben. Methylparaben. Propylparaben. Parahydroxybenzoate. The parabens are the most commonly used preservatives in the U.S. The parabens have a broad spectrum of antimicrobial activity, are safe to use—relatively nonirritating, nonsensitizing, and nonpoisonous—are stable over the pH *(see)* range in cosmetics, and are sufficiently soluble in water to be effective in liquids. The typical paraben preservative system contains 0.2 percent methyl- and 0.1 percent propylparaben. Methyl- and propylparaben are esters of parahydroxybenzoic acid. Neither occurs in nature. In foods, parabens function as preservatives that prevent the growth of molds and yeasts. They are used in baked goods, sugar substitutes, artificially sweetened jams, mincemeats, milk preparations, soft drinks, packaged fish, meat, poultry, jellies, fats, oils, and frozen dairy desserts. Methyl- and propylparabens are used at 1,000 ppm in tomato pulp, puree, catsup, pickles, and relishes. The only adverse effect of parabens reported was that methylparaben caused birth defects in offspring of mice and rats fed 550 milligrams per kilogram of body weight daily during pregnancy, and in hamsters fed 300 milligrams under the same conditions.

PARAFFIN WAX • A colorless, somewhat translucent, odorless mass with a greasy feel. Used as a defoaming component in yeast and sugar beet production. Not digested or absorbed in the intestines. Used to cover food products. A component of chewing-gum base. Used in solid brilliantines, cold creams, wax depilatories, eyelash creams and oils, eyebrow pencils, lipsticks, liquefying creams, protective creams, and mascaras; also used for extracting perfumes from flowers. Obtained from the distillate of wood, coal, petroleum, or shale oil. Easily melts over boiling water. Pure paraffin is harmless to the skin, but the presence of impurities may give rise to irritations and eczema. *See also* Wax.

PARAFORMALDEHYDE • Preservative used to control fungus in maple-tree tap holes (residue limit of 2 ppm of formaldehyde in maple syrup).

PARAMIPHOS-METHYL • A pesticide. The FDA allows a residue of 60 ppm in or on rice hulls and 50 ppm in or on rice milling fractions and in or on wheat milling fractions.

PARAQUAT • Defoliant and herbicide used in animal feed for goats, cattle, swine, and lambs. FDA limits residue to up to 0.2 ppm in dried hops, 3 in mint hay, 6 in sunflower seed hulls. Paraquat is in the EPA Genetic Toxicology Program *(see)*. Poison by ingestion and skin contact. Causes ulceration of the digestive tract, diarrhea, vomiting, renal damage, jaundice, edema, hemorrhage, lung damage, and death from suffocation. When heated to decomposition, emits toxic fumes.

PARATHION • A deep brown to yellow liquid, it is an organophosphate *(see)* insecticide and acaricide. Highly toxic by skin contact, inhalation, or ingestion. It interferes with the transmission of nerve signals. Repeated exposure may, without warning, be increasingly hazardous. *See* Organophosphates.

PARMESAN CHEESE, REGGIANO CHEESE • A hard, dry cheese with a sharp flavor that is cured for several years. It is used as a flavoring.

PARSLEY, LEAVES, OIL, and OLEORESIN • The aromatic leaves of the annual herb *Petroselinum* ssp., cultivated everywhere, are used in spice flavorings for beverages, meats, soups, baked goods, and condiments. Parsley oil is obtained by steam distillation of the ripe seeds of the herb. The *oleoresin (see)* is used in spice flavorings for condiments. Used as a preservative, perfume, and flavoring in cosmetics, it is obtained by steam distillation of the ripe seeds of the herb. Yellow to light brown with a harsh odor. Parsley may cause the skin to break out with a rash, redden, and swell when exposed to light. It may also cause an allergic reaction in the sensitive. GRAS.

PARSLEY SEED OIL • *See* Parsley, Leaves, Oil, and Oleoresin.

PARTIALLY DELACTOSED WHEY (PDW) • Used increasingly as a substitute for nonfat dry milk, which is more expensive. PDW is used in processed cheese foods and spreads. It is the result of the partial removal of lactose *(see)* from the milk ingredient whey *(see)*.

PARTIALLY DEMINERALIZED and DELACTOSED WHEY • Removal of some minerals as well as lactose from whey. *See* Partially Delactosed Whey.

PARVE • *See* Kosher.

PASSIONFLOWER • Extract of the various species of *Passiflora incamata*. Indians used passionflower for swellings, relieving sore eyes, and to induce vomiting. It is used as a flavoring. It has been shown that an extract of the plant depresses the motor nerves of the spinal cord.

PATCHOULI OIL • Patchouly Oil. Essential oil obtained from the leaves of an East Indian shrubby mint, *Pogostemon* spp. Yellowish to greenish brown liquid, with the pleasant fragrance of summer flowers. Used in cola, fruit, nut, and spice flavorings for beverages, ice cream, ices, candy, baked goods, and chewing gum. Used in perfume formulations to impart a long-lasting oriental-type aroma in soaps and cosmetics. May produce allergic reactions.

PCBs • *See* Polychlorinated Biphenyls.

PEACH ALDEHYDE • *See* y-Undecalactone.

PEACH EXTRACT • *See* Peach Juice Extract.

PEACH JUICE EXTRACT • The liquid obtained from the pulp of the peach, *Prunus persica*. It is used as a natural flavoring and as an emollient. Nontoxic.

PEACH KERNEL OIL • Persic Oil. A light yellow liquid expressed from the seed. Smells like almonds. Used as a natural flavoring in conjunction with other natural flavorings. Used as an oil base in emollients, eyelash creams, and brilliantines. GRAS.

PEACH LEAVES • Flavoring for alcoholic beverages only. *See* Peach Juice Extract.

PEANUT OIL • Arachis Oil. Greenish yellow, with a pleasant odor. Prepared by pressing shelled and skinned seeds of the peanut. A solvent in salad oil, shortening, mayonnaise, and confections. Also used in conjunction with natural flavorings. Peanut butter is about 50 percent peanut oil suspended in peanut fibers. It may migrate from cotton in dried food packaging. Used in the manufacture of soaps, baby preparations, hair-grooming aids, nail driers, shampoos, and as a solvent for ointments and liniments; also in night creams and emollients. It is used as a substitute for almond and olive oils in cosmetic creams, brilliantines, antiwrinkle oils, and sunburn preparations. Has been reported to be a mild irritant in soap, but considered harmless to the skin. The oil acts as a mild cathartic and as a protective for the gastrointestinal tract when corrosive poisons have been swallowed. The final report to the FDA of the Select Committee on GRAS Substances stated in 1980 that it should continue its GRAS status with no limitations other than good manufacturing practices. A study done by the Department of Nutrition, University of California, Davis, found in 1997 that crude peanut oil caused allergic reactions in 10 percent of allergic subjects studied and should be avoided. Refined peanut oil did not pose a risk to the subjects. Check with your physician before trying if you are allergic to peanut oil.

PEANUT STEARINE • Natural flavoring. GRAS. *See* Peanut Oil.

PEANUTAMIDEMEA • Loramine Wax. *See* Peanut Oil.

PEANUTAMIDEMIPA • A mixture of isopropanolamides of the fatty acids derived from peanut oil *(see)*.

PECAN SHELL POWDER • A coloring agent used in cosmetics. Employed medicinally by the American Indians. It is the nut from a hickory of the southern central U.S. with rough bark and hard but brittle wood. Edible. No known toxicity.

PECTINS • Pectin is found in roots, stems, and fruits of plants and forms an integral part of such structures. It is a coarse or fine powder, practically odorless, with a gluey taste. Richest source of pectin is lemon or orange rind, which contains about 30 percent of this polysaccharide. Used as a stabilizer, thickener, and bodying agent for artificially sweetened beverages, syrups for frozen products, ice cream, ice milk, confections, fruit sherbets, water ices, French dressing, fruit jelly, preserves, and jams to compensate for a deficiency in natural pectin. Used in foods as a "cementing agent." Used in cosmetics as a gelling and thickening agent. Emulsifying agent used in place of various gums in toothpaste, hair-setting lotions, and protective creams. It is soothing and mildly acidic. Also used as an antidiarrheal medicine. No known toxicity. The final report to the FDA of the Select Committee on GRAS Substances stated in 1980 that it should continue its GRAS status with no limitations other than good manufacturing practices.

PECTINASE • An enzyme used as a clarifying agent *(see)* in wine and juice.

PEGU CATECHU EXTRACT • *See* Catechu Extract.

PELARGONALDEHYDE • *See* Nonanal.

PELARGONIC ACID • Nonanoic Acid. A synthetic flavoring agent that occurs naturally in cocoa and oil of lavender. Used in berry, fruit, nut, and spice flavorings. Used in peeling solution for fruits and vegetables. A strong irritant.

PELARGONIC ALDEHYDE • *See* Pelargonic Acid.

PELARGONYL VANILLYLAMIDE • *See* Pelargonic Acid.

PENDARE • *Couma macrocarpa barb. Couma utilis.* A flavoring from tropical South American trees. *See* Coumarin.

PENDIMETHALIN • Prowl. Stomp. An herbicide. FDA tolerance is 0.1 ppm as a residue in or on corn fodder or forage, grain, potatoes, sorghum, soybeans, or sunflower seeds.

PENICILLINASE FROM *BACILLUS SUBTILIS* • An enzyme from a mold used in processing.

PENICILLINS • Amoxicillin. Ampicillin. Azlocillin. Bacampicillin. Carbenicillin. Cloxacillin. Dicloxacillin. Methicillin. Mezlocillin. Nafcillin. Oxacillin. Penicillin G, V. Piperacillin. Ticarcillin. A group of beta-lactam antibiotics produced by several species of mold and/or semisynthetically. There are many kinds and they offer a broad clinical spectrum of activity. They act by inhibiting bacterial enzymes involved in making cell walls. Used to treat animal infections and in animal feed to prevent infections and to encourage growth, particularly in chickens, lamb, swine, turkey, pheasants, and quail. FDA limits residues to 0.05 ppm in cattle. Limitation of zero in chickens, pheasant, quail, swine, sheep, eggs, milk, and foods in which milk has been used. Limitation of 0.01 ppm in turkeys. In EPA Genetic Toxicology Program *(see)*. Human reproductive effects by ingestion: abortion. Human systemic effects by intramuscular route: skin rash. Has been implicated in aplastic anemia.

PENICILLIUM ROQUEFORTII • Mold used to make cheeses.

PENNYROYAL OIL • Squaw Mint. Hedeoma. An extract of the flowering herb *Mentha pulegium.* Used since ancient days as a medicine, scent, flavoring, and food. Obtained from the dried flower tops and leaves, it contains tannin, which is soothing to the skin. Used in mint flavorings for beverages, ice cream, ices, candy, and baked goods. Formerly used as an aromatic perspirant, to stimulate menstrual flow, for flatulence, as an abortion inducer, and as a counteractant for painful menstruation. Brain damage has been reported following doses of less than one teaspoon. Nausea, vomiting, bleeding, circulatory collapse, confusion, restlessness, and delirium have been reported.

PENTACHLOROPHENOL • Chloropben. Santophen. Dark-colored flakes with a characteristic odor used as a preservative in packaging materials. FDA limit of 50 ppm in treated wood. International Agency for Research on Cancer (IARC) *(see)* review and on EPA Extremely Hazardous List, Community Right-To-Know List, and EPA Genetic Toxicology Program *(see all)*. Human poison by ingestion. A suspected human cancer-causing agent. Causes birth defects in experimental animals. Skin irritant. Acute poisoning causes weakness with difficult breathing and changes in blood pressure and urinary output. Can cause death.

PENTADECALACTONE • Angelica Lactone. Exaltolide. It is obtained from the fruit and root of a plant grown in Europe and Asia. A synthetic berry, fruit, liquor, wine, nut, and vanilla flavoring agent for beverages, ice cream, ices, candy, baked goods, gelatin desserts, and alcoholic beverages. Used as a cosmetic fragrance.

PENTADECANOLIDE • *See* Pentadecalactone.

PENTADESMA BUTTER • Kanya Butter. The vegetable fat extracted from the nut of Pentadesma butyracea. *See* Shea Butter.

PENTAERYTHRITOL ESTER OF MALEIC ANHYDRIDE MODIFIED WOOD ROSIN • Coating on citrus fruit. Pentaerythritol is a resin made by treating acetaldehyde *(see)* with formaldehyde *(see)* in a solution of calcium hydroxide.

PENTAERYTHRITOL ESTER OF PARTIALLY HYDROGENATED WOOD ROSIN • Hard, amber-colored solid used as a coating for citrus fruits and in chewing-gum bases. *See* Rosin.

PENTANAL • *See* Valeraldehyde.

PENTANE • The aliphatic hydrocarbon derived from petroleum. Used as a solvent. Narcotic in high doses.

2,3-PENTANEDIONE • A synthetic flavoring agent that occurs naturally in coffee. Used in strawberry, chocolate, butterscotch, butter, caramel, fruit, rum, and cheese flavorings for beverages, ice cream, ices, candy, baked goods, gelatin desserts, and puddings. No known toxicity.

2-PENTANETHIOL • *n*-Amyl Mercaptan. A liquid with a strong, unpleasant odor used in the manufacture of food additives. Mild irritant to skin and mucous membranes.

PENTANOIC ACID • *See* Valeric Acid.

I-PENTANOL • Pentyl Alcohol. *n*-Amyl Alcohol. Liquid with a mild, pleasant odor, slightly soluble in water. Used as a solvent. Irritating to the eyes and respiratory passages, and absorption may cause a lack of oxygen in the blood.

2-PENTANONE • A synthetic flavoring that occurs naturally in apples. Used in fruit flavorings for beverages, ice cream, ices, candy, and baked goods. Moderately toxic by ingestion. Mildly toxic by skin contact and inhalation. In humans, inhalation may cause headache, nausea, and irritation of the respiratory passages, eyes, and skin.

4-PENTENOIC ACID 9 • A synthetic butter and fruit flavoring agent for beverages, ice cream, ices, candy, baked goods, and margarine.

PENTYL ALCOHOL • *See* Amyl Alcohol.

PENTYL BUTYRATE • *See* Amyl Butyrate.

PEPPER, BLACK • A pungent product obtained from the dried, unripe berries of the East Indian pepper plant, *Piper nigrum.* Used in sausage and spice flavorings for beverages, baked goods, condiments, meats, soups, and pickles. Black pepper *oil* is used in meat and spice flavorings for beverages, ice cream, ices, candy, baked goods, condiments, and meats. Black pepper *oleoresin (see)* is used in sausage and pepper flavorings for beverages, ice cream, ices, candy, baked goods, condiments, and meats. Pepper was formerly used as a carminative to break up intestinal gas, to cause sweating, and as a gastric agent to promote gastric secretion. Has insecticidal properties. GRAS.

PEPPER, RED • GRAS. *See* Cayenne Pepper.

PEPPER TREE OIL • *See Schinus Molle* Oil.

PEPPER, WHITE • The pungent product obtained from the undecorticated (with the outer covering intact) ripe berries of the pepper plant. Used in sausage and spice flavorings for beverages, baked goods, condiments, meats, and soups. White pepper oil is used in spice flavorings for baked goods. White pepper *oleoresin (see)* is used in spice flavorings for meats. *See* Pepper, Black. GRAS.

PEPPERMINT EXTRACT • *See* Peppermint Oil.

PEPPERMINT LEAVES • *See* Peppermint Oil.

PEPPERMINT OIL • The oil made from the dried leaves and tops of a plant common to Asian, European, and American gardens, *Mentha piperita.* Used in chocolate, fruit, cordial, crème de menthe, peppermint, nut, and spice flavorings for beverages, ice cream, ices, candy (1,200 ppm), baked goods, gelatin desserts, chewing gum (8,300 ppm), meats, liquors, icings, and toppings. Peppermint has been used as a carminative to break up intestinal gas and as an antiseptic. Used in toothpaste and tooth powders, eye lotions, shaving lotions, and toilet waters. It can cause allergic reactions such as hay fever and skin rash. Two patients who consumed large quantities of peppermint candy over a long period developed irregular heart rhythms. GRAS.

PEPSIN • A digestive enzyme found in gastric juice that helps break down protein. Allowed up to 0.1 percent by weight in enriched farina. The product, also used to aid digestion, is obtained from the glandular layer of the fresh stomach of a hog. Slightly acid taste and a mild odor.

PEPTIDE • Two or more amino acids chained together in head-to-tail links. Generally larger than simple amino acids or the monoamines, the largest peptides discovered thus far have 44 amino acids. Neuropeptides signal the body's endocrine glands to balance salt and water. Opiate peptides can help control pain and anxiety. The peptides work with amino acids.

PEPTONES • Secondary protein derivatives formed during digestion—the result of gastric and pancreatic juices acting upon protein. Peptones are used as a foam stabilizer for beer and as a processing aid in baked goods, confections, and frostings. There is reported use of the chemical; it has not yet been assigned for toxicology literature. Determined to be GRAS in 1982.

PERACETIC ACID • Peroxyacetic Acid. A starch modifier prepared from acetaldehyde *(see)*. It is 40 percent acetic acid and highly corrosive. Acrid odor; explodes violently on heating to 110 degrees.

PERFLUOROHEXANE • Used to cool or freeze chickens.

PERILLALDEHYDE • Isolated from *Perilla arguta,* it is used as a sweet flavoring agent.

PERILLA OIL • Light yellow oil derived from the seeds of *Perilla ocimodes,* grown in Japan and Korea. It is used as a substitute for linseed oil and as an edible oil in Asia. It is also used in the manufacture of varnishes. There is reported use of the chemical, it has not yet been assigned for toxicology literature.

PERLITE • A filtering aid. The final report to the FDA of the Select Committee on GRAS Substances stated in 1980 it should continue its GRAS status with no limitations other than good manufacturing practices.

PEROXIDE • Benzoyl, Calcium, and Hydrogen. *Benzoyl peroxide* is used as a bleaching agent for flours, oils, and cheese. Has been used as a paste for treating poison ivy and for burns. May explode when heated. *Calcium peroxide or dioxide is* odorless, almost tasteless. Used as a dough conditioner and oxidizing agent for bread, rolls, and buns. Formerly used as an antiseptic. *Hydrogen peroxide or dioxide* is used as a bleaching and oxidizing agent, a modifier for food starch, and a preservative and bactericide for milk and cheese. Bitter taste. May decompose violently if traces of impurities are present. A strong oxidant that can injure skin and eyes. Chemists are cautioned to wear rubber gloves and goggles when handling it. Used in hair bleaches. May cause hair breakage and is an irritant. On the FDA list of additives to be studied for mutagenic, teratogenic, subacute, and reproductive effects.

PERSIC OIL • *See* Apricot and Peach Kernel Oil.

PERUVIAN BALSAM • *See* Balsam Peru. GRAS.

PESTICIDE • A broad class of crop protection chemicals including four major types: insecticides used to control insects; herbicides used to control weeds; rodenticides used to control rodents; and fungicides used to control mold, mildew, and fungi. In addition consumers use pesticides in the home or yard to control termites and roaches, clean mold from shower curtains, stave off crabgrass on the lawn, kill fleas and ticks on pets, and disinfect swimming pools, to name just a few "specialty" pesticide uses. Some pesticides are immediately toxic to humans. Others take a long time to produce cancer and other illnesses. *See* Appendix D.

PETITGRAIN OIL • Used extensively in perfumes. It is the volatile oil obtained from the leaves and twigs and unripe fruit of the bitter-orange tree. Brownish to yellow with a bittersweet odor. Used in loganberry, violet, apple, banana, berry, grape, peach, pear, honey, muscatel, nut, ginger, and ginger ale flavorings for beverages, ice cream, ices, candy, baked goods, gelatin desserts, chewing gum, and condiments. Supposedly dissolves in sweat, and under the influence of sunlight becomes an irritant. May cause allergic skin reactions. There is reported use of the chemical, it has not yet been assigned for toxicology literature. GRAS.

PETITGRAIN OIL (LEMON, MANDARIN, TANGERINE) • Fragrant essential oils from a variety of citrus trees. Used in citrus and fruit flavorings for beverages, ice cream, ices, candy, and baked goods. There is reported use of the chemical; it has not yet been assigned for toxicology literature. GRAS.

PETROLATUM • Crude or Mineral Oil. Vaseline. Petroleum Jelly. Paraffin Jelly. A purified mixture of semisolid hydrocarbons from petroleum. Yellowish to light amber or white, unctuous mass, practically odorless and tasteless, almost insoluble in water. A releasing agent and sealant for confections. A coating for fruits, vegetables, and cheese. A defoaming agent in yeast and beet sugar production. Used in baking products, as a lubricant in meatpacking plants, and used in dried-egg albumin. Defoaming agent, lubricant, polishing agent, protective coating, release (nonstick) agent, and sealing agent in bakery products, beet sugar, confectionery, egg-white solids, dehydrated fruits, and dehydrated vegetables. FDA limits petrolatum to 0.15 percent in bakery products, 0.2 percent in confectionery, 0.02 percent in dehydrated fruits and vegetables, 0.1 percent in egg white. May contain FDA-approved antioxidants. Petrolatum helps to soften and smoothe the skin in the same way as any other emollient and is less expensive. The oily film helps prevent evaporation of moisture from the skin and protects the skin from irritation. However, petrolatum does cause allergic skin reactions in the hypersensitive. When ingested, it produces a mild laxative effect. Not absorbed but may inhibit digestion. It is generally nontoxic.

PETROLEUM • Hydrocarbons, Naphtha, Waxes. A highly complex mixture of paraffinic, naphthalenic, and aromatic hydrocarbons containing some sulfur and trace amounts of nitrogen and oxygen compounds. Believed to have originated from both plant and animal sources millions of years ago. By cracking petroleum into fractions, the gases butane, ethane, and propane are obtained, as well as naphtha, gasoline, kerosene, fuel oils, gas oil, lubricating oils, paraffin wax, and asphalt. A defoaming agent in processing beet sugar and yeast and a coating on cheese and raw fruits and vegetables. Used as a coating on eggshells; in froth-flotation cleaning of vegetables; as a float on fermentation fluids as in the manufacture of vinegar, wine, and pickle brine; as a component of pesticide formulations; in modified hops extract of beer; and in many other formulations. Formerly used for bronchitis, tapeworms, and externally for arthritis and skin problems. Many petroleum products are reported to be cancer-causing agents. Others, presumably those used on food are inert.

PETROLEUM NAPTHA • Solvent used as coating on fresh citrus. *See* Petroleum.

PETROLEUM WAX • Antifoaming agent used in beet sugar and yeast. Used in chewing-gum base and other foods, as a coating on cheese, fruits, and vegetables, and as a component of microcapsules for spice flavor for frozen pizza. *See* Petroleum.

PETROLEUM WAX, SYNTHETIC • Coating on cheese and raw fruits and vegetables. Also used as an antifoaming agent in beet sugar and yeast.

pH • The scale used to measure acidity and alkalinity. pH is the hydrogen (H) ion concentration of a solution; *p* stands for the power of hydrogen ion. The pH of a solution is measured on a scale of 14. A truly neutral solution, neither acidic nor alkaline, such as water, is 7. Acid is less than 7. Alkaline is more than 7. The pH of blood is 7.3; vinegar is 2.3.; lemon juice is 8.2; and lye is 13. Skin and hair are naturally acidic. Soap and detergents are alkaline.

a-PHELLANDRENE • A synthetic flavoring agent that occurs naturally in all-spice, star anise, angelica root, bay, dill, sweet fennel, black pepper, peppermint oil, and pimenta. Isolated from the essential oils of the eucalyptus plant. Used in citrus and spice flavorings for beverages, ice cream, ices, candy, and baked goods. Can be irritating to, and is absorbed through, the skin. Ingestion can cause vomiting and diarrhea.

PHENETHYL ALCOHOL • 2-Phenethyanol. It occurs naturally in oranges, raspberries, and tea. A synthetic fruit flavoring agent that is used in strawberry, butter, caramel, floral, fruit, and honey flavorings for beverages, ice cream, ices, candy, baked goods, chewing gum, and gelatin desserts. Practically all rose perfumes contain it. It is also used as a preservative in cosmetics. It is a sensitizer. It is a strong local anesthetic and has caused central nervous system injury in mice.

PHENETHYL ANTHRANILATES • A synthetic butter, caramel, fruit, honey, and grape flavoring agent for beverages, ice cream, ices, candy, and baked goods. *See* Coal Tar.

PHENETHYL BENZOATE • A synthetic fruit and honey flavoring agent for beverages, ice cream, ices, candy, chewing gum, and baked goods. *See* Coal Tar.

PHENETHYL BUTYRATE • A synthetic butter, strawberry, caramel, floral, apple, peach, pineapple, and honey flavoring agent for beverages, ice cream, ices, candy, and baked goods. *See* Coal Tar.

PHENETHYL CINNAMATE • A synthetic fruit flavoring agent for beverages, ice cream, ices, candy, puddings, and baked goods. *See* Coal Tar.

PHENETHYL FORMATE • Formic Acid. A synthetic berry, apple, apricot, banana, cherry, peach, pear, plum, and honey flavoring agent for beverages, ice cream, ices, candy, and baked goods. *See* Coal Tar.

PHENETHYL ISOBUTYRATE • A synthetic flavoring agent, slightly yellow, with a rose odor. Used in strawberry, floral, rose, apple, peach, pineapple, honey, and cheese flavorings for beverages, ice cream, ices, candy, and baked goods. Mildly toxic by ingestion. *See* Coal Tar.

PHENETHYL ISOVALERATE • A synthetic apple, apricot, peach, pear, and pineapple flavoring agent for beverages, ice cream, ices, candy, baked goods, and chewing gum. Mildly toxic by ingestion. *See* Coal Tar.

2-PHENETHYL 2-METHYL BUTYRATE • Colorless liquid with a floral-fruity odor used as a flavoring agent in various foods.

PHENETHYL PHENYLACETATE • A synthetic fruit and honey flavoring agent for beverages, ice cream, ices, candy, maraschino cherries, and baked goods. *See* Coal Tar.

PHENETHYL PROPIONATE • A synthetic fruit and honey flavoring agent for beverages, ice cream, ices, candy, and baked goods. *See* Coal Tar.

PHENETHYL SALICYLATE • A synthetic apricot and peach flavoring agent for beverages, ice cream, ices, candy, and baked goods. *See* Coal Tar.

PHENETHYL SENECIOATE • A synthetic liquor and wine flavoring agent for beverages, ice cream, ices, candy, and alcoholic beverages. *See* Coal Tar.

PHENETHYL TIGLATE • A synthetic fruit and nut flavoring agent for beverages, ice cream, ices, candy, and baked goods. *See* Coal Tar.

PHENOL • Obtained from coal tar *(see)*, it is used in the manufacture of many food additives and processing aids. Ingestion of even small amounts of phenol may cause nausea, vomiting, circulatory collapse, paralysis, convulsions, coma, respiratory failure, and cardiac arrest. It is an antiseptic and general disinfectant.

PHENOL-FORMALDEHYDE • Used in treatment of food or potable water. *See* Formaldehyde and Phenol.

PHENOXYACETIC ACID • A synthetic fruit and honey flavoring agent for beverages, ice cream, ices, candy, and baked goods. Used to soften calluses and corns and other hard surfaces. A mild irritant.

2-PHENOXYETHYL ISOBUTYRATE • A synthetic fruit flavoring, colorless, with a roselike odor. Used in beverages, ice cream, ices, candy, and baked goods.

PHENYL ACETATE • A synthetic flavoring agent prepared from phenol and acetic chloride. Used in berry, butter, caramel, floral, rose, fruit, honey, and vanilla flavorings for beverages, ice cream, ices, candy, and baked goods. Phenol is highly toxic. Death from 1.5 grams has been reported.

4-PHENYL-2-BUTANOL • A synthetic fruit flavoring for beverages, ice cream, ices, candy, and baked goods.

4-PHENYL-3-BUTEN-2-OL • A synthetic fruit flavoring for beverages, ice cream, ices, candy, and baked goods.

4-PHENYL-3-BUTEN-2-ONE • A synthetic chocolate, cocoa, fruit, cherry, nut, and vanilla flavoring agent for beverages, ice cream, ices, candy, baked goods, gelatin desserts, and shortenings.

4-PHENYL-2-BUTYL ACETATE • A synthetic fruit and peach flavoring agent for beverages, ice cream, ices, candy, and baked goods. *See* Acetic Acid for toxicity.

PHENYL DIMETHYL CARBONYL ISOBUTYRATE • *See* a-a-Dimethylbenzyl Isobutyrate.

PHENYL 2-FUROATE • A synthetic chocolate and mushroom flavoring agent for beverages, candy, and gelatin desserts.

I-PHENYL-3-METHYL-3-PENTANOL • A synthetic fruit flavoring agent for beverages, candy, and gelatin desserts.

PHENYL PELARGONATE • Liquid, insoluble in water. Used in flavors, perfumes, bactericides, and fungicides.

I-PHENYL-1-PROPANOL • A synthetic fruit and honey flavoring agent for beverages, ice cream, ices, candy, and baked goods.

3-PHENYL-1-PROPANOL • A synthetic flavoring that occurs naturally in tea. Used in strawberry, apricot, peach, plum, hazelnut, pistachio, cinnamon, and walnut flavorings for beverages, ice cream, ices, candy, baked goods, liqueurs, and chewing gum.

PHENYLACETALDEHYDE • An oily, colorless liquid with a harsh odor. Upon dilution, emits the fragrance of lilacs and hyacinths. Derived from phenethyl alcohol *(see)*. A synthetic raspberry, strawberry, apricot, cherry, peach, honey, and spice flavoring for beverages, ice cream, ices, candy, baked goods, and chewing gum. Used also in perfumes. Less irritating than formaldehyde *(see)*, but a stronger central nervous system depressant. In addition, it sometimes produces fluid in the lungs upon ingestion. Because it is considered an irritant, it is not used in baby-cosmetic preparations.

PHENYLACETALDEHYDE 2,3-BUTYLENE GLYCOL ACETAL • A synthetic floral and fruit flavoring agent for candy *See* Phenylacetaldehyde for toxicity.

PHENYLACETALDEHYDE DIMETHYL ACETAL • A colorless liquid with a strong odor used as a synthetic fruit, apricot, cherry, honey, and spice flavoring agent for beverages, ice cream, ices, candy, baked goods, and chewing gum. Moderately toxic by ingestion.

PHENYLACETALDEHYDE GLYCERYL ACETAL • A synthetic floral and fruit flavoring agent for beverages, candy, ice cream, and ices. *See* Phenylacetaldehyde and Acetic Acid for toxicity.

PHENYLACETIC ACID • A synthetic flavoring agent that occurs naturally in Japanese mint, oil of neroli, and black pepper. A glistening, white solid with a persistent, honeylike odor. Used in butter, chocolate, rose, honey, and vanilla flavorings for beverages, ice cream, ices, candy, baked goods, gelatin desserts, chewing gum, liquors, and syrups. Used as a starting material in the manufacture of perfumes and soaps. Also used in the manufacture of penicillin. Moderately toxic by ingestion. Causes birth defects in experimental animals.

PHENYLALANINE • L form. An essential amino acid *(see)* considered essential for growth in normal human beings and not synthesized by the body. It is associated with phenylketonuria (PKU), an affliction that, if not detected soon after birth, leads to mental deterioration in children. Restricting phenylalanine in diets results in improvement. Whole egg contains 5.4 percent and skim milk 5.1 percent. Used to improve penetration of emollients. The FDA asked for further study of this amino acid as a food additive in 1980.

p-PHENYLENEDIAMINE • Most permanent home and beauty parlor dyes contain this chemical or a related one such as 4-nitro-*o*-phenylenediamine. Also called oxidation dyes, amino dyes, para dyes, or peroxide dyes. PPD was first introduced in 1890 for dyeing furs and feathers. It comes in about thirty shades and is used as an intermediate in coal tar dyes. May produce eczema, bronchial asthma, gastritis, skin rash, and death. Can crossreact with many other chemicals, including azo dyes used for temporary hair colorings. Can also produce photosensitization. It has reportedly caused cancer in some animal experiments and not in others.

2-PHENYLETHYL ISOVALERATE • *See* Phenethyl Isovalerate.

2-PHENYLPROPIONALDEHYDE • A synthetic berry, rose, apricot, cherry, peach, plum, and almond flavoring agent for beverages, ice cream, ices, candy, and baked goods.

3-PHENYLPROPIONALDEHYDE • A synthetic flavoring agent, slightly yellow, with a strong floral odor. Used in berry, rose, apricot, cherry, peach, plum, and almond flavorings for beverages, ice cream, ices, candy, and baked goods.

2-PHENYLPROPIONALDEHYDE DIMETHYL ACETAL • A synthetic berry, floral, rose, fruit, honey, mushroom, nut, and spice flavoring agent for beverages, ice cream, ices, candy, baked goods, chewing gum, and condiments. *See* Acetic Acid for toxicity.

3-PHENYLPROPYL ACETATE • A synthetic flavoring, colorless, with a spicy floral odor. Used in berry, fruit, and spice flavorings for beverages, ice cream, ices, candy, baked goods, chewing gum, and condiments. Propyl acetate may be irritating to skin and mucous membranes and narcotic in high concentrations.

2-PHENYLPROPYL BUTYRATE • A synthetic flavoring used in beverages, ice cream, ices, candy, and baked goods. No specific flavorings listed.

3-PHENYLPROPYL CINNAMATE • A synthetic butter, caramel, chocolate, cocoa, coconut, grape, and spice flavoring agent for beverages, ice cream, ices, candy, and baked goods.

3-PHENYLPROPYL FORMATE • Formic Acid. A synthetic currant, raspberry, butter, caramel, apricot, peach, and honey flavoring agent for beverages, ice cream, ices, candy, and baked goods. *See* Formic Acid for toxicity.

3-PHENYLPROPYL HEXANOATE • A synthetic fruit flavoring for beverages, ice cream, ices, candy, and baked goods. No known toxicity.

2-PHENYLPROPYL ISOBUTYRATE • A synthetic fruit flavoring for beverages, ice cream, ices, and candy. No known toxicity.

3-PHENYLPROPYL ISOBUTYRATE • A synthetic apple, apricot, peach, pear, pineapple, and plum flavoring agent for beverages, ice cream, ices, candy, and baked goods. No known toxicity.

3-PHENYLPROPYL ISOVALERATE • A synthetic butter, caramel, apple, pear, and nut flavoring agent for beverages, ice cream, ices, candy, and baked goods.

3-PHENYLPROPYL PROPIONATE • A synthetic apricot flavoring for beverages, ice cream, ices, candy, and baked goods.

2-3(3-PHENYLPROPYL) TETRAHYDROFURAN • A synthetic fruit, honey, and maple flavoring agent for beverages, ice cream, ices, candy, gelatin, puddings, and chewing gum.

PHORATE • Thimet. Vegfru. An insecticide used in animal feed. On EPA Extremely Hazardous Substances List and EPA Genetic Toxicology Program *(see both)*. Poison by ingestion. Causes mutations in experimental animals and interferes with nerve signals.

PHOSALONE • An insecticide used to kill insects and mites. FDA residue tolerance resulting from application on dried apple pomace is 85 ppm; on dried prunes, 40 ppm; on raisins, 20 ppm; on dried citrus pulp, 12 ppm; on dried grape pomace, 45 ppm; and on tea, 8 ppm. *See* Organophosphates.

PHOSPHATE • A salt of ester of phosphoric acid *(see)*. Used as an emulsifier and texturizer and sequestering agent *(see)* in foods. Sodium phosphate is used in evaporated milk up to 0.1 percent of weight. A carbonated beverage contains phosphoric acid. Without sufficient phosphate there is abnormal parathyroid (gland) function, bone metabolism, intestinal absorption, malnutrition, and kidney malfunction. Chemicals that interfere with phosphate action include detergents, mannitol (an alcohol used as a dietary supplement, the basis of dietetic sweets), vitamin D, and aluminum hydroxide *(see),* a leavening agent. Ingestion of large amounts of phosphates can cause kidney damage and may adversely affect the absorption of other minerals.

PHOSPHATE, AMMONIUM • Dibasic and Monobasic. *See* Ammonium Phosphate.

PHOSPHATE, CALCIUM HEXAMETA- • *See* Calcium Hexametaphosphate.

PHOSPHATE, CALCIUM, MONOBASIC and TRIBASIC • *See* Calcium Phosphate.

PHOSPHATE, POTASSIUM • Monobasic and Dibasic. *See* Potassium Phosphate.

PHOSPHATED DISTARCH PHOSPHATE • The final report to the FDA of the Select Committee on GRAS Substances stated in 1980 that there is no available evidence that it is a hazard to the public when used as it is now and it should continue its GRAS status with limitations on amounts that can be added to food. *See* Modified Starches.

PHOSPHOLIPIDS • Phosphatides. Complex fat substances found in all living cells. Lecithin is an example. It is used in hand creams and lotions. Phospholipids contain phosphoric acid and nitrogen and are soluble in the usual fat solvents, with the exception of acetone *(see).* They are used in moisturizers because they bind water and hold it in place. No known toxicity.

***n*-(PHOSPHONOMETHYL)GLYCINE** • An herbicide used in animal feed, imported olives, palm oil, soybean oil, dried tea, and instant tea. FDA's residue allowances: 30 ppm in molasses, sugarcane; 0.1 ppm in palm oil; 0.1 ppm in olives; 1 ppm in dried tea; 4 ppm in instant tea. Moderately toxic by ingestion.

PHOSPHORIC ACID • A colorless, odorless solution made from phosphate rock. Mixes with water and alcohol. A sequestering agent *(see)* for rendered animal fat or a combination of such fat with vegetable fat. Also used as an acidulant and flavoring in soft drinks, jellies, frozen dairy products, bakery products, candy, cheese products, and in the brewing industry. It is also used as a sequestrant and antioxidant in hair tonics, nail polishes, and skin fresheners. Concentrated solutions are irritating to the skin and mucous membranes. The final report to the FDA of the Select Committee on GRAS Substances stated in 1980 that it should continue its GRAS status with no limitations other than good manufacturing practices.

PHOSPHOROUS CHLORIDE • Phosphate derivative used as a starch modifier and a chlorinating agent. Intensely irritating to the skin, eyes, and mucous membranes. Inhalation may cause fluid in the lungs.

PHOSPHOROUS OXYCHLORIDE • Phosphoryl Chloride. Colorless, clear, strongly fuming vapors, used as a starch modifier and as a solvent and chlorinating agent. Inhalation may cause pulmonary edema.

PHOSPHOROUS SOURCES • Calcium Phosphate, Magnesium Phosphate, Potassium Glycerophosphate, and Sodium Phosphate. Mineral supplements for cereal products, particularly breakfast foods such as farina. They are also used in incendiary bombs and tracer bullets. Phosphorus was formerly used to treat rickets and degenerative disorders. *See* Phosphate.

PHOTOSENSITIVITY • A condition in which the application or ingestion of certain chemicals, such as propylparaben *(see)*, causes skin problems—including rash, hyperpigmentation, and swelling—when the skin is exposed to sunlight.

PHTHALATES • Salts of phthalic acid *(see)* used to make food packaging. Their use has increased steadily since the 1950s. By the mid-1980s, worldwide production was estimated at 2.7 million tons per year. They are now widespread environmental pollutants and concern about their use has been mounting because some of the phthalates have been shown to damage the testes and decrease sperm production. Butyl benzyl phthalate (BBP) and di-n-butyl phthalate (DBP) also act like estrogens. Phthalates in the environment are regarded as endocrine disrupters. The British Ministry of Agriculture, Fisheries and Food found that there were phthalates in infant formulae but below tolerable daily intakes (TDI) but that as "a matter of prudence phthalate levels should be reduced in infant formulae." May be cancer causing. In 1998, a panel including a former surgeon general was formed to study the safety of phthalates.

PHTHALIC ACID • Obtained by oxidation of various benzene derivatives, it can be isolated from the fungus *Gibberella fujikuroi*. It is used in the manufacture of plastics, dyes, and nail polishes. Moderately irritating to the skin and mucous membranes. *See* Phthalates.

PHTHALIC ANHYDRIDE • White crystalline needles derived from naphthalene *(see)*. Used as a hardener for resins and a plasticizer. Also used in many dyes, chlorinated products, insecticides, and polyesters. A skin irritant. *See* Phthalates.

PHTHALIMIDOMETHYL-O,O-DIMETHYL PHOSPHORODITHIOATE • APPA. Kemolate. Prolate. Smidan. A widely used insecticide in cottonseed oil. FDA residue tolerance is 0.2 ppm in cottonseed. EPA Extremely Hazardous Substance List *(see)*. A human poison by ingestion. *See* Phthalates.

PHYTIC ACID • Occurs in nature in the seeds of cereal grains and is derived commercially from corn. It is used to chelate heavy metals, as a rust inhibitor, in metal cleaning, and in the treatment of hard water. Nontoxic, although those allergic to corn may have a reaction.

PHYTOCHEMICAL • Phytochemicals are substances found in edible fruits and vegetables that may be ingested by humans daily in gram quantities and that exhibit a potential for modulating the human metabolism in a manner favorable for reducing risk of cancer.

PICHIA PASTORIS YEAST • *See* Yeast.

PICLORAM • Crystalline solid made from picolinic acid, it is used as an herbicide and defoliant. It is toxic by ingestion and inhalation. Its use has been restricted in the U.S. The FDA permits tolerances of 3 ppm in milled fractions (except flour) of barley, oats, and wheat resulting from application to the growing crop; 1 ppm in flour of barley and wheat; 0.2 ppm as residue in fat, meat byproducts, and meat of cattle, goats, hogs, and sheep; 0.05 ppm as residue in milk and eggs; and 0.5 as residue in oat, barley, and wheat grains.

PICRAMIC ACID • 4,6-Dinitro-2-Aminophenol. A red crystalline acid obtained from phenol *(see)* and used chiefly in making azo dyes *(see)*. Highly toxic material. Readily absorbed through intact skin. Vapors absorbed through respiratory tract. Produces marked increase in metabolism and temperature, profuse sweating, collapse, and death. May cause skin rash, cataracts, and weight loss.

PILEWORT EXTRACT • An extract of *Ranunculus ficaria,* the coarse, hairy, perennial figwort of the eastern and central U.S. It was once used to treat tuberculosis. No known toxicity.

PIMARICIN • Natamycin. An antibiotic from *Streptomyces chattanoogensis* used as a fungicide and mold inhibitor in cheese and wine. It is used in human medicine to treat fungal infections of the eye or eyelid. Potential adverse reactions include swelling around the eyes. Moderately toxic by ingestion.

PIMENTA LEAF OIL • Jamaica Pepper. Allspice. Derived from the dried ripe fruit of the evergreen shrub grown in the West Indies and Central and South America. Used in raspberry, fruit, nut, and spice flavorings for beverages, ice cream, ices, candy, baked goods, gelatin desserts, chewing gum, condiments, and meat products. Moderately toxic by ingestion. A severe skin irritant. GRAS.

PINE BARK, WHITE, SOLID EXTRACT • Extract from *Pinus strobus,* used as a flavoring.

PINE CONE EXTRACT • An extract from the cones of *Pinus sylvestris. See* Pine Needle Oil.

PINE MOUNTAIN OIL • *See* Pine Needle Oil and Pine Needle Dwarf Oil.

PINE NEEDLE DWARF OIL • Pine Mountain Oil. The volatile oil obtained by steam distillation from a variety of pine trees, *Pinus mugo turra* var. Colorless with a pleasant pine smell. Used in citrus, pineapple, and liquor flavorings for beverages, ice cream, ices, candy, and baked goods. There is reported use of the chemical, it has not yet been assigned for toxicology literature.

PINE NEEDLE OIL • Pine Mountain Oil. An extract of various species of Pinus used as a natural flavoring in pineapple, citrus, and spice flavorings. Also used to scent bath products. Ingestion of large amounts can cause intestinal hemorrhages.

PINE SCOTCH OIL • Volatile oil obtained by steam distillation from the needles of a pine tree. Colorless or yellowish, with an odor of turpentine. Used in various flavorings for beverages, candy, and baked goods. *See* Turpentine for toxicity.

PINE TAR • A product obtained by distillation of pinewood. A blackish brown, viscous liquid, slightly soluble in water. Used as an antiseptic in skin diseases. May be irritating to the skin.

PINE TAR OIL • The extract from a variety of pine trees. A synthetic flavoring obtained from a species of pinewood. Used in licorice flavorings for ice cream, ices, and candy. Also used as a solvent, disinfectant, and deodorant. As a *pine tar,* it is used in hair tonics; also a solvent, disinfectant, and deodorant. As an *oil* from twigs and needles, it is used in pine bath-oil emulsions, bath salts, and perfumery. Irritating to the skin and mucous membranes. *Bomyl acetate,* a substance obtained from various pine needles, has a strong pine odor and is used in bath oils. It can cause nausea, vomiting, convulsions, and dizziness if ingested. In general, pine oil in concentrated form is an irritant to human skin and may cause allergic reactions. In small amounts it is nontoxic.

PINEAPPLE EXTRACT • *See* Pineapple Juice.

PINEAPPLE JUICE • The common juice from the tropical plant. Contains a protein-digesting and milk-clotting enzyme, bromelin *(see)*. An anti-inflammatory enzyme, it is used in cosmetic treatment creams. It is also used as a texturizer. No known toxicity.

a-**PINENE** • A synthetic flavoring agent that occurs naturally in angelica root oil, anise, star anise, asafetida oil, coriander, cumin, fennel, grapefruit, juniper berries, oils of lavender and lime, mandarin orange leaf, black pepper, peppermint, pimenta, and yarrow. It is the principal ingredient of turpentine *(see)*. Used chiefly in the manufacture of camphor. Used in lemon and nutmeg flavorings for beverages, ice cream, ices, candy, baked goods, and condiments. Also used as a chewing-gum base. Readily absorbed from the gastrointestinal tract, the skin, and the respiratory tract. It is a local irritant, central nervous system depressant, and an irritant to the bladder and kidney. Has caused benign skin tumors from chronic contact.

2-PINENE • *See a*-Pinene.

b-**PINENE** • A synthetic flavoring that occurs naturally in black-currant buds, coriander, cumin, black pepper, and yarrow herb. Used in citrus flavorings for beverages, ice cream, ices, candy (600 ppm), and baked goods (600 ppm). Also cleared for use in chewing-gum base. *See a*-Pinene for toxicity.

PINUS PUMILO OIL • *See* Pine Needle Dwarf Oil.

PIPERAZINE • Adipate and Citrate. Entacyl. Antepar. Bryrel. Pin-Tega Tabs. Pipril. Ta-Verm. Vermirex. Vermizine. An anthelmintic ingredient that paralyzes worms, causing their expulsion by normal movement of the human intestines. Adverse reactions include incoordination, numbness, seizures, memory problems, headache, dizziness, eye problems, nausea, vomiting, diarrhea, abdominal cramps, hives, skin rashes, joint pain, fever, bronchospasm, and anemia.

PIPERIDINE • A synthetic flavoring that occurs naturally in black pepper. Used in beverages, candy, baked goods, meats, soups, and condiments. Soapy texture. Has been proposed for use as a tranquilizer and muscle relaxant.

PIPERINE • Celery Soda. A synthetic flavoring agent that occurs naturally in black pepper, it is used as a pungent brandy flavoring. It is also used as a nontoxic insecticide. Believed to be more toxic than the commercial pyrethrins.

PIPERITONE • A synthetic flavoring agent that occurs naturally in Japanese mint. Used in beverages, ice cream, ices, candy, and baked goods. Used to give dentifrices a minty flavor and to give perfumes their peppermint scent.

PIPERONAL • Heliotropin. A synthetic flavoring and perfume agent that occurs naturally in vanilla and black pepper. White crystalline powder with a sweet floral odor. Used in strawberry, cola, cherry, rum, maple, nut, and vanilla flavorings in beverages, ice cream, ices, baked goods, gelatin puddings, and chewing gum. Used chiefly in perfumery. Ingestion of large amounts may cause central nervous system depression. Has been reported to cause skin rash. In lipsticks, said to produce marking of the skin. Not recommended by some cosmetic chemists because of its ability to produce skin irritation.

PIPERONYL ACETATE • A synthetic fruit flavoring agent for beverages, ice cream, ices, candy, and baked goods. *See* Piperonal for toxicity.

PIPERONYL ALDEHYDE • *See* Piperonal.

PIPERONYL BUTOXIDE • Butoxide. Pyburthrin. Butocide. A light brown liquid, a widely used insecticide in animal feed, dried foods, milled fractions derived from cereal grains, and packaging materials. It is used in combination with pyrethrins *(see)* in oil solutions, emulsions, powders, or aerosols. FDA permits residues of up to 10 ppm in milled fractions derived from cereal grains, in dried foods, and in animal feed. International Agency for Research on Cancer (IARC) review and on the Community Right-To-Know List. No evidence, as yet, that it is a cancer-causing agent, but it is poisonous by skin contact. Moderately toxic by ingestion. Large doses have caused vomiting and diarrhea in humans. Has shown adverse reproductive effects in experimental animals.

PIPERONYL ISOBUTYRATE • A synthetic fruit and cheese flavoring for beverages, ice cream, ices, candy, and baked goods. *See* Piperonal for toxicity.

PIPERONYL PIPERIDINE • *See* Piperine.

PIPSISSEWA LEAVES EXTRACT • Love-in-Winter. Prince's Pine. Extracted from the leaves of an evergreen shrub. Used in root beer, sarsaparilla, wintergreen, and birch beer flavorings for beverages and candy. Its leaves have been used as an astringent, diuretic, and tonic. The Cree name means "to break up"—bladder stones, that is. GRAS. There is reported use of the chemical, it has not yet been assigned for toxicology literature.

PLANT ESTROGENS • A host of estrogens have been identified in plants. Although they are considerably less active than those in animals, chronic exposure may lead to the accumulation of levels that are active in humans.

PLANT STEROLS • Vitamin D precursors found in broccoli, cabbage, cucumbers, squash, yams, tomatoes, eggplant, peppers, soy products, and whole grains. They cause cells to differentiate.

PLANTAIN EXTRACT • The extract of various species of plantain. The starchy fruit is a staple throughout the tropics and is used for bladder infections by herbalists. It is a natural astringent and antiseptic with soothing and cooling effects on blemishes and burns.

PLANTAROME • *See* Yucca Extract.

PLUM EXTRACT • The extract of the fruit of the plum tree, *Prunus domestica*. The Indians boiled the wild plum and gargled with it to cure mouth sores.

POLOXALENE • Therabloat. Bloat Guard. An animal-feed drug derived from ethylene oxide and propylene oxide used to prevent bloat, an excessive accumulation of gas in the stomachs of cattle. Severe bloat can be fatal. No known toxicity.

POLOXAMER 331 • A thick liquid used as a dough conditioner, foam control agent, solubilizing agent in flavor concentrates, as a detergent, and in a wash for poultry. FDA limits it to equal weight in flavor concentrations and to 0.5 percent in poultry baths; 5 grams per hog in dehairing machines; and 0.5 percent by weight of flour. No known toxicity, but when heated to decomposition, it emits acrid smoke and irritating fumes.

POLY- • A prefix meaning "many."

POLYACRYLAMIDE • The polymer of acrylamide monomers, it is a white solid, water soluble, that is used as a thickening agent, suspending agent, and as an additive to adhesives. In modified form it is used to clarify (*see* Clarifying Agent) cane sugar. Used as a film former in the imprinting of soft-shell gelatin capsules. Used in washing fruits and vegetables. Used in the manufacture of plastics used in nail polishes. Highly toxic and irritating to the skin. Causes central nervous system paralysis. Can be absorbed through unbroken skin.

POLYACRYLIC ACID • *See* Acrylic Resins.

POLYALKYL ACRYLATE • Used in the production of petroleum wax. *See* Petroleum.

POLYAMINO SUGAR CONDENSATE • The condensation product of the sugars fructose, galactose, glucose, lactose, maltose, mannose, rhamnose, ribose, or xylose, with a minute amount of amino acids such as alanine, arginine, aspartic acid, glutamic acid, glycine, histidine, hydroxyproline, isoleucine, leucine, lysine, methionine, phenylalanine, prolinee, pyroglutamic acid, serine, threonine, tyrosine, or valine. *See* Amino Acids.

POLYBUTENE • Indopol. Polybutylene. A plasticizer. A polymer *(see)* of one or more butylenes obtained from petroleum oils. Used in lubricating oil, adhesives, sealing tape, cable insulation, films, and coatings. May asphyxiate.

POLYCHLORBIPHENYLS (PCB) • Clear, amber-colored, or dark oily liquids. They may have a faint smell like motor oil, and some contain chlorobenzenes, which make them smell like mothballs. Widely used since the 1930s because of their excellent electrical and insulating abilities, PCBs were banned in 1978 by the Environmental Protection Agency. The toxic effects were first noted when over twelve hundred people in Japan were poisoned by eating food cooked in oil heavily contaminated with PCBs. Soon afterward, studies showed that PCBs caused cancer in test animals. PCBs, unfortunately, remain in the environment for a long time because they do not break down. Research at the University of Maryland reported in 1998 said children exposed to dioxins *(see)* and PCBs prenatally or during infancy can suffer behavioral, memory, and learning problems. The Maryland investigators suggest that the underlying mechanism may be thyroid hormone disruption. Even moderate impairment of thyroid hormone function has been associated with various problems in behavior and intellectual development, and certain thyroid diseases are associated with attention deficit hyperactivity disorder and language disorders. Studies of adults exposed to dioxin and PCBs show no marked neurological effects. The Maryland research was funded by the University and by the American Thyroid Association.

POLYDEXTROSE • A reduced-calorie bulking agent developed by Pfizer, Inc., and approved for use in foods by the FDA in June 1981. The FDA says it is not a substitute for saccharin *(see)* nor a general sweetener but that it can replace sucrose *(see)* as a bulking agent in frozen desserts, cakes, and candies and reduce calories in some products as much as 50 percent. According to Pfizer, it is a one-calorie-per-gram bulking agent capable of replacing higher calorie—four to nine calories per gram—ingredients such as sucrose, carbohydrates, and fats in many food products.

POLYETHOXYLATED ALKYLPHENOL • Dodecyl, Nonyl, and Octyl. Components of a commercial detergent for raw foods, followed by water rinsing. The only symptoms shown in animals poisoned with this substance is gastrointestinal irritation.

POLYETHYLENE • A polymer *(see)* of ethylene; a product of petroleum gas or dehydration of alcohol. One of a group of lightweight thermoplastics that have a good resistance to chemicals, low moisture absorption, and good insulating properties. Used as a chewing-gum base ingredient and as a film former and sheets for packaging. Also used as roughage replacement in feedlot rations for cattle. Used in hand lotions. No known skin toxicity, but implants of large amounts in rats caused cancer. Ingestion of large oral doses has produced kidney and liver damage.

POLYETHYLENE GLYCOL • 400–2,000 molecular weight. PEG. Defoaming agent in processed beet sugar and yeast. Used in hair straighteners, antiperspirants, baby products, fragrances, polish removers, hair tonics, lipsticks, and protective creams. It is a binder, plasticizing agent, solvent, and softener widely used for cosmetic cream bases and pharmaceutical ointments. Improves resistance to moisture and oxidation. At this writing, the FDA was doing a toxicology search.

POLYETHYLENE GLYCOL (600) DIOLEATE • Polyethylene glycol esters of mixed fatty acids from tall oil; polyethylene glycol (400 through 6,000). An agent in nonnutritive artificial sweeteners; a component of coatings and binders in tablet food; improves resistance to oxidation and moisture. *See* Polyols.

POLYGLYCERATE 60 • *See* Glycerides.

POLYGLYCEROL • Prepared from edible fats, oils, and esters of fatty acids. Derived from corn, cottonseed, palm, peanut, safflower, sesame, and soybean oils, lard, and tallow. Used as an emulsifier in cosmetics. No known toxicity.

POLYGLYCEROL ESTER • One of several partial or complete esters of saturated and unsaturated fatty acids with a variety of derivatives of polyglycerols.

POLYGLYCERYL-4 COCOATE • *See* Coconut Oil and Polyglycerol.

POLYGLYCERYL-10 DECALINOLEATE • *See* Polyglycerol and Linoleic Acid.

POLYGLYCERYL-10 DECAOLEATE • *See* Oleic Acid and Polyglycerol.

POLYGLYCERYL-2 DIISOSTEATE • *See* Isostearic Acid and Polyglycerol.

POLYGLYCERYL-6 DIOLEATE • *See* Oleic Acid and Glycerin.

POLYGLYCERYL-6 DISTEARATE • *See* Stearic Acid and Glycerin.

POLYGLYCERYL-3 HYDROXYLAURYL ETHER • *See* Fatty Alcohols and Glycerin.

POLYGLYCERYL-4 ISOSTEARATE • *See* Isostearic Acid and Glycerin.

POLYGLYCERYL-2 LANOLIN ALCOHOL ETHER • *See* Lanolin and Glycerin.

POLYGLYCERYL-LAURYL ETHER • *See* Fatty Alcohols and Glycerin.

POLYGLYCERYL-3, -4 OLEATE • Oily liquid prepared by adding alcohol to coconut oil or other triglycerides with a polyglyceryl. Used in foods, drugs, and cosmetics as fat emulsifiers in conjunction with other emulsifiers to prepare creams, lotions, and other emulsion products. In addition, they may also be used as lubricants, plasticizers, gelling agents, and dispersants. No known toxicity.

POLYGLYCERYL-3, -4, or -8 OLEATE • An ester of oleic acid and glycerin *(see both)*.

POLYGLYCERYL-2 or -4 OLEYL ETHER • The ether of oleyl alcohol and glycerin *(see both)*.

POLYGLYCERYL-3-PEG-2 COCOAMIDE • *See* Coconut Oil and Glycerin.

POLYGLYCERYL-2-PEG-4 STEARATE • An ether of peg-4 stearate and glycerin. *See* Stearic Acid and Glycerin.

POLYGLYCERYL-2-SESQUIISOSTEARATE • A mixture of esters of isostearic acid and glycerin *(see both)*.

POLYGLYCERYL-2-SESQUIOLEATE • A mixture of ester of oleic acid and glycerin *(see both)*.

POLYGLYCERYL SORBITOL • A condensation product of glycerin and sorbitol *(see both)*.

POLYGLYCERYL-3, -4, or -8 STEARATE • An ester of stearic acid and glycerin *(see both)*.

POLYGLYCERYL-10 TETRAOLEATE • An ester of oleic acid and glycerin *(see both)*.

POLYGLYCERYL-2 TETRASTEARATE • *See* Stearic Acid and Glycerin.

POLYISOBUTENE • *See* Polybutene.

POLYISOBUTYLENE • Soft to hard, elastic, light, white solid, odorless and tasteless. Used as a chewing substance in gum. *See* Resin, Isobutylene.

POLYISOBUTYLENE 317 • Ranging from diglycerol to triacontaglycerol. Prepared from edible fats, oils, and fatty acids, hydrogenated or nonhydrogenated *(see* Hydrogenation). Derived from corn, cottonseed, palm, peanut, safflower, sesame, and soybean oils, lard, and tallow. Used as lubricants, plasticizers, gelling agents, humectants, surfactants, dispersants, and emulsifiers in foods and cosmetic preparations.

POLYLIMONENE • A general fixative derived from citrus oils. It is used in candy (4,500 ppm), chewing gum, and baked goods (1,000 ppm). It can be a skin irritant and sensitizer. Although allowed as a food additive, there is no current reported use of the chemical, and therefore, although toxicology information may be available, the FDA is not updating it. *See* Limonene.

POLYMER • A substance or product formed by combining many small molecules (monomers). The result is essentially recurring long-chain structural units that have tensile strength, elasticity, and hardness. Examples of polymers (literally, "having many parts") are plastics, fibers, rubber, and human tissue.

POLYMIXIN B • A generic term for antibiotics obtained from fermentation of various media by strains of *Bacillus polymyxa*. Used as a bactericide in yeast culture for beer. May cause renal irritation and damage.

POLYOLS • Alcohol compounds that absorb moisture. They have a low molecular weight: polyols with a weight above 1,000 are solids and less toxic than those with weight 600 or below. The latter are liquid, and although higher in toxicity, large doses are required to kill animals. Such deaths in animals have been found to be due to kidney damage. *See* Propylene Glycol and Polyethylene Glycol as examples.

POLYOXYALKALENE GLYCOL • Defoaming agent in beet sugar production. No known toxicity.

POLYOXYETHYLENE COMPOUNDS • Nonionic emulsifiers used in hand creams and lotions. Usually oily or waxy liquids. No known toxicity.

POLYOXYETHYLENE GLYCOL • Ester of edible cottonseed oil and fatty acids. Solubilizing agent in pickles. No known toxicity.

POLYOXYETHYLENE GLYCOL (600) MONORICINOLEATE • Defoaming component used in processing beet sugar and yeast. No known toxicity.

POLYOXYETHYLENE (40) MONOSTEARATE • Defoaming agent in processed foods; emulsifier for frozen desserts. Application to the skin of mice has been shown to cause skin tumors. The compound has been fed to animals and does not appear to produce tumors on its own, but there is a suggestion that it allows cancer-causing agents to penetrate more quickly. On the FDA list for further study for long- and short-term effects since 1980.

POLYOXYETHYLENE (20) SORBITAN MONOOLEATE • Emulsifier and defoamer in the production of beet sugar; a dietary vitamin and mineral supplement. Used in dill oil in spiced green beans, icing, frozen custard, iced milk, fruit, and sherbet. The FDA asked for short-term, mutagenic, teratogenic, subacute, and reproductive effects in 1980 and has not reported any findings since.

POLYOXYETHYLENE (20) SORBITAN MONOPALMITATE • An emulsifier, flavor-dispersing agent, and defoaming agent. Used in whipped cream, beverages, confectionery, and soup. The FDA asked for further study of the safety of this additive in 1980 and has reported nothing about it since.

POLYOXYETHYLENE (20) SORBITAN MONOSTEARATE • Polysorbate 60. An emulsifier and flavor-dispersing agent in shortening and edible oils. Used in whipped vegetable-oil topping, cake, and cake mixes; cake icing or filling; sugar-type confection coatings; coconut spread; beverage mixes; confectionery; chicken bases; gelatin desserts; dressings made without egg yolks; solid-state, edible vegetable-fat water emulsions used in substitutes for milk or cream; dietary vitamin supplements; foaming agents in nonalcoholic beverage mixes to be added to alcoholic beverages; and a wetting and dispersing agent for powdered processed foods. The FDA asked for further study of this additive in 1980.

POLYOXYETHYLENE (20) SORBITAN TRISTEARATE • An emulsifier, defoaming agent, and flavor-dispersing agent. Used in cakes and cake mixes, including doughnuts, whipped mixes, whipped vegetable-oil toppings, cake icings and fillings, ice cream, frozen custard, ice milk, fruit sherbet, and nonstandardized frozen desserts; solid-state, edible vegetable fat-water emulsions used as substitutes for milk or cream in coffee; and a wetting and dispersing agent in processed powdered food. No known toxicity.

POLYOXYETHYLENE STEARATE • A mixture of stearate (*see* Stearic Acid) and ethylene oxide, it is a waxy solid once added to bread to make it "feel fresh."

It was fed to rats as one-fourth of their diets and resulted in the formation of bladder stones, and subsequently a number of tumors. Banned in 1952.

POLYOXYPROPYLENE GLYCOL • Defoaming agent for yeast and beet sugar. No known toxicity.

POLYSACCHARIDES • Carbohydrates that are organic compounds consisting of carbon, hydrogen, and oxygen. The polysaccharides include starch, dextrin, glycogen, and cellulose.

POLYSORBATE 60 and POLYSORBATE 80 • Both are emulsifiers that have been associated with the contaminant 1,4 dioxane, known to cause cancer in animals. The 60 is a condensate of sorbitol with stearic acid, and the 80 is a condensate of sorbitol and oleic acid *(see all)*. The 60 is waxy, soluble in solvents, and is used as an emulsifier, stabilizer, wetting, and dispersing agent for powdered processed foods, and a foaming agent for beverage mixes. It is added to chocolate coatings to prevent cocoa-butter substitutes from tasting greasy. It is found in frozen and gelatin desserts, cakes, cake mixes, doughnuts, and artificial chocolate coatings, nondairy whipped cream and creamers, powdered convenience foods, salad dressings made without egg yolks, and vitamin supplements. The 80 is a viscous liquid with a faint caramel odor and is used as an emulsifier, stabilizer, and humectant. It prevents oil from separating from nondairy whipped cream and helps nondairy coffee whiteners to dissolve. It is also found in baked goods, ice cream, frozen custard, shortenings, and vitamin and mineral supplements. FDA residue tolerances in various products are from less than 0.1 percent to 4.5 percent. Polysorbate 80 is also widely used in baby lotions, cold creams, cream deodorants, antiperspirants, suntan lotions, and in bath oil products. *Polysorbate 40* is also widely used as an emulsifier in cosmetic creams and lotions and as a stabilizer of essential oils in water.

POLYSORBATE 80 WITH CARRAGEENAN • *See* Polysorbates and Carrageenan.

POLYSORBATES • 1 through 85. These are widely used emulsifiers and stabilizers. For example, *polysorbate 20* is a viscous, oily liquid derived from lauric acid. Used in vitamins, pickle products, mineral preparations, in special diet foods, along or in combination with sorbitan. They are also used as dispersing agents in gelatin desserts and mixes; and up to 10 ppm in finished table salt: They are used in creaming mixtures for cottage cheese and low-fat cottage cheese and as a surfactant and wetting agent for natural and artificially colored barbecue sauces. It is an emulsifier used in cosmetic creams and lotions and a stabilizer of essential oils in water. It is used as a nonionic surfactant *(see)*.

POLYSTYRENE • Used in the manufacture of cosmetic resins. Reported to be an unintentional additive when tea and coffee are drunk from polystyrene cups. Colorless to yellowish, oily liquid with a penetrating odor. Obtained from ethylbenzene by removing the hydrogen or by chlorination. Sparingly soluble in water; soluble in alcohol. May be irritating to the eyes and mucous membranes and, in high concentrations, may be narcotic.

POLYUNSAT FAT • Listing on food labels for polyunsaturated fats *(see)*.

POLYUNSATURATED FATS • The saturation of fat refers to the chemical structure of its constituent fatty acids. Polyunsaturates are liquid at room temperature and consist mainly of fatty acids that can hold four or more additional hydrogen atoms. *See* Monounsaturated Fats.

POLYVINYL ACETATE • Used in chewing-gum base.

POLYVINYL ALCOHOL 9 • Synthetic resins used to dilute the color of eggshells and used in lipstick, setting lotions, and various creams. A polymer is prepared from polyvinyl acetates by replacement of the acetate groups with the hydroxyl groups. Dry, unplasticized polyvinyl-alcohol powders are white to cream colored and have different viscosities. Solvent in hot and cold water but certain ones require alcohol-water mixtures. FDA requires no penetration of polyvinyl alcohol through eggshell. An experimental cancer-causing and tumor-inducing agent. International Agency for Research on Cancer (IARC) *(see)* review.

POLYVINYL BUTYRAL • The condensation of polyvinyl alcohol and butyraldehyde *(see both)*. It is a synthetic flavoring found in coffee and strawberry and is used in the manufacture of rubber and synthetic resins and plasticizers. May be an irritant and narcotic.

POLYVINYL CHLORIDE (PVC) • Chloroethylene Polymer. Derived from vinyl chloride *(see),* it consists of a white powder or colorless granules that are resistant to weather, moisture, acids, fats, petroleum products, and fungus. It is widely used for everything from plumbing to raincoats. The use of PVC as a plastic wrap for food, including meats, and for human blood, has alarmed some scientists. Human and animal blood can extract potentially harmful chemicals from the plastic. The chemicals are added to polyvinyl chloride to make it flexible, and they migrate from the plastic into the blood and into the meats in amounts directly proportional to the length of time of storage. The result can be contamination of the blood, causing lung shock, a condition in which the patient's blood circulation to the lungs is impeded. PVC is also used in cosmetics and toiletries in containers, nail enamels, and creams. PVC has caused tumors when injected under the skin of rats in doses of one hundred milligrams per kilogram of body weight.

POLYVINYL ETHYL ETHER • *See* Polyvinyl Alcohol.

POLYVINYL IMIDAZOLINIUM ACETATE • The polymer of vinyl imidazolinium aceta. *See* Polyvinylpyrrolidone.

POLYVINYL METHYL ETHER • *See* Polyvinyl Alcohol.

POLY(2-VINYLPYRIDICINE-CO-STYRENE) • A coating for nutrients for cattle. *See* Polyvinylpyrrolidone and Styrene.

POLYVINYLPYRROLIDONE (PVP) • A faintly yellow, solid plastic resin resembling albumin. Used in dietary products. Also a clarifying agent in vinegar, beer, and wine. Limitation of six pounds per thousand gallons in wine. FDA requires that it be removed by filtration. The FDA residue tolerance is less than 10 ppm in beer, less than 40 ppm in vinegar and 60 ppm in wine from use as a clarifying agent; and less than 60 ppm as a tableting adjuvant in nonnutritive sweeteners and in flavor, vitamin, and mineral concentrates in tablet form. Ingestion may produce gas and fecal impaction or damage to lungs and kidneys. It may last in the system several months to a year. Strong circumstantial evidence indicates thesaurosis—foreign bodies in the lung—may be produced in susceptible individuals from concentrated exposure to PVP in hairsprays. Modest intravenous doses in rats caused them to develop tumors.

POMEGRANATE BARK EXTRACT • A flavoring from the dried bark, stem, or root of the tree _Punica granatum,_ in the Mediterranean region and elsewhere. Contains about 20 percent tannic acid _(see);_ rind of fruit contains 30 percent. Formerly used to expel tapeworms. Overdose can cause nausea, vomiting, and diarrhea. GRAS. There is reported use of the chemical; it has not yet been assigned for toxicology literature.

POPLAR EXTRACT • Balm of Gilead. Extract of the leaves and twigs of _Populus nigra._ In ancient times, the buds were mashed to make a soothing salve that was spread on sunburned areas, scalds, scratches, inflamed skin, and wounds. They were also simmered in lard for use as an ointment and for antiseptic purposes. The leaves and bark were steeped by American colonists to make a soothing tea. It supposedly helped allergies and soothed reddened eyes. Used as a flavoring in alcoholic beverages only.

POPPY SEED • The seed of the poppy, _Papaver somniferum._ Used as a natural spice for flavoring for baked goods (8,600 ppm). Also used in the manufacture of paints, varnishes, and soaps. GRAS.

POT MARIGOLD • _See_ Marigold, Pot. GRAS.

POT MARJORAM • _See_ Marjoram, Pot. GRAS.

POTASSIUM • The healthy human body contains about nine grams of potassium. Most of it is found inside body cells. Potassium plays an important role in maintaining water balance and acid-base balance. It participates in the transmission of nerve impulses and in the transfer of messages from nerves to muscles. It also acts as a catalyst in carbohydrate and protein metabolism. Potassium is important for the maintenance of normal kidney function. It has a major effect on the heart and all the muscles of the body.

POTASSIUM ACETATE • Colorless, water-absorbing crystals or powder, odorless or with a faint acetic aroma and a salty taste. Used as a buffer and antimicrobial preservative. Very soluble in water. Also used medicinally to treat irregular heartbeat and as a diuretic. The GRAS designation was removed by the FDA in the 1990s.

POTASSIUM ACID TARTRATE • The salt of tartaric acid. Colorless with a pleasant odor. An acid and buffer, it is the acid constituent of some baking powders. Used in effervescent beverages. It is also used in some confectionery products. Formerly a cathartic.

POTASSIUM ALGINATE • A stabilizer _(see)._ GRAS. _See_ Alginates.

POTASSIUM ALUM • _See_ Alum.

POTASSIUM ASPARTAME • _See_ Aspartame.

POTASSIUM ASPARTATE • The potassium salt of aspartic acid _(see)._

POTASSIUM BENZOATE • A preservative used in margarine and wine. FDA limits the amount to 0.1 percent or if used in combination with sorbic acid _(see)_ to 0.2 percent in margarine and 0.1 percent in wine. _See_ Benzoic Acid.

POTASSIUM BICARBONATE • Carbonic Acid, Monopotassium Salt. Colorless, odorless, transparent crystals or powder, slightly alkaline, salty taste. Considered a miscellaneous and/or general-purpose food additive, it is present in fluids and tissues of the body as a product of normal metabolic processes. Soluble in water. It is used in baking, soft drinks, and in low-pH liquid detergents. The final report to the FDA of the Select Committee on GRAS Substances stated in 1980 that it should continue its GRAS status with no limitations other than good manufacturing practices.

POTASSIUM BISULFITE • Same uses as for sodium sulfite *(see)* in ale, beer, and fruit-pie mix. Not to be used in foods containing vitamin B_1, raw fruit and vegetables including fresh potatoes (not frozen, canned or dehydrated). The final report to the FDA of the Select Committee on GRAS Substances stated in 1980 that there is no evidence in the available information that it is a hazard to the public when used as it is now and it should continue its GRAS status with limitations on the amounts that can be added to food. *See* Sulfites.

POTASSIUM BROMATE • The compound is added as an improving agent in bread. The expected result is to obtain a fine spongelike quality with the action of oxygen. This method is used in Great Britain, the United States, and Japan. Legal allowance of potassium bromate is below 50 ppm in white flour and 75 ppm in whole wheat flour. Antiseptic and astringent in toothpaste, mouthwashes, and gargles as 3 to 5 percent solution. Colorless or white crystals. Very toxic when taken internally. Burns and skin irritation have been reported from its industrial uses. In toothpaste it has been reported to have caused inflammation and bleeding of gums. In 1980, the Ames Test *(see)* found it to be a mutagen. The FAO-WHO Expert Committee on Food Additives said in 1993 that new data about potassium bromate showed long-term toxicity and carcinogenicity including kidney tumors, tumors of the lining of the stomach, and thyroid tumors in rats and slightly increased kidney tumors in hamsters. On the basis of the new safety data and the new data on residual bromate in bread, the Committee concluded the use of potassium bromate, as a flour treatment agent was not appropriate. The previous acceptable level of treatment of flours for bread-making was therefore withdrawn.

POTASSIUM BROMIDE • A preservative used in washing fruits and vegetables. Used medicinally as a sedative and antiepileptic. In large doses it can cause central nervous system depression. Prolonged intake may cause bromism. Bromism's main symptoms are headache, mental inertia, slow heartbeat, gastric distress, skin rash, acne, muscular weakness, and occasionally violent delirium. Bromides can cross the placental barrier and have caused skin rashes in the fetus.

POTASSIUM CARBONATE • Salt of Tartar. Pearl Ash. Inorganic salt of potassium. Odorless, white powder soluble in water but practically insoluble in alcohol. Used as an alkali in combination with potassium hydroxide *(see)* for extracting color from annatto seed *(see)*. Also used in confections and cocoa products. Used in freckle lotions, liquid shampoos, vanishing creams, setting lotions, and permanent-wave lotions; also in the manufacture of soap, glass, pottery, and to finish leather. Formerly employed as a diuretic to reduce body water and as an alkalizer. Irritating and caustic to human skin and may cause dermatitis of the scalp, forehead, and hands. The final report to the FDA of the Select Committee on GRAS Substances stated in 1980 that it should continue its GRAS status with no limitations other than good manufacturing practices.

POTASSIUM CASEINATE • The potassium salt of milk proteins used in ice cream, frozen custard, ice milk, and fruit sherbets. *See* Casein.

POTASSIUM CHLORIDE • A colorless, crystalline, odorless powder with a salty taste. A yeast food used in the brewing industry to improve brewing and fermentation and in the jelling industry. Small intestinal ulcers may occur with oral administration. Large doses ingested can cause gastrointestinal irritation, purging, weakness, and circulatory collapse. Used as a substitute for sodium chloride *(see)* in low-sodium dietary foods. The final report to the FDA of the Select Committee on GRAS Substances stated in 1980 that it should continue its GRAS status with no limitations other than good manufacturing practices.

POTASSIUM CITRATE • A transparent or white powder, odorless, with a cool, salty taste. Used as a buffer in confections and in artificially sweetened jellies and preserves. It is a urinary alkalizer and gastric antacid. No known toxicity. The final report to the FDA of the Select Committee on GRAS Substances stated in 1980 that it should continue its GRAS status with no limitations other than good manufacturing practices.

POTASSIUM COCOATE • *See* Coconut Oil.

POTASSIUM COCO-HYDROLYZED PROTEIN • *See* Proteins.

POTASSIUM CORNATE • The potassium salt of fatty acids derived from corn oil. *See* Corn Oil.

POTASSIUM CYCLAMATE • Nonnutritive sweetener removed from the GRAS list in 1969 and is now illegal in foods.

POTASSIUM GIBBERELLATE • The salt of gibberellic acid, a plant growth-promoting hormone. White crystalline powder that absorbs water. Used as an enzyme activator in fermented malt beverages. FDA limits it to 2 ppm in treated barley malt and 0.5 ppm in the finished beverage.

POTASSIUM GLUCONATE • The potassium salt of gluconic acid *(see)* used as a buffering agent that helps keep soda water bubbling. Mildly toxic by ingestion. The final report to the FDA of the Select Committee on GRAS Substances stated in 1980 that it should continue its GRAS status with no limitations other than good manufacturing practices.

POTASSIUM GLYCEROPHOSPHATE • Nutrient additive. *See* Glycerides. GRAS.

POTASSIUM HYDROXIDE • Caustic Potash. An alkali used to extract color from annatto seed, a peeling agent for tubers and fruits, also in cacao products. Occasionally used to prevent the growth of horns in calves. It is used as an emulsifier in hand lotions, as a cuticle softener, and as an alkali in liquid soaps, protective creams, shaving preparations, and cream rouges. Prepared industrially by electrolysis of potassium chloride *(see)*. White or slightly yellow lumps. It may cause irritation of the skin in cuticle removers. Extremely corrosive, and ingestion may cause violent pain, bleeding, collapse, and death. When applied to the skin of mice, moderate dosages cause tumors. May cause skin rash and burning.

Concentrations above 5 percent can destroy fingernails as well. Good-quality toilet soaps do not contain more than 0.25 percent free alkali. The FDA banned household products containing more than 10 percent potassium hydroxide. GRAS.

POTASSIUM HYPOPHOSPHATE • The final report to the FDA of the Select Committee on GRAS Substances stated in 1980 that it should continue its GRAS status with no limitations other than good manufacturing practices. *See* Phosphate.

POTASSIUM IODATE • *See* Iodine Sources. GRAS.

POTASSIUM IODIDE • Potassium Salt. A dye remover and an antiseptic. Used in table salt as a source of dietary iodine. It is also in some drinking water. May cause allergic reactions. GRAS.

POTASSIUM LACTATE • Flavoring. *See* Lactic Acid. GRAS.

POTASSIUM LAURATE • The potassium salt of lauric acid *(see)*.

POTASSIUM LAURYL SULFATE • A water softener used in shampoos. *See* Sodium Lauryl Sulfate.

POTASSIUM METABISULFITE • Potassium Pyrosulfite. White or colorless, with an odor of sulfur dioxide *(see),* it is an antioxidant, preservative, and antifermentative in breweries and wineries. Should not be used in meats or foods recognized as sources of vitamin B_1. Also used for bleaching straw and as an antiseptic, preservative, antioxidant, and a developing agent in dyes. Low toxicity. The final report to the FDA of the Select Committee on GRAS Substances stated in 1980 that there is no available evidence that it is a hazard to the public when used as it is now and it should continue its GRAS status with limitations on the amounts that can be added to foods. *See* Sulfites.

POTASSIUM-*n*-METHYLDITHIO-CARBAMATE • A bacteria-killing component in controlling microorganisms in sugar cane mills. Carbamates are used to prevent sprouting in potatoes and other products by stopping cell division, something we call mutations. Carbamate mutations may lead to birth defects and to cancer. The final report to the FDA of the Select Committee on GRAS Substances stated in 1980 that there is no available evidence that it is a hazard to the public when used as it is now and it should continue its GRAS status with limitations on the amounts that can be added to food. FDA residue tolerances are less than 3.5 ppm in sugarcane being processed, less than 4.1 ppm. in terms of weight of raw cane or beets, and less than 200 ppm in cured cod roe.

POTASSIUM MYRISTATE • The potassium salt of myristic acid *(see)*. There is reported use of the chemical, it has not yet been assigned for toxicology literature.

POTASSIUM NITRATE • There is reported use of the chemical, it has not yet been assigned for toxicology literature. *See* Nitrate.

POTASSIUM NITRITE • There is reported use of the chemical, it has not yet been assigned for toxicology literature. *See* Nitrite.

POTASSIUM OCTOXYNOL-12 PHOSPHATE • The potassium salt of a mixture of esters of phosphoric acid and octoxynol *(see both)*.

POTASSIUM OLEATE • Miscellaneous additive. *See* Potassium and Oleic Acid.

POTASSIUM PALMITATE • The potassium salt of palmitic acid *(see)*.

POTASSIUM PERMANGANATE • Dark purple or bronzelike, odorless crystals with a sweet, antiseptic taste, used as a starch modifier. Dilute solutions are mildly irritating; highly concentrated solutions are caustic. There is reported use of the chemical; it has not yet been assigned for toxicology literature.

POTASSIUM PERSULFATE • White crystals, soluble in water or alcohol. Derived from potassium sulfate. Used as a flour-maturing agent, for modification of starch, and as an antiseptic. Sprayed on fresh citrus as a coating. Strong irritant.

POTASSIUM PHOSPHATE • Monobasic, Dibasic, and Tribasic. Used as a yeast food in the brewing industry and in the production of champagne and other sparkling wines. Used in frozen eggs as a color preservative. Has been used medicinally as a urinary acidifier. No known toxicity. The final report to the FDA of the Select Committee on GRAS Substances stated in 1980 that it should continue its GRAS status with no limitations other than good manufacturing practices.

POTASSIUM POLYMETAPHOSPHATE • The final report to the FDA of the Select Committee on GRAS Substances stated in 1980 that it should continue its GRAS status with no limitations other than good manufacturing practices. *See* Potassium Phosphate for uses.

POTASSIUM PYROPHOSPHATE • Colorless, deliquescent crystals or granules, used as a sequestering, peptizing, and dispersing agent and in soaps and detergents. Low toxicity. The final report to the FDA of the Select Committee on GRAS Substances stated in 1980 that it should continue its GRAS status with no limitations other than good manufacturing practices.

POTASSIUM SALTS OF FATTY ACIDS • In foods as binders, emulsifiers, and anticaking agents. *See* Fatty Acids.

POTASSIUM SILICATE • Soluble Potash Glass. Colorless or yellowish, translucent to transparent, glasslike particles. It is used for inorganic protective coatings, for phosphorous on television tubes, in detergents, as a catalyst, and in adhesives. Used as a binder in cosmetics and in soap manufacturing. Also used as a detergent and in the glass and ceramics industries. Usually slowly soluble in cold water. No known toxicity. The final report to the FDA of the Select Committee on GRAS Substances stated in 1980 that it should continue its GRAS status with no limitations other than good manufacturing practices.

POTASSIUM SORBATE • Sorbic Acid Potassium Salt. White crystalline powder used as a preservative; a mold and yeast inhibitor; and a fungistat in beverages, baked goods, chocolate, and soda fountain syrups, fresh fruit cocktail, tangerine puree (sherbet base), salads (potato, macaroni, coleslaw, gelatin), cheesecake, pie fillings, cake, cheeses in consumer-size packages, and artificially sweetened jellies and preserves. Low oral toxicity but may cause irritation of the skin. GRAS.

POTASSIUM STEARATE • Stearic Acid Potassium Salt. White powder with a fatty odor. Used as a chewing-gum base. Strongly alkaline. A defoaming agent in brewing. Also used in the manufacture of soap, hand creams, emulsified fragrances, lotions, and shaving creams. No known toxicity.

POTASSIUM SULFATE • Does not occur free in nature but is combined with sodium sulfate. Colorless or white crystalline powder, with a bitter taste. Used as a flavoring in foods. A water corrective used in the brewing industry. Used as a reagent *(see)* in cosmetics and as a salt substitute; also used as a fertilizer and a cathartic. Large doses can cause severe gastrointestinal bleeding. No known toxicity to the skin. GRAS. There is reported use of the chemical, it has not yet been assigned for toxicology literature.

POTASSIUM SULFITE • See Sulfites.

POTASSIUM TRICHLOROISOCYANURATE • A sanitizer. *See* Arsenic.

POTASSIUM TRIPOLYPHOSPHATE • A white crystalline solid that is used in water-treating compounds, cleaners, and fertilizers; widely used as a sequestering agent *(see)* in processed foods. The final report to the FDA of the Select Committee on GRAS Substances stated in 1980 that it should continue its GRAS status with no limitations other than good manufacturing practices.

POTATO STARCH • A flour prepared from potatoes ground to a pulp and washed of fibers. Swells in hot water to form a gel on cooling. A demulcent used in dusting powder; an emollient in dry shampoos and baby powders. With glycerin forms soothing, protective applications for eczema, skin rash, and chapped skin. May cause allergic skin reactions and stuffy nose in the hypersensitive. The final report to the FDA of the Select Committee on GRAS Substances stated in 1980 that it should continue its GRAS status with no limitations other than good manufacturing practices.

POTENTIATOR • A flavor ingredient with little flavor of its own that augments or alters the flavor response, such as sodium glutamate and sodium inosinate.

PPB • Abbreviation for *parts per billion.*

PPG • Abbreviation for *propylene glycol (see).*

PPG BUTETH-260 THROUGH 5100 • Emulsifiers. See Butyl Alcohol.

PPG BUTETH ETHER-200 • Emulsifier. Polymer *(see)* prepared from butyl alcohol with propylene glycol *(see both).*

PPG-4-CETETH-1, -5, or -10 • *See* Cetyl Alcohol.

PPG-8-CETETH-5, -10, or -20 • *See* Cetyl Alcohol.

PPG-10-CETYL ETHER • *See* Cetyl Alcohol.

PPG-30-CETYL ETHER • A liquid nonionic surfactant *(see)*. No known toxicity. *See* Cetyl Alcohol.

PPG-20-DECYLTETRADECETH-10 • *See* Decanoic Acid.

PPG-24 or -66 GLYCERETH-24 or -12 • *See* Glycerin.

PPG-27 and -55 GLYCERYLETHER • *See* Glycerin and Propylene Glycol.

PPG-ISOCETYL ETHER • *See* Cetyl Alcohol.

PPG-3-ISOSTEARETH-9 • *See* Stearyl Alcohol and Propylene Glycol.

PPG-2, -5, -10, -20, or -30 LANOLIN ALCOHOL ETHERS • *See* Lanolin Alcohol.

PPG-30 LANOLIN ETHER • Derived from lanolin alcohols *(see)*.

PPG-9 LAURATE • *See* Lauric Acid.

PPG-20-METHYL GLUCOSE ETHER • *See* Propylene Glycol and Glucose.

PPG-3-MYRETH-11 • *See* Polyethylene Glycol and Myristic Acid.

PPG-4 MYRISTYL ETHER • *See* Fatty Alcohols.

PPG-10 OLEYL ETHER • *See* PPG-26 Oleate.

PPG-30 or -50 OLEYL ETHER • *See* Oleic Acid.

PPG-6-C12-18 PARETH • A mixture of synthetic alcohols. *See* Fatty Alcohols.

PPG-9-STEARETH-3 • *See* Stearyl Alcohol.

PPG-11 or -15 STEARYL ETHER • *See* Propylene Glycol and Stearyl Alcohol.

PPM • Abbreviation for *parts per million.*

PRECIPITATE • To separate out from solution or suspension. A deposit of solid separated out from a solution or suspension as a result of a chemical or physical change, as by the action of a reagent *(see)*.

PRECURSOR • A biologic process in which a substance turns into another active or more mature substance. Beta-carotene is a precursor of vitamin A, because the body can use it to make vitamin A.

PREDNISOLONE • Metacortandrolone. Cortalone. Delta-Cortef. Introduced in 1955, prednisolone is related chemically to cortisol. It is used to treat inflammation in cattle. FDA residue tolerance for milk is zero. It is used to treat severe inflammation, as an immunosuppressant, in the treatment of ulcerative colitis, and in proctitis in humans. Most adverse reactions are the result of dose or length of time of administration. Should be taken with food or milk to reduce GI irritation. Potential adverse reactions include euphoria, insomnia, psychotic behavior, high blood pressure, swelling, cataracts, glaucoma, peptic ulcer, GI irritation, increased appetite, high blood sugar, growth suppression in children, delayed wound healing, acne, skin eruptions, muscle weakness, pancreatitis, hairiness, decreased immunity, and acute adrenal gland insufficiency. When withdrawn, there may be rebound inflammation, fatigue, weakness, joint pain, fever, dizziness, lethargy, depression, fainting, a drop in blood pressure upon arising from a seated or prone position, shortness of breath, loss of appetite, and high blood sugar.

PREDNISONE • Deltacortisone. Introduced in 1955 and related chemically to cortisone, a hormone secreted by the adrenal gland, prednisone is widely used to treat severe inflammation, as an immunosuppressant, and to treat acute attacks of multiple sclerosis, arthritis, and irritable-bowel syndrome in humans. It is used to treat cattle and horses for inflammation. FDA has a zero limitation in milk. International Agency for Research on Cancer (IARC) *(see)* review. Most adverse reactions are the result of dose or length of time of administration. In humans, potential adverse reactions from medication include euphoria, insomnia, psychotic behavior, high blood pressure, swelling, cataracts, glaucoma, peptic ulcer, GI irritation, increased appetite, high blood sugar, growth suppression in children, delayed wound healing, acne, skin eruptions, muscle weakness, pancreatitis, hairiness, decreased immunity, irregular menstruation, male infertility, and acute adrenal gland insufficiency. When withdrawn, there may be rebound inflammation, fatigue, weakness, joint pain, fever, dizziness, lethargy, depression, fainting, a drop in blood pressure upon arising from a seated or prone position, shortness of breath, loss of appetite, and high blood sugar. Sudden withdrawal may be fatal. Contraindicated in systemic fungal infections. Should be used cautiously in patients with GI ulceration or kidney disease, high blood pressure, diabetes, chicken pox, or osteoporosis. Prednisone has been implicated in aplastic anemia and is an experimental tumor inducer.

PREDONIN • *See* Prednisone.

PREEMPT • *See* CF-3.

PREGELATINIZED STARCH • When starch and water are heated, the starch molecules burst and form a gelatin. The final report to the FDA of the Select Committee on GRAS Substances stated in 1980 that it should continue its GRAS status with no limitations other than good manufacturing practices.

PRESERVATIVES • About one hundred "antispoilants," which retard or prevent food from going "bad," are in common use. Preservatives for fatty products are called antioxidants. Preservatives used in bread are labeled mold or rope inhibitors. They include sodium propionate and calcium propionate (*see both*). Preservatives to prevent mold and fungus growth on citrus fruits are called fungicides. Among the most commonly used preservatives are sodium benzoate (*see*) to prevent the growth of microbes on cheese and syrups, sulfur dioxide (*see*) to inhibit discoloration in fruit juice concentrates, and nitrates and nitrites that are used to "cure" processed meats. In many instances a product might show no visible evidence of microbial contamination and yet contain actively growing, potentially harmful germs.

PRICKLY ASH BARK • A natural cola, maple, and root beer flavor extract from a prickly aromatic shrub or small tree, *Zanthoxylum* spp., bearing yellow flowers. Used in beverages, candy, and baked goods. GRAS.

PRIMATOL • Prometon. Aatrex. Zeazine. Weedex A. Widely used herbicide on cropland. Moderately toxic by ingestion. Induces tumors and causes adverse reproductive effects in experimental animals. A skin and severe eye irritant.

PRIMULA EXTRACT • The extract of various species of *Primula* taken from the rhizome and roots of the primrose or cowslip. It has been used as an expectorant, diuretic, and worm medicine. In some sensitive persons, it may cause a rash.

PROCAINE PENICILLIN • An antibiotic used as an injection in animals. FDA tolerance in uncooked edible tissue of cattle is 0.05 ppm, and in uncooked edible tissue of turkey, 0.01 ppm. Zero tolerance in milk and uncooked edible tissue of chicken, pheasants, quail, swine, sheep, and eggs.

PROFENOFOS • A pesticide used in feed. FDA tolerances are 6 ppm in or on cottonseed hulls; 15 ppm in soap stocks. As a residue in meat by products of goats, cattle, hogs, poultry, and sheep, the FDA allows a residue of 0.05 ppm.

PROFLURALIN • Yellow-orange crystals used as an herbicide. FDA residue tolerances are 0.3 as a residue in or on soybean hay; 0.1 ppm in or on cottonseed, pod vegetables, and sunflower seeds; and 0.02 ppm as residue in or on eggs or milk, meat, fat, and meat byproducts of cattle, hogs, goats, poultry, and sheep.

PROGESTERONE • Corlutin. Cyclogest. Luteal Hormone. Synovex. Gesterol 50. Progestaject. A progestin drug that suppresses ovulation, possibly by inhibiting pituitary gonadotropin secretion. It forms a thick cervical mucus. Used to treat absent menstruation or abnormal uterine bleeding in humans. Used in beef and lamb to regulate reproductive cycles. Not allowed in veal calves. Potential adverse reactions in humans include nausea, vomiting, depression, high blood pressure, dizziness, migraine, lethargy, blood clots, swelling, bloating, and abdominal cramps. May cause breakthrough bleeding, altered menstrual flow, painful or absent menstruation, enlargement of benign tumors of the uterus, cervical erosion, abnormal secretions, and vaginal candidiasis. There may be jaundice; high blood sugar; dark spots appearing on the skin; breast tenderness, enlargement, or secretion; and decreased libido. Contraindicated in persons with blood-clot disorders, cancer of the breast, undiagnosed abnormal vaginal bleeding, and in pregnancy. The FDA limits residues from progesterone treatment in animals to 3 ppb in muscle, 12 ppb in fat, 9 ppb in kidney, and 6 ppb in liver of steers and calves, and 3 ppb in muscle and 15 ppb for fat, kidney, and liver of lambs. International Agency for Research on Cancer (IARC) *(see)* review. A cancer and tumor inducer in experimental animals. May cause birth defects.

PROLINA • A soy protein that can be made into fat-free whipped cream. *See* Soybeans.

PROLINE • L Form. An amino acid *(see)* used as a food supplement but classified as nonessential. Usually isolated from wheat or gelatin. L-Proline is the naturally occurring form and DL-Proline is the synthetic. GRAS.

PROMOTION • An intermediate stage of cancer development during which initiated *(see)* cells, in the presence of promoters, move further along the pathway to cancer. The promotion stage may take several decades in humans.

PROPANE • A gas heavier than air; odorless when pure. It is used as a fuel and refrigerant. Cleared for use in combination with octafluorocyclobutane in a spray propellant and as an aerating agent for foamed and sprayed foods. Cleared for use in a spray propellant and as an aerating agent for cosmetics in aerosols. May be narcotic in high concentrations. The final report to the FDA of the Select Committee on GRAS Substances stated in 1980 that it should continue its GRAS status with no limitations other than good manufacturing practices.

1,2-PROPANEDIOL • *See* Propylene Glycol.

PROPANOIC ACID • *See* Propionic Acid.

PROPARQUITE • A pesticide applied to growing crops to kill mites. FDA residue tolerance is 80 ppm in dried apple pomace and 40 ppm in dried citrus pulp and dried grape pulp. Less than 100 ppm can kill fish if it gets in water.

PROPAZINE • Propasin. Prozinex. An herbicide used on animal feed to control weeds. Moderately toxic by ingestion. Caused tumors in experimental animals.

PROPELLANT • A compressed gas used to expel the contents of containers in the form of aerosols. Chlorofluorocarbons were widely used because of their non-flammability. The strong possibility that they contribute to depletion of the ozone layer of the upper atmosphere has resulted in prohibition of their use for this purpose. Other propellants used are hydrocarbon gases, such as butane and propane, carbon dioxide, and nitrous oxide. The materials dispersed include shaving cream, whipping cream, and cosmetic preparations.

PROPETAMPHOS • A pesticide used as a spot, crack, and crevice treatment to kill parasites.

PROPIOMAZINE • Propionylpromethazine. A sedative and hypnotic used in human medicine. A tranquilizer used to treat stress in pigs. *See* Appendix C.

PROPIONALDEHYDE • Propanal. A synthetic flavoring agent that occurs naturally in apples and onions. Used in fruit flavorings for beverages, ice cream, ices, candy, and baked goods. Suffocating odor. May cause respiratory irritation. Moderately toxic by ingestion.

PROPIONIC ACID • Propanoic Acid. Occurs naturally in apples, strawberries, tea, and violet leaves. An oily liquid with a slightly pungent, rancid odor. Can be obtained from wood pulp, waste liquor, and by fermentation. Used in butter and fruit flavorings for beverages, ice cream, ices, candy, baked goods, and cheese flavorings for beverages, ice cream, ices, candy, baked goods, and cheese (600 ppm). Also used as an inhibitor and preservative to prevent mold in baked goods and processed cheeses. Also used in perfume bases and as a mold inhibitor, antioxidant, and preservative in cosmetics. Its salts have been used as antifungal agents to treat skin mold. May cause migraine in those susceptible to migraines, and contact with the chemical may cause skin irritations in bakery workers. Large oral dose in rats is lethal. GRAS.

PROPYL ACETATE • Colorless liquid, soluble in water, derived from propane and acetate *(see both)*. It has the odor of pears. A synthetic currant, raspberry, strawberry, apple, cherry, peach, pineapple, and rum flavoring agent for beverages, ice cream, ices, candy, and baked goods. Also used in the manufacture of perfumes and as a solvent for resins. It may be irritating to the skin and mucous membranes and narcotic in high doses.

PROPYL ALCOHOL • Obtained from natural gas and fusel oil. Alcoholic and slightly overpowering odor. Occurs naturally in cognac green oil, cognac white oil, and onion oil. A synthetic fruit flavoring for beverages, ice cream, ices, candy, and baked goods. Used instead of ethyl alcohol as a solvent for shellac, gums, resins, and oils; as a denaturant *(see)* for alcohol in perfumery. Not a primary irritant, but because it dissolves fat, it has a drying effect on the skin and may lead to cracking, fissuring, and infections. No adverse effects have been reported from local application as a lotion, liniment, mouthwash, gargle, or sponge bath. Mildly irritating to the eyes and mucous membranes. Ingestion may cause symptoms similar to that of ethyl alcohol *(see)*.

p-**PROPYL ANISOLE** • A synthetic flavoring agent, colorless to pale yellow, with an anise odor. Used in licorice, root beer, spice, vanilla, wintergreen, and birch beer flavoring for beverages, ice cream, candy, and baked goods. Moderately toxic by ingestion. Caused mutations in experimental animals.

PROPYL BENZOATE • A synthetic fruit flavoring agent for beverages, ice cream, ices, candy, and baked goods.

PROPYL BUTYRATE • Contains propyl alcohol and butyric acid. A synthetic strawberry, banana, pineapple, plum, tutti-frutti, liquor, and rum flavoring agent for beverages, ice cream, ices, candy, and baked goods. *See* Propyl Alcohol and Butyric Acid for toxicity.

PROPYL CINNAMATE • Cinnamic Acid. A synthetic berry, floral, rose, apple, grape, and honey flavoring agent for beverages, ice cream, ices, candy, baked goods, and gelatins.

PROPYL FORMATE • Formic Acid. A synthetic berry, apple, and rum flavoring agent for beverages, ice cream, ices, candy, and baked goods. *See* Formic Acid for toxicity.

PROPYL 2-FURANACRYLATE • A synthetic coffee and honey flavoring agent for beverages and candy.

PROPYL 2-FUROATE • A synthetic chocolate and mushroom flavoring agent for candy, baked goods, and condiments.

PROPYL GALLATE • A fine, white, odorless powder with a bitter taste used as an antioxidant for foods, fats, and oils and for potato flakes, mashed potatoes, and mayonnaise. Also used in lemon, lime, fruit, and spice flavorings for beverages, ice cream, ices, candy, baked goods, and gelatin desserts. Used as an antioxidant in creams and lotions. Used in pressure-sensitive adhesives as the food contact surface of labels and or tapes applied to food. Can cause stomach or skin irritation especially in people who suffer from asthma or are sensitive to aspirin. Reaffirmed as GRAS in the FDA's reevaluation in the following amounts: 0.02 percent maximum in fat or oil content of food; maximum of 0.015 percent in food prepared by the manufacturer.

PROPYL HEPTANOATE • A synthetic berry, coffee, fruit, cognac, and rum flavoring agent for beverages, ice cream, ices, candy, liqueurs, and baked goods.

PROPYL HEXANOATE • A synthetic pineapple flavoring agent for beverages, ice cream, ices, and candy.

PROPYL-*p*-HYDROXYRENZOATE • Propylparaben. A preservative used in beverages, candy, baked goods, and artificially sweetened jellies and preserves. Also used in fruit flavorings for beverages, ice cream, ices, candy, and baked goods. Less toxic than benzoic acid *(see)* or salicylic acid *(see)*. Experimental animals showed no kidney or liver damage. On the FDA list for further study for short-term mutagenic, subacute, teratogenic, and reproductive effects. GRAS.

PROPYL ISOVALERATE • A synthetic strawberry, apple, banana, and peach flavoring agent for beverages, ice cream, ices, candy, and baked goods.

PROPYL MERCAPTAN • A synthetic berry and onion flavoring agent for baked goods and pickles.

PROPYL METHOXYBENZENE • *See p-Propyl Anisole.*

PROPYL PHENYLACETATE • A synthetic butter, caramel, rose, fruit, and honey flavoring agent for beverages, ice cream, ices, candy, and baked goods.

PROPYL PROPIONATE • Propyl alcohol and propionic acid. A synthetic banana, cherry, melon, peach, prune, apple, plum, and rum flavoring agent for beverages, ice cream, ices, candy, and baked goods. Colorless, thick liquid prepared from glycerol *(see* Glycerin) and used as an anticaking agent, antioxidant, dough conditioner, humectant, solvent, stabilizer, detergent, texturizer, thickener, and wetting agent. Used in alcoholic beverages, confections, flavorings, frostings, frozen dairy products, pork, nut products, poultry, seasonings, and wine. FDA limits it to 5 percent in alcoholic beverages; 24 percent in confections and frostings; 2.5 percent in frozen dairy products; 97 percent in seasonings and flavorings; 5 percent in nuts and nut products; and 2 percent in all other foods when used in accordance with good manufacturing practices. Limitation of 40 ppm in wine. EPA Genetic Toxicology Program. Caused birth defects in experimental animals.

PROPYLENE GLYCOL • 1,2-Propanediol. A clear, colorless, viscous liquid, slightly bitter tasting. In food, it is used in confectionery, chocolate products, ice cream emulsifiers, shredded coconut, beverages, baked goods, toppings, icings, and meat products to prevent discoloration during storage. Defoaming agent in processed beet sugar and yeast. Used in antifreeze in breweries and dairy establishments. It is the most common moisture-carrying vehicle other than water itself in cosmetics. It is being reduced and being replaced by safer glycols such as butylene and polyethylene glycol. Large oral doses in animals have been reported to cause central nervous system depression and slight kidney changes. The final report to the FDA of the Select Committee on GRAS Substances stated in 1980 that it should continue its GRAS status with no limitations other than good manufacturing practices.

PROPYLENE GLYCOL ALGINATE • Kelcloid. The propylene glycol ester of alginic acid *(see),* derived from seaweed. Used as a stabilizer, filler, and defoaming agent in food. Cleared for use in French dressing and salad dressing under the food standard regulations. Used as a stabilizer in ice cream, frozen custard, ice milk, fruit sherbet, and water ices, it is permitted up to 0.5 percent of the weight of the finished product. Can cause allergic reactions. The final report to the FDA of the Select Committee on GRAS Substances stated in 1980 that there is no available evidence that it is a hazard to the public when used as it is now and it should continue its GRAS status with limitations on amounts that can be added to food.

PROPYLENE GLYCOL MONOSTEARATE • Cream-colored wax that disperses in water and is soluble in hot alcohol. It is used as a lubricating agent and emulsifier; also a dough conditioner in baked goods. Employed as a stabilizer of essential oils. Slightly more toxic than propylene glycol *(see)* in animals and in large doses produces central nervous system depression and kidney injury. The final report to the FDA of the Select Committee on GRAS Substances stated in 1980 that it should continue its GRAS status with no limitations other than good manufacturing practices.

PROPYLENE OXIDE • Propene Oxide. Colorless, liquid starch modifier. FDA tolerance residues are less than 25 percent for treatment of starch; 700 ppm as propylene glycol in dried prunes and glacéd fruit; and 300 ppm in cocoa gums and processed nut meats (except peanuts).

3-PROPYLI DENEPHTHALI DE • A synthetic fruit and spice flavoring agent for beverages, ice cream, ices, candy, and baked goods. No known toxicity.

PROPYLPARABEN • Propyl-*p*-Hydroxybenzoate. Developed in Europe, the esters of *p*-hydroxybenzoic acid are widely used in the cosmetics industry as preservatives and bacteria and fungus killers. They are active against a variety of organisms, are neutral, low in toxicity, slightly soluble, and active in all solutions, alkaline, neutral, or acid. Used in shampoos, baby preparations, foundation creams, beauty masks, dentifrices, eye lotions, hair-grooming aids, nail creams, and wave sets. Used medicinally to treat fungus infections. Can cause contact dermatitis. Less toxic than benzoic or salicylic acid *(see both).* GRAS.

PROPYLPARASEPT • *See* Propyl-*p*-Hydroxybenzoate.

a-PROPYLPHENETHYL ALCOHOL • A synthetic fruit flavoring agent for beverages, ice cream, ices, candy, and puddings. Toxicity similar to ethanol *(see).*

PROSTAGLANDINS • PGA, PGB, PGC, PGD. Taglandin F2-a. Lutalyse. A group of extremely potent hormonelike substances present in many tissues. There are more than sixteen known with effects such as dilating or constricting blood vessels, stimulation of intestinal or bronchial smooth muscle, uterine stimulation, and antagonism to hormones and influencing fat metabolism. Various prostaglandins in the body can cause fever, inflammation, and headaches. Prostaglandins or drugs that affect prostaglandins are used medically in humans to induce labor, prevent and treat peptic ulcers, control high blood pressure, in the treatment of bronchial asthma, and to induce delayed menstruation. They are used in animals to induce labor and to induce abortion.

PROTEASE • An enzyme used as a meat tenderizer and in sausage curing, dough conditioning, and beer-haze removal.

PROTECTIVE COATINGS • Antioxidants and preservatives that are used in goat cheeses and fresh fruits and vegetables to retard spoilage. The coatings may expose consumers to hidden antibiotics or coal-tar products. Among the coating additives used are anoxomer, calcium disodium and disodium EDTA, cournarone-indene resin, ethoxyquin, morpholine, natamycin, petroleum naphtha, polyacrylamide, synthetic paraffin and succinic derivatives, and terpene resin *(see all)*. Citrus fruits, squash, grapes, sweet potatoes, asparagus, melons, papaya, plantain, turnips, watermelons, and nuts are commonly coated.

PROTEIN • Chemically, a protein is a complex nitrogenous compound made up of amino acids in peptide linkages. Dietary proteins are involved in the synthesis of tissue protein and other special metabolic functions. In anabolic processes they furnish the amino acids required to build and maintain body tissues. As an energy source, proteins are equivalent to carbohydrates in providing 4 calories per gram. Proteins perform a major structural role in all body tissues and in the formation of enzymes, hormones, and various body fluids and secretions. Proteins participate in the transport of some lipids, vitamins, and minerals and help maintain the body's homeostasis.

PROTEIN CONCENTRATE, WHOLE FISH • Dietary supplement.

PROTEIN FATTY ACID CONDENSATES • *See* Amides.

PROTEIN HYDROLYSATES • Used as flavor enhancers, particularly in meat products. *See* Proteins and Hydrolyzed.

PROTEIN, VEGETABLE, HYDROLYZED • *See* Hydrolyzed Vegetable Proteins.

PROVITAMIN A • *See* Carotene.

PRUSSIATE OF SODA, YELLOW • Salt of hydrocyanic acid derived from ammonia. Anticaking agent in salt. Hydrocyanic acid is toxic by ingestion, inhalation, and skin absorption.

PSEUDOPINENE • A synthetic flavoring agent used in various foods. Mildly toxic by ingestion. *See* a-Pinene.

PSYLLIUM • *Plantago psyllium* is a cultivated weed and has been used as a laxative since the early 1930s. It absorbs water and expands to increase bulk and moisture content of the stool to encourage bowel movement. Psyllium contains a soluble fiber that studies have shown can lower cholesterol levels.

General Mills introduced the first psyllium cereal, Benefit, in April 1989. Heartwise was introduced in August of that year. Procter and Gamble, which makes the psyllium laxative Metamucil, had asked the FDA to prohibit General Mills from making claims that its cereal could reduce cholesterol. Procter and Gamble contended psyllium was a drug, not a food, and thus the cereal could only be marketed after extensive tests to prove to regulators that it is safe and effective in performing as claimed. Procter and Gamble is barred from making claims about Metamucil's ability to reduce cholesterol.

General Mills withdrew Benefit from the market in December 1989 citing poor sales. Heartwise is the only major brand of cereal containing a significant amount of psyllium, 3 grams in a one-ounce serving. Bran Buds is made by Kellogg but has less psyllium. Allergic reactions occurred in some people who ate the cereal Heartless, made by the Kellogg company; reactions ranged from itchy eyes and runny noses to severe difficulty in breathing. In September 1989 the FDA sent a letter to Kellogg raising new questions about its use of psyllium which has been used for decades in bulk laxatives like Metamucil and Fiberall. On Oct 30, 1990, the FDA published proposed regulations in the Federal Register that would require a warning label on over-the-counter drugs containing water-soluble fibers, including psyllium, which is not absorbed systemically. The FDA ruled in February 1998 that labels on food containing soluble fiber from psyllium seed, including some breakfast cereals, may claim that these products may reduce the risk of coronary artery disease when eaten as part of a diet low in saturated fat and cholesterol. As psyllium can be hard to swallow, the new labels are also required to recommend that people eating these types of foods drink plenty of liquid.

PSYLLIUM SEED HUSK • A stabilizer from the seed of the fleaseed plant used in frozen desserts up to 0.5 percent of the weight of the finished product. *See* Psyllium.

PTEROYLGLUTAMIC ACID • Dietary supplement. Isolated from yeast.

PTWI • Provisional Tolerable Weekly Intake.

PULEGONE • Found in oils of plants, principally the pennyroyal. Pleasant odor, midway between camphor and peppermint. Used in peppermint flavorings for beverages, ice cream, ices, candy, and baked goods. *See* Pennyroyal Oil for toxicity.

PULPS • From wood, straw, bagasse, or other natural sources. A source of cellulose in food. The wood is treated with a mixture containing mainly sodium hydroxide *(see)*. Treatment removes the fibrous lignin—the resinous substance that binds the fiber that lines the cells of wood. An indirect human food additive from packaging. The FDA's reevaluation in 1976 labeled pulps GRAS.

PURINES • Components of nucleic acid, they are widely distributed in nature. Inportant purines are uric acid, adenine, guanine, and xanthine. Uric acid is the form of purines excreted in human urine. Caffeine is a stimulant purine. Some of the richest food sources of purines are anchovies, asparagus, organ meats, mushrooms, and sardines. Foods with low purines include bread, cereals, fats, cheese, eggs, fruits, milk, and nuts.

PYCNOGENOL • An extract of the French maritime pine tree, it is a rich source of antioxidant flavonoids *(see)*. It reported reduces free radicals *(see)* in the body.

PYRANTEL TARTRATE • An antiworm medicine used in feed and as a veterinary medicine. The FDA's residue tolerance is 10 ppm in swine liver and kidney and 1 ppm in swine muscle.

PYRAZINE ETHANETHIOL • *See* Piperazine.

PYRETHRINS • Thick liquids from the pyrethrum flowers. Used in household insecticidal sprays and powders and deodorant sprays. Also used in paper bags for shipping cereals. Residues from packaging materials and equipment and storage areas may be only 1 ppm on dried foods, cereal grains, and dried prunes. Insecticides labeled nontoxic to human beings and pets usually contain pyrethrins.

PYRIDINE • Occurs naturally in coffee and coal tar. Disagreeable odor; sharp taste. Used in chocolate flavorings for beverages, ice cream, ices, candy, and baked goods. Also used as a solvent for organic liquids and compounds. Once used to treat asthma, but may cause central nervous system depression and irritation of the skin and respiratory tract. After prolonged administration, kidney and liver damage may result. Pyridine is absorbed from the respiratory and gastrointestinal tract. Small oral doses in humans have produced loss of appetite, nausea, fatigue, and mental depression.

PYRIDOXINE • *See* Pyridoxine Hydrochloride.

PYRIDOXINE DIOCTENCIATE • Vitamin B_6 Hydrochloride. Texturizer. A colorless or white crystalline powder present in many foodstuffs. A coenzyme that helps in the metabolism of amino acids *(see)* and fats. Also soothing to the skin. Nontoxic.

PYRIDOXINE HYDROCHLORIDE • Vitamin B_6. A colorless or white crystalline powder added to evaporated milk base in infant foods. Present in many foodstuffs. Especially good sources are yeast, liver, and cereals. A coenzyme that helps in the metabolism of amino acids *(see)* and fat. Permits normal red blood cell formation. The final report to the FDA of the Select Committee on GRAS Substances stated in 1980 that it should continue its GRAS status with no limitations other than good manufacturing practices. The FDA is doing a toxicology search on this additive.

PYRIDOXINE TRIPALMITATE • Vitamin B_6 Tripalmitate. *See* Pyridoxine Hydrochloride.

PYRIDOXOL HYDROCHLORIDE • Vitamin B_6. Dietary supplement and nutrient used in baked goods, beverages and beverage bases, cereals, dairy products, meat products, plant-protein products, and snack foods.

PYROLIGNEOUS ACID and EXTRACT • A yellow acid. Consists of 6 percent acetic acid *(see)* and small concentrations of creosote, methyl alcohol, and acetone *(see)*. It is obtained by the destructive distillation of wood. Used as a synthetic flavoring in butter, butterscotch, caramel, rum, tobacco, smoke, and vanilla flavorings for beverages, ice cream, ices, candy, baked goods, puddings, and meats (300 ppm). The extract is used largely for smoking meats (300 ppm) and in smoke flavorings for baked goods (200 ppm) and alcoholic beverages. It is corrosive and may cause epigastric pain, vomiting, circulatory collapse, and death. There is reported use of the chemical, it has not yet been assigned for toxicology literature.

PYROMUCIC ALDEHYDE • *See* Furfural.

PYROPHOSPHATE • Salt of pyrophosphoric acid. It increases the effectiveness of antioxidants in creams and ointments. In concentrated solutions it can be irritating to the skin and mucous membranes.

PYROPHYLLITE • Aluminum Silicate Monohydrate. Obtained naturally from clay or synthesized, it is used as an anticaking and coloring agent in powders. Used as a carrier or pelleting aid in animal feed. Nontoxic.

PYRORACEMIC ACID • *See* Pyruvic Acid.

PYRROLE • Colorless liquid with a mild, nutty odor used as a flavoring agent in various foods. GRAS when used at a level not in excess of the amount reasonably required to accomplish the intended effect.

PYRUVALDEHYDE • A synthetic flavoring, yellowish, with a pungent odor. Formed as an intermediate in the metabolism or fermentation of carbohydrates and lactic acid *(see)*. Used in coffee, honey, and maple flavorings for beverages, ice cream, ices, candy, and baked goods.

PYRUVIC ACID • An important intermediate in fermentation and metabolism, it occurs naturally in coffee and when sugar is metabolized in muscle. It is reduced to lactic acid *(see)* during exertion. Pyruvic acid is isolated from cane sugar. It is a synthetic flavoring used in coffee and rum flavorings for beverages, ice cream, ices, candy, chewing gum, and baked goods. Has been used as a paste in the treatment of deep burns.

Q

QUACK GRASS • A couch grass, a pernicious weed in cultivated fields. *See* Dog Grass Extract.

QUASSIA EXTRACT • Bitter Ash. Bitterwood. Yellowish white to bright yellow chips. Bitter alkaloid obtained from the wood of *Quassia amara,* a tree bearing bright scarlet flowers grown in Jamaica, the Caribbean Islands, and South America. Named for a black slave who discovered its medicinal value in the mid-eighteenth century. Slight odor, bitter taste. Used in bitters, citrus, cherry, grape, liquor, root beer, sarsaparilla, and vanilla flavorings for beverages, baked goods, and liquors. In cosmetics, it is used chiefly as a denaturant for ethyl alcohol. Used to poison flies, to imitate hops, and as a bitter tonic and remedy for roundworms in children. Toxic to humans. There is reported use of the chemical, it has not yet been assigned for toxicology literature.

QUATERNARY AMMONIUM COMPOUNDS • A wide variety of preservatives, surfactants, germicides, sanitizers, antiseptics, and deodorants. They are used in processing sugarcane and in beet sugar mills. Benzalkonium chloride *(see)* is one of the most popular. Quaternary ammonium compounds are synthetic derivatives of ammonia, a natural product that occurs in animal metabolism.

QUEBRACHO BARK EXTRACT • Extract of a native Argentine tree, used in fruit, rum, and vanilla flavorings for beverages, ice cream, candy, ices, and baked goods. Closely related to the tranquilizer reserpine. Once promoted as an aphrodisiac, it can cause low blood pressure, nausea, abdominal distress, weakness, and fatigue. There is reported use of the chemical, it has not yet been assigned for toxicology literature.

QUERCETIN • Widely distributed in the plant kingdom especially in rinds and barks and in clover blossoms and ragweed pollen. Used therapeutically to protect blood vessels. Used in food additives to form epoxy resins.

QUERCITRON • The inner bark of a species of oak tree common in North America. Its active ingredient, isoquercitrin, is used in forming resins and in dark brown hair-dye shades mainly for dyeing artificial hairpieces. Allergic reactions have been reported. *See* Rutin.

QUERCUS ALBA • *See* Oak Bark Extract.

QUICK GRASS • Triticum. *See* Dog Grass Extract.

QUILLAIA • China Bark Extract Soap Bark. *See* Quillaja Extract.

QUILLAJA EXTRACT • Soapbark. Quillay Bark. Panama Bark. China Bark. The extract of the inner dried bark of a tree grown in South America, *Quillaja saponaria*. Used in fruit, root beer, and spice flavorings for beverages, ice cream, and candy. Formerly used to treat bronchitis and externally as a detergent and local irritant.

QUINCE SEED • The seed of a plant, *Cydonia* spp., grown in southern Asia and Europe for its fatty oil. Thick jelly produced by soaking seeds in water. Used in fruit flavorings for beverages, ice cream, ices, and baked goods. Used as a suspension in setting skin creams and lotions, as a thickening agent in depilatories, and as an emulsifier for fragrances, hand creams, lotions, rouges, and wave sets. Used medicinally as a demulcent. Has been largely replaced by cheaper substitutes. It may cause allergic reactions. GRAS.

QUININE BISULFATE • Most important alkaloid of cinchona extract *(see)* from trees that grow wild in South America and are cultivated in Java. Very bitter. Used in bitters flavoring for beverages and not to exceed 83 ppm in soda. Used to treat fever and as a local anesthetic and analgesic. No known toxicity. *See* Quinine Extract.

QUININE EXTRACT • An extract of cinchona bark (*see* Cinchona Extract), which grows wild in South America. White crystalline powder, almost insoluble in water. It is used as a local anesthetic in hair tonics and sunscreen preparations. Used in bitters in limited amounts as flavoring for beverages When taken internally, it reduces fever. It is also used as a flavoring agent in numerous over-the-counter cold and headache remedies as well as "bitter lemon" and tonic water, which may contain as much as five milligrams per hundred milliliters. Cinchonism, which may consist of nausea, vomiting, disturbances of vision, ringing in ears, and nerve deafness, may occur from an overdose of quinine. If there is a sensitivity to quinine, such symptoms can result from drinking tonic water. Quinine more commonly causes a rash. The FAO/WHO said the amount of quinine in drinks was not of concern to most, but that some consumers show a hyperreactivity to quinine, and therefore, its presence in foods and beverages should be noted.

QUININE HYDROCHLORIDE • A synthetic flavoring agent derived from cinchona bark *(see)* and used in bitters, citrus, and fruit flavorings for beverages. Some medical use as quinine sulfate *(see)*. *See* Quinine Extract for toxicity.

QUININE SULFATE • A synthetic flavoring agent derived from cinchona bark *(see)* and used in bitters flavoring for beverages. Also used medicinally to treat malaria, as an analgesic, and as a local anesthetic.

QUINOLINE • A coal tar derivative used in the manufacture of cosmetic dyes. Also a solvent for resins. Made either by the distillation of coal tar, bones, and alkaloids or by the interaction of aniline *(see)* with acetaldehyde and formaldehyde *(see both)*. Absorbs water, has a weak base. Soluble in hot water. Also used as a preservative for anatomical specimens. *See* Coal Tar for toxicity. *See also* FD and C Colors.

QUIZALOFOPETHYL • White crystals used as an herbicide in animal feed. FDA residue tolerances are: 0.2 ppm in soybean hulls; 0.5 ppm in soybean meal; 1.0 ppm in soybean soap stock; 0.5 on soybeans; 0.2 ppm in eggs; 0.1 in eggs; 0.05 ppm in milk fat; 0.05 in fat of cattle, goats, hogs, and sheep; 0.02 ppm in meat of cattle, goats, hogs, and sheep; 0.05 ppm; 0.05 ppm as residues in fat, meat, and meat byproducts of cattle, goats, hogs, and sheep; and 1.0 as residues on cotton seed.

R

RACEMIC ACID • *See* Tartaric Acid.

RADISH EXTRACT • Extract of *Raphanus sativus*. The small seeds of the radish remain viable for years. Has been used as a food since ancient times. Used as a counterirritant *(see)* in herbal cosmetics.

RAISIN-SEED OIL • Dried grapes or berries used in lubricating creams. *See* Grape-Seed Oil.

RALGRO • Zeranol. Used to increase growth in beef and lamb. FDA limits residue to zero in cattle and sheep. Has adverse reproductive effects in experimental animals.

RAPESEED OIL, HYDROGENATED • Brownish yellow oil from a turniplike annual herb of European origin. Widely grown as a forage crop for sheep in the United States. Canada sought clearance to sell rapeseed in the U.S. market, but it was barred because it contains erucic acid, which was cited in the early 1970s as a possible source of heart problems based on the results of tests on rats. New varieties of the seeds, canola, have been developed that have low erucic acid levels. Now, rapeseed oil is used in American salad oils, peanut butter, and some cake mixes. A distinctly unpleasant odor. It is used chiefly as a lubricant, an illuminant, and in rubber substitutes; also used in soft soaps. Can cause acnelike skin eruptions. When rats were fed a diet high in rapeseed oil over a lifetime, they showed significantly greater degenerative changes in the liver and a higher incidence of kidney damage than animals fed other vegetable oils. GRAS. *See* Erucic Acid.

RAPESEED OIL, FULLY HYDROGENATED • A stabilizer used in peanut butter. GRAS.

RAPESEED OIL, FULLY HYDROGENATED, SUPERGLYCERINATED • An emulsifier used in shortenings for cake mixes. *See* Rapeseed Oil, Hydrogenation, and Glycerin. GRAS.

RAPESEED OIL, LOW ERUCIC ACID • A miscellaneous additive that may be used in many products except in infant formula. May be declared on the label as *canola oil*. *See* Erucic Oil.

RAPESEED OIL, UNSAPONIFIABLES • The fraction of rapeseed oil *(see)* that is not changed into a fatty alcohol when it is saponified (heated with an alkali and acid). GRAS except in infant formula.

RASPBERRY EXTRACT • *See* Raspberry Juice.

RASPBERRY JUICE • Juice from the fresh ripe fruit grown in Europe, Asia, the United States, and Canada. Used as a flavoring for lipsticks, food, and medicines. It has astringent properties.

rBST • Abbreviation for Recombinant Bovine Somatotropin. *See* Bovine Somatotropin and IGF-I.

RDA • *Recommended Dietary Allowances* of the Food and Nutrition Board, National Academy of Sciences, National Research Council. The Recommended Daily Dietary Allowance was started in the 1940s to safeguard the public's health. The RDA were estimates of the nutritional needs of adults and children developed by the FDA to be used as the legal standards for labeling foods in regard to nutritional content.

U.S. RDA (Recommended Daily Allowances) for Adults and Children (Four Years and Over)

Vitamin A	800–1,000 mg	Vitamin B_6	2.0 mg
Vitamin C		Folic Acid	4 mg
(ascorbic acid)	60 mg	Vitamin B_{12}	6 mcg
Vitamin B_1		Phosphorus	1.0 g
(thiamine)	1.5 mg	Iodine	150 mcg
Vitamin B_2		Magnesium	400 mg
(riboflavin)	1.7 mg	Zinc	15 mg
Niacin	20 mg	Copper	2 mg
Calcium	1.0 g		
Iron	18 mg	Biotin	3 mg
Vitamin D	400 IU	Pantothenic Acid	10 mg
Vitamin E	30 IU	*See* Appendixes E and F.	

REAGENT • A chemical that reacts or participates in a reaction; a substance that is used for the detection or determination of another substance by chemical or microscopical means. The various categories of reagents are colorimetric—to produce color-soluble compounds; fluxes—to lower melting point; oxidizers—used in oxidation; precipitants—to produce insoluble compounds; reducers—used in reduction *(see);* solvents—used to dissolve water-insoluble compounds.

RECOMBINANT DNA • The DNA formed by combining segments of DNA from different types of organisms. Recombinant DNA technology is one technique of genetic engineering.

RECOMBINANT DNA TECHNOLOGY • A broad range of techniques involving the manipulation of genetic material of organisms, including technologies by which scientists isolate genes from one organism and insert them into another. The term is often used synonymously with *genetic engineering* and to describe DNA sequences isolated from and transferred between organisms by genetic engineering techniques.

RECOMMENDED DIETARY ALLOWANCES (RDA) • The former listing of amounts of certain of nutrients needed to maintain health. These have been replaced by Daily Values (*see* page 5 in introduction) on labels. *See* RDA.

RED • *See* FD and C Red (Nos. 3, 4, 40, and Citrus Red).

RED ALGAE • Seaweed. GRAS. *See* Algae, Red.

RED PEPPER • Cayenne Pepper. A condiment made from the pungent fruit of the plant. Used in sausage and pepper flavorings. Also used as a stimulant in hair tonics but may be an irritant and also cause allergic reactions.

RED RASPBERRY LEAF EXTRACT • An extract of the leaves of the red raspberry. Used as a flavoring.

RED SAUNDERS • Red Sandalwood. Flavoring in alcoholic beverages only. No known toxicity.

REDUCED • Product has been nutritionally altered and contains at least 25 percent less of a nutrient such as fat or salt or 25 percent fewer calories than the regular product.

REDUCED-LACTOSE WHEY • GRAS. *See* Whey and Reducing Agent.

REDUCED-MINERALS WHEY • Obtained by removing a portion of the minerals from whey. Used as a texturizer, nutritional extender, nutritive sweetener, formulation, and processing aid. GRAS. *See* Whey and Reducing Agent.

REDUCING AGENT • A substance that decreases, deoxidizes, or concentrates the volume of another substance. For instance, a reducing agent is used to convert a metal oxide to the metal itself. It also means a substance that adds hydrogen agents to another; for example, when acetaldehyde is converted to alcohol in the final step of alcoholic fermentation. It is used in foods to keep metals from oxidizing and affecting the taste or color of fats, oils, salad dressings, and other foods containing minerals.

REDUCTION • The process of reducing by chemical or electrochemical means. The gain of one or more electrons by an ion or compound. It is the reverse of oxidation.

REGENERATED CELLULOSE • Miscellaneous use with resins. *See* Cellulose.

RELEASING AGENT • A compound such as butter or an oil that prevents a product from sticking to the sides of a container. Also refers to a chemical that permits easy removal of the meat of a clam or other crustacean.

RENNET • Rennin. Enzyme from the lining membranes of the stomach of suckling calves. Used for curdling milk in cheese making and in junket. Sometimes as a digestant. Reaffirmed GRAS in 1982.

RESIN, ACRYLAMIDE—ACRYLIC ACID • A clarifying agent in beet sugar and sugarcane juice. The acid is used in the synthesis of this acrylic resin. No known toxicity.

RESIN, COUMARONE—INDENE • A chewing-gum base and protective coating for citrus fruit. Coumarone is derived from coal tar and is used with a mixture of indene chiefly in the synthesis of coumarone resins. No known toxicity.

RESIN, ISOBUTYLENE • Polyisobutylene. A chewing-gum base made from the chemical used chiefly in manufacturing synthetic rubber. No known toxicity.

RESIN, METHACRYLIC and DIVINYL BENZENE • A compound of fine particle size, weakly acidic. Used as an absorbent for Vitamin B_{12} in nutritional supplement products. No known toxicity.

RESIN, PETROLEUM HYDROCARBON • A chewing-gum base synthesized from fuel oil. No known toxicity.

RESINS • The brittle substance, usually translucent or transparent, formed from the hardened secretions of plants. Among the natural resins are dammar, elemi, and sandarac. Synthetic resins include polyvinyl acetate, various polyester resins, and sulfonamide resins. Resins have many uses in cosmetics. They contribute depth, gloss, flow adhesion, and water resistance. Toxicity depends upon ingredients used. *See* Gums.

RESIN, TERPENE • Alpha and Beta Pinene. A chewing-gum base and coating for fresh fruits and vegetables. Pinene *(see)* has the same toxicity as turpentine.

RESORCINOL • A preservative, antiseptic, antifungal agent, astringent, and anti-itching agent, particularly in dandruff shampoos. Also used in hair dyes, lipsticks, and hair tonics; in tanning, explosives, printing textiles, and the manufacture of resins. Obtained from various resins. Resorcinol's white crystals become pink on exposure to air. A sweetish taste. Irritating to the skin and mucous membranes. May cause allergic reactions, particularly of the skin. The FDA issued a notice in 1992 that resorcinol has not been shown to be safe and effective for stated claims in OTC products.

RETINOIDS • Derived from retinoic acid, vitamin A, it is used to treat acne and other skin disorders. *See* Vitamin A.

RETINOL • Vitamin A *(see)*.

RETINYL PALMITATE • The ester of vitamin A and palmitic acid sometimes mixed with vitamin D *(see all)*.

RHAMNOSE • Occurs in poison sumac, *Rhus toxicodendron*. Combined with sugar in many other plants. It is used in the manufacture of food additives.

RHATANY ROOT • A flavoring. The dried root of *Krameria triandra R.* from Peru and Brazil. A flavoring additive. Used as a cosmetic astringent. *See* Krameria

Extract. There is reported use of the chemical; it has not yet been assigned for toxicology literature.

RHIZOPUS ORYZAE • An enzyme used in production of dextrose (sugar) from starch.

RHODENAL • *See* Citronellal.

RHODINOL • A synthetic flavoring agent isolated from geranium rose oil *(see)*. It has the strong odor of rose and consists essentially of geraniol and citronellol *(see both)*. Used in strawberry, chocolate, rose, grape, honey, spice, and ginger ale flavorings for beverages, ice cream, ices, candy, baked goods, gelatin desserts, chewing gum, and jelly. Used also in perfumes, especially those of the rose type.

RHODINYL ACETATE • Acetic Acid. An acidulant and synthetic flavoring, colorless to slightly yellow, with a light, fresh, roselike odor. Used in berry, coconut, apricot, floral, rose, and honey flavorings for beverages, ice cream, ices, candy, and baked goods. A skin irritant.

RHODINYL BUTYRATE • Butyric Acid. A synthetic raspberry, strawberry, and fruit flavoring agent for beverages, ice cream, ices, candy, baked goods, and chewing gum. No known toxicity.

RHODINYL FORMATE • Formic Acid. A synthetic flavoring, colorless to slight yellow, with a roselike odor. Used in raspberry, rose, apple, cherry, plum, pear, and pineapple flavorings for beverages, ice cream, ices, candy, baked goods, and gelatin desserts. *See* Formic Acid for toxicity.

RHODINYL ISOBUTRYATE • Isobutyric Acid. A synthetic raspberry, floral, rose, apple, pear, pineapple, and honey flavoring agent for beverages, ice cream, ices, candy, baked goods, and gelatin desserts.

RHODINYL ISOVALERATE • Isovaleric Acid. A synthetic berry, floral, rose, and fruit flavoring agent for beverages, ice cream, ices, candy, and baked goods.

RHODINYL PHENYLACETATE • Phenylacetic Acid. A synthetic flavoring used in beverages, ice cream, ices, candy, and baked goods.

RHODINYL PROPIONATE • Propionic Acid. A synthetic berry, rose, plum, and honey flavoring agent for beverages, ice cream, ices, candy, and baked goods.

RHODYMENIA PALMATA • *See* Dulse.

RHUBARB • The garden root of *Rheum rhaponticum,* used as a flavoring in alcoholic beverages only. Has been used as a laxative.

RHYNCHOSIA PYRAMIDALIS • A large, tropical twining plant with yellow flowers. Used as a flavoring. No known toxicity.

RIBOFLAVIN • Vitamin B_2. Lactoflavin. Formerly called vitamin G. Riboflavin is a factor in the vitamin B complex and is used in emollients. Every plant and animal cell contains a minute amount. Good sources are milk, eggs, and organ meats. It is necessary for healthy skin and respiration, protects the eyes from sensitivity to light, and is used for building and maintaining human body tissues. A deficiency leads to lesions at the corner of the mouth and to changes in the cornea. Recommended Daily Requirements for infants is 4,000 micrograms per day and for adults 1,300 micrograms. Its yellow to orange-yellow color is used to dye eggshells. It is permanently listed as a food color. It does not require certification.

Riboflavin and its more soluble form, riboflavin-5-phosphate, are added as enrichment to dry baby cereals, poultry stuffing, peanut butter, prepared breakfast cereals, enriched flour, enriched cornmeal, enriched corn grits, enriched macaroni, and enriched breads and rolls. GRAS. There is reported use of the chemical, it has not yet been assigned for toxicology literature.

RIBOFLAVIN-5-PHOSPHATE • A more soluble form of riboflavin *(see)*. The final report to the FDA of the Select Committee on GRAS Substances stated in 1980 that it should continue its GRAS status with no limitations other than good manufacturing practices.

RIBONUCLEIC ACID (RNA) • Found in both the nucleus and cytoplasm of the cell, it is the material that contains directions for the genetic code of the cell, DNA.

D-RIBOSE • Prepared by hydrolysis of yeast *(see)*.

RIBOTIDE • A flavor enhancer developed by the Japanese.

RICE BRAN OIL • Oil expressed from the broken coat of rice grain. Used as a coating for candy. Nontoxic.

RICE BRAN WAX • The wax obtained from the broken coat of rice grain. Used as a coating agent, as a chewing-gum base, and a releasing agent *(see)*.

RICE STARCH • The finely pulverized grains of the rice plant used as an anticaking agent, thickener, and gelling agent. Also used in baby powders, face powders, and dusting powders. It is a demulcent and emollient and forms a soothing, protective film when applied. May cause mechanical irritation by blocking the pores and putrefying. May also cause an allergic reaction. The final report to the FDA of the Select Committee on GRAS Substances stated in 1980 that it should continue its GRAS status with no limitations other than good manufacturing practices.

RICINOLEIC ACID • A mixture of fatty oils found in the seeds of castor beans. Castor oil contains 80 to 85 percent ricinoleic acid. The oily liquid is used in soaps, flavorings, antifungal agents, and in contraceptive jellies. It is believed to be the active laxative in castor oil. Also used externally as an emollient. No known toxicity.

RICINOLEATE • Salt of ricinoleic acid found in castor oil. Used in the manufacture of soaps. No known toxicity.

RIGHT-TO-KNOW • *See* Community Right-To-Know List established by the Environmental Protection Agency and other government and civic organizations.

RNA • (Ribonucleic Acid). A nucleic acid that is found in the cytoplasm and also in the nucleus of some cells. One function of RNA is to direct the manufacture of proteins.

ROBENIDINE • Crystals from ethanol *(see)*. Used to treat parasites in chickens. FDA limits 0.2 ppm in skin and fat of chickens and 0.1 ppm in other chicken tissues. Moderately toxic by ingestion.

ROCHELLE SALT • Potassium Sodium Tartrate. Used in the manufacture of baking powder and in the silvering of mirrors. Translucent crystals or white crystalline powder with cooling saline taste. Slight efflorescence in warm air. Probably used in mouthwashes, but use not identified in cosmetics. No known toxicity.

RONNEL • Used in cattle feed. A systemic pesticide. *See* Organophosphates.

ROSA ALBA • *See* Rose Absolute.

ROSA CANINA • *See* Rose Hips Extract.

ROSA CENTIFOLIA • *See* Rose, Absolute.

ROSE, ABSOLUTE • Same origin as for rose Bulgarian *(see)*. Used as a berry, rose, fruit, and nut flavoring agent for beverages, ice cream, ices, candy, and baked goods. No known toxicity except for allergic reactions. GRAS. There is reported use of the chemical, it has not yet been assigned for toxicology literature.

ROSE BENGAL • A bluish red, fragrant liquid taken from the rose of the Bengal region of the Asian subcontinent. Used to scent perfumes and as an edible color product to make lipstick dyes. Nontoxic.

ROSE BUDS, FLOWERS, FRUITS (HIPS), LEAVES • Flavoring. *See* Rose Extract. GRAS.

ROSE BULGARIAN • True Otto Oil. Attar of Roses. Rose Otto Bulgaria. One of the most widely-used perfume ingredients, it is the essential oil, steam-distilled from the flowers of *Rosa damascena*. The rose flowers are picked early in the morning when they contain the maximum amount of perfume and are distilled quickly after harvesting. Bulgaria is the main source of supply, but Russia, Turkey, Syria, and Indochina also grow it. The liquid is pale yellow and has warm, deep floral, slightly spicy, and extremely fragrant red-rose smell. It is used as a flavoring agent in loganberry, raspberry, strawberry, orange, rose, violet, cherry, grape, peach, honey, muscatel, maple, almond, pecan, and ginger ale flavorings for beverages, ice cream, ices, candy, baked goods, gelatin desserts, chewing gum, and jellies. Also used in mucilage, coloring matter, and as a flavoring in pills. May cause allergic reactions. GRAS.

ROSE EXTRACT • An extract of the various species of rose, it is used in raspberry and cola beverages and in fragrances. No known toxicity except for allergic reactions. GRAS.

ROSE GERANIUM • Distilled from any of several South African herbs grown for their fragrant leaves. Used in perfumes, and to scent toothpaste and dusting powders. May cause allergic reactions. GRAS.

ROSE HIPS EXTRACT • Hip berries. Extract of the fruit of various species of wild roses, it is rich in vitamin C and is used as a natural flavoring. Widely used by organic food enthusiasts GRAS. There is reported use of the chemical, it has not yet been assigned for toxicology literature.

ROSE LEAVES EXTRACT • Derived from the leaves of the genus *Rosa*. Used in raspberry and cola beverages.

ROSE OIL • Attar of Roses. The fragrant, volatile, essential oil distilled from fresh flowers. Colorless or yellow with a strong fragrant odor and taste of roses. Used in perfumes, toilet waters, and ointments. Nontoxic but may cause allergic reactions. *See* Rose Bulgarian.

ROSE OTTO BULGARIA • *See* Rose Bulgarian.

ROSELLE • *Hibiscus sabdariffa*. An herb cultivated in the East Indies, it is used for making tarts and jellies, and gives a tart taste to acid drinks. It is also used as a natural red food coloring for soft drinks, tea-type products, punches, apple jelly, and pectin jelly, but it is not stable in carbonated beverages. No known toxicity. GRAS.

ROSEMARY EXTRACT • Garden Rosemary. A flavoring and perfume from the fresh aromatic flowering tops of the evergreen shrub, *Rosemarinus officinalis l.* grown in the Mediterranean region. Light blue flowers and gray-green leaves. Used for beverages, condiments, and meat. It is also used in citrus, peach, and ginger flavorings for beverages, ice cream, ices, candy, baked goods, condiments, and meats. Also being studied as a natural antioxidant. A teaspoonful of the oil may cause illness in an adult, and an ounce may cause death. GRAS. There is reported use of the chemical, it has not yet been assigned for toxicology literature.

ROSIDINHA • Sideroxylon. A large green genus of tropical trees, family Sapotaceae having hard wood and somewhat bell-shaped flowers with a few seeded berries. Used as a flavoring.

ROSIN • Colophony. Softener for chewing gum. Also used as a coating for citrus fruit. It is a pale yellow residue left after distilling off the volatile oil from the oleoresin obtained from various species of pine trees chiefly produced in the United States. Also used in the manufacture of varnishes and fireworks. It can cause contact dermatitis.

ROSIN, GUM, GLYCEROL ESTER • A softener for chewing gum. *See* Rosin and Glycerol.

ROSIN, METHYL ESTER, PARTIALLY HYDROGENATED • Used in the manufacture of food additives and as a softener for chewing gum.

ROSIN, PARTIAL DIMERIZED, CALCIUM SALT, or PARTIALLY (CAT-ALYTICALLY) HYDROGENATED • A coating for fresh citrus fruit. *See* Rosin and Hydrogenated.

ROSIN, POLYMERIZED GLYCEROL ESTER, PARTIALLY HYDROGENATED GLYCEROL ESTER, or PARTIALLY DIMERIZED GLYCEROL ESTER • A softener for chewing gum. *See* Rosin and Glycerol.

ROSIN, WOOD, PENTAERYTHRITOL ESTER OF MALEIC ANHYDRIDE • A coating for fresh citrus fruit. *See* Rosin and Maleic Acid.

ROSMARIN OFFICINALIS • *See* Rosemary.

ROXARSONE • An antibacterial for control of enteric infections and to improve growth and feed efficiency. Used in chicken and swine feeds, in drinking water of chickens, turkey, and swine.

RUBBER • Rubber as well as rubber-based adhesives are common causes of contact dermatitis. The natural gum obtained from the rubber tree is not allergenic; the offenders are the chemicals added to natural rubber gum to make it a useful product. Such chemicals are accelerators, antioxidants, stabilizers, and vulcanizers, many of which can cause allergies.

RUBBER, BUTADIENE STYRENE • Latex. A chewing-gum base. No known toxicity.

RUBBER, SMOKED SHEET • A chewing-gum base. No known toxicity.

RUBEFACIENT • Helps to stimulate blood circulation to the scalp and the activity of the oil-secreting glands. Pilocarpine *(see)* is an example.

RUE OIL • A spice agent obtained from the fresh aromatic blossoming plants grown in southern Europe and Asia. The oil has a fatty odor and is used in baked goods. It is obtained by steam distillation and is used in fragrances and in blueberry, raspberry, coconut, grape, peach, rum, cheese, spice flavorings for beverages, ice cream, ices, candy, baked goods, and condiments. Formerly used in medicine to treat disorders and hysteria. It is on the FDA list for study of mutagenic, teratogenic, subacute, and reproductive effects. It may cause photosensitivity. In 1976 the FDA confirmed rue as GRAS in all categories of food at a maximum use level of 2 ppm. The final report to the FDA of the Select Committee on GRAS Substances stated in 1980 that there is no evidence in the available information that it is a hazard to the public when used as it is now and it should continue its GRAS status with limitations on amounts that can be added to food.

RUM • An alcoholic beverage from fermented molasses. Flavoring for candied fruits.

RUM ETHER • A synthetic flavoring, consisting of water, ethanol, ethyl acetate, methanol, ethyl formate, acetone, acetaldehyde, and formaldehyde *(see all)*. Used in butter, liquor, and rum flavorings for beverages, ice cream, ices, candy, baked goods, gelatin, chewing gum, and alcoholic beverages (1,600 ppm).

RUTIN • Pale yellow crystals found in many plants, particularly buckwheat. Used as a dietary supplement for blood or lymph vessel fragility. There is reported use of the chemical; it has not yet been assigned for toxicology literature.

RYE FLOUR • Used in powders. Flour made from hardy annual cereal grass. Seeds are used for feed and in the manufacture of whiskey and bread. May cause allergic reactions.

S

SACCHARIDE HYDROLYSATE • A mixture of sugars derived from using an alkali and water on a mixture of glucose and lactose *(see)*.

SACCHARIDE ISOMERATE • *See* Saccharide Hydrolysate.

SACCHARIN • An artificial sweetener in use since 1879. It is three hundred times as sweet as natural sugar. Used as a sweetener for mouthwashes, dentifrices, and lipsticks. It sweetens dentifrices and mouthwashes in a 0.05 to 1 percent concentration. On the FDA's top-priority list to retest for mutagenic, subacute, and reproductive effects. White crystals or crystalline powder. Odorless or with a faint aromatic odor. It was used with cyclamates in the experiments that led to the ban on cyclamates. The FDA proposed restricting saccharin to fifteen milligrams per day for each kilogram of body weight or one gram a day for a 150-pound person. Then, on March 9, 1977, the FDA announced the use of saccharin in foods and beverages would be banned because the artificial sweetener had been found to cause malignant bladder tumors in laboratory animals. The ban was based on the findings of a study sponsored by the Canadian government that found that seven out of thirty-eight animals developed tumors, three of them malignant. In addition, one hundred offspring were fed saccharin, and fourteen of them developed bladder tumors. In contrast, one hundred control rats were not fed saccharin and only two developed tumors. At the time of the FDA's announcement, five million pounds of saccharin were being consumed per year, 74 percent of it in diet soda, 14 percent in dietetic food, and 12 percent as a tabletop replacement for sugar. There was an immediate outcry, led vociferously by the Calorie Control Council, an organization made up of commercial producers and users of saccharin. The FDA, urged by Congress, then delayed the ban. The moratorium on prohibiting the use of saccharin has been extended indefinitely. Since 1977, however, saccharin containers carry labels warning that saccharin may be hazardous to your health.

Saccharin has exhibited mutagenic activity (genetic changes) in the early-warning Ames Test *(see)* for carcinogens. When administered orally to mice, mutagenic activity was demonstrated in the urine of these animals as well as in tissue tests. Highly purified saccharin was not mutagenic in tissue tests, but the urine of mice fed saccharin was. Congress's Office of Technology Assessment, in view of the evidence to date, strongly endorsed the scientific basis of the FDA's proposed ban. "This review of animal studies leads to the conclusion that saccharin is a carcinogen for animals," the FDA panel said. Clouding the degree of risk, however, is that up to 20 ppm of unknown chemical impurities contaminated those doses fed the rats in the Canadian study that led to the FDA's original move. The impurities themselves proved mutagenic in the Ames Test.

On November 6, 1978, the Committee of the Institute of Medicine and National Research Council concluded that saccharin is a potential carcinogen in humans. The extremely low potency of saccharin as a carcinogen was emphasized by the Committee. However, they expressed special concern that children under ten years of age were consuming diet sodas and other saccharin-containing products in increasing amounts. Exposure in children, the Committee noted, may have special significance because of the long time required for some cancers to develop. There were some "worrisome data" regarding consumption by women of child-bearing age, children, and teenagers. The concern about fetal exposure grew out of earlier findings of increased bladder cancers in male rats fed high-saccharin diets or born to mothers that were on high-saccharin diets during pregnancy. The Committee concluded that it is most likely that saccharin itself is the carcinogenic agent, rather than any impurities that may be associated with its manufacture. The fight to keep saccharin on the market spotlighted the Delaney Amendment, which prohibits known carcinogens from being added to food, and a move to weaken that amendment persists. In 1969, Britain banned saccharin except as an artificial sweetener. In 1950, France banned it except as a nonprescription drug. Germany restricts its use to certain foods and beverages, which must state on the label that it is in the product. In 1997, the Caloric Control Council, a trade group, successfully requested the National Toxicology Program to review new data to lead to a delisting of saccharin as a carcinogen.

SAFFLOWER GLYCERIDE • *See* Safflower Oil.

SAFFLOWER OIL • The edible oil expressed from the seed of an Old World herb that resembles a thistle, with large, bright red or orange flowers. Widely cultivated for its oil, which thickens and becomes rancid on exposure to air. It is used in salad oils and shortenings, and as a vehicle for medicines. As a dietary supplement it is alleged to be a preventative in the development of atherosclerosis—fat-clogged arteries. A drug consisting of the dried flowers of safflower is used in medicine in place of saffron *(see)*. Used in creams and lotions to soften the skin. No known toxicity. American safflower (American saffron) is no longer authorized for use.

SAFFRON • Crocus. Vegetable Gold. Spanish or French Saffron. The dried stigma of the crocus, *Crocus sativus,* cultivated in Spain, Greece, France, and Iran. Orange-brown; strong, peculiar aromatic odor; bitterish, aromatic taste. Almost entirely employed for coloring and flavoring. It has been permanently listed for use in foods since 1966. It does not require certification. Used in bitters, liquors, and spice flavorings for beverages, baked goods, meats, and liquors. Cleared by the USDA Meat Inspection Department for coloring sausage casing, oleomargarine, shortening, and for marking ink. The extract is used in honey and rum flavorings for beverages, ice cream, ices, candy, baked goods, and condiments, and it goes into yellow coloring. Formerly used to treat skin diseases. GRAS.

SAFROLE and ANY OIL CONTAINING SAFROLE • Illegal. Found in certain natural oils such as star anise, nutmeg, ylang-ylang, it is a stable, colorless to brown liquid with an odor of sassafras and root beer. Used in the manufacture of heliotropin *(see)* and in expensive soaps and perfumes. Used as a beverage flavoring until it was banned in 1960. The toxicity of this fragrance ingredient is being questioned by the FDA. It is an animal liver carcinogen.

SAFROLE-FREE EXTRACT OF SASSAFRAS • A flavoring in food. *See* Sassafras.

SAGE • Spanish. Greek. The flowering tops and leaves of the shrubby mints. Spices include Greek sage and Spanish sage. The genus is *Salvia,* so named for the plant's supposed healing powers. *Greek sage* is used in fruit and spice flavorings for beverages, baked goods, and meats (1,500 ppm). *Greek sage oil,* obtained by steam distillation, is used in berry, grape, liquor, meat, crème de menthe, nutmeg, and sage flavorings for beverages, ice cream, ices, candy, baked goods, chewing gum, condiments, meats, and pickles. *Greek sage oleoresin (see)* is used in sausage and spice flavorings for condiments and meats. *Spanish sage oil* is used in fruit and spice flavorings for beverages, ice cream, ices, candy, baked goods, condiments, and meats. It is also used as a meat preservative. Greek sage is used in medicine. Used by herbalists to treat sore gums, mouth ulcers, and to remove warts. The Arabs believed that it prevents dying. No known toxicity. GRAS.

SAIGON CINNAMON • *See* Cinnamon.

SAIGON CINNAMON LEAF OIL • *See* Cinnamon.

SAINT JOHN'S BREAD • *See* Locust Bean Gum. GRAS.

SAINT JOHN'S WORT FLOWERS, LEAVES, and CAULIS • *Hypericum perforatum.* Amber. Blessed. Devil's Scourge. God's Wonder Herb. Grace of God. Goatweed. Hypericum. Klamath Weed. A perennial native to Britain, Europe, and Asia, it is now found throughout North America. The plant contains volatile oil, tannin, resin, pectin *(see all),* and glycosides. It was believed to have infinite healing powers derived from the saint, the red juice representing his blood. It was used as an antivenereal. It is used to treat pains and diseases of the nervous system, arthritic pains, and injuries. An infusion made from its leaves is used for stomach disorders, diarrhea, depression, and bladder problems, and to remove threadworms in children. A salve made from the flowers is used by herbalists to treat scratches, swellings, and small wounds. The oil is used for burns. A spray has been used for colds. It reputedly also eases fibrositis, sciatica, and varicose veins. It is now being studied by researchers from the National Cancer Institute and universities as a potential treatment for cancer and AIDS. The FDA listed Saint John's wort as an "unsafe herb" in 1977. The FDA issued a notice in 1992 that Saint John's wort has not been shown to be safe and effective as claimed in OTC digestive-aid products. That does not mean, however, that it cannot be used for other purposes.

SALAD OIL • Any edible vegetable oil. Dermatologists advise rubbing salad oils or fats on the skin, particularly on babies and older persons. Vegetable oils are used in commercial baby preparations, cleansers, emollient creams, face powders, hair-grooming preparations, hypoallergenic cosmetics, lipsticks, nail creams, shampoos, shaving creams, and wave sets. Nontoxic.

SALATRIM • Short and Long Chain Acid Triglyceride Molecules. This is a family of reduced-calorie fats that are only partially absorbed in the body. It contains 5 calories per gram. It is used in such products as Hershey's reduced-fat, semi-sweet chocolate flavor baking chips. GRAS.

SALICARIA EXTRACT • Spiked Loose Strife. Extract of the flowering herb *Lythrum salicaria,* which has purple or pink flowers. Used since ancient Greek times as an herb that calms nerves and soothes skin.

SALICIN • A chemical derived from the bark of several species of willows and poplar trees. Aspirin and other salicylates are derived from salicin or made synthetically.

SALICYLALDEHYDE • Salicylic Aldehyde. A synthetic flavoring made by heating phenol (very toxic) and chloroform. Occurs naturally in cassia bark. Clear, bitter, almondlike odor, burning taste. White to slightly pink, crystalline, bitter powder. Gives a sensation of warmth on the tongue. Soluble in hot water. Used in butter flavorings for beverages, ice cream, ices, candy, baked goods, chewing gum, condiments, and liqueurs. Used chiefly in perfumery. Used as an analgesic, fungicide, and anti-inflammatory agent to soothe the skin. Lethal dose in rats is one gram per kilogram of body weight.

SALICYLATES • Amyl. Phenyl. Benzyl. Menthyl. Glyceryl. Dipropylene Glycol Esters. Salts of Salicylic Acid. Those who are sensitive to aspirin may also be hypersensitive to FD and C Yellow No. 5, a salicylate, and to a number of foods that naturally contain salicylate, such as almonds, apples, apple cider, apricots, blackberries, boysenberries, cherries, cloves, cucumbers, currants, gooseberries, grapes, nectarines, oil of wintergreen, oranges, peaches, pickles, plums, prunes, raisins, raspberries, strawberries, and tomatoes. Foods with added salicylates for flavoring may be ice cream, bakery goods (except bread), candy, chewing gum, soft drinks,

Jell-O, jams, cake mixes, and wintergreen flavors. The salts are used as sunburn preventatives and antiseptics.

SALICYLIC ACID • Occurs naturally in wintergreen leaves, sweet birch, and other plants and has a sweetish taste. Synthetically prepared by heating phenol with carbon dioxide, it is used as a preservative in food products. It is also used as a fungicide in the treatment of animals. Residues are prohibited in milk. EPA Genetic Toxicology Program *(see)*. It is also used as a preservative and antimicrobial at 0.1 to 0.5 percent in skin softeners, face masks, hair tonics, deodorants, dandruff preparations, protective creams, hair dye removers, and suntan lotions and oils. It is antipuretic (anti-itch) and antiseptic. In fact, in medicine, it is used as an antimicrobial at 2 to 20 percent concentration in lotions, ointments, powders, and plasters. It is also used in making aspirin. It can be absorbed through the skin. Absorption of large amounts may cause vomiting, abdominal pain, increased respiration, acidosis, mental disturbances, and skin rashes in sensitive individuals. It is poisonous by ingestion. Causes birth defects in experimental animals.

SALICYLIC ETHER • *See* Ethyl Salicylate.

SALICYLIDES • Any of several crystalline derivatives of salicylic acid *(see)* from which the water has been removed.

SALINOMYCIN • Coxistac. An antiparasite drug used in chicken feed.

SALMONELLA • Named for the American veterinarian, Dr. D. E. Salmon, it is a bacteria that occurs in the intestinal tract and tissues of infected humans and animals. Many of the more than twelve hundred different types can cause food poisoning, entering the food supply through meats or animal products from infected animals or from contamination by an infected animal or person. One of the most common foodborne illnesses in the United States, the symptoms are diarrhea, abdominal cramps, fever, and sometimes vomiting, which occur six to forty-eight hours after eating. Infections range from moderate, with recovery in three to four days, to fatal. Salmonella bacteria grow rapidly in cooked foods such as meat, eggs, custards, and salads that have been left unrefrigerated for several hours. It may also be transmitted by infected poultry and by sewage-polluted water. The National Academy of Science's Institute of Medicine estimated that doses of antibiotics in livestock promote growth or prevent infection for less than 2 percent of the human deaths due to food-borne, antibiotic-resistant Salmonella. In 1989, according to a "new risks" assessment made for the FDA by the National Academy of Science's Institute of Medicine (IOM), the group "was unable to find data directly implicating subtherapeutic doses of antibiotics in livestock with illnesses in people" or to come up with a "numerical answer" about the risk of animal medication posed to humans. The IOM estimated that the doses of antibiotics given to livestock to promote growth or prevent infection would account for less than 2 percent of the human deaths due to foodborne, antibiotic-resistant salmonella. The Committee felt that stopping the use of antibiotics to promote growth in livestock might reduce the total number of human deaths due to salmonella poisoning, but that such results could not be supported scientifically. Since 1989, of course, the incidences of salmonella resistant to antibiotics has been increasing, according to another government agency, the Centers for

Disease Control. Salmonella has contaminated almost every chicken sent to market and has led the U.S. government to require warning labels on poultry products.

SALT • A compound formed by the interaction of an acid and a base. Sodium chloride, or common table salt, is an example. Sodium is the alkali or base and chloride provides the acidic factor.

SALTPETER • Potassium Nitrate. Niter. *See* Nitrate, Potassium. Acute intoxication is unlikely because a large dose causes vomiting and because it is rapidly excreted. Potassium poisoning disturbs the rhythm of the heart, and orally poisoned animals die from respiratory failure. Prolonged exposure to even small amounts may produce anemia, methemoglobinemia (lack of oxygen in the blood), and kidney damage.

SALT OF STEARIC ACID • *See* Stearic Acid.

SALTS OF FATTY ACIDS • Aluminum, calcium, magnesium, potassium, and sodium salts of capric, caprylic, myristic, oleic, palmitic, and stearic acids *(see all)* manufactured from fats and oils derived from edible sources. Used as anticaking agents, binders, and emulsifiers in various foods.

SALVIA • *See* Sage.

SAMBUCUS EXTRACT • *See* Elder Flowers.

SANDALWOOD OIL, EAST INDIAN • The pale yellow, somewhat viscous volatile oil obtained by steam distillation from the dried ground roots and wood of the plant. A strong, warm, persistent odor; soluble in most fixed oils. Used in floral, fruit, honey, and ginger ale flavorings for beverages, ice cream, ices, candy, baked goods, and chewing gum. Used in perfume. Also used for incense and as a fumigant. May produce skin rash in the hypersensitive, especially if present in high concentrations in expensive perfumes.

SANDALWOOD OIL, WEST INDIAN • Less soluble than the East Indian variety. *See* Amyris Oil.

SANDALWOOD OIL, YELLOW • Arheol. Same origin as East Indian sandalwood oil *(see)*. A floral, fruit, honey, and ginger ale flavoring agent for beverages, ice cream, ices, candy, baked goods, and chewing gum. No known toxicity.

SANDARAC • Used in alcoholic beverages only. Resin, from a plant grown in Morocco, is light yellow, brittle, insoluble in water. Used in tooth cements, varnishes, and for gloss and adhesion in nail lacquers. There is reported use of the chemical, it has not yet been assigned for toxicology literature.

SANITIZING SOLUTIONS • For use on food processing equipment followed by adequate draining. The FDA sets limits on uses and concentrations for many compounds. *See,* for example, Quaternary Ammonium Compounds or Butoxy Monoether of mixed (ethylene) prolyalkylene glycol.

SANTALOL • Alcohol from sandalwood used in fragrances. There is reported use of the chemical; it has not yet been assigned for toxicology literature. *See* Sandalwood Oil.

SANTALUM ALBUM • *See* Sandalwood Oil.

SANTALYL ACETATE • Acetic Acid. A synthetic flavoring agent obtained from sandalwood oils *(see)*. Used in floral, pear, and pineapple flavorings for beverages, ice cream, ices, candy, baked goods, and chewing gum.

SANTALYL PHENYLACETATE • Phenylacetic Acid. A synthetic flavoring obtained from sandalwood oils *(see)*. Used in butter, caramel, fruit, and honey flavorings for beverages, ice cream, ices, candy, and baked goods.

SANTOQUIN • Ethoxyquin. A yellow liquid antioxidant and herbicide. It has been found to cause liver tumors in newborn mice. *See* Sodium Acid Pyrophosphate (SAP). A questionable additive. *See* Ethoxyquin.

SAPONIN • Any of numerous glycosides—natural or synthetic compounds derived from sugars—that occur in many plants such as soapbark, soapwort, or sarsaparilla. Characterized by their ability to foam in water. Yellowish to white, acrid, hygroscopic. In powder form they can cause sneezing. Extracted from soapbark or soapwort and used chiefly as foaming and emulsifying agents and detergents; also to reduce surface tensions, produce fine bubble lather in shaving creams, shampoos, bath oils, and dry shampoos. No known skin toxicity.

SARSAPARILLA EXTRACT • The dried root from tropical American plants, *Smilax* spp. Used in cola, mint, root beer, sarsaparilla, wintergreen, and birch beer flavorings for beverages, ice cream, ices, candy, and baked goods. Still used for psoriasis; formerly used for syphilis. There is reported use of the chemical, it has not yet been assigned for toxicology literature.

SASSAFRAS BARK EXTRACT • Safrol. Safrol-free. It is the yellow to reddish yellow volatile oil obtained from the roots of the sassafras, *Sassafras albidum*. It is 80 percent safrole *(see)* and has the characteristic odor and taste of sassafras. Used in rum and root beer flavorings for beverages, ice cream, ices, candy, and baked goods. Used in dentifrices, perfumes, soaps, and powders to correct disagreeable odors. Applied to insect bites and stings to relieve symptoms; also a topical antiseptic and used medicinally to break up intestinal gas. May produce dermatitis in hypersensitive individuals. There is reported use of the chemical, it has not yet been assigned for toxicology literature.

SASSAFRAS LEAVES • Safrol-free. Same origin as the bark extract. Used in soups (30,000 ppm). There is no reported use of the chemical and no toxicology information is available. *See* Sassafras Bark Extract for toxicity.

SAT FAT • Abbreviation for *saturated fat* on food labels.

SAT FAT CAL • Abbreviation for *satured fat calories* on food labels.

SAUNDERS WHITE OIL • *See* Sandalwood Oil.

SAVORY EXTRACT • An extract of *Satureia hortensis,* an aromatic mint known as summer or winter savory. The dried leaves of summer savory is a spice used in baked goods, condiments, and meats. *Summer savory oil* is obtained from the dried whole plant. It is used as a spice in condiments, candy, and baked goods. *Summer savory oil oleoresin (see)* is a spice used in candy, baked goods, and condiments. *Winter savory oil and oleoresin* spices are used in candy, baked goods, and condiments. Poisonous by skin contact. Moderately toxic by ingestion. A severe skin irritant. GRAS.

SCALAREOLIDE • There is reported use of the chemical; it has not yet been assigned for toxicology literature.

SCURVY GRASS EXTRACT • The extract of the leaves and flower stalks of

Cochlearia officinalis. The bright green leaves of this northerly herb were collected and eaten in large quantities by European seamen to prevent scurvy. The plant has the strong odor of horseradish, to which it is related. No known toxicity.

SCHINUS MOLLE OIL • A natural flavoring extract from the tropical pepper tree, *Schinus molle.* Used in candy, baked goods, and condiments. GRAS. There is reported use of the chemical, it has not yet been assigned for toxicology literature.

SEBACIC ACID • Decanedioic acid. Colorless leaflets, sparingly soluble in water and soluble in alcohol. Manufactured by heating castor oil with alkalies or by distillation of oleic acid *(see).* The esters of sebacic acid are used as stabilizers. No known toxicity.

SELENIUM • Yellow solid or brownish powder, insoluble in water. Discovered in 1807 in the earth's crust. Used as a nutrient. Used in antidandruff shampoos. Can severely irritate the eyes if it gets into them while hair is being washed. Occupational exposure causes pallor, nervousness, depression, garlic odor of breath, gastrointestinal disturbances, and skin rash. Liver injury in experimental animals.

SELENIUM AS SODIUM SELENITE or SELENATE • Used as a feed additive. The FDA limits it to less than 0.1 ppm in complete feed for chickens, swine, turkeys, sheep, beef, cattle, dairy cattle, and ducks.

SENNA, ALEXANDRIA • Flavoring from the dried leaves of *Cassia senna* grown in India and Egypt. Has been used as a cathartic. There is reported use of the chemical; it has not yet been assigned for toxicology literature.

SENSITIVITY • Hypersensitivity. An increased reaction to a substance that may be quite harmless to nonallergic persons.

SENSITIZE • To administer or expose to an antigen provoking an immune response so that, on later exposure to that antigen, a more vigorous secondary response will occur.

SEQUESTERING AGENT • A preservative that prevents physical or chemical changes affecting color, flavor, texture, or appearance of a product. Ethylenediamine tetraacetic acid (EDTA) is an example. It is used in carbonated beverages. It also prevents adverse effects of metals in shampoos.

SERINE • L form only. An amino acid *(see),* nonessential, taken as a dietary supplement. It is a constituent of many proteins. *See* Proteins. On the FDA list requiring further information since 1980.

SEROTONIN • A neurotransmitter thought to play a role in temperature regulation, mood, and sleep. It is believed that it can be raised by eating carbohydrates, inhibits secretions in the digestive tract, and stimulates smooth muscles. It is an important regulator of both mood and affects appetite. It may be useful for victims of seasonal depression, people who want to stop smoking, and others.

SERPENTARIA EXTRACT • Snakeroot. Snakeweed. Virginia Snakeroot. Extracted from the roots of *Rauwolfia serpentina,* its yellow rods turn red upon drying. Used in the manufacture of resins and as a bitter tonic. It is permitted in alcoholic beverages only. No known toxicity when applied to the skin but can affect heart and blood pressure when ingested. Related to black cohosh and echinacea *(see both).*

SERUM ALBUMIN • The major protein component of blood plasma derived from bovines. Used as a moisturizing ingredient.

SERUM PROTEINS • *See* Serum Albumin.

SERV SIZE • Abbreviation on labels for *serving size*.

SERVINGS • Label listing for servings per container.

SESAME • Seeds and Oils. The edible seeds of an East Indian herb, *Sesamum indicum,* which has a rosy or white flower. The seeds, which flavor bread, crackers, cakes, confectionery, and other products, yield a pale yellow, bland-tasting, almost odorless oil used in the manufacture of margarine. The oil has been used as a laxative and skin softener and contains elements active against lice. May cause allergic reactions, primarily contact dermatitis. GRAS.

SESQUITERPENE LACTONES • In recent years, more than six hundred plants have been identified as containing these substances, and more than fifty are known to cause allergic contact dermatitis. Among them are arnica, chamomile, and yarrow *(see all)*.

SHADDOCK EXTRACT • An extract of *Citrus grandis* and named for a seventeenth-century sea captain who brought the seeds back from the East Indies to Barbados. Shaddock is a large, thick-rinded, pear-shaped citrus fruit related to and largely replaced by the grapefruit. No known toxicity.

SHARK-LIVER OIL • A rich source of vitamin A, believed to be beneficial to the skin. A brown, fatty oil obtained from the livers of the large predatory fish. Used in lubricating creams and lotions. No known toxicity.

SHEA BUTTER • The natural fat obtained from the fruit of the karite tree, *Butyrosperum parkii.* Also called karite butter, it is chiefly used as a food but also in soap and candies. No known toxicity.

SHEA BUTTER UNSAPONIFIABLES • The fraction of shea butter that is not saponified during processing, that is, not turned into fatty alcohol.

SHELLAC • A resinous excretion of certain insects feeding on appropriate host trees, usually in India. As processed for marketing, the lacca, which is formed by the insects, may be mixed with small amounts of arsenic trisulfide for color and with rosin. White shellac is free of arsenic. Shellac is used as a candy glaze and polish up to 0.4 percent. Also used in hair lacquer and on jewelry and accessories. May cause allergic contact dermatitis. There is reported use of the chemical, it has not yet been assigned for toxicology literature.

SHELLAC WAX • Bleached, refined shellac. *See* Shellac.

SHORTENINGS • A fat such as butter, lard, or vegetable oil used to make cake, pastry, bread, etc., light and flaky. *See* Salad Oil.

SIBERIAN FIR OIL • *See* Pine Needle Oil.

SILICA • A white powder, slightly soluble in water, that occurs abundantly in nature and is 12 percent of all rocks. Sand is a silica. Upon drying and heating in a vacuum, hard transparent porous granules are formed that are used in absorbent and adsorbent material in toilet preparations, particularly skin protectant creams. Also used as a coloring agent.

SILICA AEROGEL • A fine, white powder, slightly soluble in water, that occurs abundantly in nature and is 12 percent of all rocks. Sand is a silica. Chemically and biologically inert, it is used as an antifoaming agent in beverages and as a surfactant. Used chiefly in the manufacture of glass. Upon drying and heating in a vacuum, hard, transparent, porous granules are formed that are used in absorbents and adsorbent material in toilet preparations, particularly skin-protectant creams. Also used as a coloring agent. The final report to the FDA of the Select Committee on GRAS Substances stated in 1980 that it should continue its GRAS status with no limitations other than good manufacturing practices. There is reported use of the chemical, it has not yet been assigned for toxicology literature. *See* Silicones.

SILICATES • Salts or esters derived from silicic acid *(see)*. Any of numerous insoluble complex metal salts that contain silicon and oxygen that constitute the largest group of minerals and that with quartz make up the greater part of the earth's crust (as rocks, soils, and clays). Contained in building materials such as cement, concrete, bricks, and glass. No known toxicity. The simplest silicate is sand, a molecule formed by joining one silicon atom with two oxygen atoms.

SILICIC ACID • Silica Gel. White, gelatinous substance obtained by the action of acids on sodium silicate *(see)*. Odorless, tasteless, inert, white, fluffy powder when dried. Insoluble in water and acids. Absorbs water readily. Used in face powders, dentifrices, creams, and talcum powders as an opacifier. Soothing to skin. No known toxicity.

SILICON DIOXIDE • Silica. Transparent, tasteless crystals or powder, practically insoluble in water. Occurs in nature as agate, amethyst, chalcedony, cristobalite, flint, quartz, sand, and tridymite. Used as a defoamer in beer production. Cleared for use as a food additive and as an anticaking agent at a level not to exceed 2 percent in salt and salt substitutes, in BHT (*see* Butylated Hydroxytoluene), in vitamins up to 3 percent, in urea up to 1 percent, and in sodium propionate up to 1 percent *(see all)*. In feed and feed components it is also used as an anticaking or grinding agent and is limited to 1 percent by weight of finished food. In dried egg products with moisture it is limited to less than 5 percent of weight. It is used as an absorbent for some vitamin E and vitamin B in tableted foods for special dietary use. It is also a component of microcapsules for flavoring oil and it migrates to food from paper and paperboard products. Prolonged inhalation of the dust can injure lungs. The final report to the FDA of the Select Committee on GRAS Substances stated in 1980 that it should continue its GRAS status with no limitations other than good manufacturing practices. *See* Silica Aerogel.

SILICONES • Any of a large group of fluid oils, rubbers, resins, and compounds derived from silica *(see)* that are water repellent, skin adherent, and stable over a wide range of temperatures. Used as anticaking agents in foods and in waterproofing and lubrication. Used in aftershave preparations, hair-waving preparations, nail driers, hair straighteners, hand lotions, and protective creams. No known toxicity when used externally.

SIMARUBA BARK • A flavoring for use in alcoholic beverages only. It is from a southern American tree or shrub with a bitter bark.

SIMAZINE • A herbicide. The tolerance is 1 ppm in molasses for animal feed. The tolerance is 0.01 ppm in drinkable water as a result of spray aquatic plants.

SIMPLESSE • A fat substitute developed by the same company that brought you NutraSweet. It is made from egg and milk protein. It can be used, according to the company, in margarine, ice cream, salad dressings, and yogurt. It cannot be used in baked food. Its introduction was delayed by the FDA, which said in 1988 that even though Simplesse was made from natural food, it should be premarket-tested for safety.

SITOSTANOL • A substance in some Finnish margarines, it cut LDL cholesterol (the bad kind) by 20 percent. It reportedly inhibits cholesterol absorption, while statins, the medications used for that purpose prevent cholesterol manufacture. Researchers speculate that sitostanol may be especially effective in people with high cholesterol-absorption rates who may not respond to statin therapy.

SKATOLE • Used in perfumery as a fixative (see). A constituent of beet root, feces, and coal tar. Gives a violet color when mixed with iron and sulfuric acid.

SKIM MILK • See Milk.

SLOE BERRIES • Blackthorn Berries. The fruit of the common juniper. The extract is a natural flavoring used in berry, plum, and liquor flavorings for beverages, ice cream, ices, candy, baked goods, and cordials (up to 43,000 ppm). Sloe gin is flavored with sloe berries. GRAS. There is reported use of the chemical; it has not yet been assigned for toxicology literature.

SMALLAGE • See Lovage.

SMELLAGE • See Lovage.

SMOKE FLAVORING SOLUTIONS • Condensates from burning hardwood in a limited amount of air. The solutions are used to flavor various foods, primarily meats, and as antioxidants to retard bacterial growth. Also permitted in cheese- and smoke-flavored fish. The Select Committee of the Federation of American Societies for Experimental Biology (FASEB), under contract to the FDA, concluded that smoke flavorings in general pose no hazard to the public when used at current levels and under present procedures, but uncertainties exist that require further study. The committee also said there are insufficient data upon which to base an evaluation of smoked-yeast flavoring, produced by exposing food-grade yeast to wood smoke. It is used to flavor soups, cheese, crackers, dip, pizza, and seasoning mixes.

SMOKED SHEET RUBBER • A chewing-gum base. No known toxicity.

SNAKEROOT OIL • Canadian Oil. Wild Ginger. Derived from the roots of the plant *Asarum canadense,* which had a reputation for curing snakebites. Grown from Canada to North Carolina and Kansas. Used in ginger, ginger ale, wintergreen, and birch beer flavorings for beverages, ice cream, ices, candy, baked goods, and condiments. There is reported use of the chemical, it has not yet been assigned for toxicology literature. See Black Cohosh and Echinacea.

SOAP • Sodium Oleate and Sodium Palmitate. Any salt of a fatty acid usually made by saponification of a vegetable oil with caustic soda. The oldest cleanser, usually a mixture of sodium salts of various fatty acids. In liquid soaps, potassium instead of sodium salts are used. Bar soaps vary in contents from brand to brand, depending on the fats or oils used. Sodium hydroxide makes a strong soap; fatty acids, a mild soap. So-called neutral soaps are actually alkaline, with pH around 10 (compared to skin, which is 5 to 6.5 pH) when dissolved in water. Soaps are usually in toothpastes, tooth powder, and shaving creams. Hard soap consists largely of sodium oleate or sodium palmitate and is used medicinally as an antiseptic, detergent, or suppository. Many people are allergic to soaps. They may also be drying to the skin, irritate the eyes, and cause rashes, depending upon ingredients. GRAS for food packaging.

SOAPBARK • *See* Quillaja Extract.

SODIUM • A metallic element that is soft, silvery, and oxidizes easily in air. It is waxlike at room temperature and brittle at low temperature. It has many uses in combination with other chemicals. Sodium chloride *(see)* is common table salt.

SODIUM ACETATE • Sodium Salt of Acetic Acid. Transparent crystals highly soluble in water. Used as a preservative, flavoring, and pH control agent in candy, cereals, fats, grain products, jams, jellies, meat products, oils, pasta, snack foods, soup mixes, soups, and sweet sauces. Also migrates from cotton and cotton fabrics used in dry food packaging. In industrial forms, it is used in photography, dyeing processes, and in foot warmers because it retains heat. Medicinally it is used as an alkalizer and as a diuretic. EPA Genetic Toxicology Program *(see)*. Moderately toxic by ingestion. A skin and eye irritant. The final report to the FDA of the Select Committee on GRAS Substances stated in 1980 that it should continue its GRAS status with no limitations other than good manufacturing practices.

SODIUM ACID PHOSPHATE • A sequestrant in cheeses and frozen desserts. GRAS.

SODIUM ACID PYROPHOSPHATE (SAP) • A white mass or free-flowing powder used as a buffer. It is a slow-acting acid constituent of a leavening mixture for self-rising and prepared cakes, doughnuts, waffles, muffins, cupcakes, and other types of flours and mixes. Also used in canned tuna fish. The U.S. Department of Agriculture has proposed that SAP be added to hot dogs and other sausages to accelerate the development of a rose-red color, thus cutting production time by some 25 to 40 percent. It is related to phosphoric acid, which is sometimes used as a gastric acidifier. No known toxicity. The final report to the FDA of the Select Committee on GRAS Substances stated in 1980 that it should continue its GRAS status with no limitations other than good manufacturing practices.

SODIUM ACID SULFITE • *See* Sodium Bisulfite.

SODIUM ALGINATE • Dissolves in water to form a viscous, colloidal solution and is used in cosmetics as a stabilizer, thickener, and emulsifier. Used in frozen desserts, fruit jelly preservatives, and jams. An emollient used in baby lotions, hair lacquers, wave sets, and shaving creams. It is the sodium salt of alginic acid extracted from brown seaweed. Occurs as a white to yellowish, fibrous or granular powder, nearly odorless and tasteless. No known toxicity. GRAS.

SODIUM ALUM • *See* Alum.

SODIUM ALUMINATE • A strong alkaline employed in the manufacture of lake colors used in foods (*see* FD and C Lakes). Also used in water softening and printing. The final report to the FDA of the Select Committee on GRAS Substances stated in 1980 that it should continue its GRAS status with no limitations other than good manufacturing practices. Migrates to food from paper and paperboard products.

SODIUM ALUMINOSILICATE • Sodium Silicoaluminate. Anticaking agent used in dried whole eggs and egg yolks and grated cheese. A chemical substance used in dental compounds, colored lakes (*see* FD and C Lakes) for foods, and in washing compounds. The final report to the FDA of the Select Committee on GRAS Substances stated in 1980 that it should continue its GRAS status with no limitations other than good manufacturing practices.

SODIUM ALUMINUM PHOSPHATE • A white, odorless powder, insoluble in water, used as a buffer in self-rising flour. Used with sodium bicarbonate (*see*). Used also in various cheeses. No known toxicity. The final report to the FDA of the Select Committee on GRAS Substances stated in 1980 that it should continue its GRAS status with no limitations other than good manufacturing practices.

SODIUM ALUMINUM SULFATE • A flour-bleaching agent alone or in combination with potassium aluminum, calcium sulfate, and other compounds. Used in cereal flours. *See* Aluminum. GRAS.

SODIUM ARSANILATE • Used in animal feed. *See* Arsenic.

SODIUM ASCORBATE • Vitamin C. Sodium. Aside from its use in vitamin C preparations, it can serve as an antioxidant in chopped meat and other foods to retard spoiling; also used in curing meat. No known toxicity. The final report to the FDA of the Select Committee on GRAS Substances stated in 1980 that it should continue its GRAS status with no limitations other than good manufacturing practices. *See* Ascorbic Acid.

SODIUM BENZOATE • White, odorless powders or crystals; sweet, antiseptic taste. Works best in slightly acid media. Used as a preservative in margarine, codfish, bottled soft drinks, maraschino cherries, mincemeat, fruit juices, pickles, confections, fruit jelly preserves, and jams. Also used in the ice for cooling fish. An antiseptic and preservative used in eye creams, vanishing creams, and toothpastes. Once used medicinally for rheumatism and tonsillitis. No known toxicity for external use. Moderately toxic by ingestion. Caused birth defects in experimental animals. Larger doses of eight to ten grams by mouth may cause nausea and vomiting. Small doses have little or no effect. GRAS.

SODIUM BICARBONATE • Bicarbonate of Soda. Baking Soda. An alkali prepared by the reaction of soda ash with carbon dioxide and used in prepared pancake, biscuit, and muffin mixes; a leavening agent in baking powders; in various crackers and cookies; to adjust acidity in tomato soup, ices, and sherbets; in pastes and beverages; in syrups for frozen products; in confections and self-rising flours. Also used in cornmeals and canned peas. Also used in effervescent bath salts, mouthwashes, and skin-soothing powders. Its white crystals or powder are used as a gastric antacid, as an alkaline wash, and to treat burns. Used also as a neutralizer for butter, cream, milk, and ice cream. Essentially harmless to the skin, but when used on very dry skin in preparations that evaporate, it leaves an alkaline residue that may cause irritation. It may alter the urinary excretion of other drugs, thus making those drugs either more toxic or less effective. GRAS.

SODIUM BISULFATE • Sodium Acid Sulfite. Sodium Hydrogen Sulfite. Colorless or white crystals fused in water, with a disagreeable taste. It is used as a disinfectant in the manufacture of soaps, and in perfumes, foods, and pickling compounds. GRAS. *See* Sodium Bisulfite.

SODIUM BISULFITE • Sodium Acid Sulfite. An inorganic salt. It is a white powder with a disagreeable taste, used as a bleaching agent in ale, wine, beer, and other food products. Used as a preservative in canned shrimp but not recognized as a source of vitamin B_1. Commercial bisulfite consists chiefly of sodium metabisulfite *(see)*. It is used as an antiseptic, as an antifermentative in cosmetic creams, mouthwashes, bleaches, perfumes, and hair dyes, to treat parasitic skin diseases, and to remove warts. In its aqueous solution, it is an acid. Concentrated solutions are highly irritating to the skin and mucous membranes. Sodium bisulfite can cause changes in the genetic material of bacteria and is a suspect mutagen. Not permitted in meats and other sources of vitamin B_1; strong irritant to the skin and tissue. The Select Committee on GRAS Substances found it did not present a hazard at present use levels but that additional data would be needed if higher use occurred. The Committee said in 1980 that it should continue as GRAS with limitations on the amounts that can be added to food. *See* Sulfites.

SODIUM BORATE • Used as a preservative and emulsifier. Used in freckle lotions, nail whiteners, liquefying (cleansing) creams, and eye lotions. Hard, odorless powder insoluble in water, it is a weak antiseptic and astringent for mucous membranes. Used also in bath salts, foot preparations, scalp lotions, permanent-wave solutions, and hair-setting lotions. Has a drying effect on the skin and may cause irritation. Continued use of a shampoo containing it will cause the hair to become dry and brittle.

SODIUM BOROHYDRIDE • Prepared from methyl borate and sodium hydride, it is used as a reducing agent *(see)* for various food additive chemicals. It scavenges for traces of aldehyde, ketones, and peroxides in organic chemicals. It is used as a modifier for hop extract. There is reported use of the chemical, it has not yet been assigned for toxicology literature.

SODIUM BROMATE • Inorganic salt. Colorless, odorless crystals that liberate oxygen. Used as a solvent. *See* Potassium Bromate for toxicity.

SODIUM BROMIDE • A sanitizing agent that requires adequate drainage, according to the FDA.

SODIUM CALCIUM ALUMINOSILICATE • Used to prevent salt and dry mixes from caking. No known toxicity. The final report to the FDA of the Select Committee on GRAS Substances stated in 1980 that it should continue its GRAS status with no limitations other than good manufacturing practices.

SODIUM CAPRYL LACTYLATE • *See* Palm Oil.

SODIUM CAPRYLATE • *See* Palm Oil.

SODIUM CARBONATE • Soda Ash. Small, odorless crystals or powder that occur in nature in ores and in lake brines or seawater. Absorbs water from the air. Used as a neutralizer for butter, cream, fluid milk, and ice cream; in the processing of olives before canning; and in cocoa products. Used in cocoa products and canned peas as an optional ingredient in standardized foods *(see)*. Has an alkaline taste and is used as an antacid and reagent in permanent-wave solutions, soaps, mouthwashes, shampoos, foot preparations, bath salts, and vaginal douches. A strong alkali used like lye. It is used to treat skin rashes and as a water softener. It caused scalp, forehead, and hand rashes when the hypersensitive used cosmetics containing it. Ingestion of large quantities may produce corrosion of the gastrointestinal tract, vomiting, diarrhea, circulatory collapse, and death. The final report to the FDA of the Select Committee on GRAS Substances stated in 1980 that it should continue its GRAS status with no limitations other than good manufacturing practices.

SODIUM CARBOXYMETHYLCELLULOSE • Made from a cotton byproduct, it occurs as a white powder or granules. Used as a stabilizer, thickener, gelling agent, and nonnutritive bulking aid. Used to prevent water loss, make food opaque, and to texturize food. Found in ice cream, beverages, confections, baked goods, icings, toppings, chocolate milk, chocolate-flavored beverages, gassed cream (pressure-dispensed whipped cream), syrup for frozen products, variegated mixtures, cheese spreads, and in certain cheeses. Also used in French dressing, artificially sweetened jellies, preserves, gelling ingredients, and mix-it-yourself and powdered drinks. Medicinally used as a laxative (1.5 grams orally), antacid (15–30 milligrams of 5 percent solution), and in pharmacies for preparing suspensions. Used in setting lotions, it is an artificial gum that dries and leaves a film on the hair. Prepared by treating alkali cellulose with sodium chloroacetate. Can cause digestive disturbances. *See* Cellulose Gums.

SODIUM CARRAGEENAN • Sodium salt of carrageenan *(see)*.

SODIUM CASEINATE • Casein. The soluble form of milk protein in which casein is partially neutralized with sodium hydroxide and used as a texturizer in ice cream, frozen custard, ice milk, and sherbet. Cleared by the USDA Meat Inspection Department for use in imitation sausage, soups, and stews. No known toxicity. GRAS. The final report to the FDA of the Select Committee on GRAS Substances stated in 1980 that it should continue its GRAS status with no limitations other than good manufacturing practices.

SODIUM CASTORATE • The sodium salt of the fatty acids derived from castor oil *(see)*.

SODIUM CHLORIDE • Common table salt. In addition to seasoning it is used as a pickling agent, a preservative for meats, vegetables, and butter. Prevents browning in cut fruit. Used as an astringent and antiseptic in mouthwashes, dentifrices, bubble baths, soap, bath salts, and eye lotions. It consists of opaque white crystals. Odorless, with a characteristic salty taste, and absorbs water. Used topically to treat inflamed lesions. Diluted solutions are not considered irritating, but upon drying, water is drawn from the skin and may produce irritation. Salt workers have a great deal of skin rashes. Also reported to irritate the roots of the teeth when used for a long time in dentifrices. Not considered toxic but can adversely affect persons with high blood pressure and kidney disease. The final report to the FDA of the Select Committee on GRAS Substances stated in 1980 that it should continue its GRAS status with no limitations other than good manufacturing practices.

SODIUM CHLORITE • A powerful oxidizer prepared commercially and used to modify food starch (*see* Modified Starch) up to 0.5 percent. Used as a bleaching agent for textiles and paper pulp and in water purification. Toxicity depends on concentration. There is reported use of the chemical, it has not yet been assigned for toxicology literature.

SODIUM CHOLATE • *See* Cholic Acid.

SODIUM CITRATE • White, odorless crystals, granules, or powder with a cool salty taste. Stable in air. Prevents "cream plug" in cream and "feathering" when cream is used in coffee; an emulsifier in ice cream, processed cheese, and evaporated milk; a buffer to control acidity and retain carbonation in beverages, in frozen fruit drinks, confections, fruit jellies, preserves, and jams. It attaches itself to trace metals present in water and inhibits their entering the living cell. Proposed as a replacement for phosphates in detergents, but also causes algae growth and removes the necessary trace metals from water as well as the toxic ones. Used as a sequestering agent *(see)* to remove trace metals in solutions and as an alkalizer in cosmetic products. Can alter urinary excretion of other drugs, thus making those drugs either less effective or more toxic. The final report to the FDA of the Select Committee on GRAS Substances stated in 1980 that it should continue its GRAS status with no limitations other than good manufacturing practices.

SODIUM CLOXACILLIN • A penicillin antibiotic. The FDA tolerance for residues in milk is 0.01 ppm. *See* Cloxacillin.

SODIUM COCOATE • *See* Coconut Oil.

SODIUM COCO-HYDROLYZED ANIMAL PROTEIN • The sodium salt of the condensation product of coconut acid chloride and hydrolyzed animal protein. *See* Hydrolyzed Protein.

SODIUM COCOYL GLUTAMATE • A softener. *See* Glutamate.

SODIUM DECYLBENZENESULFONATE • An additive with miscellaneous uses but generally used in coatings for fresh citrus fruits. *See* Benzoic Acid.

SODIUM DEHYDROACETATE • Dehydroacetic Acid. A preservative; white, odorless, powdered, with an acrid taste. Used in cut or peeled squash and as a plasticizer, fungicide, and bactericide in antienzyme toothpaste. Used as a plasticizer, fungicide, and bacteria killer in cosmetics; as an antienzyme ingredient in dentifrices, allegedly prevents decay; a kidney-tube blocking agent. Can cause impaired kidney function. Large doses can cause vomiting, ataxia, and convulsions. There are no apparent allergic skin reactions. There is reported use of the chemical; it has not yet been assigned for toxicology literature.

SODIUM DIACETATE • A compound of sodium acetate and acetic acid *(see)*; a white, crystalline solid. Smells like vinegar. Used as a preservative. Inhibits molds and rope-forming bacteria in baked goods. No known toxicity. The final report to the FDA of the Select Committee on GRAS Substances stated in 1980 that it should continue its GRAS status with no limitations other than good manufacturing practices.

SODIUM DIALKYLPHENOXYBENZENEDISULFONATE • Used in lye mixtures for peeling fruits and vegetables.

SODIUM 2,2-DICHLOROPROPIONATE • Dalapon. A pesticide. The FDA tolerance is 20 ppm in dehydrated citrus pulp for cattle feed from application to citrus during growing season. It is a strong irritant to the eyes and skin. *See* Propionic Acid.

SODIUM DIHYDROGEN PHOSPHATE • White, odorless powder or granules used as a buffer, dietary supplement, emulsifier, nutrient, and in poultry wash. Used in beverages, cheese, meat products, poultry, and soft drinks. In meat food products, where allowed, limited to 5 percent. Mildly toxic by ingestion. A human eye irritant.

SODIUM N, *n*-DIMETHYLDITHIOCARBAMATE • Vinstop. Sta-Fresh 615. An antimicrobial agent used on beets and sugarcane. FDA limits the additive to 3 ppm based on weight of raw product. Moderately toxic by ingestion. Has caused mutations in experimental animals.

SODIUM DODECYLBENZENESULFONATE • An anionic detergent, it is used to treat raw food products and in cosmetic bath products and creams. It may irritate the skin. Will cause vomiting if swallowed.

SODIUM ERYTHORBATE • Sodium Isoascorbate. A white, odorless powder used as an antioxidant in pickling brine up to 7.5 ounces per 100 gallons and in meat products up to three-quarters of an ounce per 100 pounds. Also used in beverages and baked goods; in cured cuts and cured, pulverized products to accelerate color fixing in curing. No known toxicity. The final report to the FDA of the Select Committee on GRAS Substances stated in 1980 that it should continue its GRAS status with no limitations other than good manufacturing practices.

SODIUM 2-ETHYL 1-HEXYLSULFATE • A component of a commercial detergent for washing raw foods.

SODIUM FERRIC EDTA • Prepared from disodium ethylenediaminetetraacetic acid and ferric nitrate. Used as an iron source. The final report to the FDA of the Select Committee on GRAS Substances stated in 1980 that there were insufficient biological and other studies upon which to base an evaluation of it when it is used as a food ingredient. Nothing new has been reported by the FDA since. *See* Iron Salts.

SODIUM FERRICITROPYROPHOSPHATE • A white powder used in food enrichment. It is less prone to induce rancidity than other orthophosphates. The final report to the FDA of the Select Committee on GRAS Substances stated in 1980 that there were insufficient biological and other studies upon which to base an evaluation of it when it is used as a food ingredient. *See* Iron Salts.

SODIUM FERROCYANIDE • Yellow crystals or crystalline powder used as an anticaking agent for table salt and as a processing aid in wine. FDA limits residue to 1 ppm in finished wine.

SODIUM FLUORIDE • Used in toothpastes to prevent tooth decay and an insecticide, disinfectant, and preservative. It is used to fluoridate municipal water, as a wood preservative, rodenticide, for chemical cleaning, electroplating, and glass manufacture as well as a preservative for adhesives. Can cause nausea and vomiting when ingested, and even death, depending upon the dose. Strong irritant to the tissues. Fluorides added to water to reduce the incidence of dental caries is 1 ppm. The concentration used has been established to be far below the permissible level of toxicity. The program has been in existence for more than thirty years, yet there are still some scientists and citizens who worry about its adverse effects. Chronic endemic fluorosis due to high concentration of natural fluoride in local water supplies involves mottling of the teeth, bone changes, and, rarely, brain and nerve involvement. Acute fluoride poisoning can cause heart, brain, nerve, and gastrointestinal damage. This is a substance for which a petition has been filed but the FDA has not allowed it a as a nutrient additive because "it has not been proven safe."

SODIUM FORMATE • White, deliquescent crystals used in paper packaging. Moderately toxic by ingestion.

SODIUM GLUCONATE • Gluconic Acid. Sodium Salt. A pleasant-smelling compound, it is used as a sequestering agent *(see)*. The final report to the FDA of the Select Committee on GRAS Substances stated in 1980 that it should continue its GRAS status with no limitations other than good manufacturing practices.

SODIUM GLUTAMATE • The monosodium salt of the L-form of glutamic acid *(see)*.

SODIUM GLYCERYL OLEATE PHOSPHATE • *See* Glyceryl Monostearate.

SODIUM HEXAMETAPHOSPHATE • Sodium Polymetaphosphate. Graham's Salt. An emulsifier, sequestering agent *(see),* and texturizer. Used in breakfast cereals, angel food cake, flaked fish, ice cream, ice milk, beer, bottled beverages, reconstituted lemon juice, puddings, processed cheeses, and artificially sweetened jellies. Used in foods and potable water to prevent scale formation and corrosion. Because it keeps calcium, magnesium, and iron salts in solution, it is an excellent water softener and detergent. Used in bath salts, bubble baths, permanent-wave neutralizers, and shampoos. Phosphorus is an essential nutrient, but it has to be in balance with other minerals such as calcium in the diet. Too much phosphorus in foods could lead to an imbalance and adversely affect bones, kidney, and heart. Lethal dose in dogs is 140 milligrams per kilogram of body weight. Used in Calgon, Giltex, and other such products. The final report to the FDA of the Select Committee on GRAS Substances stated in 1980 that it should continue its GRAS status for packaging with no limitations other than good manufacturing practices.

SODIUM HYALURONATE • The sodium salt of hyaluronic acid. From the fluid in the eye; it is used as a gelling agent. No known toxicity.

SODIUM HYDROSULFATE • Sodium Dithionate. A bacterial inhibitor and antifermentative. Slight odor. White or grayish white, crystalline powder that oxidizes in air. No known toxicity to the skin.

SODIUM HYDROSULFITE • A bacterial inhibitor and antifermentative in the sugar and syrup industries. Slight odor. No known toxicity. The final report to the FDA of the Select Committee on GRAS Substances stated in 1980 that it should continue its GRAS status with no limitations other than good manufacturing practices. There is reported use of the chemical, it has not yet been assigned for toxicology literature. *See* Sulfites.

SODIUM HYDROXIDE • Caustic Soda. Soda Lye. An alkali and emulsifier. Readily absorbs water. Used as a modifier for food starch, a glazing agent for pretzels, and a peeling agent for tubers and fruits. An alkali and emulsifier in liquid face powders, soaps, shampoos, cuticle removers, hair straighteners, shaving soaps, and creams. The FDA banned use of more than 10 percent in household liquid drain cleaners. If too much alkali is used, dermatitis of the scalp may occur. Its ingestion causes vomiting, prostration, and collapse. Inhalation causes lung damage. The final report to the FDA of the Select Committee on GRAS Substances stated in 1980 that it should continue its GRAS status for packaging with no limitations other than good manufacturing practices.

SODIUM HYDROXIDE GELATINIZED STARCH • Starch *(see)* that has been gelatinized with sodium hydroxide. The final report to the FDA of the Select Committee on GRAS Substances stated in 1980 that there were insufficient biological and other studies upon which to base an evaluation of it when it is used as a food ingredient. Nothing new has been reported since.

SODIUM HYPOCHLORITE • A preservative used in the washing of cottage cheese curd. Also used medically as an antiseptic for wounds. Ingestion may cause corrosion of mucous membranes, esophageal or gastric perforation. The aqueous solutions are Eau de Javelle, Clorox, Dazzle.

SODIUM HYPOPHOSPHATE • White crystals, soluble in water, used as a sequestering agent *(see)*. The final report to the FDA of the Select Committee on GRAS Substances stated in 1980 that it should continue its GRAS status with no limitations other than good manufacturing practices.

SODIUM IODATE • A source of iodine in animal feed. GRAS. *See* Iodine.

SODIUM IODIDE • A source of iodine in animal feed. GRAS. *See* Iodine.

SODIUM INOSINATE • *See* Inosinate.

SODIUM IRON EDTA • A dietary supplement for use in supervised food fortification programs in populations in which iron-deficiency anemia is widespread. The FAO/WHO Expert Committee on Food Additives was asked to comment on this additive that is supposed to be restricted to specific supervised applications. The Committee was concerned about overfortification or misuse and did not recommend its availability for general use by individuals. It recommended it be used only as a supervised dietary supplement.

SODIUM IRON PYROPHOSPHATE • *See* Sodium Pyrophosphate.

SODIUM ISCISTEROYL LACTYLATE • The sodium salt of isostearic acid and lactyl lactate. *See* Stearic Acid and Lactic Acid.

SODIUM ISOASCORBATE • *See* Erythrobic Acid.

SODIUM LACTATE • Plasticizer substitute for glycerin. Colorless, thick, odorless liquid miscible with water, alcohol, and glycerin. It is used as an antioxidant, bodying agent, and humectant. Solution is neutral. Used medicinally as a systemic and urinary alkalizer. GRAS.

SODIUM LAURATE • *See* Sodium Lauryl Sulfate.

SODIUM LAURETH SULFATE • The sodium salt of sulfated ethoxylated lauryl alcohol, widely used as a water softener, and in baby and other nonirritating shampoos as a wetting agent and cleansing agent. *See also* Surfactants.

SODIUM LAUROYL GLUTAMATE • A softener. *See* Glutamate.

SODIUM LAURYL SULFATE (SLS) • A detergent, wetting agent, and emulsifier. It is used to treat raw foods, followed by a water rinsing. It is employed as a whipping aid in cake mixes and dried-egg products. In frozen and liquid egg whites the FDA allows up to 125 ppm; in egg white solids, 0.1 percent; 5,000 ppm by weight of gelatin as a whipping agent used in preparing marshmallows; 25 ppm in finished product. It is also used as a surfactant in fumaric acid-acidulated dry beverage base and fruit juice drinks unless precluded by food standards *(see)*. The FDA allows 10 ppm in crude vegetable oils and animal fats. Also used in bubble baths, emollient creams, cream depilatories, hand lotions, cold permanent waves, soapless shampoos, and toothpastes. Prepared by sulfation of lauryl alcohol followed by neutralization with sodium carbonate. Faint fatty odor; also emulsifies fats. May cause drying of the skin because of its degreasing ability and is an irritant to the skin. On the FDA list for further studies on the safety of this widely used additive.

SODIUM LIGNOSULFONATE • The sodium salt of polysulfonated lignin derived from wood. It is used as a dispersing agent. A tan, free-flowing powder, it is also used as an emulsifier, stabilizer, and cleaning agent.

SODIUM MAGNESIUM SILICATES • *See* Silicates.

SODIUM METABISULFITE • An inorganic salt. A bacterial inhibitor in wine, ale, and beer; an antifermentative in sugar and syrups; a preservative for fruit and vegetable juices; antibrowning agent in cut fruits, frozen apples, dried fruits, prepared fruit-pie mix, peeled potatoes, and maraschino cherries. The final report to the FDA of the Select Committee on GRAS Substances stated in 1980 that the additive did not present a hazard when used at present levels but that increased use would require additional safety data. *See* Sulfites.

SODIUM METAPHOSPHATE • Graham's Salts. A dough conditioner. Used in dental polishing agents, detergents, water softeners, sequestrants, emulsifiers, food additives, and textile laundering. The final report to the FDA of the Select Committee on GRAS Substances stated in 1980 that it should continue its GRAS status with no limitations other than good manufacturing practices. *See* Sodium Hexametaphosphate.

SODIUM METASILICATE • An alkali usually prepared from sand and soda ash. Used as a peeling solution for peaches and as a denuder for tripe "in amounts sufficient for the purpose." Used in detergents. Caustic substance, corrosive to the skin, harmful if swallowed, and cause of severe eye irritations. Preserves eggs in egg shampoos. GRAS.

SODIUM METHYL COCOYL TAURATE • *See* Ox Bile.

SODIUM METHYL OLEYL TAURATE • *See* Ox Bile.

SODIUM *n*-METHYL-*n*-OLEYL TAURATE • *See* Ox Bile.

SODIUM METHYL SULFATE • Used in processing pectin *(see)*. No known toxicity.

SODIUM MONOALKYLPHENOXYBENZENEDISULFONATE • Used in lye for peeling fruits and vegetables. No known toxicity.

SODIUM MONO- and DIMETHYL NAPHTHALENE SULFONATE • Anticaking agent and lye peeling agent used in cured fish and meats, and potable water. Also used in sodium nitrite in cured fish and meat.

SODIUM MONOHYDROGEN PHOSPHATE • Dibasic Sodium Phosphate. Used as a buffer, to retain juices, as a dietary supplement, emulsifier, hog wash, poultry wash, and in evaporated milk, poultry, instant pudding, and whipped products. Limited by FDA to 0.5 percent of total poultry product. Mildly toxic by ingestion. A skin and eye irritant.

SODIUM MYRISTATE • *See* Myristic Acid and Fatty Acids.

SODIUM MYRISTOYL ISETHIONATE • *See* Myristic Acid.

SODIUM NICOTINATE • This was used for what the FDA termed "deceptive use in ground meat for color retention." The FDA has banned it despite the request by producers for extension of its use.

SODIUM NITRATE • *See* Nitrate, Sodium.

SODIUM NITRITE • *See* Nitrite, Sodium.

SODIUM OLEATE • Sodium Salt of Oleic Acid. White powders, fatty odor, alkaline. Used in soaps.

SODIUM PALMITATE • Sodium salt of palmitic acid *(see)*. *See also* Fatty Acids.

SODIUM PANTOTHENATE • A member of the B-vitamin family. It is important as a constituent of coenzyme A. Its name is derived from the Greek word *pantothen* meaning "everywhere." Used as a dietary supplement. The final report to the FDA of the Select Committee on GRAS Substances stated in 1980 that it should continue its GRAS status with no limitations other than good manufacturing practices.

SODIUM PECTINATE • A stabilizer and thickener for syrups for frozen products, ice cream, ice milk, confections, fruit sherbets, French dressing and other salad dressings, fruit jelly, preserves, and jams. Used in quantities that reasonably compensate for the deficiency, if any, of natural pectin content of the fruit ingredients. GRAS.

SODIUM PHOSPHATE (DIBASIC) • Disodium Phosphate. Used in frozen desserts, enriched farina, and macaroni and noodle products. GRAS. *See* Sodium Phosphate.

SODIUM PHOSPHATE (MONO-, DI-, and TRIBASIC) • Buffer and effervescent used in the manufacture of nail enamels and detergents. White crystalline or granular powder, stable in air. Without water, it can be irritating to the skin but has no known skin toxicity. The final report to the FDA of the Select Committee on GRAS Substances stated in 1980 that it should continue its GRAS status with no limitations other than good manufacturing practices. *See* Phosphorous Sources.

SODIUM PHOSPHOALUMINATE • The acid salt of phosphoric acid. An ingredient of baking powders and other leavening mixtures. GRAS for packaging. *See* Phosphoric Acid for toxicity.

SODIUM POLYACRYLATE • Used in boiler water to inhibit mineral scale in beet and cane sugar production. The FDA allows up to 3.6 ppm of raw juice weight. *See* Acrylates.

SODIUM POLYACRYLATE-ACRYLAMIDE RESIN • A miscellaneous additive used in beet sugar or cane sugar juice to control organic mineral scale. The FDA says it can be up to 2.5 percent by weight of juice or liquor. *See* Acrylates and Acrylamide.

SODIUM POTASSIUM TARTRATE • Rochelle Salt. A buffer for confections, fruit jelly preserves, and jams. For each hundred pounds of saccharin in these products, three ounces of sodium potassium tartrate is used. Also used in cheese. Used medicinally as a cathartic. GRAS.

SODIUM PROPIONATE • Colorless or transparent, odorless crystals that gather water in moist air. Used as a preservative in cosmetics and foodstuffs to prevent mold and fungus. Used in baked goods, frostings, confections, and gelatin. It has been used to treat fungal infections of the skin, but can cause allergic reactions. GRAS.

SODIUM PYROPHOSPHATE • Used to decrease the amount of cooked-out juices in canned hams, pork shoulders, and bacon at 5 percent phosphate in pickle; 0.5 percent phosphate in product (only clear solution may be injected into hams). It is also used in cold-water puddings and processed cheese. It is an emulsifier salt and a texturizer as well as a sequestrant. The FDA labeled it GRAS for use as a sequestrant.

SODIUM RIBOFLAVIN PHOSPHATE • A B vitamin containing sodium phosphate *(see)*.

SODIUM SACCHARIN • An artificial sweetener in dentifrices, mouthwashes, and lipsticks. In use since 1879. Pound for pound it is three hundred times as sweet as natural sugar but leaves a bitter aftertaste. It was used along with cyclamates in the experiments that led to their ban in 1969. The FDA has proposed restricting saccharin to fifteen milligrams per day for each kilogram of body weight or one gram a day for a 150-pound person. On the FDA's priority list for further safety testing.

SODIUM SALT • *See* Sodium Benzoate.

SODIUM SALTS OF FATTY ACIDS • *See* Sodium and Fatty Acids.

SODIUM SESQUICARBONATE • Lye. White crystals, flakes, or powder produced from sodium carbonate. Soluble in water. Used as a neutralizer for butter, cream, fluid milk, and ice cream, in the processing of olives before canning, cacao products, and canned peas. Used as an alkalizer in bath salts, shampoos, tooth powders, and soaps. Irritating to the skin and mucous membranes. May cause an allergic reaction in the hypersensitive. The final report to the FDA of the Select Committee on GRAS Substances stated in 1980 that it should continue its GRAS status with no limitations other than good manufacturing practices. There is reported use of the chemical; it has not yet been assigned for toxicology literature.

SODIUM SILICATE • Water Glass. Soluble Glass. An anticaking agent for preserving eggs, detergents in soaps, depilatories, and protective creams. Consists of colorless to white or grayish white, crystalline pieces or lumps. These silicates are almost insoluble in cold water. Strongly alkaline. As a topical antiseptic can be irritating and caustic to the skin and mucous membranes. If swallowed, it causes vomiting and diarrhea. The final report to the FDA of the Select Committee on

GRAS Substances stated in 1980 that it should continue its GRAS status with no limitations other than good manufacturing practices.

SODIUM SILICOALUMINATE • Anticaking agent used in table salt up to 2 percent; dried egg yolks up to 2 percent; in sugar up to 1 percent; and in baking powder up to 5 percent. Slightly alkaline. No known toxicity. *See* Silicates. GRAS.

SODIUM SOAP • *See* Sodium Stearate.

SODIUM SORBATE • A food preservative used in cheeses alone or in combination with potassium sorbate or sorbic acid *(see both)*. It is also used in fruit butter, artificially sweetened fruit jelly, preserves, jams, and margarines. Also migrates from packaging into food. The final report to the FDA of the Select Committee on GRAS Substances stated in 1980 that it should continue its GRAS status with no limitations other than good manufacturing practices.

SODIUM STEARATE • Alkaline; 92.82 percent stearic acid *(see)*. Used as an emulsifier in foods. A fatty acid used as a chewing-gum base. It was approved in 1998 as an anticaking agent in animal feed. Also used in deodorant sticks, stick perfumes, toothpastes, soapless shampoos, and shaving lather. A white powder with a soapy feel and a slight tallowlike odor. Slowly soluble in cold water or cold alcohol. Also a waterproofing agent and has been used to treat skin diseases and in suppositories. One of the least allergy-causing of the sodium salts of fatty acids. Nonirritating to the skin. There is reported use of the chemical, it has not yet been assigned for toxicology literature.

SODIUM STEAROYL LACTYLATE • Used as follows unless precluded by food standards *(see):* 0.5 percent by weight of flour as a dough strengthener, emulsifier, or processing aid in baked products, pancakes, waffles, and prepared mixes; 0.2 percent by weight of finished food as surface active agent, emulsifier, or stabilizers in icings, fillings, pudding, and toppings; 0.3 percent by weight of finished emulsion or stabilizer in liquid and solid edible-fat water emulsion used as substitutes for milk and cream in coffee; 0.5 percent of dry weight as formulation aid, processing aid, or surfactant in dehydrated potatoes; 0.2 percent by weight as an emulsifier, stabilizer, or texturizer in snack dips and cheese and cheese product substitutes and imitations; 0.25 percent by weight of finished food as an emulsifier, stabilizer, or texturizer in sauces or gravies, products containing same, and prepared mixes of same. *See* Lactic Acid.

SODIUM STEAROYL-2-LACTYLATE • The sodium salt of a lactylic ester of fatty acid. Prepared from lactic acid and fatty acids. It is used as an emulsifier, plasticizer, or surfactant in an amount not greater than that required to produce the intended physical or technical effect, and where standards of identity *(see)* do not preclude use, in the following: bakery mixes, baked products, cake icings, fillings and toppings, dehydrated fruits and vegetables, dehydrated fruit and vegetable juices, frozen desserts, liquid shortenings for household use, pancake mixes, precooked instant rice, pudding mixes, solid-state edible vegetable-fat water emulsions used as substitutes for milk or cream in coffee, and with shortening and edible fats and oils when such are required in the foods listed above. *See* Lactic Acid for toxicity.

SODIUM STEARYL FUMARATE • Fine white powder used as a dough conditioner in bakery products, cereals processed for cooking, starch-thickened flour, and dehydrated potatoes. As a stabilizing agent in nonyeast-leavening bakery products up to 1 percent of weight of flour used. FDA limits are 0.5 percent of flour for yeast-leavened baked goods; 1 percent for nonyeast-leavened baked goods; 1 percent of dehydrated potatoes; 1 percent of dry processed cereals for cooking; and 0.2 percent for starch-thickened flour.

SODIUM SULFACHLOROPYRIDAZINE MONOHYDRATE • An antibiotic used for chickens. FDA requires zero residue in uncooked edible tissues of chickens.

SODIUM SULFATE • Salt Cake. Occurs in nature as the minerals mirabilite and nardite. Used in chewing-gum base and to preserve tuna fish and biscuits. Used medicinally to reduce body water. Used chiefly in the manufacture of dyes, soaps, and detergents. It is a reagent *(see)* and a precipitant; mildly saline in taste. Usually harmless when applied in toilet preparations. May prove irritating in concentrated solutions if applied to the skin and permitted to dry and then remain. May also enhance the irritant action of certain detergents. Taken by mouth, it stimulates gastric mucous production and sometimes inactivates a natural digestive juice—pepsin. Fatally poisoned animals show only diarrhea and intestinal bloating with no gross lesions outside the intestinal tract.

SODIUM SULFIDE • Composition in chewing-gum base. Crystals or granules prepared from ammonia that easily absorb water. Also used in dehairing hides and wool pulling, engraving, and cotton printing.

SODIUM SULFITE • White to tan-pink, odorless or nearly odorless powder having a cooling, salty, sulfurlike taste. An antiseptic, preservative, and antioxidant used as a bacterial inhibitor in wine-brewing and distilled-beverage industries. Also an antifermentative in the sugar and syrup industries and a browning inhibitor in cut fruits, used in frozen apples, dried fruit, prepared fruit-pie mix, peeled potatoes, maraschino cherries, dried fruits, and glacéed fruits. Used to bleach straw, silk, and wool; a developer in photography; treats upset stomachs and combats fungus infections. Also used in hair dyes. Foods and drinks containing sulfites may release sulfur dioxide. If this is inhaled by people who suffer from asthma, it can trigger an asthmatic attack. Sulfites are known to cause stomach irritation, nausea, diarrhea, skin rash, or swelling in sulfite-sensitive people. People whose kidneys or livers are impaired may not be able to produce the enzymes that break down sulfites in the body. Sulfites may destroy thiamin and consequently are not added to foods that are sources of this B vitamin. The final report to the FDA of the Select Committee on GRAS Substances stated in 1980 that it did not present a hazard when used at present levels but that additional data would be necessary if a significant increase in consumption occurred. *See* Sulfites.

SODIUM SULFO-ACETATE DERIVATIVES • Used as emulsifiers in margarine. Up to 0.5 percent. *See* Sodium Sulfate.

SODIUM TARTRATE • A laxative, sequestrant, chemical reactant, and stabilizer in cheese and artificially sweetened jelly. *See* Tartaric Acid. GRAS.

SODIUM TAUROCHOLATE • Taurocholic Acid. The chief ingredient of the bile of carnivorous animals. Used as an emulsifier in dried egg white up to 0.1 percent. It is a lipase accelerator. Lipase is a fat-splitting enzyme in the blood, pancreatic secretion, and tissues.

SODIUM TETRAPHOSPHATE • Sodium Polyphosphate. Used as a sequestering agent. The final report to the FDA of the Select Committee on GRAS Substances stated in 1980 that it should continue its GRAS status with no limitations other than good manufacturing practices. *See* Phosphate.

SODIUM THIOSULFATE • An antioxidant used to protect sliced potatoes and uncooked french fries from browning and as a stabilizer for potassium iodide in iodized salt. Also used to neutralize chlorine and to bleach bone. It is an antidote for cyanide poisoning and has been used in the past to combat blood clots; used to treat ringworm and mange in animals. Poorly absorbed by the bowel. The final report to the FDA of the Select Committee on GRAS Substances stated in 1980 that it should continue its GRAS status with no limitations other than good manufacturing practices.

SODIUM *p*-TOLUENE-SULFOCHLORAMINE • Chloramine-T. Water-purifying agent and a deodorant used to remove weed odor in cheese. Suspected of causing rapid allergic reaction in the hypersensitive. Poisoning by chloramine-T is characterized by pain, vomiting, sudden loss of consciousness, circulatory and respiratory collapse, and death.

SODIUM TOLUENESULFONATE • Methylbenzenesulfonic Acid, Sodium Salt. An aromatic compound that is used as a solvent. *See* Benzene.

SODIUM TRIMETAPHOSPHATE • A starch modifier. *See* Sodium Metaphosphate and Modified Starch.

SODIUM TRIPOLYPHOSPHATE (STPP) • A texturizer and sequestrant cleared for use in food-starch modifiers. A water softener. Also cleared by the USDA Meat Inspection Department to preserve meat by decreasing cooked-out juices in canned hams, pork shoulders, chopped ham, and bacon. Also used as a dilutant for Citrus Red No. 2 *(see)*. It is used in angel food cake mix, beef, desserts, gelling juices, goat, canned ham, lamb, lima beans, meat loaf, meat toppings, meringues, mutton, canned peas, pork, poultry, sausage products, and veal. It may deplete the body of calcium if taken in sufficient amounts, and such a case of low calcium was reported in a patient poisoned with water softener. Used in bubble baths and as a texturizer in soaps. It is a crystalline salt, moderately irritating to the skin and mucous membranes. Ingestion can cause violent purging. The final report to the FDA of the Select Committee on GRAS Substances stated in 1980 that it should continue its GRAS status for packaging with no limitations other than good manufacturing practices. *See* Sodium Phosphate.

SODIUM XYLENESULFONATE • A composition of sanitizing solutions.

SOL FIBER • Listing on food labels for *soluble fiber*. *See* Solubilization and Fiber.

SOLUBILIZATION • The process of dissolving in water such substances as fats and liquids that are not readily soluble under standard conditions by the action of a detergent or similar agent. Technically, a solubilized product is clear because the particle size in an emulsion is so small that light is not bounced off the particle. Solubilization is used in colognes and clear lotions. Sodium sulfonates *(see)* are common solubilizing agents.

SOLUBLE ANIMAL COLLAGEN • *See* Solubilization and Collagen.

SOLUBLE COLLAGEN • The protein derived from the connective tissue of young animals.

SOLVENT • A liquid capable of dissolving or dispersing one or more substances. Methyl ethyl ketone is an example of a solvent.

SORBATE, CALCIUM • *See* Calcium Sorbate.

SORBIC ACID • Acetic Acid. Hexadienic Acid. Hexadienoic Acid. Sorbistat. A white, free-flowing powder obtained from the berries of the mountain ash. It is also made from chemicals in the factory. It is used in cosmetics as a preservative and humectant. A mold and yeast inhibitor, it is used in foods, especially cheeses and beverages. It is also used in baked goods, chocolate syrup, fresh fruit cocktail, soda-fountain-type syrups, tangerine puree (sherbet base), salads (potato, macaroni, coleslaw, gelatin), cheesecake, pie fillings, cake, cheese in consumer-size packages, and artificially sweetened jellies and preserves. Percentages range from 0.003 in beverages to 0.2 percent in cheeses. Used as a replacement for glycerin in emulsions, ointments, embalming fluids, mouthwashes, dental creams, and various cosmetic creams. A binder for toilet preparations and plasticizers. Produces a velvetlike feel when rubbed on skin. In large amounts, sticky. Practically nontoxic but may cause skin irritation in susceptible people. When injected under the skin in 2,600-milligram doses per kilogram of body weight, it caused cancer in rodents. The final report to the FDA of the Select Committee on GRAS Substances stated in 1980 that it should continue its GRAS status with no limitations other than good manufacturing practices.

SORBITAN • A compound from sorbitol that has the water removed.

SORBITAN DIISOSTEARATE • The diester of isostearic acid and hexitol *(see* Fatty Acids).

SORBITAN DIOLEATE • The diester of oleic acid and hexitol anhydrides derived from sorbitol. *See* Sorbitan Fatty Acid Esters.

SORBITAN FATTY ACID ESTERS • Mixture of fatty acids *(see)* and esters of sorbitol *(see)* and sorbitol with the water removed. Widely used in food and the cosmetics industry as an emulsifier and stabilizer. Also used to prevent irritation from other cosmetic ingredients.

SORBITAN ISOSTEARATE • *See* Sorbitan Fatty Acid Esters.

SORBITAN LAURATE • Span 20. Oily liquid, insoluble in water, soluble in alcohol and oils. An emulsifier in cosmetic creams and lotions; a stabilizer of essential oils in water. No known toxicity.

SORBITAN MONOOLEATE • Polysorbate 80. An emulsifying agent for special dietary products and pharmaceuticals, a defoamer in yeast production, and a chewing gum plasticizer. An unintentionally administered daily dose of 19.2 grams per kilogram of body weight for two days to a four-month-old baby caused no harm except loose stools.

SORBITAN MONOPALMITATE • An emulsifier and flavor-dispersing agent used as an alternate for sorbitan monostearate *(see)* in cake mixes. No known toxicity.

SORBITAN MONOSTEARATE • An emulsifier, defoamer, and flavor dispersing agent. Used in cakes and cake mixes, whipped vegetable-oil toppings, cookie coatings, cake icings and fillings, solid-state edible vegetable fat–water emulsions used as substitutes for milk or cream in coffee, coconut spread, beverages, confectionery, baked goods. Percentages range from 1 to 0.66 percent. No single dose is known to be lethal in animals, and man has been fed a daily single dose of twenty grams without harm.

SORBITAN OLEATE • Sorbitan Monooleate. An emulsifying agent, defoaming agent, and plasticizer. No known toxicity.

SORBITAN PALMITATE • Span 40. Derived from sorbitol *(see)*. An emulsifier in cosmetic creams and lotions, a solubilizer of essential oils in water. Light yellow wax, insoluble in water, soluble in solvents. No known toxicity.

SORBITAN SESQUIOLEATE • An emulsifier. *See* Sorbitol and Oleic Acid.

SORBITAN SEQUISTEARATE • *See* Sorbitan Stearate.

SORBITAN STEARATE • Sorbitan Monostearate. An emulsifier in cosmetic creams and lotions, a solubilizer of essential oils in water. Used in antiperspirants, deodorants, cake makeup, hand creams, hair tonics, rouge, and suntan creams. Manufactured by reacting edible commercial stearic acid with sorbitol *(see both)*. Light cream to tan-colored, hard, waxy solid, with a bland odor and taste. Soluble at temperatures above its melting point in toluene, ethanol, methanol, and other alcohols. No known toxicity.

SORBITAN TRIISOSTEARATE • *See* Stearic Acid.

SORBITAN TRIOLEATE • *See* Sorbitol.

SORBITAN TRISTEARATE • An emulsifier and alternate for sorbitan stearate *(see)*. No known toxicity.

SORBITOL • An alcohol first found in the ripe berries of the mountain ash; it also occurs in other berries (except grapes), and in cherries, plums, pears, apples, seaweed, and algae. Consists of white, hygroscopic powder, flakes, or granules with a sweet taste. A sugar substitute for diabetics. Used as a thickener in candy, a sequestrant in vegetable oils, a stabilizer and sweetener in frozen desserts for special dietary purposes, and a humectant and texturizing agent in shredded coconut and dietetic fruits and soft drinks. Gives a velvety feel to skin. Used as a replacement for glycerin in emulsions, ointments, embalming fluid, mouthwashes, dental creams, and various cosmetic creams. A binder for toilet preparations and a plasticizer. Also used in hairsprays, beauty masks, cuticle removers, foundation cake makeup, hand lotions, liquid powders, dentifrices, aftershave lotions, deodorants, antiperspirants, shampoos, rouge, in writing inks to ensure a smooth flow from the point of the pen, and in pharmaceutical preparations to increase the absorption of vitamins. Medicinally used to reduce body water and for intravenous feedings. No known toxicity if it is applied to the skin. However, if ingested in excess, it can cause diarrhea and gastrointestinal disturbances.

Eating as little as ten grams of sorbitol can cause diarrhea in some children, according to Dr. Laurel Prestridge, a gastroenterologist and assistant professor of pediatrics at the University of Texas Southwestern Medical Center at Dallas. One piece of hard, sugar-free candy contains about 2.6 grams of sorbitol, and one thin, sugar-free chocolate bar contains about ten grams. In adults and children, sorbitol may alter the absorption of other drugs, making them less effective or more toxic.

SORBOSE • Derived from sorbitol *(see)* by fermentation. Used in the manufacture of vitamin C—accounts for nearly a thousand tons of ascorbic acid *(see)* produced yearly. No known toxicity. The final report to the FDA of the Select Committee on GRAS Substances stated in 1980 that it should continue its GRAS status for packaging with no limitations other than good manufacturing practices.

SORBUS EXTRACT • Service Tree Extract. The extract of *Sorbus domestica*. An extract was used by the Indians to make a wash for sore and blurred eyes from the sun, as from climbing and hiking or from dust.

SORGHUM • The second most widely grown feed grain in the U.S. Only 2 to 3 percent of the crop is used for human food in America, but it is the reverse in Africa and Asia. However, a new sorghum plant has been developed that is twice as nutritious in protein as the common variety and is 50 percent richer in lysine, an essential amino acid. The *syrup,* produced by evaporation from the stems and the juice, resembles cane sugar but contains a high proportion of invert sugars *(see)* as well as a starch and dextrin *(see both).* Very sweet, it is used as a texturizer and sweetener in foods. No known toxicity.

SORGHUM GRAIN SYRUP • Produced from dried sorghum juice. *See* Sorghum.

SORREL EXTRACT • Rumex Extract. An extract of the various species of *Rumex.* The Europeans imported this to America and the Indians adopted it. Originally the root was used as a laxative and as a mild astringent. It was also used for scabs on the skin and as a dentifrice. It was widely used by American medical circles in this century to treat skin diseases.

SOY EXTRACT • *See* Soybean Oil.

SOY FLOUR • *See* Soybean Oil.

SOY PROTEIN ISOLATES • *See* Soybean.

SOY SAUCE • Fermented or Hydrolyzed. A hydrolysis product of soybeans. A combination of mold fermentation and acid hydrolysis is used. The molds employed are *Aspergillus flavus, A. niger,* and *A. oryzae.* Soy sauce consists of a mixture of amino acids, peptides, polypeptides, peptones, simple proteins, purines, carbohydrates, and other organic compounds suspended in an 18 percent sodium chloride solution. In 1983, some manufacturers began producing soy sauce with a lower salt content. Used directly on food as a flavoring. The final report to the FDA of the Select Committee on GRAS Substances stated in 1980 that there is no available evidence that it is a hazard to the public when used as it is now and it should continue its GRAS status with limitations on the amounts that can be added to food.

SOY STEROL • *See* Soybean Oil.

SOY STEROL ACETATE • *See* Soybean Oil and Acetate.

SOYA FATTY ACIDS HYDROXYLATED • *See* Soybean and Hydroxylate.

SOYA HYDROXYETHYL IMIDAZOLINE • *See* Ethylenediamine and Urea.

SOYAMIDE DEA • *See* Soybean Oil.

SOYAMINE • *See* Soybean Oil.

SOYBEAN • An erect, bushy, hairy legume, *Glycine max,* native to Asia and extensively cultivated in China, Japan, and elsewhere, whose seeds yield valuable products. Contains glycerides of linoleic, oleic, linolenic, and palmitic acids. *See* Soybean Oil.

SOYBEAN OIL • Flour. Extracted from the seeds of plants grown in eastern Asia, especially Manchuria, and the midwestern U.S. The oil is made up of 40 percent protein, 17 percent carbohydrates, 18 percent oil, and 4.6 percent ash. It contains ascorbic acid, vitamin A, and thiamine. Pale yellow to brownish yellow. Also used in the manufacture of margarine. Debittered soybean flour contains practically no starch and is widely used in dietetic foods. Soybean oil is used in defoamers in the production of beet sugar and yeast, and in the manufacture of margarine, shortenings, candy, and soap. Soybean is used in many products including MSG, dough mixes, Lea and Perrins sauce, Heinz's Worcestershire sauce, soy sauce, salad dressings, pork link sausages, luncheon meats, hard candies, nut candies, and milk and coffee substitutes. It is made into soybean milk, soybean curd, and soybean cheese. Used in the manufacture of soaps, shampoos, and bath oils. About 300 million bushels of soybeans are grown yearly in the U.S., one-third more than in China. May cause allergic reactions, including hair damage and acnelike pimples. The final report to the FDA of the Select Committee on GRAS Substances stated in 1980 that it should continue its GRAS status with no limitations other than good manufacturing practices. There is reported use of the chemical, it has not yet been assigned for toxicology literature.

SOYBEAN OIL UNSAPONIFIABLES • The fraction of soybean oil that is not saponified (turned into fatty alcohol) in the refining of soybean oil fatty acids.

SPANISH HOPS • *See* Ditanny of Crete.

SPANISH ORIGANUM • *See* Origanum Oil.

SPEARMINT • Garden Mint. Green Mint. It is the essential volatile oil obtained by steam distillation from the fresh aboveground parts of the flowering plant *Mentha spicata,* grown in the United States, Europe, and Asia. It is colorless, yellow, or yellow-green with the characteristic taste and odor of spearmint. The principal active constituent of the oil contains at least 50 percent carvone *(see).* The fresh ground parts of the aromatic herb are used in spearmint flavoring for beverages, meats, and condiments (1,000 ppm). Widely cultivated in the U.S., it is used in butter, caramel, citrus, fruit, garlic, soy, and spice flavorings for beverages, ice cream, ices, candy, baked goods, condiments (100,000 ppm), fats, oils, and icings (50,000 ppm). Has been used to break up intestinal gas. Used in perfumes, perfumed cosmetics, and toothpaste. May cause allergic reactions such as skin rash. GRAS. There is reported use of the chemical, it has not yet been assigned for toxicology literature.

SPECTINOMYCIN • A veterinary antibacterial agent. The FDA tolerance for its residue in edible tissues of chicken and in drinking water is 0.1 ppm.

SPERMACETI • Cetyl Palmitate. Derived as a wax from the head of the sperm whale. Used to make creams glossy and increase their viscosity. Generally nontoxic but may become rancid and cause irritations.

SPERM OIL • Hydrogenated *(see)*. Obtained from the sperm whale. Yellow, thin liquid; slightly fishy odor if not of good quality. Used as a releasing agent or lubricant in baking pans and as a coating on fresh citrus fruits. Also used as an industrial lubricant.

SPICE OLEORESINS • Derived from spices and contain the total odors and related characteristics. They are produced by extraction of the spice with a solvent or by distillation. Spice oleoresins are frequently used with added food-grade diluents, preservatives, and antioxidants, and other substances that must be listed on the label in accordance with current U.S. regulations or with the regulations of other countries. *See* Oleoresins.

SPIKE LAVENDER OIL • French Lavender. Used in perfumes. A pale yellow, stable oil obtained from a flower grown in the Mediterranean region. A lavender-like odor. Used in fruit, floral, mint, and spice flavorings for beverages, ice cream, ices, candy, and baked goods. Used in cologne, toilet water, blended with lavender oil, soaps, and varnishes. Used also for fumigating to keep moths from clothes and in food and beverage flavorings. Moderately toxic by ingestion. GRAS.

SPIKENARD EXTRACT • *Nardostachys jatamansi.* An East Indian aromatic plant. The dried roots and young stems are used for a soothing ointment and as an ingredient in flavorings and perfumes. There is reported use of the chemical, it has not yet been assigned for toxicology literature.

SPINACH EXTRACT • An extract of the leaves of spinach, *Spinacea oleracea.*

SPIRAEA EXTRACT • Queen Meadow. An extract from the flowers of *Spiraea ulmaria.* Contains an oil similar to wintergreen oil *(see)*. The roots are rich in tannic acid *(see)*.

SPIRAL FLAG OIL • *See* Costus Root Oil.

SPIRIT of NITROUS ETHER • *See* Ethyl Nitrite.

SPLENDA • *See* Sucralose.

SPRUCE NEEDLES and TWIGS • Extract of *Picea* spp. used in flavorings. *See* Spruce Oil.

SPRUCE OIL • Colorless to light yellow, pleasant-smelling oil obtained from the needles and twigs of various spruces and hemlocks. Used chiefly in scenting soaps and cosmetics but also used as a flavoring. *See* Hemlock Oil.

SQUALENE • Obtained by hydrogenation of shark-liver oil. Stable in air and oxygen. Occurs in smaller amounts in olive oil, wheat germ oil, and rice bran oil. A faint agreeable odor, tasteless, miscible with vegetable and mineral oils, organic solvents, and fatty substances. Insoluble in water. A lubricant and perfume fixative. A bactericide, an intermediate *(see)* in hair dyes, and used in surfactants. No known toxicity.

STABILIZER • A substance added to a product to give it body and to maintain a desired texture or consistency. Chocolate milk needs a stabilizer to keep the particles of chocolate from settling to the bottom of the container. Calcium *(see* Calcium Acetate) is used as a stabilizer in canned tomatoes to keep them from falling apart. Among the most widely used stabilizers are the gums, such as gum arabic and agar-agar *(see both)*.

STANDARDS OF COMPOSITION • Regulate the amounts of cooked meat and poultry that processed products must contain. These standards dictate how much chicken goes into a chicken pot pie along with the peas and gravy. When shopping, you can compare foods for overall content. In "beef with noodles," beef is the main ingredient. In "noodles with beef," noodles are the main ingredient.

STANDARDS OF FILL • Guarantee that a minimum amount of food is placed in its container and prohibits excessive amounts of air or water.

STANDARDS OF IDENTITY • The FDA and USDA previously established a "recipe" for about three hundred foods such as peanut butter and mayonnaise, fixing the ingredients by law. Many of these foods were exempted from the need for ingredient listing. The new labeling law effective in 1994 requires manufacturers to give full ingredient listings for all foods.

STANDARDS OF QUALITY • Ensure that only those fruits and vegetables of high quality, free of defects, are used. Products of lesser quality might be so labeled (mandarin orange pieces instead of segments, for example).

STANILO • Spectinomycin. An antibiotic used on chickens. FDA limits residues to 0.1 ppm. in chickens. Used to treat syphilis in humans. Potential adverse reactions in humans include hives, decreased urine output, fever, and chills.

STANNIC CHLORIDE • Tin Tetrachloride. A thin, colorless, fuming caustic liquid, soluble in water, used in cosmetics. May be highly irritating to the eyes and mucous membranes.

STANNOUS CHLORIDE • Tin Dichloride. An antioxidant, soluble in water, and a powerful reducing agent, used in canned asparagus, canned soda (11 ppm), and other foods. Used to revive yeast. Low systemic toxicity but may be irritating to the skin and mucous membranes. On the FDA list for further study of mutagenic, teratogenic, subacute, and reproductive effects since 1980. GRAS.

STAPHYBIOTIC • Bactopen. Cloxacillin. Tegopen. A penicillin antibiotic used on cattle. FDA permits residue of 0.01 ppm in uncooked edible tissue of cattle and in milk. Mildly toxic by ingestion but can cause allergic reactions.

STAR ANISE • Chinese Anis. Fruit of *Illicium verum* from China, called star because of the fruit's shape. The *extract* is used in fruit, licorice, anise, liquor sausage, root beer, sarsaparilla, vanilla, wintergreen, and birch beer flavorings for beverages, ice cream, ices, candy, meats (1,000 ppm), and liqueurs. The *oil* is used in blackberry, peach, licorice, anise, liquor, meat, root beer, spice, winter green, and birch beer flavorings for beverages, ice cream, ices, candy, baked goods, meats, syrups, and liqueurs. The *fruit* is a source of anise oil (*see* Anise). Star anise has been used as an expectorant and carminative. Japanese star anise is *Illicium anisatum* and contains a toxic lactone called anisatin, unknown in the Chinese variety. No known toxicity. GRAS.

STARCH • Acid Modified. Pregelatinized and Unmodified. Starch is stored by plants and is taken from grains of wheat, potatoes, rice, corn, beans, and many other vegetable foods. Insoluble in cold water or alcohol but soluble in boiling water. Comparatively resistant to naturally occurring enzymes, and this is why processors "modify" starch to make it more digestible. Starch is modified with propylene oxide, succinic anhydride, 1-octenyl succinic anhydride, aluminum sulfate, or sodium hydroxide *(see all)*. Starch is a major component of cereals and many vegetables. The average U.S. diet has about 180 grams per person daily. Modified starch contributes about a gram per person per day. The source of starch and the type of modification are not usually identified on the label, since the FDA does not require it. The modified starches used in foods are most often bleached starch, acetylated distarch adipate, distarch phosphate, acetylated distarch phosphate, and hydroxypropyl distarch phosphate. The later three are commonly used in baby foods. Starch is also used in dusting powders, dentifrices, hair colorings, rouge, dry shampoos, baby powders, emollients, and bath salts. Soothing to the skin and used to treat rashes. Used internally to alleviate diarrhea. Allergic reaction to starch in toilet goods includes stuffy nose and other symptoms due to inhalation. Absorbs moisture and swells, causing blocking and distension of the pores leading to mechanical irritation. Particles remain in pores and putrefy, accelerated by sweat. The final report to the FDA of the Select Committee on GRAS Substances said there was no information that starch acetate was hazardous to the public when used as it is now and it should continue its GRAS status with limitations on amounts that can be added to food. On the other hand, starch sodium succinate, starch sodium octenyl succinate, and starch sodium hypochlorite oxidized were said not to demonstrate a hazard to the public at current use levels, but uncertainties do exist, requiring additional studies. However, GRAS status continues while tests are being completed and evaluated. Acid-modified and pregelatinized starches were said in the final report to be GRAS, requiring no limitations other than good manufacturing practices.

STARCH/ACRYLATES/ACRYLAMIDE COPOLYMER • *See* Starch and Acrylic Acid.

STARCH DIETHYLAMINCIETHYL ETHER • *See* Starch.

STARTER DISTILLATE • Butter Starter Distillate. Steam distillate of *Streptococcus lactis, S. cremoris, S. lactis* subsp. *diacetylactic, Leuconostoc citrovorum,* and *L. dextronicum.* Used as a flavoring agent in margarine. GRAS.

STEARAMIDE • An emulsifier. Colorless leaflets, insoluble in water. No known toxicity. *See* Stearic Acid.

STEARAMINE • *See* Stearic Acid.

STEARAMINE OXIDE • *See* Stearyl Alcohol.

STEARATES • *See* Stearic Acid.

STEARETH-2 • A polyoxyethylene *(see)* ether of fatty alcohol. The oily liquid is used as a surfactant *(see)* and emulsifier *(see)*. No known toxicity.

STEARETH-4 THROUGH -100 • The polyethylene glycol ethers of stearyl alcohol. The number indicates the degree of liquidity; the higher, the more solid. *See* Steareth-2.

STEARIC ACID • Octadecanoic Acid. Occurs naturally in some vegetable oils, cascarilla bark extract, and as a glyceride *(see)* in tallow and other animal fats and oils. A white, waxy, natural fatty acid, it is the major ingredient used in making bar soap and lubricants. Prepared synthetically by hydrogenation *(see)* of cottonseed and other vegetable oils. Slight tallowlike odor. Used in butter and vanilla flavorings for beverages, baked goods, and candy (4,000 ppm). Also a softener in chewing-gum base. Also used in deodorants and antiperspirants, liquid powders, foundation creams, hand creams, hand lotions, liquefying creams, hair straighteners, protective creams, and shaving creams. A large percentage of all cosmetic creams on the market contain it. It gives pearliness to hand creams. It is also used for suppositories. It is a possible sensitizer for allergic people. Caused tumors in experimental animals. A human skin irritant. The final report to the FDA of the Select Committee on GRAS Substances stated in 1980 that it should continue its GRAS status with no limitations other than good manufacturing practices. In 1988, University of Texas researchers reported in the *New England Journal of Medicine* that it did not raise blood cholesterol levels as much as other saturated fats. *See* Fatty Acids.

STEARYL ACETATE • The ester of stearyl alcohol and acetic acid *(see both)*.

STEARYL ALCOHOL • Stenol. A mixture of solid alcohols prepared from sperm whale oil. White flakes, insoluble in water, soluble in alcohol and ether. Used as a coating agent, emulsifier, lubricant, solvent, and texturizing agent in baked goods, cake, desserts, fruits, ice cream, nuts, peanut butter, puddings, shortening, and whipped topping. A substitute for cetyl alcohol *(see)* to obtain a firmer product at ordinary temperatures. Used in pharmaceuticals, cosmetic creams, for emulsions, as an antifoam agent, and lubricant; also in depilatories, hair rinses, and shampoos.

STEARYL BETAINE • *See* Surfactants and Stearic Acid.

STEARYL CAPRYLATE • The ester of stearyl alcohol and citric acid *(see both)*.

STEARYL CITRATE • The ester of stearyl alcohol and citric acid *(see both)*. A metal scavenger to prevent adverse effects of trace metals in foods and an antioxidant to prevent rancidity in margarine. The final report to the FDA of the Select Committee on GRAS Substances stated in 1980 that it should continue its GRAS status with no limitations other than good manufacturing practices.

STEARYL DIMETHYLAMINE • *See* Stearyl Alcohol.

STEARYL ERUCATE • *See* Stearyl Alcohol and Erucic Acid.

STEARYL GLYCYRRHETINATE • The ester of stearyl alcohol and glycyrrhetinic acid *(see both)*.

STEARYL HEPTANOATE • Ester of stearyl alcohol and heptanoic acid *(see both)*. Used as a wax.

STEARYL LACTATE • An emulsifier that occurs in tallow and other animal fats as well as vegetable oils. Used to emulsify shortening in nonyeast-leavened bakery products and pancake mixes. Also used to emulsify cakes, icing, and fillings. No known toxicity.

STEARYL MONOGLYCERIDYL CITRATE • The soft, practically tasteless, off-white, waxy solid used as an emulsion stabilizer in shortening with emulsifiers.

Not over 0.15 percent in food. It is prepared by the chemical reaction of citric acid on monoglycerides of fatty acids *(see)*. Although allowed as a food additive, there is no current reported use of the chemical, and therefore, although toxicology information may be available, the FDA is not updating it.

STEARYL OCTANOATE • The ester of stearyl alcohol and 2-ethylhexanoic acid. *See* Stearyl Alcohol.

STEARYL STEARATE • The ester of stearyl alcohol and stearic acid *(see both)*.

STEARYL STEAROYL STEARATE • *See* Stearyl Alcohol.

STERCULEN • Sterculia. *See* Karaya Gum.

STERCULIA GUM • GRAS. *See* Karaya Gum.

STEROIDS • Class of compounds that includes certain compounds of hormonal origin, such as cortisone, and used to treat the inflammations caused by allergies. Cholesterol, precursors of certain vitamins, bile acids, alcohols, and many plant derivatives such as digitalis are steroids. Steroids can reduce white blood cell production, and reduce prostaglandins and leukotrienes. Natural and synthetic steroids have four rings of carbon atoms but have different actions according to what is attached to the rings. Cortisone and oral contraceptives are steroids.

STEROL • Any class of solid complex alcohols from animals and plants. Cholesterol is a sterol and is used in hand creams. Sterols are lubricants in baby preparations, emollient creams and lotions, emulsified fragrances, hair conditioners, hand creams, and hand lotions. No known toxicity.

STEROYL MONOGLYCERIDYL CITRATE • A stabilizer in shortenings. *See* Monoglycerides and Citric Acid.

STEVIOSIDE • A candidate for approval as an artifical sweetener at this writing. It is six hundred times as sweet as sugar and contains calories. It would be used as a tabletop sweetener, in soft drinks, gum, sauces, and syrups if approved by the FDA. It is already approved in ten countries.

STONEROOT • Horse Balm. Used for its constituents of resin, saponin, and tannic acid *(see all)*. An erect, smooth perennial; a strong-scented herb of eastern North America with pointed leaves. It produces a chocolate-colored powder with a peculiar odor and bitter, astringent taste. Soluble in alcohol. No known toxicity.

STORAX • Styrax. Sweet Asian gum from *Liquidambar* spp. Used in perfumes. It is the resin obtained from the bark of an Asiatic tree. Grayish brown, fragrant semiliquid, containing also styrene and cinnamic acid *(see both)*. Once used in medicine as a weak antiseptic and as an expectorant. Used in strawberry, fruit, and spice flavorings for beverages, ice cream, ices, candy, baked goods, chewing gum, and toppings. Moderately toxic when ingested. Can cause urinary problems when absorbed through the skin. Can cause skin irritation, welts, and discomfort when applied topically. A common allergen. There is reported use of the chemical, it has not yet been assigned for toxicology literature.

STPP • *See* Sodium Tripolyphosphate.

STRAWBERRY ALDEHYDE • Synthetic flavoring. GRAS.

STRAWBERRY EXTRACT • *See* Strawberry Juice.

STRAWBERRY JUICE • Flavoring. Fresh ripe strawberries are reputed to contain ingredients that soften and nourish the skin. Widely used in natural cosmetics today. No scientific evidence of benefit or harm.

STRAWFLOWER EXTRACT • The extract of *Helichrysum italicum,* grown for its bright yellow, strawlike flowers. Used in coloring.

STREPTOMYCIN • An aminoglycoside antibiotic, it is given by injection and is active against streptococcal endocarditis, an infection of the heart in humans. It is used as an animal antibiotic in chickens, swine, and turkeys. FDA limits residue to zero in these products, including eggs. EPA Genetic Toxicology Program *(see).* Potential adverse reactions in humans to streptomycin include ear problems, muscle problems, kidney dysfunction, local pain, irritation, and sterile abscesses at the site of injection and skin disorders. Has been implicated in aplastic anemia.

STRONTIUM HYDROXIDE • Used chiefly in making soaps and greases in cosmetics. Colorless, water-absorbing crystals or white powder. Absorbs carbon dioxide from the air. Very alkaline in solution. Also used in refining beet sugar and separating sugar from molasses. Irritating when applied to the skin.

STYRACIN • *See* Cinnamyl Cinnamate.

STYRAX • *See* Storax.

STYRENE • Obtained from ethylbenzene by taking out the hydrogen. Colorless to yellowish oil with a penetrating odor. Used in the manufacture of paper and paperboard and used as a chewing substance in chewing gum. May be irritating to the eyes and mucous membranes, and in high concentrations it is narcotic.

STYRYLCARBINOL • *See* Cinnamyl Alcohol.

STYRYLPYRIDINIUM CHLORIDE, DIETHYL CARBAMAZINE • Used in animal feed to combat worms.

SUBACUTE • A zone between acute and chronic or the process of a disease that is not overt. Subacute endocarditis, for example, is an infection of the heart. It is usually due to a "strep germ" and may follow temporary infection after a tooth extraction.

SUBSTITUTE • Means the product is equivalent to the food it resembles. *See* Imitation.

SUCCINIC ACID • Occurs in fossils, fungi, lichens, etc. Prepared from acetic acid *(see).* Odorless; acid taste. The acid is used as a plant-growth retardant. A buffer and neutralizing agent in food processing. A germicide and mouthwash; used in perfumes and lacquers; also a buffer and neutralizing agent. Has been employed medicinally as a laxative. No known toxicity in cosmetic use. Large amounts injected under the skin of frogs kills them. The final report to the FDA of the Select Committee on GRAS Substances stated in 1980 that it should continue its GRAS status with no limitations other than good manufacturing practices. There is reported use of the chemical, it has not yet been assigned for toxicology literature.

SUCCINIC ANHYDRIDE • A starch modifier up to 4 percent. *See* Succinic Acid.

SUCCINISTEARIN • Stearoyl Propylene Glycol Hydrogen Succinate. Emulsifier in or with shortenings and edible oils used in cakes, cake mixes, fillings, icings, pastries, and toppings. *See* Succinic Acid.

SUCCINYLATED GELATIN • Used for making microcapsules for flavoring oils.
SUCCINYLATED MONOGLYCERIDES • Surfactants *(see)* used as dough conditioners to add loaf volume and firmness. *See* Glycerides and Succinic Acid.
SUCRALOSE • Splenda. An artifical sweetener made from sugar. It is about six hundred times sweeter than sugar but does not contain calories. Producers claim it has no aftertaste and is more stable. It can be used in cooking and is already sold in Canada and Latin America. Among its users are Cadbury Beverages and Corby Distilleries in liqueurs. Johnson and Johnson plans to make it another NutraSweet in the United States by aggressively marketing it when it is approved. It had been waiting for U.S. approval since 1987 in fifteen food categories. The FDA approved it in April 1998. It will be used as a tabletop sweetener, in baked goods, fruit spreads, desserts, and confections, but its biggest use is expected to be in diet drinks.
SUCROSE • Sugar. Cane Sugar. Saccharose. A sweetening agent and food, a starting agent in fermentation production, a preservative and antioxidant in pharmaceuticals, a demulcent, and a substitute for glycerin *(see)*. Table sugar can stimulate the production of fat in the body, apart from its calorie content in the diet, and may be particularly fat-producing in women on the "pill." Workers who handle raw sugar often develop rashes and other skin problems. When it oxidizes with sweat sugar draws water from the skin and causes chapping and cracking. Infections, erosions, and fissures around the nails can occur. No known toxicity in cosmetics. The final report to the FDA of the Select Committee on GRAS Substances stated in 1980 that it should continue its GRAS status with no limitations other than good manufacturing practices.
SUCROSE ACETATE ISOBUTYRATE • A mixture of esters *(see)* of sucrose with acetic and isobutyric acids *(see both)*. Sucrose acetate isobutyrate produced liver damage in dogs but not in mice or rats. Three studies involving a total of seventy-one human volunteers did not respond the same way as dogs did and did not seem to have any adverse effects. The Committee decided to use the NOEL *(see)* of 2 grams per kg of body weight per day for rats—the lowest obtained in long-term toxicity studies—to allocate a temporary ADI of 0–10 mg per kg of body weight using a safety factor of 200. They also asked for further data that would explain the disparate effects of sucrose acetate isobutryate on the liver functions in dogs compared to other species, in particular the human. There is reported use of the chemical; it has not yet been assigned for toxicology literature.
SUCROSE BENZOATE • *See* Benzoic Acid.
SUCROSE DISTEARATE • A mixture of sucrose and stearic acid *(see both)*.
SUCROSE FATTY ACID ESTERS • Sucrose Esters. Derived from sucrose *(see)* and edible tallow, the FDA gave permission in 1982 for their use as components of protective coatings for fruits. They are also used as emulsifiers, stabilizers, and texturizers. No known toxicity.
SUCROSE LAURATE • A mixture of sucrose and lauric acid *(see both)*.
SUCROSE OCTAACETATE • Prepared from sucrose *(see)*. A synthetic flavoring used in bitters, spice, and ginger ale flavorings for beverages. Used in adhesives; a denaturant for alcohol.

SUCROSE POLYESTER • *See* Olestra.

SUCROSE STEARATE • A mixture of sucrose and stearic acid *(see both)*.

SUGAR • A carbohydrate product made up of one, two, or more saccharose groups. The monosaccharide sugars—often called simple sugars—are composed of chains of 207 carbon atoms. Chief among the monosaccharides are glucose, dextrose, fructose, and levulose. Among the disaccharides are sucrose—cane or beet sugar—lactose found in milk, maltose found in starch, and cellobiose from cellulose *(see)*. High polymer sugars occur as water-soluble gums such as Arabic and tragacanth. Sugar is an important source of metabolic energy in foods and its formation in plants is an essential factor in the life process. It has many uses as a food additive other than just sweetening. It acts as a tenderizer by absorbing water and inhibiting flour gluten development, as well as slowing down starch gelling. It mixes air into shortening in the creaming process and caramelizes under heat, to provide cooked and baked foods with pleasing color and aroma. It speeds the growth of yeast by providing nourishment and helps to keep beaten eggs whipped. It delays coagulation of egg proteins in custards and helps the gelling of fruit jellies and preserves. It also helps prevent them from spoiling and keeps canned and frozen fruits looking appetizing and tender. It helps to make a wide variety of candies through varying degrees of recrystallization and enhances the smoothness and flavor of ice cream. Most people think of table sugar or sucrose when the word is mentioned. It contains only sixteen calories per teaspoon, something to consider when considering a sugar substitute.

SUGAR ALC • Listing on food labels for *sugar alcohols (see)*.

SUGAR ALCOHOLS • These are monosaccharides. One of the most important is glycerol *(see)* while others include inositol, mannitol, sorbitol, and xylitol *(see all)*.

SUGAR BEET EXTRACT FLAVOR BASE • A flavoring in foods. *See* Sucrose.

SUGAR BEET FIBER • Beet Fiber. Sugar Beet Pulp. The natural, light-brown colored fiber of sugar beets remaining after water extraction of the sugar from the mechanically sliced sugar beets. It exists in various grades from coarse fibrous flakes to fine powders. It is used as an anticaking agent, binding agent, bulking agent, dietary supplement, dispersing agent, nutrient, stabilizing agent, texturizing agent, and thickening agent. No known toxicity.

L-SUGARS • Candidate for artificial sweeteners. No specific use given as yet.

SUGAR SOLID EXTRACT • *See* Sucrose.

SULFA ANTIBIOTICS • More than fifty compounds that contain both sulfur and nitrogen with a specificity for certain bacteria. Because of their toxicity and often serious side effects, their use in treating disease is limited, at least intentionally in humans. They are widely used, however, in treating animals and animal feeds.

SULFABROMOMETHAZINE SODIUM • 5-Bromosulfamethazine. A widely used sulfa antibacterial to treat cattle. FDA limits residue to 0.1 ppm in uncooked edible tissues of cattle and 0.01 ppm in milk. Sulfa drugs can cause sensitivity to the sun. Mildly toxic by ingestion. Caused tumors and birth defects in experimental animals.

SULFACHLORPYRIDAZINE • A veterinary antibiotic. The FDA allows 0.1 ppm as residue in uncooked edible tissue of calves and swine. *See* Sulfa Antibiotics.

SULFADIMETHOXINE PLUS ORMETOPRIM • A feed additive, the FDA allows 0.1 ppm sulfa residue in uncooked edible tissues of chickens, turkeys, cattle, ducks, salmon, and catfish. The agency allows 0.01 ppm in milk. Ormetoprim residue is allowed at 0.1 ppm in edible tissues of chickens, turkeys, ducks, salmon and catfish. *See* Sulfa Antibiotics.

SULFAETHOXYPYRIDAZINE • A feed additive. The residues allowed in edible tissues of cattle are 0.1 ppm and zero in milk and uncooked edible tissue of swine. It is used in the drinking water of cattle and swine. *See* Sulfa Antibiotics.

SULFAMERAZINE • Used in fish feed on fish farms. The FDA tolerance is zero in edible tissues of trout as residue. *See* Sulfa Antibiotics.

SULFAMETHAZLINE • An antibiotic used in cattle. The FDA permits 0.1 ppm as residue in the edible tissues of cattle, swine, turkeys, and chicken. *See* Sulfa Antibiotics.

SULFAMETHAZINE A (WITH CHLORTETRACYCLINE and PENICILLIN) or SULFAMETHAZINE B (WITH TYLOSIN) • Antibiotics used in animal feed. The FDA permits 0.1 ppm in uncooked edible tissues of chickens, turkeys, cattle, and swine. *See* Sulfa Antibiotics, Tetracyclines, Penicillin, and Tylosin.

SULFAMETHAZINE SODIUM • *See* Sulfa Antibiotics.

SULFAMIC ACID • A strong, white crystalline acid used chiefly as a weed killer, in cleaning metals, and as a softening agent. Used as a plasticizer and fire retardant for paper and other cellulose products; as a stabilizing agent for chlorine and hypochlorite, bleaching paper pulp; and as a catalyst for urea formaldehyde resin. A cleaning agent in cosmetics and used in the manufacture of hair dyes and lakes (*see* FD and C Lakes). Moderately irritating to the skin and mucous membranes. The final report to the FDA of the Select Committee on GRAS Substances stated in 1980 that it should continue its GRAS status with no limitations other than good manufacturing practices. There is reported use of the chemical; it has not yet been assigned for toxicology literature.

6-SULFANILAMIDO-2,4-DIMETHOXYPYRIMIDINE. ABCID • Agribon. Albon. Bactrovet. A widely used sulfa antibacterial drug to treat cattle, poultry, and in animal feed. It is also used in catfish farming to prevent infections. FDA limits residues to 0.1 ppm in chickens, turkeys, cattle, ducks, salmon, and catfish. Caused birth defects in experimental animals. Sulfa drugs can cause sensitivity to sunlight and allergic reactions.

SULFANITRAN • A sulfa antibiotic used to treat chickens. FDA residue limit is zero in chickens. Sulfa drugs can cause sensitivity to light and allergic reactions in humans.

SULFAQUINOXALINE • A sulfa drug used in animal feed. Moderately toxic by ingestion. Sulfa drugs can cause sensitivity to light and allergic reactions in humans.

SULFATE • A salt or ester of sulfuric acid (*see*). A chemical is "sulfated" to help control the acid-alkali balance.

SULFATED BUTYL OLEATE • An emulsion used to dehydrate grapes to raisins. Made from oleic acid with butanol. *See* Oleic Acid and Butyl Alcohol.

SULFATED GLYCERYL OLEATE • Produced by adding sulfuric acid to glyceryl oleate. *See* Sulfonated Oils.

SULFATED OIL • Sulfated Oil. A compound to which a salt of sulfuric acid has been added to help control the acid-alkali balance.

SULFATED TALLOW • Fat from fatty tissues of sheep and cattle that becomes solid at 40 to 46°F. It is a defoaming agent in yeast and beet sugar production in "amounts reasonably required to inhibit foaming." *See* Tallow Flakes for toxicity.

SULFATHIAZOLE COMBINED WITH CHLORTETRACYCLINE and PENI-CILLIN • Antibiotic compound used in animal feeds. *See* Sulfa Antibiotics, Tetracyclines, and Penicillin.

SULFIDES • Inorganic sulfur compounds that occur free or in combination with minerals. They are salts of weak acid and are used in dyes and hair-dissolving agents in depilatories. They are skin irritants.

SULFITE DIOXIDE • *See* Sulfites.

SULFITES • Sodium, Potassium, and Ammonium. Preservatives, antioxidants, and antibrowning agents used in foods. Sulfites are also used for bleaching food starches and as a preventive against rust and scale in boiler water used in making steam that will come in contact with food. Some sulfites are used in the production of cellophane for food packaging. The FDA prohibits the use of sulfites in foods that are important sources of thiamine (vitamin B_1), such as enriched flour, because sulfites destroy the nutrient. There are six sulfiting agents that are currently listed as GRAS chemical preservatives. They are sulfur dioxide, sodium sulfite, sodium and potassium bisulfite, and sodium and potassium metabisulfite *(see all)*. Under the current listing, sulfiting agents may be used as preservatives in any food except recognized sources of vitamin B_1. These agents have been used in many processed foods and in cafeterias and restaurants to prevent fruits, green vegetables, potatoes, and salads from turning brown, as well as to enhance their crispness.

The FDA had sulfiting agents under review. As part of this review, a proposal to affirm the GRAS status of sulfur dioxide, sodium bisulfite, and sodium and potassium metabisulfite, with specific use limitations, was published in the *Federal Register* of July 9, 1982. The agency did not propose to affirm the GRAS status of sodium sulfite and potassium bisulfite because it had no evidence to indicate their current use in food.

Reactions to sulfites can include acute asthma attacks, loss of consciousness, anaphylactic shock, diarrhea, and nausea occurring soon after ingesting sulfiting agents. There have been seventeen deaths that the FDA has determined were "probably or possibly" associated with sulfites. The FDA banned the use of the preservative on fresh fruits and vegetables and at this writing is reviewing a proposal to prohibit it on fresh, precut potatoes. The FDA decided in 1988 against extending its ban on the use of sulfites to a variety of foods sold in supermarkets and served in restaurants, including wine, dried fruit, some seafood, and condiments. Sulfites must be declared on the labels of wine and packaged foods sold in supermarkets when they are added in excess of 10 ppm.

A citizens' petition was submitted by the Center for Science in the Public Interest, Washington, D.C., on October 28, 1982, that asked the agency to restrict the use of sulfiting agents to a safe residue level in food or require labels on those food products in which sulfiting agents must be used at higher levels to perform essential public health functions. In the meantime, the California Grape and Tree Fruit League recommended that the Food and Drug Administration affirm as GRAS sulfiting agents used in sulfur dioxide fumigation within specific limitations and include its use as an ingredient to treat fresh grapes. Stating that the compound is essential to the marketing, transport, storage, and export of table grapes, the group claimed lack of any known substitute for the gaseous compound effective in preventing mold-rot and other storage fungi and in prolonging storage life. A spokesperson for the Wine Institute, which represents 460 domestic wine makers, said that many of the sulfur compounds in wine are natural parts of fermentation, but they are also added to many wines.

Sulfites are still used in processed foods, dried fruits, wines, and beers. When dining in a restaurant, you have to have a lot of faith in your waiter if you are allergic to sulfites. Foods, especially potato products and some canned foods served in restaurants, could contain sulfites. You can ask, but you may not receive an informed answer.

You have to be cautious about "prepared" products in general if you are sulfite sensitive. For example, lemon juice from a lemon may be fine, but from a bottle it may contain sodium bisulfite. The following are food categories with common levels of sulfur dioxide residues.[1]

baked goods	30 ppm
beer	25
canned vegetables	30
condiments & relishes	30
dairy products	200
dehydrated potatoes	500
dehydrated vegetables	200
dried fruit	2000
filled crackers	75
frozen potatoes	50
fruit juices (regular strength)	300
fruit juices (concentrates)	1000
gelatin	40

---

[1] Judith Foulke, "A Fresh Look at Food Preservatives," *FDA Consumer,* October 1993, p. 26.

glacéed fruit	150
grain products	200
gravies & sauces	75
jams & jellies	30
lobster, frozen	100
maraschino cherries	150
molasses	300
nut products	25
plant protein isolates	110
processed seafood (other than dried or frozen)	25
shrimp, fresh or frozen	100
soup mixes (dry)	20
sugar	20
sweet sauces & syrups	60
tea	90
vegetable juice	100
vinegar	75

The FAO-WHO Expert Committee on Food Additives concluded in June 1998 that "the potential exists for high consumers of sulfites to exceed the ADI, but the available data were insufficient to estimate the number of high consumers or the magnitude and duration of intake above the ADI." The Committee is reviewing this additive's levels in dried fruits, jams, jellies, marmalades, fruit preparations including pulp and fruit toppings, dried vegetables, vegetables, nut and seed purees and spreads, white and semiwhite sugar, concentrates for fruit juice, wines, and fruit wines.

SULFOACETATE DERIVATIVES OF MONOGLYCERIDES and DIGLYC-ERIDES • Used as emulsifiers. The final report to the FDA of the Select Committee on GRAS Substances stated in 1980 that there were insufficient biological and other studies upon which to base an evaluation of them when they are used as food ingredients.

SULFOMYXIN • A sulfa drug used to combat bacteria in chickens and turkeys. FDA limits residue to zero in uncooked edible tissues of chickens and turkeys. Sulfa drugs can cause sensitivity to light and allergic reactions in humans.

SULFONATED OILS • Sulfated. Prepared by reacting oils with sulfuric acid. Used in soapless shampoos and hair sprays as an emulsifier and wetting agent.

SULFO-p-TOLUENE • Sodium Chloramine. A water-purifying agent and a deodorant used to remove onion and weed odors in cheese. Toluene may cause mild anemia and is narcotic in high concentrations.

SULFUR DIOXIDE • A gas formed when sulfur burns. Used to bleach vegetable colors and to preserve fruits and vegetables; a disinfectant in breweries and food factories; a bleaching agent in gelatin, glue, and beet sugars; an antioxidant, preservative, and antibrowning agent in wine, corn syrup, table syrup, jelly, dried fruits, brined fruit, maraschino cherries, beverages, dehydrated potatoes, soups, and condiments. Should not be used on meats or on foods recognized as a source of vitamin A because it destroys the vitamin. Poisonous, highly irritating. Often cited as an air pollutant. EPA Extremely Hazardous Substances List and EPA Genetic Toxicology Program *(see both)*. Inhalation produces respiratory irritation and death when sufficiently concentrated. The final report to the FDA of the Select Committee on GRAS Substances stated in 1980 that there is no available evidence that it is a hazard to the public when used as it is now and it should continue its GRAS status with limitations on amounts that can be added to food. Sulfur dioxide is also a preservative, but not to be used in meats or in foods recognized as a source of vitamin b_1. The following are food categories with common levels of sulfur dioxide:

baked goods	30 ppm
beer	25
canned vegetables	30
condiments & relishes	30
dairy products	200
dehydrated potatoes	500
dehydrated vegetables	200

SULFURIC ACID • Oil of Vitriol. A clear, colorless, odorless, oily acid used to modify starch and to regulate acid-alkalinity balance in the brewing industry. It is corrosive and produces severe burns on contact with the skin and other body tissues. Inhalation of the vapors can cause serious lung damage. Dilute sulfuric acid has been used to stimulate appetite and to combat overalkaline stomach juices. It is used as a topical caustic in cosmetic products. If ingested undiluted, it can be fatal. The final report to the FDA of the Select Committee on GRAS Substances stated in 1980 that it should continue its GRAS status with no limitations other than good manufacturing practices.

SULFUROUS ACID • A solution of sulfur dioxide in water. It is toxic by ingestion and inhalation and very irritating to tissue. It is used in bleaching, paper manufacturing, wine manufacturing, brewing, and as a preservative for fruits, nuts, foods, and wines. There is reported use of the chemical; it has not yet been assigned for toxicology literature.

SUNETTE • *See* Acesulfame.

SUNFLOWER SEED OIL • Oil obtained by milling the seeds of the large flower produced in Russia, India, Egypt, and Argentina. A bland, pale yellow oil, it contains vitamin E (*see* Tocopherols) and forms a "skin" after drying. Used in food, salad oils, and in resin and soap manufacturing. No known toxicity.

SUNFLOWER SEED OIL GLYCERIDE • *See* Sunflower Seed Oil and Glycerides.

SUPERGLYCERINATED FULLY HYDROGENATED RAPESEED OIL • Used in some margarines and emulsions. *See* Rapeseed Oil, Glycerin, and Hydrogenation.

SUPER-OV • Derived from pig pituitary glands, it is used for the induction of superovulation in cows for procedures requiring the production of multiple eggs at a single estrus. Follicle-stimulating hormone is not orally active; therefore residues of this drug are said to be safe for human consumption, and therefore "no toxicological studies were required" by the U.S. government.

SURFACE-ACTIVE AGENT • *See* Surfactants.

SURFACTANTS • These are wetting agents. They lower water's surface tension, permitting water to spread out and penetrate more easily. These surface-active agents are classified by whether or not they ionize in solution and by the nature of their electrical charges. There are four major categories—anionic, nonionic, cationic, and amphoteric. *Anionic surfactants,* which carry a negative charge, have excellent cleaning properties. They are stain and dirt removers in household detergents, powders, and liquids and in toilet soaps. *Nonionic surfactants* have no electrical charge. Since they are resistant to hard water and dissolve in oil and grease, they are especially effective in spray-on oven cleaners. *Cationic surfactants* have a positive charge. These are primarily ammonia derivatives and are antistatic and sanitizing agents used as friction reducers in hair rinses and fabric softeners. *Amphoteric surfactants* may be either negatively charged or positively charged depending on the acidity or alkalinity of the water. They are used for cosmetics where mildness is important, such as in shampoos and lotions. Surfactants may be classified as emulsifiers, dispersants, wetting and foaming agents, detergents, viscosity modifiers, or stabilizers. For example, in peanut butter, a surfactant keeps oil and water mixtures from separating; in cosmetics, it makes lotions more spreadable; salad dressings and cheeses are thickened by surfactants, which make them pour better.

SWEET BIRCH • *See* Methyl Salicylate.

SWEET CLOVER EXTRACT • The extract of various species of *Melilotus,* grown for hay and soil improvement. It contains coumarin *(see)* and is used as a scent to disguise bad odors.

SWEET FLAG • *See* Calamus.

SWEET MARJORAM OIL • Pot Marjoram. Used in perfumery and hair preparations. The natural extract of the flowers and leaves of two varieties of the fragrant marjoram. Also a food flavoring. No known toxicity.

SWEETENER 2000 • An artifical sweetener made by the company that brought us NutraSweet. It is not on the market, as of this writing. *See* Aspartame.

SYLVIC ACID • *See* Abietic Acid.

SYNTHETIC • Made in the laboratory and not by nature. For example, vanillin, made in the laboratory may be identical to vanilla extracted from the vanilla bean, but vanillin cannot be called "natural."

SYNTHETIC BEESWAX • A mixture of alcohol esters.

SYNTHETIC FATTY ALCOHOLS • Made from fatty alcohols *(see)* obtained by distillation. Used as substitutes for naturally derived fatty acids *(see)*.

SYNTHETIC GLYCERIN • *See* Glycerin.

SYNTHETIC IRON OXIDE • For coloring sausage casings and for cat and dog food. Limited to 0.1 percent of weight of finished human food and 0.25 percent of weight of finished food for dogs and cats. Exempt from color certification.

SYNTHETIC JOJOBA OIL • *See* Jojoba Oil.

SYNTHETIC PARAFFIN and SUCCINIC DERIVATIVES • Used as a coating on fresh citrus, muskmelons, and sweet potatoes. *See* Paraffin Wax and Succinic Acid.

SYNTHETIC SPERMACETI • *See* Spermaceti.

SYNTHETIC WAX • A hydrocarbon wax derived from various oils.

T

TAGETES • *Meal, Extract, and Oil. Marigold.* The *meal* is the dried, ground flower petals of the Aztec marigold, a strong-scented, tropical American herb, mixed with no more than 0.3 percent ethoxyquin, an herbicide and antioxidant. The *extract* is taken from tagetes peels. Both the meal and the extract are used to enhance the yellow color of chicken skin and eggs. They are incorporated in chicken feed, supplemented sufficiently with yellow coloring xanthophyll. The coloring has been permanently listed since 1963 but is exempt from certification. The *oil* is extracted from the Aztec flower and used in fruit flavorings for beverages, ice cream, ices, candy, baked goods, gelatin, desserts, and condiments.

TALC • French Chalk. Magnesium Silicate. The lumps are known as soapstone of steatite. An anticaking agent added to vitamin supplements to render a free flow; also to chewing-gum base. Gives a slippery sensation to powders and creams. Talc is finely powdered native magnesium silicate, a mineral. The main ingredient of baby and bath powders, face powders, eye shadows, liquid powders, protective creams, dry rouges, face masks, foundation cake makeups, skin fresheners, foot powders, and face creams. It usually has small amounts of other powders such as boric acid or zinc oxide added as a coloring agent. Prolonged inhalation can cause lung problems because it is similar in chemical composition to asbestos, a known lung irritant and cancer-causing agent. There is no known acute toxicity, but there is a question about it being a cancer-causing agent upon ingestion. It is suspected that the high incidence of stomach cancer among the Japanese is due to the fact that the Japanese prefer that their rice be treated with talc. Talc is not considered food grade by the FDA as it contains asbestiform minerals. GRAS.

TALLAMIDE DEA • *See* Tall Oil.

TALLAMPHOPROPIONATE • *See* Tall Oil.

TALL OIL • Liquid Rosin. A byproduct of the wood pulp industry. *Tall* is Swedish for "pine." Dark brown liquid. Acrid odor. A fungicide and cutting oil. It may be a mild irritant and sensitizer. The final report to the FDA of the Select Committee on GRAS Substances stated in 1980 that it should continue its GRAS status with no limitations other than good manufacturing practices.

TALL OIL BENZYL HYDROXYETHYL IMIDAZOLINIUM CHLORIDE • *See* Quaternary Ammonium Compounds and Tall Oil.

TALL OIL ROSIN, GLYCEROL ESTER • Softener for chewing-gum base. *See* Tall Oil.

TALLOW ACID • *See* Tallow Flakes.

TALLOW AMIDE • *See* Tallow Flakes.

TALLOWAMIDE DEA and MEA • *See* Tallow Acid.

TALLOW AMIDOPROPYLAMINE OXIDE • *See* Tallow Acid.

TALLOW AMINE • *See* Tallow Flakes.

TALLOW AMINE OXIDE • *See* Tallow Flakes.

TALLOWETH-6 • *See* Tallow Flakes.

TALLOW FATTY ACIDS • *See* Tallow Flakes and Fatty Acids.

TALLOW FLAKES • Suet. Dripping. The fat from the fatty tissue of bovine cattle and sheep in North America. White, almost tasteless when pure, and generally harder than grease. Used as a defoaming agent in yeast and beet sugar production. In miniature pigs in one year, feeding tallow caused moderate-to-severe atherosclerosis (clogging of the aeries) similar to that in humans. Used in shaving creams, lipsticks, shampoos, and soaps. May cause eczema and blackheads. The final report to the FDA of the Select Committee on GRAS Substances stated in 1980 that it should continue its GRAS status for packaging with no limitations other than good manufacturing practices.

TALLOW GLYCERIDES • A mixture of triglycerides (fats) derived from tallow.

TALLOW, HYDROGENATED, OXIDIZED, or SULFATED • Antifoaming agent. *See* Tallow Flakes and Hydrogenation. Used in defoaming agents.

TALLOW HYDROXYETHYL IMIDAZOLINE • *See* Tallow and Imidazoline.

TALLOW IMIDAZOLINE • *See* Tallow Flakes.

TAMARIND EXTRACT • The extract of *Tamarindus indica,* a large tropical tree grown in the East Indies and Africa. Preserved in sugar or syrup, it is used as a natural fruit flavoring. The pulp contains about 10 percent tartaric acid *(see).* Has been used as a cooling laxative drink. GRAS. There is reported use of the chemical, it has not yet been assigned for toxicology literature.

TANGERINE OIL • The oil obtained by expression from the peels of the ripe fruit from several related tangerine species. Reddish orange, with a pleasant orange aroma. Used in blueberry, mandarin, orange, tangerine, and other fruit flavorings for beverages, ice cream, ices, candy, baked goods, gelatin desserts, and chewing gum. A skin irritant. GRAS.

TANNIC ACID • Occurs in the bark and fruit of many plants, notably in the bark of the oak and sumac, and in cherries, coffee, and tea. It is used to clarify beer and wine, and as a refining agent for rendered fats. As a flavoring it is used in butter, caramel, fruit, brandy, maple, and nut flavorings for beverages, ice cream, ices, candy, baked goods, and liquor (1,000 ppm). Used medicinally as a mild astringent and when applied it may turn the skin brown. Used in sunscreen preparations, eye lotions, and antiperspirants. Tea contains tannic acid, and this explains its folk use as an eye lotion. Excessive use in creams or lotions in hypersensitive persons may lead to irritation, blistering, and increase pigmentation. Low toxicity orally, but large doses may cause gastric distress. Can cause tumors and death by injection, but not, evidently, by ingestion. IARC review and EPA Genetic Toxicology Program *(see both)*. The final report to the FDA of the Select Committee on GRAS Substances stated in 1980 that there is no evidence in the available information that it is a hazard to the public when used as it is now and it should continue its GRAS status with limitations on the amount that may be added to food.

TANNIN • Used in alcoholic beverages only. *See* Tannic Acid.

TANSY • A common herb, *Tanacetum vulgara,* which the Greeks believed prolonged life. Strong aromatic odor and bitter taste. Flavoring used in alcoholic beverages only.

TAPIOCA STARCH • A preparation of cassava, the tapioca plant. Used for thickening liquid foods such as puddings, juicy pies, and soups. No known toxicity. The final report to the FDA of the Select Committee on GRAS Substances stated in 1980 that it should continue its GRAS status with no limitations other than good manufacturing practices.

TAR OIL • The volatile oil distilled from wood tar, generally from the family Pinaceae. Used externally to treat skin diseases, the principle toxic ingredients are phenols (very toxic) and other hydrocarbons such as the naphthalenes. Toxicity estimates are hard to make because even the U.S. Pharmacopoeia does not specify the phenol content of official preparations. However, if ingested, it is estimated that one ounce would kill. *See* Pine Tar Oil, which is a rectified tar oil used as a licorice flavoring.

TARA GUM • Peruvian Carob. Obtained by grinding the endosperms of the seeds of an evergreen tree common to Peru. The whitish yellow, nearly odorless powder that is produced is used as a thickening agent and stabilizer. No known toxicity. *See also* Locust Bean Gum.

TARAXACUM ERYTHROSPERUMUM • *See* Dandelion Leaf and Root.

TARDIVE DYSKINESIA • Abnormal grimacing about the mouth occurring as a side effect of some antipsychotic medication.

TARRAGON • Derived from the dried leaves of a small European perennial wormwood herb. Pale yellow oil grown for its aromatic, pungent foliage. Used in making pickles and vinegar. Also used in perfumery. GRAS.

TARS • An antiseptic, deodorant, and bug killer. Any of the various dark brown or black bituminous, usually odorous, viscous liquids or semiliquids obtained by the destructive distillation of wood, coal, peat, shale, and other organic materials. Used in hair tonics and shampoos and as a licorice food flavoring. May cause allergic reactions.

TARTARIC ACID • Sodium Tartrate. Sodium Potassium Tartrate. Rochelle Salts. Described in ancient times as being a residual of grape fermentation. Widely distributed in nature in many fruits but usually obtained as a byproduct of wine making. Consists of colorless or translucent crystals or a white fine-to-granular crystalline powder, which is odorless and has an acid taste. It is the acidic constituent of some baking powders and is used to adjust acidity in frozen dairy products, jellies, bakery products, beverages, confections, dried egg whites, food colorings, candies, artificially sweetened preserves up to 4 percent. Used as a sequestrant, especially in wines, as an emulsifier, and as a grape and sour flavoring for candies, canned sodas and colas, preserves, baked goods, dried egg white, lemon meringue pie mix, pasteurized processed cheese, cheese food and cheese spread, and some types of baking powder. Effervescent acid used in bath salts, denture powders, nail bleaches, hair-grooming aids, hair rinses, depilatories, and hair coloring. Large amounts may have a laxative effect. GRAS.

TARTRATE, SODIUM POTASSIUM • The final report to the FDA of the Select Committee on GRAS Substances stated in 1980 that it should continue its GRAS status with no limitations other than good manufacturing practices. *See* Sodium Potassium Tartrate.

TARTRAZINE • FD and C Yellow No. 5. Bright orange-yellow powder used in foods, drugs, and cosmetics and as a dye for wool and silk. Those allergic to aspirin are often allergic to tartrazine. Allergies have been reported in persons eating sweet corn, soft drinks, and cheese crackers—all colored with Yellow No. 5. It is derived from coal tar.

TAURINE • An amino acid found in almost every tissue of the body and high in human milk. Most infant soy protein formulas are now supplemented with taurine. It is also used as a nutritional supplement in feed for growing chicks. Taurine is almost absent from vegetarian diets. It is believed necessary for healthy eyes and it is an antioxidant. Irregular heartbeat is characteristic of lack of blood to the heart and may be partly due to loss of intracellular taurine, some researchers theorize. Much like magnesium, taurine affects membrane excitability by normalizing potassium flux in and out of the heart muscle cells. Supplementation may prevent digitalis-induced arrhythmias. Taurine may also lower blood pressure. In a group of nineteen young patients with borderline high blood pressure, some received six grams daily of taurine and others a placebo. After seven days, systolic and diastolic blood pressure fell significantly in patients receiving taurine. Epinephrine, which stimulates heartbeat, was blunted by taurine, suggesting that its anti–high blood pressure effect may be mediated by reduction in signals from the nervous system.

TAUROCHOLIC ACID • Cholic Acid. Cholyltaurine. Occurs as a sodium salt in bile. It is formed by the combination of the sulfur-containing amino acid, taurine, and cholic acid. It aids digestion and absorption of fats. It is used as an emulsifying agent in foods. The final report to the FDA of the Select Committee on GRAS Substances stated in 1980 that it should continue its GRAS status with no limitations other than good manufacturing practices.

TBHQ • *See* Tertiary Butylhydroquinone.

TBS • *See* Tribromsalan.

TCC • *See* Triclocarban.

TEA- • The abbreviation for triethanolamine *(see)*.

TEA • The leaves, leaf buds, and internodes of plant and fragrant white flowers prepared and cured to make an aromatic beverage. Cultivated principally in China, Japan, Ceylon, and other Asian countries. Tea is a mild stimulant and its tonic properties are due to the alkaloid caffeine; tannic acid *(see)* makes it astringent. There is tremendous interest among researchers worldwide to identify those nutraceuticals in tea that may help prevent malignancies. Cultivated principally in China, Japan, Sri Lanka, and other Asian countries, tea leaves come from an evergreen of the Camellia family, *Camellia sinensis,* and are processed in different ways to produce green, black, and oolong tea. Each emerges with different chemical properties. To produce black tea, which most Americans drink, leaves are subjected to warmth for a few hours and heated to 200°F to finish the drying process. Green tea is popular in Asia and is not heated but simply steamed, rolled, and crushed. Oolong tea is less heated than black, but just enough to give it a different character from green. Green tea, which has been used in Japan for more than one thousand years, is now believed to have the most beneficial effects. No known toxicity. GRAS.

TEA-ABIETOYL HYDROLYZED ANIMAL PROTEIN • The salt of the condensation product of abietic acid and hydrolyzed animal protein *(see both)*.

TEA-C12-15 ALCOHOLS SULFATE • *See* Triethanolamine, Alcohol, and Sulfate.

TEA-COCO-HYDROLYZED ANIMAL PROTEIN • *See* Hydrolyzed Animal Protein and Surfactants, anionic.

TEA-COCO-HYDROLYZED PROTEIN • *See* Proteins.

TEA-COCYL GLUTAMATE • A softener. *See* Glutamate.

TEA-EDTA • *See* Ethylenediamine Tetraacetic Acid.

TEA EXTRACT • Essential oil. *See* Tea. GRAS.

TEA-HYDROGENATED TALLOW GLUTAMATE • A softener. *See* Glutamate.

TEA-LAUROYL GLUTAMATE • A softener. *See* Glutamate.

TEA-SORBATE • *See* Triethanolamine and Sorbic Acid.

TEA-STEARATE • *See* Triethanolamine and Stearic Acid.

TEA-SULFATE • *See* Triethanolamine and Sulfuric Acid.

TEA TREE OIL • *Melaleuca altemifolia.* Any of various shrubs or trees so named because their leaves are used as a substitute for tea leaves. The essential oil is obtained from the leaves and used as a germicide.

TECHNICAL WHITE MINERAL OIL • A mineral supplement for animals. The ratio is 0.06 percent in total feed.

TERA JAPONICA • *See* Catechu Extract.

TERATOGENIC • From the Greek *terat* (monster) and Latin *genesis* (origin): the origin or cause of a monster—or defective fetus.

TERGITOL • Tergemist. Sodium Etasulfate. Lye peeling agent, poultry scald agent, washing water agent used on fruits, poultry, and vegetables. FDA limits residue to 0.2 percent in wash water. Moderately toxic by ingestion and skin contact. A skin and eye irritant.

TERPENELESS OILS • An essential oil from which the terpene components have been removed by extraction and fractionation, either alone or in combination. The terpeneless grades are more highly concentrated than the original oil. Removal of the terpenes is necessary to inhibit spoilage, particularly of oils derived from citrus. It also makes the compound more soluble in alcohol. *See* Terpenes.

TERPENE RESINS • Moisture barrier on soft gelatin capsules and on powders of ascorbic acid *(see)* or its salts. Also used as a component of chewing-gum bases. *See* Terpenes.

TERPENES • A class of unsaturated hydrocarbons *(see)*. Its removal from products improves their flavor and gives them a more stable stronger odor. However, some perfumers feel that the removal of terpenes destroys some of the original odor. Has been used as an antiseptic.

TERPINEOL • A colorless, viscous liquid with a lilaclike odor, insoluble in mineral oil and slightly soluble in water. It is primarily used as a flavoring agent but is also employed as a denaturant to make alcohol undrinkable. It has been used as an antiseptic. It can be a sensitizer.

TERPINOLENE • A synthetic citrus and fruit flavoring agent for beverages, ice cream, ices, candy, and baked goods. *See* Turpentine for toxicity.

TERPINYL ACETATE • Colorless liquid, odor suggestive of bergamot and lavender occurs naturally in cardamom. Slightly soluble in water and glycerol. Derived by heating terpineol with acetic acid *(see both)*. Used in berry, lime, orange, cherry, peach, plum, and meat flavorings for beverages, ice cream, ices, candy, and baked goods. *See* Turpentine for toxicity.

TERPINYL ANTHRANILATE • A synthetic fruit flavoring agent. Derived by heating terpineol with anthranilic acid *(see both)*. Used as a synthetic fruit flavoring agent for beverages, ice cream, ices candy, and baked goods. *See* Turpentine for toxicity.

TERPINYL BUTYRATE • A synthetic fruit flavoring agent. Derived by heating terpineol with butyric acid *(see both)*. Used as a synthetic fruit flavoring agent for beverages, ice cream, ices, candy, chewing gum, and baked goods. *See* Turpentine for toxicity.

TERPINYL CINNAMATE • A synthetic fruit flavoring agent. Derived by heating terpineol with cinnamic acid *(see both)*. Used as a synthetic fruit flavoring agent for beverages, ice cream, ices, candy, and baked goods. *See* Turpentine for toxicity.

TERPINYL FORMATE • Formic Acid. A synthetic fruit flavoring agent. Derived by heating terpineol with formic acid *(see both)*. Used as a synthetic fruit flavoring agent for beverages, ice cream, ices, candy, liqueurs, and baked goods. *See* Turpentine for toxicity.

TERPINYL ISOBUTYRATE • A synthetic fruit flavoring agent. Derived by heating terpineol with isobutyric acid *(see both)*. Used as a synthetic fruit flavoring agent for beverages, ice cream, ices, candy, and baked goods. *See* Turpentine for toxicity.

TERPINYL ISOVALERATE • A synthetic fruit flavoring agent. Derived by heating terpineol with isovaleric acid *(see both)*. Used as a synthetic fruit flavoring agent for beverages, ice cream, ices, candy, and baked goods. *See* Turpentine for toxicity.

TERPINYL PROPIONATE • A synthetic fruit flavoring agent, colorless with a lavender odor. Derived by heating terpineol with propionic acid *(see both)*. Used as a synthetic fruit flavoring agent for beverages, ice cream, ices, candy, and baked goods. *See* Turpentine for toxicity.

TERTIARY BUTYLHYDROQUINONE (TBHQ) • This antioxidant was put on the market after years of pushing by food manufacturers to get it approved. It contains petroleum-derived butane and is used either alone or in combination with the preservative-antioxidant butylated hydroxyanisole (BHA) and/or butylated hydroxytoluene (BHT) *(see both)*. Hydroquinone combines with oxygen very rapidly and becomes brown when exposed to air. The FDA said that TBHQ must not exceed 0.02 percent of its oil and fat content. Death has occurred from the ingestion of as little as 5 grams. Ingestion of a single gram (a thirtieth of an ounce) has caused nausea, vomiting, ringing in the ears, delirium, a sense of suffocation, and collapse. Industrial workers exposed to the vapors—without obvious systemic effects—suffered clouding of the eye lens. Application to the skin may cause allergic reactions.

TESTOSTERONE PROPIONATE • Agovirin. Androgen. Androsan. Testoviron. TP. Uniteston. Vulvan. The male hormone, a steroid *(see)* produced by cells of the testicles. It is used to increase growth in cattle. FDA limits residue to 0.60 ppb in muscle, 2.6 ppb in fat, 1.9 ppb in kidney, and 1.3 ppb in liver of heifers. IARC review *(see)* and EPA Genetic Toxicology Program *(see)*. Moderately toxic by ingestion. Given by injection or tablet, it stimulates target tissues to develop normally in androgen-deficient men. It is used to treat eunuchs and male hormonal-change symptoms. It is used for breast engorgement in nonnursing mothers and to treat breast cancer in women one to five years postmenopausal. Potential adverse reactions in women include acne, edema, oily skin, weight gain, hairiness, hoarseness, clitoral enlargement, changes in libido, flushing, sweating, and vaginitis with itching. In males, used to treat in prepuberty, premature epiphyseal closure, priapism, growth of body and facial hair, phallic enlargement; in postpuberty, testicular atrophy, scanty sperm, decreased ejaculatory volume, impotence, enlargement of breasts, and epididymitis. In both sexes, edema, gastroenteritis, nausea, vomiting, diarrhea, constipation, changes in appetite, bladder irritability, jaundice, liver toxicity, and high levels of calcium in the blood.

2,4,4,4-TETRACHLORODIPHENYL SULFONE • Tetradifon. Tedion. A pesticide. A white crystalline powder. The FDA allows a residue of 10 ppm in dried figs from use on growing crops; 120 ppm in dried hops; 8 ppm in dried tea.

TETRACHLOROETHYLENE • Perchlorethylene. Tetrachloroethane. Ethylene Tetrachloride. 1,1,2,2-Tetrachloroethylene. Perchlor. Carbon Dichloride. A clear, colorless, nonflammable liquid with an etherlike smell, it is the main solvent used in the dry-cleaning process. It is also used in metal degreasing and during the production of fluorocarbons. It is used in some adhesives, aerosols, paints, and coatings. Used in food packaging. FDA limits residue to 0.3 percent in finished foamed polyethylene. IARC review *(see)*. This chemical enters your body when you breathe its vapors in the air. Liquid "perc" can be absorbed through your skin, to a limited extent. The most common effects of overexposure are irritation of the eyes, nose, throat, or skin. Like most organic solvents, it affects the brain the same way as drinking alcohol does. The symptoms of short-term overexposure usually clear up within hours after exposure stops. The mildest effects may start occurring at exposure levels of about 1,090 ppm. Effects occur more quickly and become more noticeable and serious as the exposure levels increase. Effects of this chemical on the nervous system include feeling "high," dizziness, headache, nausea, vomiting, fatigue, weakness, confusion, slurred speech, loss of balance, and poor coordination. At very high exposure (above 5,000 to 10,000) it can cause loss of consciousness and even death. Some studies, according to the California State Hazard Evaluation and Information System, show that overexposure to organic solvents over months or years may have long-lasting and possibly permanent effects on the nervous system. The symptoms of these long-term effects include fatigue, poor muscle coordination, difficulty in concentrating, loss of short-term memory, and personality changes such as increased anxiety, nervousness, and irritability. Tetrachloroethylene causes cancer in laboratory animals at exposure levels close to the level of what is legally allowed in the workplace. Contamination of drinking water with this chemical in Massachusetts and New Jersey has been implicated in clusters of leukemia and birth defects among residents. In any case, do not use perc around an open flame or intense ultraviolet light. Like most solvents containing chlorine, perc can break down into very hazardous compounds such as phosgene, hydrochloric acid, and chlorine.

TETRACHLOROISOPHTHALONITRILE • Bravo. Termil. TCPN. A fungicide used on broccoli, cabbage, cantaloupe, carrots, cauliflower, celery, citrus oil, cucumber, lettuce, onions, potatoes, tomatoes, and watermelon. Fungicide residue tolerance of 10 ppm in citrus oil. IARC review *(see)*. Cyanide products are on the Community Right-To-Know List *(see)* and the EPA Genetic Toxicology Program *(see)*. Causes cancer in experimental animals. Mildly toxic by ingestion.

TETRACHLORVINPHOS • A white powder that inhibits the transmission of nerve signals, it is used as an insecticide. Used as a feed additive for cattle and swine. FDA limits residue to 0.00015 lb per 100 lb of body weight of cattle and horses when used in animal feed. Limitation of 0.00011 lb per 100 lb of body weight of swine when used in animal feed. Found to be carcinogenic in feed by the National Cancer Institute. On the Community Right-To-Know List *(see)*. Poisonous by ingestion. Also caused reproductive problems in experimental animals.

TETRACYCLINE • Achromycin. Antibiotic introduced in 1953, tetracycline antibiotics are among the most widely prescribed. Used to treat cattle, chickens, lambs, swine, and turkeys. FDA limits residues to 0.25 ppm in calves, swine, sheep, chickens, and turkeys. In humans, tetracyclines are used to treat acne, bronchitis, pneumonia, syphilis, gonorrhea, inflammation of the tube that carries urine, and to prevent chest infections. Also used to treat Rocky Mountain spotted fever, brucellosis, relapsing fever, cholera, trachoma, and arthritis due to infection, syphilis, gonorrhea, chlamydia, trachoma, brucellosis, shigellosis, rickettsia, and *Mycoplasma*. Tetracyclines are also used to prevent and treat eye infections. Potential adverse effects of oral tetracyclines include nausea, vomiting, and diarrhea, drop in white blood cells, dizziness, headache, pressure on the brain, sore throat, sore tongue, trouble swallowing, loss of appetite, colitis, inflammation around the anus, liver problems, kidney problems, and diarrhea. Tetracyclines may cause sensitivity to sunlight and result in a rash and discoloration of the skin. If tetracycline is taken during pregnancy, a child may have discolored teeth. Oral tetracyclines must be used with extreme caution if kidney or liver problems are present. The effects of antibiotics such as tetracycline in meat eaten by humans is a matter of controversy. It is believed by many scientists that it causes resistance to antibiotics used by humans and may cause allergic reactions in sensitive persons, even in minute amounts.

TETRADECANAL • *See* Myristaldehyde.

TETRADECANOIC ACID • *See* Ethyl Myristate.

TETRADECYL ALDEHYDE • *See* Myristaldehyde.

TETRAETHYLENE GLYCOL • Colorless, pale yellow liquid used as a finishing agent on twine used to tie meat. Mildly toxic by ingestion. *See* Glycols.

TETRAHYDROFURAN • Butylene oxide. Oxolane. A colorless liquid with an etherlike odor, it is used as a solvent for packaging materials. FDA limits it to 1.5 percent of film. Moderately toxic by ingestion. Causes mutations in experimental animals. Human systemic effects by inhalation. Affects consciousness. Irritating to eyes and mucous membranes.

TETRAHYDROFURFURYL ACETATE • *See* Furfural.

TETRAHYDROFURFURYL ALCOHOL • A liquid that absorbs water and is flammable in air. A solvent for cosmetic fats, waxes, and resins. Mixes with water, ether, and acetone. Mildly irritating to the skin and mucous membranes. *See* Furfural.

TETRAHYDROFURFURYL BUTYRATE • Butyric Acid. A synthetic chocolate, honey, and maple flavoring agent for beverages, ice cream, ices, candy, and baked goods. May be irritating to the skin and mucous membranes.

TETRAHYDROFURFURYL PROPIONATE • Propionic Acid. A synthetic chocolate, honey, and maple flavoring agent for beverages, ice cream, ices, candy, and baked goods. Also used as a solvent for intravenous drugs. Moderately irritating to skin and mucous membranes.

TETRAHYDROGERANYL HYDROXYL STEARATE • *See* Stearic Acid and Hydroxylation.

TETRAHYDROLINALOOL • Colorless liquid with a floral odor used as a flavoring agent in various foods. *See* Linalool.

TETRAHYDROXYPROPYL ETHYLENEDIAMINE • Clear, colorless, thick liquid, a component of the bacteria-killing substance in sugarcane. It is strongly alkaline and is used as a solvent and preservative. It may be irritating to the skin and mucous membranes and may cause skin sensitization.

TETRAIODOFLUORESCEIN SODIUM • FD and C Red No. 3. Brown powder used as a color additive for candy, cherries, and confections. EPA Genetic Toxicology Program *(see)*. Moderately toxic by ingestion. *See* FD and C Red No. 3.

TETRAKIS (HYDROXYMETHYL) PHOSPHONIUM CHLORIDE • Catalyst, humectant, emulsifier, and plasticizer. No known toxicity.

TETRAMETHYL DECYNEDIOL • *See* Fatty Alcohols.

TETRAMETHYL PYRAZINE • White crystals or powder with a fermented soybean odor. Used as a flavoring agent in various foods. Moderately toxic by ingestion. GRAS.

2,4,5,8-TETRAMETHYL-1,2,5,6-TETROXOCANE • Metason. Slug-Tox. A pesticide to kill slugs and other parasites on strawberries. Human poison by ingestion. Can cause convulsions. Causes mutations in experimental animals.

TETRAMETHYLTHIURAM • Sprayed on some bananas. Seed disinfectant. fungicide; bacteriostat in soap. Can cause contact dermatitis. Irritating to mucous membranes.

TETRA POTASSIUM PHOSPHATE (TKPP) • An emulsifier. *See* Tetrasodium Pyrophosphate.

TETRA POTASSIUM PYROPHOSPHATE • An emulsifier used in cheese and as a sequestering agent in cheese and ice cream. Also used in cleaning compounds, oil-well drilling, water treatment, and as a general sequestering agent to remove rust stains. A sequestering agent, clarifying agent, and buffering agent for shampoos. Produced by molecular dehydration of dibasic sodium phosphate. Insoluble in alcohol. A water softener in bath preparations. It is alkaline and irritating and ingestion can cause nausea, diarrhea, and vomiting. GRAS for packaging. *See* Tetrasodium Pyrophosphate.

TETRASODIUM EDTA • Sodium Edetate. Powdered sodium salt that reacts with metals. A sequestering agent and chelating agent *(see both)* used in cosmetic solutions. Can deplete the body of calcium if taken internally. *See* Ethylenediamine Tetraacetic Acid. No known toxicity on the skin.

TETRASODIUM PYROPHOSPHATE (TSPP) • Used in cheese emulsification and as a sequestering agent in cheese and ice cream. Also used in cleansing compounds, oil-well drilling, water treatment, and as a general sequestering agent to remove rust stains. A sequestering agent, clarifying agent, and buffering agent for shampoos. Produced by molecular dehydration of dibasic sodium phosphate. Insoluble in alcohol. A water softener in bath preparations. It is alkaline and irritating and ingestion can cause nausea, diarrhea, and vomiting. GRAS for packaging.

TEXTURIZER • A chemical used to improve the texture of various foods. For instance, canned tomatoes, canned potatoes, and canned apple slices tend to become soft and fall apart unless the texturizer calcium chloride *(see)*, for example, of its salts are added, which keep the product firm.

TFC • Abbreviation for *triclofIucarban,* a disinfectant.

THALOSE • A blend of food-grade acidulants *(see)* that contains propylene glycol and citric, lactic, phosphoric, and tartaric acids *(see all),* and water and salt. Adding this compound to sugar permits a reduction in the amount required to achieve a desired sweetness (one ounce of liquid Thalose added to thirty-two pounds of sugar causes the perceived sweetness to be increased by 90 percent). One pint added to sugar will result in a saving of five hundred pounds of sugar without reducing sweetness. Thalose itself is not sweet and does not alter the flavor or aroma of the foods to which it is added. It does not contribute calories but will reduce the caloric level of the end product by lowering the amount of carbohydrates in the compound. Thalose can be used in beverages, bakery and confectionery products, and in ice cream, as long as the physical properties of the sugar are not needed (sugar is often used as a thickening agent and texturizer). All of the substances contained in this extender are GRAS and comply with the FDA provision for food-grade ingredients.

THAMNIDIUM ELEGANS • A grayish white mold used for aging meat. It is related to the tropical bread mold. No known toxicity.

THAUMATIN • A mixture of intensely sweet-tasting proteins extracted from the fruit of a West African plant, *Thaumatococcus daniellii.* It has about 2,000 to 3,000 times the sweetness of sugar. It does contain calories. The fruits of the plant have been used for centuries by the West Africans as a source of sweetness. It is also sold in Japan. Because of problems with stability, taste profile, and compatibility, thaumatin is used primarily as a flavor enhancer, at levels below the sweet-taste threshold. It is awaiting approval in the United States. There is reported use of the chemical, it has not yet been assigned for toxicology literature.

THBP • *See* 2,4,5-Trihydroxybutyrophenone. Antioxidant in fats and oils.

THEINE • *See* Caffeine.

THEOBROMA OIL • Cacao Butter. Cocoa Butter. Yellowish white solid with chocolatelike taste and odor. Derived from the cacao bean. Widely used in confections, suppositories, pharmaceuticals, soaps, and cosmetics. No known toxicity but may cause allergic reactions in the sensitive.

THEOBROMINE • The alkaloid found in cocoa, cola nuts, tea, and chocolate products, closely related to caffeine. It is used as a diuretic, smooth muscle relaxant, heart stimulant, and blood vessel dilator. In 1992, the FDA proposed a ban on theobromine sodium salicylate in oral menstrual drug products because it has not been shown to be safe and effective for its stated claims.

THIABENDAZOLE HYDROCHLORIDE • A mold retardant used on animal feed, apples, bananas, beef, citrus fruit, lamb, milk, pears, pheasants, pork, potato processing waste, rice hulls. FDA limits are 0.1 ppm in cattle, goats, sheep, pheasant, and swine; 0.05 ppm in milk; 33 ppm in dried apple pomace; 150 ppm in dry or wet grape pomace; 30 ppm in potato processing waste; and 8 ppm in rice hulls when used for animal feed. Moderately toxic by ingestion.

THIAMIN HYDROCHLORIDE • A co-enzyme of vitamin B_1. A white crystalline powder used as a dietary supplement in prepared breakfast cereals, peanut butter, poultry, stuffing, baby cereals, skimmed milk, bottled soft drinks, enriched flours, enriched farina, cornmeal, enriched macaroni and noodle products, and enriched bread and rolls. Acts as a helper in important energy-yielding reactions in the body. Practically all B_1 sold is synthetic. The vitamin is destroyed by alkalies and alkaline drugs such as phenobarbital. GRAS.

THIAMIN MONONITRATE • A co-enzyme of vitamin B_1. A white crystalline powder used as a diet supplement and to enrich flour. GRAS.

THIAMUTILIN • Tiamulin. Crystals from acetone *(see)* used in animal feed and as an animal drug to combat bacterial infections. Moderately toxic by ingestion and injections under the skin.

THIAZOLE • Colorless or pale yellow liquid. Used in organic synthesis of fungicides, dyes, and rubber accelerators.

2-(THIAZOL-4-YL)BENZIMIDAZOLE • Thiabendazole. Arbotect. TBDZ. Mycozol. White to tan odorless compound used as a fungicide in animal feed and for citrus fruit and to control fungal diseases in seed potatoes. Used therapeutically in animals to combat worms and fungus infections. EPA Genetic Toxicology Program. Poisonous by ingestion. Caused birth defects in experimental animals.

THIAZOLYLSULFANILAMIDE • Sulzol. Thiazamide. An antibiotic used to treat infections in swine. EPA Genetic Toxicology Program. Human poison.

THIBETOLIDE • *See* Pentadecalactone.

THICKENERS • Many natural gums and starches are used to add body to mixtures. Pectin *(see),* for instance, which is used in fruits naturally low in this gelling agent, enables manufacturers to produce jams and jellies of a marketable thickness. Algin (*see* Alginates) is used to make salad dressings that will not be runny. Also used to add body to lotions and creams. Those usually employed include such natural gums as sodium alginate and pectins.

THIDIAZURON • A pesticide used on cottonseed hulls. The FDA residue tolerance is 0.05 ppm in milk; 0.1 ppm in eggs; and 0.2 ppm as residue in meat, fat, and meat byproducts of cattle, sheep, and poultry. As residue in or on cottonseed, the limit is 0.4 ppm.

2-THIENYL MERCAPTAN • A synthetic flavoring agent that occurs naturally in coffee. Used in coffee flavoring for candy and baked goods. No known toxicity.

THIETHYL CITRATE • An antioxidant used primarily in dried egg whites. *See* Citric Acid. GRAS.

THIOALLYL ETHER • *See* Allyl Sulfide.

THIOBIS (DODECYL PROPIONATE) • White crystalline flakes with a sweet odor used as an antioxidant in fats, oils, and packaging materials. FDA regulations limit to 0.005 percent migrating from food package. An eye irritant.

THIOCYANATE • Colorless or white crystals derived from cyanide. Used in animal feeds as a growth stimulant.

THIODICARB • An insecticide used on cottonseed and soybean hulls. FDA permits 0.8 ppm on cottonseed hulls and 0.4 ppm on soybean hulls. *See* Carbamate.

THIODIPROPIONIC ACID • An acid freely soluble in hot water, alcohol, and acetone. Used as an antioxidant in general food use. Percent of fat or oil, including essential oil, content of food is up to .02. Used also for soap products and polymers *(see)* of ethylene. The final report to the FDA of the Select Committee on GRAS Substances stated in 1980 that there is no evidence in the available information that it is a hazard to the public when used as it is now and it should continue its GRAS status with limitations on the amounts that can be added to food.

THIOPHANATE, METHYL • A fungicide. The FDA residue tolerance in or on dried apple pomace feed to animals is 40 ppm.

THIOUREA • A banned antioxidant.

THISTLE, BLESSED • Holy Thistle. Extract of the prickly plant, *Cnicus benedictus*. Cleared for use as a natural flavoring in alcoholic beverages only. Also called cardin, it is an annual herb. The plant is a native of the south of Europe and is cultivated in gardens all over the world. It has been used in medicine since A.D. 100. Once believed to be a panacea, it has been credited with reducing excess fluid. There is reported use of the chemical; it has not yet been assigned for toxicology literature.

THREONINE • L form only. An essential amino acid *(see);* the last to be discovered (1935). Prevents the buildup of fat on the liver. Occurs in whole eggs, skim milk, casein, and gelatin. On the FDA list for further study. GRAS.

4-THUJANOL • An alcohol from thuja oil *(see)*.

THUJA OIL • A constituent of many essential oils. Usually derived from the leaves of the white cedar. Colorless liquid, almost insoluble in water. Ingestion may cause convulsions. It is used in flavorings and perfumery.

THYME OIL • A seasoning from the dried leaves and flowering tops of the wild creeping thyme grown in Eurasia and throughout the United States, *Thymus vulgaris* and *Thymus zygis*. Colorless, yellow, or red, with a pleasant odor. Used in sausage, spice, and thyme flavorings for beverages, ice cream, ices, candy, baked goods, chewing gum, condiments, meats, and soups. Used to flavor toothpaste, mouthwashes, and to scent perfumes, aftershave lotions, and soap. Used as a flavoring in cough medicines. May cause contact dermatitis and hay fever. GRAS.

THYME, WHITE OIL • Obtained from the plant and used in fruit, liquor, and thyme. Used in fruit, peppermint, and spice flavorings for beverages, ice cream, ices, candy, baked goods, and chewing gum. Oral dose as medicine is .067 grams. It can cause vomiting, diarrhea, dizziness, and cardiac depression when taken in sufficient amounts. GRAS. *See* Thyme Oil.

THYMOL • Obtained from the essential oil of lavender, origanum oil, and other volatile oils. It destroys mold, preserves anatomical specimens, and is a topical antifungal agent with a pleasant aromatic odor. Used in fruit, peppermint, and spice flavorings for beverages, ice cream, ices, candy, baked goods, and chewing gum. Used in mouthwashes, and to scent perfumes, aftershave lotions, and soap. It is omitted from hypoallergenic cosmetics because it can cause allergic reactions. Oral dose as medicine is .067 grams. It can cause vomiting, diarrhea, dizziness, and cardiac depression when taken in sufficient amounts. GRAS.

THYMOL IODIDE • A dietary supplement. In animal feed a source of trace mineral. GRAS.

THYMUS CAPITATUS • Spanish Origanum. Flavoring. *See* Organum Oil.

THYROID • The thyroid is a butterfly-shaped gland located in the neck with a "wing" on either side of the windpipe. The gland produces thyroxine, which controls the rates of chemical reactions in the body. Generally, the more thyroxine, the faster the body works. Thyroxine needs iodine to function.

TIAMULIN • *See* Thiamutilin.

TIGLIC ACID • *See* Allyl Tiglate.

TIN CHLORIDE • Colorless crystals used as an antioxidant and reducing agent *(see)* in asparagus, and carbonated beverages. FDA limits it to 20 ppm in asparagus packed in glass. EPA Genetic Toxicology Program *(see)*. Poison by ingestion.

TINCTURE • A solution in alcohol of the flavors derived from plants obtained by mashing or boiling.

TIPA • The abbreviation for *triisopropanolamine (see)*.

TIPA-STEARATE • *See* Stearic Acid.

TITANIUM DIOXIDE • Occurs naturally in minerals. Used chiefly as a white pigment and as an opacifier; also a white pigment for candy, gum, and marker ink. A pound has been ingested without apparent ill effects. The greatest covering and tinting power of any white pigment used in bath powders, nail whites, depilatories, eyeliners, white eye shadows, antiperspirants, face powders, protective creams, liquid powders, lipsticks, hand lotions, and nail polish. In high concentrations the dust may cause lung damage. It has been permanently listed for use as a food color with a limit of 1 percent by weight of finished food since 1966.

TITANIUM HYDROXIDE • *See* Titanium Dioxide.

TITANIUM OXIDE • *See* Titanium Dioxide.

TOASTED PARTIALLY DEFATTED COOKED COTTONSEED FLOUR • Used as a food coloring. It is exempt from certification.

TOCOPHEROL ACETATE • A dietary supplement. GRAS. *See* Tocopherols.

TOCOPHEROLS • Vitamin E. Obtained by the vacuum distillation of edible vegetable oils. Protects fat in the body's tissues from abnormal breakdown. Experimental evidence shows vitamin E may protect the heart and blood vessels and retard aging. Used as a dietary supplement and as an antioxidant for essential oils, rendered animal fats, or a combination of such fats with vegetable oils. Helps form normal red blood cells, muscle, and other tissues. The final report to the FDA of the Select Committee on GRAS Substances stated in 1980 that it should continue its GRAS status with no limitations other than good manufacturing practices.

TOCOPHERYL SUCCINATE • Vitamin E Succinate. Obtained by the distillation of edible vegetable oils and used as a dietary supplement and as an antioxidant for fats and oils. No known toxicity.

TOLERANCE • The ability to live with an allergen.

a-TOLUALDEHYDE • *See* Phenylacetaldehyde.

TOLUALDEHYDE GLYCERYL ACETAL • A synthetic chocolate, fruit, cherry, coconut, and vanilla flavoring agent for beverages, ice cream, ices, candy, and baked goods. No known toxicity.

TOLUALDEHYDES (MIXED *o, m, p*) • Synthetic berry, loganberry, fruit, cherry, muscatel, peach, apricot, nut, almond, and vanilla flavorings for beverages, ice cream, ices, candy, baked goods, chewing gum, gelatin desserts, and maraschino cherries. No known toxicity.

TOLU BALSAM • Extract and Gum. Extract from the Peruvian or Indian plant, *Myroxylon* spp. Contains cinnamic acid and benzoic acid *(see both)*. Used in butter, butterscotch, cherry, and spice flavorings for beverages, ice cream, ices, candy, baked goods, and chewing gum. The gum is used in fruit, maple, and vanilla flavorings for beverages, ice cream, ices, candy, baked goods, and syrups. Mildly antiseptic and may be mildly irritating to the skin. There is reported use of the chemical; it has not yet been assigned for the toxicology literature.

TOLUENE • Toluol. Methyl Benzene. Used in water purifying agents, to remove odors in cheese, and in a number of food processing compounds. Also used as a solvent for paints, nail polish, lacquers, thinners, coatings, shellacs, adhesives, metal cleaners, rust preservatives, fuel system antifreezes, asphalt removers, flame retardants, high-octane gasoline blends, rotogravure printing processes, and glue, and is being used to replace more toxic benzene solvents in many products. Obtained from petroleum or by distilling balsam Tolu. Resembles benzene but is less volatile, flammable, or toxic. May cause mild anemia if ingested, and it is narcotic in high concentrations. Being tested at the U.S. Frederick Cancer Research Center for possible cancer-causing effects. It can cause liver damage and is irritating to the skin and respiratory tract.

While halogenated hydrocarbons like toluene are assumed responsible for health risks, long-term effects of low-level exposure to them in drinking water of at least 20 cities is unknown. There is concern about the role of toluene on the brain and nervous system because symptoms have been observed in workers chronically exposed in jobs such as spray painting. The chronic high-dose exposures seen in toluene abuse such as glue sniffers have been associated epidemiologically with sudden death secondary to irregular heartbeat, liver, and neurologic disorders. The current U.S. standard is 200 ppm in eight hours and maximum peaks up to 500 ppm for 10 minutes. NIOSH *(see)* currently recommends that toluene exposures be limited to 100 ppm. Brief exposure to 100 ppm causes statistical impairment of reflexes and thinking. Exposure to 800 ppm causes severe fatigue, confusion, and staggering that may persist for several days. Exposure to 10,000 ppm can cause loss of consciousness and death.

o-TOLUENETHIOL • Thiocresol. Cream to white, moist crystals with a musty odor. A skin irritant. Used as an intermediate *(see)* and as a germicide.

TOLYL ACETATE • Acetic Acid. A synthetic butter, caramel, fruit, honey, nut, and spice flavoring for beverages, ice cream, ices, candy, baked goods, chewing gum, and gelatin desserts.

o-TOLYL ACETATE • Acetic Acid. A synthetic butter, caramel, fruit, honey, and cherry flavoring for beverages, ice cream, ices, candy, baked goods, chewing gum, and gelatin desserts.

p-TOLYL ACETATE • Acetic Acid. A synthetic butter, caramel, fruit, honey, nut, and spice flavorings for beverages, ice cream, ices, candy, baked goods, chewing gum, and condiments.

4-(p-TOLYL)-2-BUTANONE • A synthetic fruit flavoring for beverages, ice cream, ices, candy, and baked goods.

p-TOLYL ISOBUTYRATE • A synthetic fruit flavoring for beverages, ice cream, ices, candy, and baked goods.

p-TOLYL LAURATE • Dodecanoic Acid. A synthetic butter, caramel, fruit, honey, nut flavoring for beverages, ice cream, ices, candy, and baked goods.

p-TOLYL PHENYLACETATE • A synthetic butter, caramel, fruit, honey, and nut flavoring for beverages, ice cream, ices, candy, and baked goods.

TOLYLACETALDEHYDE • A synthetic berry, loganberry, fruit, cherry, muscatel, peach, apricot, nut, almond, and vanilla flavoring agent for beverages, ice cream, ices, candy, baked goods, gelatin desserts, chewing gum, and maraschino cherries. No known toxicity.

p-TOLYALDEHYDE • Colorless liquid derived from benzene. Used in perfumes and flavoring agents.

2-(p-TOYL) PROPIONALDEHYDE • A synthetic caraway flavoring agent for beverages, ice cream, ices, candy, baked goods, and liqueurs.

TOMATO EXTRACT • Tomatine. Extract from the fruit of the tomato, *Solanum esculentum*. Used as a fungicide and as a precipitating agent. Nontoxic.

TONKA • Tonka Bean. Coumarouna Bean. Black-brownish seeds with a wrinkled surface and brittle, shining or fatty skins. A vanillalike odor and a bitter taste. Used in the production of natural coumarin *(see)*, flavoring extracts, and toilet powders. Banned from food because of it coumarin content. *See* Coumarin.

TORMENTIL EXTRACT • The extract of the roots of *Potentilla erecta*.

TORTUA YEAST • Dried *Candida utils*. Flavoring in food. *See* Yeast.

TOTAL CARB • Label listing for *total carbohydrates*. *See* Carbohydrates.

TOUCH OF NATURE • A sweetener made from both sap extracts and crushed leaves of nature's taste tree, grown in the Brazilian rain forest.

TOXAPHENE • Chlorinated camphene containing 67–69 percent chlorine. Yellow waxy solid with a pleasant pine odor, it is used as an insecticide in soybean oil. FDA regulations set a residue tolerance of 6 ppm in soybean oil from use on growing crop. Human poison by ingestion. Can be absorbed through the skin. Causes cancer and birth defects in experimental animals. Lethal amounts of toxaphene can enter the body through the mouth, lungs, and skin.

TRAGACANTH • *See* Gum Tragacanth. GRAS.

TRAILBLAZER • A fat-based replacer for fat. It is a microparticulated protein product (MPP) similar to Simplesse *(see)*. It is made from whey protein or milk and egg protein. It has about one to four calories per gram and is approved for use in frozen dessert type foods. The FDA says that whey-based MPP conforms to the definition of whey protein concentrate *(see)* such as the fat replacer Dairy-Lo, a GRAS substance. Therefore, it can be used in other foods including reduced-fat versions of butter, sour cream, cheese, yogurt, salad dressing, margarine, mayonnaise, baked goods, coffee creamers, soups, and sauces.

TRALOMETHRIN • An insecticide. FDA residue tolerance in or on cottonseed oil, 0.2 ppm; on or in cottonseed, 0.02 ppm; on or in soybeans 0.05 ppm.

TRANS FATTY ACIDS • A polyunsaturated *(see)* fatty acid in which some of the missing hydrogen atoms have been put back by hydrogenation. Trans fatty acids are the building blocks of hydrogenated fats. In the 1960s, doctors told us to eat margarine instead of butter to lower our cholesterol levels and protect our hearts. The amount of butter consumed by Americans is now half of what it was in 1961. In 1992, reports from the United States Department of Agriculture researchers and scientific institutions in Europe stated that margarines, which develop trans fatty acids during the processing to form "sticks," may be as bad or worse for our cholesterol levels and our hearts. The sale of margarine immediately plummeted after publicity about the research. Joseph T. Judd at the USDA (which funded the $1 million margarine study) then said: "At this point, we really do not have all of the evidence to relate trans fatty acids to heart disease because in cardiovascular disease there are many factors. . . . And we don't know the effect of trans fatty acids in these other risk factors; all we're looking at is blood cholesterol."

TRENBOLONE • A synthetic anabolic steroid. A male sex hormone given to cattle to "build up," to stimulate growth, weight gain, strength and appetite. Abuse of these drugs has caused problems, especially among young athletes who wish to build muscle and strength. Uncontrolled use can cause liver damage and cancer. February 27, 1991, anabolic steroids became controlled drugs requiring security ordering and record keeping for humans. Increased tumors were evident in long-term studies of rats fed trenbolone. The FDA limits residues to 50 ppb in the muscle of beef, 100 ppb in liver, 300 ppb in kidney, and 400 ppb in fat in cattle. The FAO-WHO Expert Committee on Food Additives set a marginal no-effect level at 0.1 mg/kg diet equal to approximately 2 mg/kg of body weight. The Committee set an ADI *(see)* of 0–0.02 mg/kg of body weight. The European Union will not permit United States red meat to be imported with this growth promoter.

TRENBOLONE ACETATE and ESTRADIOL • Hormones used as implants in feedlot cattle. As residues in cattle, *see* Trenbolone and Estradiol.

TRIACETIN • Glyceryl Triacetate. Primarily a solvent for hair dyes. Also a fix-ative in perfume and used in toothpaste. A colorless, somewhat oily liquid with a slight fatty odor and a bitter taste. Obtained from adding acetate to glycerin *(see both)*. Soluble in water and miscible with alcohol. No known toxicity in above use. Large subcutaneous injections are lethal to rats. GRAS.

TRIACETYL GLYCERIN • Colorless, oily liquid with a fatty odor and taste, it is used as a flavoring agent, a humectant *(see),* plasticizer, solvent, and carrier for food additives. Used in baked goods, baking mixes, beverages, candy, chewing gum, confections, fillings, frostings, frozen dairy desserts. dessert mixes, gelatins, and puddings. Poison by ingestion. An eye irritant.

TRIBASIC CALCIUM PHOSPHATE • Tricalcium Diorthophosphate. Tricalcium Phosphate. An anticaking agent and calcium supplement in grain products used in packaged cake mixes, candy, baked goods, gelatin desserts, powdered beverage mixes, seasoning mixes, powdered soups, and sugar. Too much phosphorus in the form of phosphates from processed foods could upset the body's mineral balance, particularly calcium and could adversely affect teeth, bones, and kidneys.

TRIBROMSALAN • TBS. 3,4',5-Tribromosalicylanilide. Used in medicated cosmetics; an antiseptic and fungicide. Irritating to the skin and may cause allergic reaction when skin is exposed to the sun. Salicylanilide is an antifungal compound used to treat ringworm. TBS is in the most popular soaps to kill skin bacteria. Used as a germicide, frequently replacing hexachlorophene.

TRIBUTYL ACETYLCITRATE • A synthetic fruit flavoring agent for beverages.

TRIBUTYL CITRATE • The triester of butyl alcohol and citric acid *(see both),* it is a pale yellow, odorless liquid used as a plasticizer, antifoam agent, and solvent for nitrocellulose. Low toxicity.

TRIBUTYLCRESYLBUTANE • Used as a stabilizer. *See* Phenol.

TRIBUTYRIN • Glyceryl Tributyrate. A colorless, somewhat oily liquid that occurs naturally in butter. It has a characteristic odor and bitter taste. It is soluble in alcohol. Used as a flavoring agent in beverages, ice cream, candy, baked goods, margarine, and puddings. Moderately toxic by ingestion. *See* Glycerol and Butyric Acid.

TRICALCIUM PHOSPHATE • The calcium salt of phosphate *(see).* An anticaking agent in table salt and vanilla powder, and a dietary supplement. Used as a bleaching agent in flour at not more than 6 ppm by weight alone or in combination with potassium alum, calcium sulfate *(see),* and other compounds. Also used as a polishing agent in dentifrices. No known toxicity. *See* Calcium Phosphate. GRAS.

TRICALCIUM SILICATE • Used in table salt and baking powder as an anticaking agent up to 2 percent. On the FDA list to be studied for subacute, mutagenic, teratogenic, and reproductive effects. No known toxicity. GRAS.

TRICETETH-5 PHOSPHATE • *See* Phosphoric Acid and Cetyl Alcohol.

TRICHLOROETHYLENE (TCE) • Residue in decaffeinated coffee powder. Used in spice oleoresins as a solvent. Moderate exposure can cause symptoms similar to alcohol inebriation, and its analgesic and anesthetic properties make it useful for short operations. High concentrations have a narcotic effect. Deaths have been attributed to irregular heart rhythm. Tests conducted by the National Cancer Institute showed that this chlorinated hydrocarbon caused cancer of the liver in mice. Rats failed to show significant response, a fact which may be attributed to the cancer-resistance of the strain used. Despite the species difference in cancer response, the NCI concluded that the TCE test clearly showed the compound caused liver cancer in mice. The findings are considered definitive for animal studies and serve as a warning of possible carcinogenicity in humans. IARC review *(see)*. However, the extent of the possible human risk cannot be predicted reliably on the basis of these studies alone. A related compound vinyl chloride *(see),* does cause liver cancer in humans. FDA residue tolerance in decaffeinated ground coffee, 25 ppm (0.0025 percent); decaffeinated soluble (instant) coffee extract, 10 ppm (0.001 percent); spice oleoresins, 30 ppm. In 1997, the NTP *(see)* put it on the list for review as a carcinogen.

(2,2,2-TRICHLORO-1-HYDROEXYETHYL)DIMETHYL PHOSPHONATE • Anthon. Chloroftalm. Chlorophos. Chlorofos. Dimetox. Dipterax. Dipterex. Trichlorfon. Widely used insecticide for the control of flies and roaches and also to fight worms in animals. Used in animal feed and on citrus pulp. FDA limits it to 2.5 ppm in dried citrus pulp when used for animal feed. Inhibits nerve signals. Poison by ingestion, inhalation, and other routes except skin. On skin, it is moderately toxic. Causes cancer and birth defects in experimental animals.

TRICHLOROMETAFOS • Dermaphos. Ronnel. Fenchlorphos. White powder widely used as an insecticide in animal feed. Chlorophenol compounds are on the Community Right-To-Know List *(see).* Poisonous by ingestion. Causes birth defects in experimental animals. Inhibits nerve transmission.

***n*-TRICHLOROMETHYL MERCAPTO-4-CYCLOHEXENE-1,2-DICARBOX-IMIDE •** A fumigant. *See* Captan.

TRICLOCARBAN • Prepared from aniline and chlorophenyl isocyanate, it is used as an antiseptic in soaps and other cleaning products. *See* Aniline and Phenol.

TRICLOPYR • A preemergent herbicide. FDA residue tolerance is 0.01 ppm in milk; 0.05 ppm in meat, fat, and meat byproducts of cattle, goats, hogs, and sheep; and 0.5 ppm in liver and kidneys of cattle, goats, hogs, and sheep.

TRICYCLAZOLE • A fungicide used on rice. The FDA tolerance for residues are 30 ppm in rice bran, rice hulls, and rice polishings.

TRICYCLOHEXYLTIN HYDROXIDE (TCTH) • Cyhexatin. A pesticide used on animal feed. FDA residue tolerance is 8 ppm in dried apple pomace and dried citrus pulp resulting from application to growing crops; 90 ppm in dried hops; 4 ppm in dried prunes. Irritating to the eyes.

2-TRIDECENAL • A synthetic citrus and flavoring for beverages, ice cream, ices, candy, baked goods, and chewing gum.

TRIDECYL ALCOHOL • Derived from tridecane, a paraffin hydrocarbon obtained from petroleum. Used as an emulsifier in cosmetic creams, lotions, and lipsticks. No known toxicity.

TRIETHANOLAMINE • A coating agent for fresh fruit and vegetables and widely used in surfactants *(see).* Used in flume water for washing sugar beets prior to slicing operation. Also used as a dispersing agent and detergent in hand and body lotions, shaving creams, soaps, shampoo, and bath powders. Its principal toxic effect in animals has been attributed to overalkalinity. Gross pathology has been found in the gastrointestinal tract in fatally poisoned guinea pigs. It is an irritant.

TRIETHANOLAMINE STEARATE • Made from ethylene oxide. Used in brilliantines, cleansing creams, foundation creams, hair lacquers, liquid makeups, fragrances, liquid powders, mascara, protective creams, baby preparations, shaving creams, and lathers, and preshave lotions. A moisture absorber, viscous, used in making emulsions. Cream color turns brown on exposure to air. May be irritating to the skin and mucous membranes, but less so than many other amines *(see)*.

TRIETHYL CITRATE • Citric Acid. Ethyl Citrate. Odorless, practically colorless, bitter; also used in dried egg as a sequestering agent *(see)* and to prevent rancidity. Citrates may interfere with laboratory tests for blood, liver, and pancreatic function, but no known skin toxicity. The final report to the FDA of the Select Committee on GRAS Substances stated in 1980 that it should continue its GRAS status with no limitations other than good manufacturing practices.

TRIETHYLENE GLYCOL • Used in stick perfume. Prepared from ethylene oxide and ethylene glycol *(see both)*. Used as a solvent. *See* Polyethylene Glycol for toxicity.

TRIFLUMIZOLE • Fungicide used in animal feed. FDA residue tolerances are 2 ppm in apple pomace; 25 ppm in grape pomace; and 8 ppm in raisin waste.

TRIFLUROMETHANE SULFONIC ACID • A catalyst used in the production of cocoa butter substitute. Toxic by inhalation. Slightly irritating to the skin.

TRIFORINE • White crystals used as a fungicide for animal feed and hops. FDA limits residue to 60 ppm in dried hops and in spent hops when used for animal feed.

TRIFURAN • A pesticide used in peppermint and spearmint oil. FDA residue tolerance 2 ppm.

2-4-5-TRIHYDROXYBUTYROPHENONE (THBP) • An antioxidant used alone or in combination with other antioxidants. Total antioxidant not to exceed 0.02 percent of the oil or fat content of any product. Also used in the manufacture of food packaging materials, with a limit of .005 percent in food. On the FDA list for further study of this widely used additive. May not be listed on labels.

TRIHYDROXY STEARIN • Isolated from cork and used as a thickener. No known toxicity.

TRIILAURYL CITRATE • *See* Lauryl Alcohol and Citric Acid.

TRIISOPROPANOLAMINE • A crystalline, white solid. A mild base used as an emulsifying agent. A component of a coating used for fresh fruits and vegetables. No known toxicity.

TRIISOSTEARIN • *See* Glycerin and Isostearic Acid.

TRILAURIN • *See* Lauric Acid.

TRIMETHYLAMINE • Miscellaneous use. Colorless gas at room temperature easily liquefied. Derived from the interaction of methanol and ammonia. Used in insecticides, quaternary ammonium compounds *(see)*, and plastics.

2,6,6-TRIMETHYL-2-CYCLOHEXANE-1-ONE • Nicomol. Crystals from dilute acetic acid. Odorless and tasteless. Breaks down fats.

2,4,5-TRIMETHYL DELTA-3-OXAZOLINE • Yellow to orange liquid with a strong, nutlike odor. Used as a flavoring agent in various foods. GRAS.

TRIPOLYPHOSPHATE • A phosphorus salt. A sequestering agent *(see)* in foods and a food additive. Used to soften water and as a dispersing and buffering agent in shampoos. Can be irritating because of its alkalinity. May cause esophageal stricture if swallowed. Moderately irritating to the skin and mucous membranes. Ingestion can cause violent vomiting. GRAS.

TRISODIUM-3-CARBOXY-5-HYDROXY-1-*p*-SULFOPHENYL-4-*p*-SULFO-PHENYLAZOPYRAZOLE • *See* FD and C Yellow No. 5.

TRISODIUM EDTA • *See* Tetrasodium EDTA.

TRISODIUM HEDTA • Mineral suspending agents. *See* Sequestrants.

TRISODIUM HYDROXY EDTA • *See* Tetrasodium EDTA.

TRISODIUM HYDROXYETHYL ETHLENEDIAMINETRIACETATE • *See* Tetrasodium EDTA.

TRISODIUM NTA • *See* Sequestrants.

TRISODIUM PHOSPHATE • Obtained from phosphate rock. Highly alkaline. An emulsifier, in cheese; the FDA allows residue in cheese less than 3 percent of weight. It is also used in fruit jellies. Used in shampoos, cuticle softeners, bubble baths, and bath salts for its water-softening and cleaning actions. Phosphorus was formerly used to treat rickets and degenerative disorders and is now used as a mineral supplement for foods; also in incendiary bombs and tracer bullets. Can cause skin irritation from alkalinity. GRAS.

TRISTEARIN • Present in many animal and vegetable fats, especially hard ones like tallow and cocoa butter, it is used in surfactants, quaternary ammonium compounds, and emollients. No known toxicity.

TRISTEARYL CITRATE • The triester of stearyl alcohol and citric acid *(see both)*.

TRITHION • Acarithion. Akarithion. Endyl. Trithion Miticide. Insecticide and miticide used in animal feed, grapefruit, lemons, limes, oranges, tangelos, tangerines, and dried tea. FDA's insecticide residue tolerance is 20 ppm on dried tea and 10 ppm in dehydrated citrus pulp and citrus meal when used for cattle feed. EPA Extremely Hazardous Substances List *(see)*. Poisonous by ingestion and skin contact. Inhibits nerve transmission.

TRITICALE • A manmade cross between wheat *(see* Dog Grass, Triticum) and rye (secale), but more nutritious than wheat. The protein content of bread made with it is 10 percent higher and its essential amino acid, lysine *(see)*, exceeds wheat bread by 50 percent. The crop is the result of seven years' development and is being offered both as an ingredient and as a basic food substance. A number of novel products are being made from it, including ethnic breads. Two slices of Tritibread (made with triticale) supply 12 percent of the U.S. recommended daily allowance for protein, 30 percent for thiamin, and 10 percent for riboflavin, niacin, and iron. Triticale is intended for baked goods, ready-to-eat cereals, and malt products; also as a thickener, emulsifier, fortifier, and supplement. Once accepted, triticale can be an important nutritious addition to the food supply.

TRITICUM • *See* Dog Grass. GRAS.

TROMETHAMINE • Made by the reduction *(see)* of nitro compounds, it is a crystalline mass used in the manufacture of surfactants *(see)*. Used as an emulsifying agent for cosmetic creams and lotions, mineral oil, and paraffin wax emulsions. Used medicinally to correct an overabundance of acid in the body. No known toxicity.

TRUE FIXATIVE • This holds back the evaporation of the other materials. Benzoin is an example. *See* Fixatives.

TRYPSIN • An enzyme formed in the intestine. It is administered as a drug in the treatment of indigestion.

TRYPTOPHAN • L form only. A tremendous amount of research is now in progress with this amino acid *(see)*. First isolated in milk in 1901, it is now being studied as a means to calm hyperactive children, induce sleep, and fight depression and pain. Although it is sold over the counter, it is not believed to be completely harmless and has been suspected of being a cocarcinogen and to affect the liver when taken in high doses. Like niacin, it is capable of preventing and curing pellagra. It is a partial precursor of the brain hormone serotonin and is indispensable for the manufacture of certain cell proteins. In cosmetics, it is used to increase the protein content of creams and lotions. Causes cancer in experimental animals. The FDA called for further study of this additive. GRAS.

TUBEROSE EXTRACT • Derived from a Mexican bulbous herb commonly cultivated for its spike of fragrant white single or double flowers that resemble small lilies. Used in peach flavorings for beverages, ice cream, ices, candy, and baked goods. Tuberose is used in perfumes. Can cause allergic reactions. GRAS.

TUMERIC • *See* Turmeric.

TUNG NUT OIL • Chinawood Oil. Drying oil used to waterproof packaging materials. Toxic by ingestion. Causes contact dermatitis (skin rash). Ingestion causes nausea, vomiting, cramps, diarrhea, thirst, dizziness, lethargy, and disorientation. Large doses can cause fever, irregular heartbeat, and respiratory effects.

TUNU EXTRACT • Tuno. From a Central American tree, *Castilla fallax cook,* closely related to the rubber tree. Cleared for use as a natural masticatory substance of vegetable origin in chewing-gum base.

TURMERIC • Tumeric. Derived from an East Indian herb, *Curcuma longa.* An aromatic, pepperlike but somewhat bitter taste. The cleaned, boiled, sun-dried, pulverized root is used in coconut, ginger ale, and curry flavorings for puddings, condiments, meats, soups, and pickles; also for yellow coloring used to color sausage casings, oleomargarine, shortening, and marker ink. The *extract* is used in fruit, meat, and cheese flavorings for beverages, condiments, meats, soup bases, and pickles. The *oleoresin (see)* is obtained by extraction with one or more of the solvents acetone, ethyl alcohol, ethylene dichloride *(see all),* and others. It is used in spice flavorings for condiments, meats, pickles, and brine. Both turmeric and its oleoresin have been permanently listed for coloring food since 1966. It is exempt from certification. GRAS. There is reported use of the chemical, it has not yet been assigned for toxicology literature.

TURPENTINE • Gum and Steam Distilled. Any of the various resins obtained from coniferous trees. A yellowish, viscous exudate with a characteristic smell, both forms are used in spice flavorings for baked goods. Steam-distilled turpentine is also used in candy. Also used as a solvent in hair lotions, waxes, perfume soaps, and to soothe skin. It is the oleoresin from a species of pines. Readily absorbed through the skin. Irritating to the skin and mucous membranes. In addition to being a local skin irritant, it can cause allergic reactions. It is also a central nervous system depressant. Death is usually due to respiratory failure. As little as 15 milliliters has killed children. There is reported use of the chemical, it has not yet been assigned for toxicology literature.

(TWO) 2 PERCENT MILK • *See* Milk.

TYLOSIN • Tylon. Tylan. Antibiotic from *Streptomycetes fradiae* used for beef, chicken, eggs, milk, pork, and turkey. FDA limitations are 0.2 ppm in chickens, turkeys, cattle, swine and eggs; 0.05 ppm in milk. Moderately toxic by ingestion.

TYLOSIN and SULFAMETHAZINE • Used in swine feeds. Residues of tylosin *(see)* in edible tissue of swine is tolerated by the FDA at 0.2 ppm and residues of sulfamethazine is 0.1 ppm. Both are antibiotics.

TYRAMINE • A derivative of tyrosine *(see)* it is a chemical present in mistletoe and many common foods and beverages. It raises blood pressure but usually causes no problem because enzymes in the body hold it in check. When drugs are used that inhibit the major enzyme that restrains its actions, monoamine oxidase (MAO) *(see),* the blood pressure can shoot up to dangerous levels when foods and beverages containing significant levels of tyramine are ingested. Among the foods that are high in tyramine are cheese, beer, wines, pickled herring, chicken livers, yeast extract, canned figs, raisins, bananas, avocados, chocolate, soy sauce, fava beans, meat tenderizers, egg plant, tea, cola, beef liver, and yogurt. Among the drugs that inhibit the enzyme and may lead to a serious rise in blood pressure are the MAO-inhibitors, anti-TB drugs, such as isoniazid, and anticancer drugs, such as procarbazine.

TYROSINE • L form. Widely distributed amino acid *(see),* termed nonessential because it does not seem to be necessary for growth. It is used as a dietary supplement. It is a building block of protein and is used in cosmetics to help creams penetrate the skin. The FDA has asked for further study of this additive. GRAS.

U

U • Symbol meaning "kosher" *(see)*.

UL • Abbreviation for tolerable *Upper* (intake) *Level.* The highest level of daily nutrient intake that can be consumed by individuals in the general population without posing a risk of adverse health effects.

ULTRAMARINE BLUE • A color additive occurring naturally in the mineral lapis lazuli. Used for packaging material and a salt for animal feed only. FDA limitation of 0.5 percent of salt. It is used for external use only. No longer permitted for use as a drug coloring.

2,3-UNDECADIONE • A synthetic butter flavoring agent for beverages, ice cream, ices, candy, and baked goods.

γ-UNDECALACTONE • Peach Aldehyde. Colorless to light yellow liquid with a peachy odor. Derived from undecylenic acid with sulfuric acid. A synthetic fruit flavoring, colorless or yellow, with a strong peach odor. Used for beverages, ice cream, ices, candy, baked goods, gelatin desserts, and chewing gum. Used also in perfumery.

UNDECANAL • A synthetic flavoring agent. Colorless to slightly yellow, with a sweet, fatty odor. Used in lemon, orange, rose, fruit, and honey flavorings for beverages, ice cream, ices, candy, baked goods, and chewing gum.

9-UNDECANAL • A synthetic citrus and fruit flavorings for beverages, ice cream, ices, candy, baked goods, and chewing gum. No known toxicity.

10-UNDECANAL • A synthetic citrus, floral, and fruit flavoring agent for beverages, ice cream, ices, and candy. No known toxicity.

2-UNDECANONE • A synthetic flavoring agent that occurs naturally in rue and hops oil. Used in citrus, coconut, peach, and cheese flavorings for beverages, ice cream, ices, candy, baked goods, and puddings.

1-UNDECANOL • Colorless liquid with a citrus odor used in perfumery and as a flavoring. *See* Undecylenic Acid.

2-UNDECANOL • Antifoaming agent, perfume fixative, and plasticizer. *See* Undecylenic Acid.

10-UNDECENOIC ACID • Occurs in sweat. Obtained from ricinoleic acid *(see)*. Used as an antifungal agent.

2-UNDECENOL • White to slightly yellow liquid with a sweet floral odor used as a flavoring agent in various foods.

10-UNDECEN-1-YL ACETATE • A synthetic citrus and fruit flavoring agent for beverages, ice cream, ices, candy, and baked goods.

UNDECYL ALCOHOL • A synthetic lemon, lime, orange, and rose flavoring agent for beverages, ice cream, ices, candy, and baked goods.

UNDECYLENIC ACID • 10-Undecenioc Acid. Occurs in sweat. Obtained from ricinoleic acid *(see)*. A liquid or crystalline powder, with an odor suggestive of perspiration or citrus. Used as a fungicide, in perfumes, as a flavoring, and as a lubricant additive in cosmetics. Has been given orally but it causes dizziness, headaches, and stomach upset. No known toxicity for the skin.

UNDECYLENYL ALCOHOL • Colorless liquid with a citrus odor. Used in perfumes. It is combustible but has a low toxicity.

UNDECYLIC ACID • *See* Undecylenic Acid.

UNDECYLPENTADECANOL • *See* Fatty Alcohols.

UNSAPONIFIABLE OLIVE OILS • The oil fraction that is not broken down in the refining of olive fatty acids.

UNSAPONIFIABLE RAPESEED OIL • The oil that is not broken down in the refining of rapeseed oil fatty acids. *See* Rapeseed Oil.

UNSAPONIFIABLE SHEA BUTTER • The fraction of shea butter that is not broken down during processing.

UNSAPONIFIABLE SOYBEAN OIL • The fraction of soybean oil that is not broken down in the refining recovery of soybean oil fatty acids.

UPC • Abbreviation for Universal Product Code.

UREA • Carbamide. A product of protein metabolism and excreted from human urine. Used in yeast food and wine production up to 2 pounds per gallon. It is used to "brown" baked goods such as pretzels, and consists of colorless or white odorless crystals that have a cool salty taste. An antiseptic and deodorizer used in liquid antiperspirants, ammoniated dentifrices, roll-on deodorants, mouthwashes, hair colorings, hand creams, lotions, and shampoos. Medicinally, urea is used as a topical antiseptic and as a diuretic to reduce body water. Its largest use, however, is as a fertilizer, and only a small part of its production goes into the manufacture of other urea products. The FAO-WHO Expert Committee on Food Additives considered urea for evaluation only in relation to its use in chewing gum. Chewing gum may contain up to 3 percent urea, and intake from this source could be up to three hundred mg of urea per day. Since urea is a natural end product of amino acid metabolism in humans and approximately twenty grams per day are excreted in the urine in adults (proportionately less in children), the Committee concluded that the use of urea levels of up to 3 percent in chewing gum was of no toxicological concern. The final report to the FDA of the Select Committee on GRAS Substances stated in 1980 that urea should continue its GRAS status with no limitations other than good manufacturing practices. There is reported use of the chemical; it has not yet been assigned for toxicology literature search.

UREASE • An enzyme from *Lactobacillius fermentum*. Used to inhibit urethane formation in wine. Urethane is used in pesticides and fungicides and is toxic by ingestion. Urethane was also the first cancer-causing agent demonstrated to pass through the placenta and affect the fetus. GRAS.

UROCANIC ACID • Prepared from Histidine *(see)*.

URSOLIC ACID • Bearberry. Privet Fruit. Found in leaves and berries of *Arctostaphylos uva-ursi*. Used as an emulsifying agent in foods and pharmaceuticals.

USDA • Abbreviation for the *United States Department of Agriculture*.

USNIC ACID • Antibacterial compound found in lichens. Pale yellow, slightly soluble in water. No known toxicity.

UVA-URSI • *Arctostaphylos uva*. Bearberry. An astringent used to treat bladder problems, it is believed that its action is due to the high concentration of the antiseptic arbutin. In passing through the system, arbutin yields hydroquinone, a urinary disinfectant. Leaves from the plant uva-ursi also contain anesthetic principles that numb pain in the urinary system and the herb has been shown to have antibiotic activity. Crude extracts of uva-ursi reportedly possess some anticancer property. In 1992, the FDA proposed a ban on uva-ursi in oral menstrual drug products because it had not been shown to be safe and effective for its stated claims.

V

VALBAZEN • Albendazole. Zental. A worm medicine for animals. Moderately toxic by ingestion. Causes birth defects in experimental animals.

VALERAL • *See* Valeraldehyde.

VALERALDEHYDE • Pentanal. A synthetic flavoring agent which occurs naturally in coffee extract. Used in fruit and nut flavorings for beverages, ice cream, ices, candy, and baked goods. Has narcotic properties and is a mild irritant.

VALERIAN • *Valeriana officinalis*. A perennial native to Europe and the United States, it was reputed as a love potion. Used as a flavoring. Its vapor was found to kill the bacillus of typhoid fever after forty-five minutes. The herb has been widely studied in Europe and Russia, and the major constituents, the Valepotriate, have been reported to have marked sedative, anticonvulsive, blood pressure lowering, and tranquilizing effects. It has been used for centuries to treat panic attacks. In Germany, valerian preparations have been used for more than a decade to treat childhood behavioral disorders, supposedly without the side effects experienced with pharmaceuticals for that purpose. It has been reported that it also helps concentration and energy. Prolonged use of valerian may result in side effects such as irregular heartbeat, headaches, uneasiness, nervousness, and insomnia. Very large doses may cause paralysis. There is reported use of the chemical; it has not yet been assigned for toxicology literature.

VALERIC ACID • Occurs naturally in apples, cocoa, coffee, oil of lavender, peaches, and strawberries. A synthetic flavoring agent used in butter, butterscotch, fruit, rum, and cheese flavorings for beverages, ice cream, ices, candy, and baked goods. Colorless, with an unpleasant odor. Usually distilled from valerian root. Used in the manufacture of perfumes. Some of its salts are used in medicine. Also used in peeling solution for fruits and vegetables. Moderately toxic by ingestion. A corrosive irritant to skin, eyes, and mucous membranes.

VALERIC ALDEHYDE • *See* Valeraldehyde.

VALEROLACTONE • A synthetic vanilla flavoring agent for beverages, ice cream, ices, candy, and baked goods. Moderately toxic by ingestion. A skin irritant.

VALINE • L form. An essential amino acid *(see)*. Occurs in the largest quantities in fibrous protein. It is indispensable for growth and nitrogen balance. Used in suntan lotions. No known toxicity in cosmetics but the FDA asked for further study of this ingredient as a food additive in 1980. GRAS.

VANADIUM TETRACHLORIDE • Derived from chlorination of ferrovanadium. Catalyst. Toxic by ingestion, inhalation, and skin absorption.

VANAY • *See* Triacetin.

VANILLA EXTRACT • Extracted from the full-grown unripe fruit of the vanilla plant of Mexico and the West Indies. Contains not less than 35 percent aqueous ethyl alcohol *(see)* and one or more of the following ingredients: glycerin, propylene glycol, sugar (including invert sugar) and corn syrup. Used in many food and beverages as flavorings. No known toxicity. GRAS.

VANILLAL • *See* Ethyl Vanillin.

VANILLIN • Occurs naturally in vanilla *(see)* and potato parings but is an artificial flavoring. Odor and taste of vanilla. Made synthetically from eugenol *(see);* also from the waste of the wood pulp industry. One part vanillin equals 400 parts vanilla pods. Used in butter, chocolate, fruit, root beer, and vanilla flavorings for beverages, ice cream, ices, candy, baked goods, gelatin desserts, puddings, syrups (30,000 ppm), toppings, margarine, chocolate products, and liqueurs. May migrate from paper and paperboard to food. The lethal dose in mice is three grams (thirty grams to the ounce) per kilogram of body weight. A skin irritant that produces a burning sensation and eczema. May also cause pigmentation of the skin. GRAS.

VANILLIN ACETATE • Vanillin. A synthetic spice and vanilla flavoring agent for beverages, ice cream, ices, candy, and baked goods. *See* Vanillin.

VANILLYL ETHYL ETHER • *See* Vanillin.

VEGETABLE GUMS • Includes derivatives from quince seed, karaya, acacia, tragacanth, Irish moss, guar, sodium alginate, potassium alginate, ammonium alginate, and propylene glycol alginate. All are subject to deterioration and always need a preservative. The gums function as liquid emulsions; that is, they thicken cosmetic products and make them cream. No known toxicity other than allergic reactions hypersensitive persons.

VEGETABLE JUICE • Used in food colorings consistent with good manufacturing practices. Permanently listed for coloring since 1966. Does not require certification.

VEGETABLE OILS • Peanut, sesame, olive, and cottonseed oil obtained from plants and used in many food additives and in baby preparations, cleansing creams, emollient creams, face powders, hair-grooming aids, hypoallergenic cosmetics, lipsticks, nail creams, shampoos, shaving creams, and wave sets. No known toxicity. *See* Vegetable Oils, Bromated.

VEGETABLE OILS, BROMINATED • Peanut, sesame, and cottonseed oil obtained from plants. Used in fruit-flavored beverages where not prohibited by standards. FDA tolerance, less than 15 ppm. Also used in baby preparations, cleansing creams, emollient creams, face powders, hair-grooming aids, hypoallergenic cosmetics, lipsticks, nail creams, shampoos, shaving creams, and wave sets. *See* Bromates.

VEGETARIAN • According to the Vegetarian Resource Group, less than 1 percent of Americans are true vegetarians. Such people never eat meat, fish, or poultry, although they may eat foods derived from animals such as dairy products and eggs. There are even fewer *vegans,* strict vegetarians who avoid all animal-derived foods—even honey.

VERATRALDEHYDE • A synthetic fruit, nut, and vanilla flavoring agent for beverages, ice cream, ices, candy, and baked goods, and puddings. Derived from vanillin. May have narcotic and irritant effects but no specific data.

VERATRIC ALDEHYDE • *See* Veratraldehye.

VERBENALOL • An alcohol made from *Verbena officinalis.*

VERONICA • Extract of *Veronica officinalis,* a small herb of wide distribution that has pink or white flowers. Flavoring in alcoholic beverages only.

VERVAIN, EUROPEAN • *Verbena officinalis.* A class of medicinal plants used as a flavoring in alcoholic beverages only.

VERXITE GRANULES and FLAKES • Hydrated magnesium-aluminum iron silicate. Soft and resilient. Used as an anticaking and blending agent in ruminant feeds.

VERXITE GRITS • Used as a roughage replacement in ruminant feeds.

VERY LOW SODIUM • Less than 35 mg per serving.

VETIVER OIL • Vetiverol. Khus-Khus. Stable brown to reddish brown oil from the roots of a fragrant grass. It has an aromatic to harsh woodsy odor. Used as a flavoring in alcoholic beverages only and as a scent in soaps and perfumes. There is reported use of the chemical, it has not yet been assigned for toxicology literature.

VIBURNUM EXTRACT • Haw Bark. Black Extract. Extract of the fruit of a hawthorn shrub or tree. Used in fragrances and in butter, caramel, cola, maple, and walnut flavorings for beverages. Has been used as a uterine antispasmodic. No known toxicity.

VIBURNUM PRUNIFOLIUM • *See* Viburnum Extract.

VINEGAR • Used for hundreds of years to remove lime soap after shampooing. It is a solvent for cosmetic oils and resins. Vinegar is about 4 to 6 percent acetic acid. Acetic acid occurs naturally in apples, cheese, grapes, milk, and other foods. No known toxicity but may cause an allergic reaction in those allergic to corn.

VINEGAR NAPHTHA • *See* Ethyl Acetate.

VINYL • Made from acetylene with various other substances to form plastics.

VINYL ACETATE • A starch modifier not to exceed 2.5 percent in modified starch *(see).* Vapors in high concentration may be narcotic; animal experiments show low toxicity.

VINYL CHLORIDE • Chloroethylene. Prepared from ethylene dichloride and alcoholic potassium, it is a colorless gas that becomes liquid upon freezing. It is one of the most frequently used vinyl compounds and is a very hazardous chemical by all avenues of exposure. It may be narcotic in high concentrations. If spilled on the skin, rapid evaporation causes local frostbite. It is a known cancer-causing agent, and because of that it has been banned from aerosol sprays. It is used for many polyvinyl compounds in paper coating, adhesives, and refrigerants. It is permitted by the FDA for use in adhesives, and in food contact coatings.

VINYL CHLORIDE-VINYLIDENE CHLORIDE COPOLYMER • Used as a coating on fresh citrus fruits. Vinyl chloride was banned in hair sprays because it is a cancer-causing agent. It is a proven liver cancer-causing agent in people who work with the compound. Vinylidene chloride is an irritant to mucous membranes, narcotic in high concentrations, and has caused liver and kidney injury in experimental animals.

VIOLA ODORATA • *See* Violet Extract, Leaves.

VIOLAXANTHIN • Natural orange-red coloring isolated from yellow pansies and Valencia orange peel. Soluble in alcohol. *See* Xanthophyll. No known toxicity.

VIOLET EXTRACT • Flowers and Leaves. Green liquid with typical odor of violet. It is taken from the plant widely grown in the United States. Used in berry, violet, and fruit flavorings for beverages, ice cream, ices, candy, and baked goods. Also used in face powders and for coloring inorganic pigments. May produce skin rash in the allergic. No known toxicity. GRAS.

VIOLET LEAVES, ABSOLUTE • Essential Oil of *Viola Odorata*. There is reported use of the chemical; it has not yet been assigned for toxicology literature. *See* Violet Extract. GRAS.

VIRGINIAMYCIN • Eskalin. Pristinamycin. Staphlyomycin. White powder used as an antibiotic from *Streptomyces* for chickens and swine. FDA limits residue in swine of 0.4 ppm in kidney, skin, and fat, 0.3 ppm in liver, 0.1 ppm in muscle. In broiler chickens, the limit is 0.5 ppm in kidney, 0.3 ppm in liver, 0.2 ppm in skin and fat, 0.1 ppm in muscle. Moderately toxic by ingestion.

VIRIDINE • *See* Phenyl Acetaldehyde Dimethyl Acetal.

VITAMINS • Vitamins are organic compounds that are nutritionally essential in small amounts to control metabolic processes and cannot be synthesized by the body. Vitamins are usually classified by their solubility, which to some degree determines their stability, occurrence in foodstuffs, distribution in body fluids, and tissue storage capacity. Each of the fat-soluble vitamins A, D. E, and K has a distinct and separate physiologic role. Several are among those supporting antioxidant efforts to depress the effects of metabolic byproducts called free radicals, which are thought to cause degenerative changes related to aging. Most of the water-soluble vitamins are components of essential enzyme systems. Many are involved in the reactions supporting energy metabolism. These vitamins are not normally stored in the body in appreciable amounts and are normally excreted in small quantities in the urine. Thus, a daily supply is desirable to avoid depletion and interruption of normal physiologic functions.

VITAMIN A • Acetate and Palmitate. A yellow viscous liquid insoluble in water. An anti-infective, antixerophthalmic vitamin, essential to growth and development. Deficiency leads to retarded growth in the young, diminished visual acuity, night blindness, and skin problems. Insoluble in water. Toxic when children or adults receive more than 100,000 units daily over several months. Recommended daily dietary allowance is 1,500 units for infants and 4,500 units for adults and 2,000–3,500 units for children. It is used to fortify mellorine (vegetable-fat imitation ice cream), skim milk, dietary infant formula, blue cheese, Gorgonzola cheese, milk, and oleomargarine (1 pound of margarine contains 15,000 USP units of vitamin A). Vitamin A is also used in lubricating creams and oils for its alleged skin-healing properties. Can be absorbed through the skin. The final report to the FDA of the Select Committee on GRAS Substances stated in 1980 that it should continue its GRAS status with no limitations other than good manufacturing practices.

VITAMIN B$_1$ • *See* Thiamine Hydrochloride.

VITAMIN B$_2$ • Riboflavin. Lactoflavin. Formerly called vitamin G. Riboflavin is a factor in the vitamin B complex and is used in emollients. Every plant and animal cell contains a minute amount. Helps to metabolize protein, carbohydrate, and fat; maintains healthy skin, eyes; aids formation of red blood cells and antibodies. Symptoms of deficiency include sores or cracking around the mouth, skin problems, and eye disorders. It is necessary for healthy skin and respiration, protects the eyes from sensitivity to light, and is used for building and maintaining human body tissues. A deficiency leads to lesions at the corner of the mouth and to changes in the cornea. Recommended daily allowances for infants to six months, 0.4 mg. Children one to three years, 0.8 mg. Children four to six years, 1.1 mg. Children seven to ten years, 1.2 mg. Males eleven to fourteen years, 1.5 mg. Males fifteen to eighteen years, 1.8 mg. Males nineteen to fifty years, 1.7 mg. Males fifty-one years and over, 1.4 mg. Females eleven to fifty years, 1.3 mg. Females fifty-one years and over 1.4 mg. Pregnant women 1.6 mg. Lactating women 1.7–18 mg. It is used to treat riboflavin deficiency or as an adjunct to thiamine treatment for nerve inflammation of lips secondary to pellagra. In 1992, the FDA proposed a ban on riboflavin in oral menstrual drug products because it has not been shown to be safe and effective for its stated claims.

VITAMIN B$_3$ • *See* Niacin.

VITAMIN B$_5$ • *See* Pantothenic Acid.

VITAMIN B$_6$ • Pyridoxine. Beesix. Hexa-Betalin. Hexacrest. Nestrex. Rodex. Vitabee 6. Metabolizes protein; helps produce red blood cells; maintains proper functioning of nervous system tissue. Vitamin B$_6$ is believed to act as a partner for more than one hundred different enzymes. A number of the brain chemicals that send messages back and forth between nerves depend upon it for formation. A deficiency in this vitamin is known to cause depression and mental confusion. The occurrence of seizures in experimental animals in response to vitamin B$_6$ antagonists has been observed by many. Similar seizures observed in human infants made vitamin B$_6$ deficient inadvertently when they were fed a commercial infant formula in which the vitamin had not been properly preserved. Certain substances that deplete B$_6$ also produce deficiency seizures. Vitamin B$_6$ also reportedly helps rid the body tissues of excess fluid that causes some of the symptoms of premenstrual tension. Estrogen and cortisone deplete B$_6$. Storage over a long period of time diminishes the vitamin. Recommended daily allowance for newborns and infants to six months is 0.3 mg. Children four to six years, 1.1 mg. Children seven to ten years, 1.4 mg. Males eleven to fourteen years, 1.7 mg. Males fifteen years and over, 2 mg. Females eleven to fourteen years, 1.4 mg. Females fifteen to eighteen years, 1.5 mg. Females nineteen years and over 1.6 mg. Pregnant women, 2.2 mg. Lactating women, 2.1 mg. Used to treat vitamin B$_6$ deficiency and responsive anemias. Also prevents vitamin B$_6$ deficiency during isoniazid therapy to treat tuberculosis. Patients are likely to have a deficiency of B$_6$ if they are alcoholics, or have burns, diarrhea, heart disease, intestinal problems, liver disease, overactive thyroid, or are suffering the stress of long-term illness or serious injury. Patients on dialysis or who have their stomachs removed are also probably deficient in the vitamin. Current research seems to indicate that B$_6$ enhances the immune response in the elderly and may alleviate some signs of carpal tunnel syndrome, a wrist problem. Overdosing on B_6 is unwise. A study reported in the *New England Journal of Medicine* in 1983 described the loss of balance and numbness suffered by seven young adults who took from two to six grams of pyridoxine daily for several months to a year. Other potential adverse reactions include drowsiness and a feeling of pins and needles in limbs. In 1992, the FDA proposed a ban on pyridoxine in fever blister and cold sore treatment products because it has not been shown to be safe and effective for its stated claims.

VITAMIN B₉ • *See* Folic Acid.

VITAMIN B₁₂ • Cyanocobalamin. Anacobin. Bedoce. Betalin 12. Bioglan B_{12}. Crystamine. Cyano-Gel. Dodex. Kaybovite. Poyamin. Redisol. Rubesol-1000. Rubramin. Sigamine. Alpha-Ruvite. Codroxomin. Droxomin. Helps form red blood cells; maintains healthy nervous system. Deficiency symptoms include anemia, brain damage, and nervousness. More than one in five older Americans may need to take vitamin B_{12} by injection to prevent neurological disorders, because their stomach acid does not enable them to absorb the vitamin from foods. The condition, known as atrophic gastritis, affects at least 20 percent of people over the age of sixty. Recommended daily allowance: neonates and infants to six months, 0.3 mcg. Infants six months to one year, 0.5 mcg. Children over one year to three years, 0.7 mcg. Children four to six years, 1 mcg. Adults and children eleven years and over, 2 mcg. Pregnant women, 2.2 mcg. Lactating women, 2.6 mcg. Potential adverse reactions include blood clots in veins, transient diarrhea, itching, hives, and severe allergic reactions with IV or injection. Aminoglycosides, colchicine, para-aminosalicylic acid, and chloramphenicol *(see all)* cause malabsorption of Vitamin B_{12}. Cobalt and its compounds are on the Community Right-To-Know List *(see)* and on EPA Genetic Toxicology Program *(see)*. Causes adverse reproductive effects in experimental animals.

VITAMIN B COMPLEX FACTOR • *See* Panthenol.

VITAMIN C • *See* Ascorbic Acid.

VITAMIN D₂ • Calciferol. A pale yellow, oily liquid, odorless, tasteless, insoluble in water. Nutritional factor added to prepared breakfast cereals. Mellorine (vegetable-fat imitation ice cream), vitamin D milk, evaporated and skim milks, margarine, infant dietary formulas, enriched flour, self-rising flour, enriched cornmeal and grits, enriched macaroni and noodle products (250–1,000 USP units), enriched farina and enriched bread, rolls, etc. Vitamin D speeds the body's production of calcium and has been found to cause calcium deposits and facial deformities and subnormal IQs in children of mothers given too much vitamin D. Nutritionists recommend 400 units per day for pregnant women. Some women taking vitamin pills and vitamin enriched milk and foods consume as much as 2,000 to 3,000 units daily. Used for its alleged skin-healing properties in lubricating creams and lotions. The absence of vitamin D in the food of young animals can lead to rickets, a bone-affecting condition. It is soluble in fats and fat solvents and is present in animal fats. Absorbed through the skin. Its value in cosmetics has not been proven. No known toxicity to the skin. The final report to the FDA of the Select Committee on GRAS Substances stated in 1980 that there is no evidence in the available information that it is a hazard to the public when used as it is now and it should continue its GRAS status with limitations on amounts that can be added to food.

VITAMIN D₃ • Activated 7-dehydrocholesterol. Approximately as effective as vitamin D₂ *(see)*. The final report to the FDA of the Select Committee on GRAS Substances stated in 1980 that there is no evidence in the available information that it is a hazard to the public when used as it is now and it should continue its GRAS status with limitations on the amounts that can be added to food.

VITAMIN E • *See* Tocopherols.

VITAMIN E ACETATE • *See* Tocopherols.

VITAMIN E SUCCINATE • *See* Tocopherols.

VITAMIN G • *See* Riboflavin.

VITAMIN H • *See* Biotin.

VITAMIN K • Recommended daily allowance for adults has not been established, but the safety and adequate daily dietary intake level is listed at 0.07 to 0.14 mg. It is necessary for blood clotting. Current research seems to indicate it helps maintain bone mass in the elderly and prevents osteoporosis *(see)*. Vitamin K antagonizes the action of anticoagulants and has been used as an antidote in managing overdosages or excessive responses to the latter. The excessive use of vitamin K–containing substances—drugs or dietary items such as green leafy vegetables—should be avoided in patients receiving anticoagulants.

VIVERRA CIVETTA SCHREBER • *See* Civet, Absolute.

VIVERRA ZIBETHASCHREBER • *See* Civet, Absolute.

VOLATILE FATTY ACIDS INCLUDING ISOBUTYRIC ACID; ISOVALERIC ACID; METHYL BUTYRIC ACID; M-VALERIC ACID • Used in dairy cattle feeds as source of energy. *See all.*

VOLATILE OILS • The volatillity in oils is the tendency to give off vapors, usually at room temperature. The volatile oils in plants such as peppermint or rose produce the aroma. The volatile oils in plants stimulate the tissue with which they come in contact whether they are inhaled, ingested, or placed on the skin. They can relax or stimulate, irritate or soothe, depending upon the of treatment and concentration.

W

WALNUT EXTRACT • An extract of the husk of the nut of *Juglans* spp., the English walnut tree. Used in walnut flavorings for beverages, ice cream, ices, candy, and baked goods. Also used for brown coloring. There is reported use of the chemical, it has not yet been assigned for toxicology literature.

WALNUT OIL • *See* Walnut Extract.

WALNUT SHELL POWDER • The ground shell of English walnuts, *Juglans regia. See* Walnut Extract.

WATER • Although deficiencies of other nutrients can be sustained for months or even years, a person can survive only a few days without water. Experts rank water second only to oxygen as essential for life. In addition to offering true refreshment for the thirsty, water plays a vital role in all bodily processes. It supplies the medium in which various chemical changes of the body occur, aiding in digestion, absorption, circulation, and lubrication of body joints. For example, as a major component of blood, water helps deliver nutrients to body cells and removes waste to the kidneys for excretion. Average adults need about sixty-four ounces of fluid each day for optimal health. Although experts generally advise drinking several glasses of water a day, the need for fluid can also be met by consuming a variety of foods and beverages.

WATERCRESS EXTRACT • Extract obtained from *Nasturtium officinalis.*

WAX, PARAFFIN • Component of chewing-gum base and of certain cheeses. *See* Paraffin Wax.

WAXES • Obtained from insects, animals, petroleum, and plants. Waxes made in the United States are vegetable, petroleum, or bug based. One of the most common vegetable waxes, carnauba *(see),* is made from a palm leaf. Waxes from petroleum are the same as those used as chewing-gum bases. The "shellac" used on some products is made from the secretion of the lac bug, native to Pakistan and India. More than twenty varieties of fruits and vegetables, including cantaloupes, eggplants, oranges, peaches, grapefruits, rutabagas, persimmons, squash, cucumbers, sweet potatoes, and tomatoes are being waxed. Waxing reduces the loss of moisture and keeps produce from dehydration. Some waxes are cosmetic. For example, oranges are waxed because consumers prefer a shiny surface rather than the natural dull matte of the rind. Beeswax is a substance secreted by the bee's special glands on the underside of its abdomen. The wax is glossy and hard but plastic when warm. Insoluble in water but partially soluble in boiling alcohol. Used in candy and vegetable coatings as well as for packaging. Waxes are generally nontoxic but may cause allergic reactions in the hypersensitive depending upon the source of the wax. It is also difficult to know which items have been waxed. Some foreign imports may use beef tallow, for example, which is undesirable in vegetarian or kosher diets. In many cases, pesticides and fungicides are added to waxes to help prevent decay. The wax is mainly used to keep produce fresh longer by sealing in moisture. The FDA does have regulations requiring all waxed products at the supermarket to be labeled as such, either with a card listing the specific ingredients in the wax above the bin or on the bin or container itself. (Have you seen such a listing?) Some companies, according to Cornell University professor of food science Joseph Regenstein, Ph.D., switch waxes three times a day depending on environmental conditions. If you want to reduce the waxes on fruit and vegetables, wash them with warm water, and when appropriate scrub with a brush.

WAXY MAIZE • Corn Starch. The soft, sticky material from the inside of the corn kernel. The final report to the FDA of the Select Committee on GRAS

Substances stated in 1980 that it should continue its GRAS status with no limitations other than good manufacturing practices.

WETTING AGENT • Any of numerous water-soluble agents that promote spreading of a liquid on a surface or penetration into a material such as skin. It lowers surface tension for better contact and absorption. *See* Surfactants.

WHEAT • A cereal grain that yields a fine white powder. Wheat is avoided by some allergic people. Bread, cakes, crackers, cookies, pretzels, pastries, and noodles are made of wheat; also breakfast foods such as cream of wheat, pablum, Grapenuts, Wheaties, puffed wheat, shredded wheat, and bran; sauces, soups, gravies; Postum, Ovaltine, malted milk; sausages, hamburger, and meat loaf. Nontoxic.

WHEAT BRAN • The broken coat of *Triticum aestivum*. About 14.5 percent of the kernel. In addition to indigestible cellulose, it contains 86 percent of niacin, 73 percent of pyridoxine, 50 percent of pantothenic acid, 42 percent of riboflavin, 33 percent of thiamine, and 19 percent of protein. *See* Wheat Germ.

WHEAT BRAN LIPIDS • An extract of the coat of wheat. *See* Wheat Germ.

WHEAT FLOUR • Milled from the kernels of wheat, *Triticum aestivum*. *See* Wheat Starch.

WHEAT GERM • The golden germ of the wheat is high in vitamin E. About 2.5 percent of the whole wheat kernel. The germ contains about 64 percent of thiamine, 26 percent of riboflavin, and 21 percent of pyridoxine. *See* Tocopherols.

WHEAT GERMANIDOPROPYLAMINE • *See* Tocopherols.

WHEAT GERMAMIDOPROPYL BETAINE • *See* Surfactants.

WHEAT GERMAMIDOPROPYL DIMETHYLAMINE LACTATE • *See* Tocopherols.

WHEAT GERMANIDOPROPYLAMINE • *See* Tocopherols.

WHEAT GERM EXTRACT • *See* Tocopherols.

WHEAT GERM GLYCERIDES • *See* Tocopherols.

WHEAT GERM OIL • *See* Tocopherols.

WHEAT GLUTEN • A mixture of proteins present in wheat flour and obtained as an extremely sticky, yellowish gray mass by making a dough and then washing out the starch. It consists almost entirely of two proteins, gliadin and glutenin. It contributes to the porous and spongy structure of bread. Used in powders and creams as a base.

WHEAT STARCH • A product of cereal grain. It swells when water is added. A minor part of starch production in the U.S. Used as a demulcent, emollient, and in dusting and face powders. May migrate from cotton and cotton fabrics used in dry food packaging. May cause allergic reactions such as red eyes and stuffy nose. The final report to the FDA of the Select Committee on GRAS Substances stated in 1980 that it should continue its GRAS status with no limitations other than good manufacturing practices.

WHEY • The serum that remains after removal of fat and casein *(see)* from milk. Used as a texturizer, processing aid, and nutritional extender. Fermented whey is used as a dietary source of protein and nitrogen for cattle. GRAS.

WHEY, FERMENTED, AMMONIATED, CONDENSED • Thirty percent of dietary crude protein in animal feed for cattle. Provides source of protein and nonprotein nitrogen.

WHEY PROTEIN CONCENTRATE • Milk Serum. Serum Lactis. The water part of milk remaining after the separation of casein *(see)*. Cleared by the U.S. Department of Agriculture's Meat Inspection Department to bind and extend imitation sausage, and for use in soups and stews. Also used as source of protein and nonprotein nitrogen for cattle. It is used in emollients. GRAS.

WHEY, REDUCED LACTOSE • Used in frozen desserts. GRAS.

WHITE CEDAR LEAF OIL • Oil of Arborvitae. Stable, pale yellow volatile oil obtained by steam distillation from the fresh leaves and branch ends of the eastern arborvitae. Has a strong camphoraceous and sagelike scent. Used as a perfume and scent for soaps and room sprays. Also used as a flavoring agent. Soluble in most fixed oils. *See* Cedar for toxicity.

WHITE FLAG EXTRACT • *See* Orris.

WHITE LILY EXTRACT • Extract of the bulbs of *Lilium candidum*. Edible bulbs that were made into soup by the Indians, the lily is used in perfumery.

WHITE MINERAL OIL • Obtained from petroleum and used in baked goods. *See* Mineral Oil.

WHITE NETTLE EXTRACT • Obtained from the flowers of *Lamium album*. *See* Nettles.

WHOLE FISH PROTEIN CONCENTRATE • Dietary supplement for household use only. FDA tolerance is less than twenty mg per day when consumed regularly by children up to eight years of age. When used in manufactured food, less than 8 ppm total fluoride content of finished food. For household use only. Package size, less than one pound. Less than 8 ppm total fluoride content of finished food when used in manufactured food.

WILD CHERRY • Wild Black Cherry Bark. The dried stem bark collected in autumn in North America. Used in cherry flavorings for food, lipsticks, and medicines. Also used as a sedative and expectorant medicinally. No known toxicity. GRAS.

WILD GINGER • Canadian Oil. *See* Snakeroot Oil.

WILD MARJORAM EXTRACT • Extract of the flowering ends of *Origanum vulgare*. Yellow or greenish yellow liquid containing about 40 percent terpenes *(see)*. Used in flavoring and perfumery. *See* Marjoram Oil.

WILD MINT EXTRACT • Extract of the leaves and tender twigs of *Mentha arvensis*. The Cheyenne Indians prepared a decoction of the ground leaves and stems of wild mint and drank the liquid to check nausea. Pulegone and thymol *(see)* are derived from an oil of wild mint. Its odor resembles peppermint. Used in flavoring. *See* Peppermint.

WILD THYME EXTRACT • The flowering tops of a plant grown in Eurasia and throughout the United States. The dried leaves are used as a seasoning in foods and in emollients and fragrances. Has also been used as a muscle relaxant. No known toxicity. GRAS.

WILLOW LEAF EXTRACT • The extract of the leaves of the willow tree species, *Salix*. The willow has been used for pain-relieving and fever-lowering properties since ancient Greece. The American Indians used willow baths to cool fevers, and indeed, the extract of willows contain salicylic acid, a close cousin of aspirin.

WINTERGREEN OIL • Extract and Oil. Menthyl Salicylate. Checkerberry Extract. Obtained naturally from betula, sweet birch, or teaberry oil. Present in certain leaves and bark but usually prepared by treating salicylic acid with methanol *(see both)*. Wintergreen extract is used in root beer and wintergreen flavorings for beverages and candy (5,000 ppm). The oil is used for checkerberry, raspberry, teaberry, fruit, nut, root beer, sassafras, spice, and wintergreen flavorings for beverages, ice cream, ices, candy, baked goods (1,500 ppm), and chewing gum (3,900 ppm). Used in toothpaste, tooth powder, and perfumes. Wintergreen is a strong irritant. Ingestion of relatively small amounts may cause severe poisoning and death. Average lethal dose in children is 10 milliliters and in adults 30 milliliters. It is very irritating to the mucous membranes and skin and can be absorbed rapidly through the skin. Like other salicylates, it has a wide range of interaction with other drugs, including alcohol, antidiabetic medications, vitamin C, and tranquilizers. There is reported use of the chemical, it has not yet been assigned for toxicology literature.

WOOD ROSIN • The exudate from a living Southern pine tree. Pale yellow to amber, slight turpentine odor. Used as a coating for fresh citrus fruits. No known toxicity.

WOODRUFF • Master of the Woods. Used as a flavoring in alcoholic beverages only. Made of the leaves of the herb grown in Europe, Siberia, North Africa, and Australia. It is a symbol of spring, and has clean fresh smell. There is reported use of the chemical; it has not yet been assigned for toxicology literature.

WORMWOOD • Absinthium. A European woody herb with a bitter taste, used in bitters and as a liquor flavoring for beverages and liquors. The extract is used in bitters, liquor, and vermouth flavorings for beverages, ice cream, candy, and liquors, and in making absinthe. The oil is a dark green to brown and a narcotic substance. Used in bitters, apple, vermouth, and wine flavorings for beverages, ice cream, ices, candy, baked goods, and liquors. In large doses or frequently repeated doses, it is a narcotic poison, causing headache, trembling, and convulsions. Ingestion of the volatile oil or of the liquor, absinthe, may cause gastrointestinal symptoms, nervousness, stupor, coma, and death.

X

XANTHAN GUM • A gum produced by a pure culture fermentation of a carbohydrate with *Xanthomonas campestris*. Also called corn sugar gum. The U.S. Department of Agriculture has asked for the use of xanthan gum as a necessary ingredient in packaging meat and poultry products. It is now used to thicken, suspend, emulsify, and stabilize water-based foods, such as dairy products and salad dressings.

It is also used as a "pseudo plasticizer" in salad dressings to help them pour well. In animal feeds it is used as a stabilizer, thickener, and suspending agent. FDA tolerance is 0.25 percent in liquid feeds for ruminants; 0.1 percent in calf milk replacer.

XANTHENE • Colorants are divided into acid and basic groups. They are the second largest category of certified colors. The acids are derived from fluorescein. The quinoid acid type is represented by FD and C Red No. 3, erythrosine, used frequently in lipsticks. The phenolic formulations, often called "bromo acids" is represented by D and C Red No. 2, used to "stain" lips. The only basic type certified is D and C Red No. 19, also called rhodamine B.

XANTHOPHYLL • Vegetable Lutein. A yellow coloring originally isolated from egg yolk, now isolated from petals of flowers. Occurs also in colored feathers of birds. One of the most widespread carotinoid alcohols (a group of red and yellow pigments) in nature. Provisionally listed for use in food. Although carotinoids can usually be turned into vitamin A, xanthophyll has no vitamin A activity. There is reported use of the chemical, it has not yet been assigned for toxicology literature.

XANTHOXYLUM AMERICANUM • Zanthoxylum. Ash Bark. Toothache Tree. Angelica Tree. The dried bark or berries of this tree, which grows in Canada, south of Virginia and Missouri, is used to ease the pain of toothaches, to soothe stomachs, and as an antidiarrheal medicine. No known toxicity.

XYLENOL • 2-4-Dimethylphenol. A white crystalline solid that is derived from coal tar and is toxic by ingestion and skin absorption. It is used as a disinfectant and as a solvent in pharmaceuticals, as a solvent in insecticides and rubber manufacture, and as a wetting agent for dyestuffs. It caused cancer when painted on the skin of mice.

XYLITOL • Formerly made from birch wood, but now made from waste products from the pulp industry. Xylitol has been reported to have diuretic effect but this has not been substantiated. It is used in chewing gum and as an artificial sweetener. It has been reported to sharply reduce cavities in teeth but costs more than sugar. The reason is that, unlike sugar, it doesn't ferment in the mouth. Therefore, it is sold for foods that stay in the mouth for some time, such as gum, toffee, and mints. FDA preliminary reports cited it as a possible cancer-causing agent. Xylitol is now used in eleven European countries and the United States and Canada. It is also used in large amounts in the Soviet Union as a diabetic sweetener. Xylitol was evaluated by the FAO-WHO Expert Committee on Food Additives in Geneva, April 11–20, 1983. On the basis of submitted data, the committee accepted that the adverse effects observed in British studies, in which cancer-prone rats were fed large doses of xylitol, were species-specific and could not be extrapolated to humans. Therefore, no limit on daily intake was set and no additional toxicological studies were recommended. It can cause stomach upsets when taken in large amounts. It may be of benefit to diabetics since xylitol metabolization does not involve insulin.

D-XYLOSE • Xylo-Pfan. Wood Sugar. Used for evaluating intestinal absorption and diagnosing malabsorptive states.

Y

YAM FLOUR • *See* Konjac Flour.

YARA YARA • *See b*-Naphthyl Methyl Ether.

YARROW • Milfoil. A strong-scented, spicy, wild herb, *Achillea millefolium,* used in liquor, root beer, and spice flavorings for beverages and liquor. Also used in shampoos. Its astringent qualities have caused it to be recommended by herbalists for greasy skins. According to old herbal recipes, it prevents baldness when the hair is washed regularly with it. Used medicinally as an astringent, tonic, and stimulant. May cause a sensitivity to sunlight and artificial light, in which the skin breaks out and swells.

YEAST • A fungi that is a dietary source of folic acid. It produces enzymes that will convert sugar to alcohol and carbon dioxide. It is used in enriched farina, enriched cornmeal and corn grits, and in bakery products. It is employed as a flavoring agent and flavor enhancer. It is used in hot dogs, hamburger and frankfurter buns and rolls, pretzels, milk fortified with vitamins, meat fried in cracker crumbs, mushrooms, truffles, cheeses of all kinds, vinegars, catsup, barbecue sauce, fermented brews, and all dried fruits. Any yeast is a type of one-celled fungus. Ordinary yeast produces the enzymes invertase and zymase, which eventually convert cane sugar to alcohol and carbon dioxide in the fermentation process. Some of the living organisms pressed into damp, starch, or other absorbent material give a product known as "baker's yeast," which is not as potent as brewer's yeast. No known toxicity. GRAS.

YEAST AUTOLYZATES • Concentrated soluble components of hydrolyzed brewer's or baker's yeasts, a byproduct of brewing. They provide a good source of B vitamins. The final report to the FDA of the Select Committee on GRAS Substances stated in 1980 that while no evidence on the available information on it demonstrates a hazard to the public at current use levels, uncertainties exist, requiring that additional studies be conducted. The FDA said GRAS status should continue while tests were being completed and evaluated. *See* Autolyzed Yeast.

YEAST EXTRACT • *See* Yeast.

YEAST, MALT SPROUT EXTRACT • Used as a flavor enhancer. *See* Yeast.

YEAST and TORTULA YEAST, DRIED • Dietary supplement used in food provided total folic acid content. *See* Yeast.

YELLOW BEESWAX • Obtained from bee honeycombs, it is brittle with a honeylike odor and a balsamic taste. It is used in the manufacture of wax paper, candles, cosmetics, shoe polish, and in pharmaceutical ointment and plasters. May cause allergic reactions.

YELLOW NO. 5 • All foods containing this coloring, which is the most widely used color additive in food, drugs, and cosmetics, are supposed to identify it on the label. The FDA ordered this so that those allergic to it could avoid it. *See also* Tartrazine and Salicylates.

YELLOW PRUSSIATE OF SODA • Sodium Ferrocyanide. An anticaking agent, it is used in table salt to prevent the formation of clumps and keep it free-flowing.

The additive is produced by heating sodium carbonate andiron with organic materials. The average daily diet in the United States contains 0.6 milligrams of sodium ferrocyanide per person. The FAO-WHO Expert Committee on Food Additives considers 1.5 milligrams daily an acceptable and safe intake for a 132-pound human.

YELLOW WAX • *See* Beeswax.

YERBA SANTA FLUID EXTRACT • Holy Herb. Fruit flavoring derived from evergreen shrubs, *Eriodictyon californicum,* grown in California. Used in beverages, ice cream, ices, candy, and baked goods, and to mask the bitter taste of drugs. Also used as an expectorant.

YLANG-YLANG OIL • A light yellow, very fragrant liquid obtained in the Philippines from flowers of *Canangium odoratum.* Used in raspberry, cola, violet, cherry, rum, and ginger ale flavorings for beverages, ice cream, ices, candy, baked goods, chewing gum, and icing. Used in perfumes, cosmetics, and soap. No known toxicity. GRAS.

YOGURT • A dairy product produced by the action of bacteria or yeast on milk. No known toxicity. Supposedly has emollient properties.

YUCCA EXTRACT • Mohave Extract. Joshua Tree. Adam's Needle. Derived from a southwestern U.S. plant, *Yucca* spp., and used as a base for organic cosmetics and as a root beer flavoring for beverages, ices, and ice cream.

Z

ZANTHOXYLUM • Xanthoxylum. Ash Bark. Toothache Tree. Angelica Tree. The dried bark or berries of this tree, which grows in Canada, south of Virginia, and Missouri, is used to ease the pain of toothaches, to soothe stomachaches, and as an antidiarrheal medicine. No known toxicity. A member of the Rue family.

ZEDOARY • A bark extract from the East Indies, *Curcuma zeodaria,* used as a bitters and ginger ale flavorings for beverages. GRAS. There is reported use of the chemical, it has not yet been assigned for toxicology literature.

ZEIN • It is the principal protein in corn. Contains seventeen amino acids. A byproduct of corn processing, it is used to coat food and in label varnishes and microencapsulation fibers. Also used in face masks, nail polishes, and as a plasticizer. Obtained as a yellowish powder by extracting corn gluten with an alcohol; also used to make textile fibers plastics, printing inks, varnishes, and other coatings and adhesives. GRAS. There is reported use of the chemical, it has not yet been assigned for toxicology literature.

ZERANOL • Zearalanol. A hormone used to increase growth in animals. FDA allows zero residues in uncooked edible tissues of sheep; 150 ppb in uncooked edible muscle tissue of cattle; 300 ppb as residue in uncooked kidney of cattle; 450 ppb as residues in uncooked fat of cattle; 600 ppb as an implant.

ZINC • Acetate, Carbonate, Chloride, Oxide, Sulfate. A white brittle metal insoluble in water and soluble in acids or hot solutions of alkalies. It is a mineral source and added as a nutrient to food. Widely used as an astringent for mouthwashes and as a reducing agent *(see)* and reagent *(see).* Ingestion of the salts can cause nausea and vomiting. It can cause contact dermatitis. GRAS. The FDA says some studies appeared to show zinc supplements improved immunity to disease in older people. But the studies were flawed. In larger, well-designed studies, the FDA says, in which older patients received either zinc or placebos in addition to multivitamins and mineral preparations, the greatest immune function improvement were among those taking placebos. Zinc supplementation, the FDA says, not only did not improve immune system function in the elderly at 100 mg or more a day, it actually suppressed immunity. *See* Zinc Chloride.

ZINC ACETATE • The zinc salt of acetic acid *(see)* used in medicine as a dietary supplement and as a cross-linking agent for polymers *(see)*. For toxicity, *see* Zinc. GRAS.

ZINC BACITRACIN • Used in animal feed. *See* Bacitracin.

ZINC BORATE • The inorganic salt of zinc oxide and boric oxide, it is used as a fungistat and mildew inhibitor. *See* Zinc.

ZINC CARBONATE • A cosmetic coloring agent, it is a crystalline salt of zinc occurring in nature as smithsonite. *See* Zinc for toxicity. GRAS.

ZINC CHLORIDE • Butter of Zinc. A zinc salt used as an antiseptic and astringent in shaving creams, dentifrices, and mouthwashes. Odorless and water absorbing; also a deodorant and disinfectant. Can cause contact dermatitis and is mildly irritating to the skin. Can be absorbed through the skin. GRAS.

ZINC GLUCONATE • A dietary supplement. GRAS. *See* Zinc.

ZINC GLUTAMATE • The zinc salt of glutamic acid *(see)*.

ZINC ION and MANEB • A pesticide used on raisins, flours of barley, oats, rye, and wheat. Maneb is a fungicide. FDA residue tolerances: 28 ppm in raisins; 1 ppm in flours of barley, oats, rye, and wheat; 20 ppm in bran of barley, oats, rye, and wheat as well as milled feed fractions of those grains.

ZINC METHIONINE SULFATE • A nutrient. *See* Zinc and Methionine.

ZINC OXIDE • A nutrient supplement. GRAS. *See* Zinc.

ZINC RESINATE • The zinc salt of rosin *(see)*.

ZINC RICINOLEATE • The zinc salt of ricinoleate *(see)*. Used as a fungicide, emulsifier, and stabilizer.

ZINC ROSINATE • The zinc salt of rosin *(see)*.

ZINC STEARATE • Nutrient. Should be free from chick edema factor. GRAS. *See* Zinc.

ZINC SULFATE • White Vitriol. The reaction of sulfuric acid with zinc. Mild crystalline zinc salt used as a nutrient. Migrates to food from paperboard products. Also used in shaving cream, eye lotions, astringents, styptic, as a gargle spray, skin tonic, and aftershave lotion. Used medicinally as an emetic. Irritating to the skin and mucous membranes. May cause an allergic reaction. Injection under the skin of 2.5 milligrams per kilogram of body weight caused tumors in rabbits. *See* Zinc. GRAS.

ZINGERONE • A synthetic flavoring occurring naturally in ginger. Used in fruit, root beer, sarsaparilla, spice, ginger ale, wintergreen, and birch beer flavorings for beverages, ice cream, ices, candy, baked goods, and chewing gum.

ZINGIBER OFFICINALE • *See* Ginger.

ZINGIBER ONE • *See* Zingerone.

ZOALENE • Dinitolmide. Used in chicken and turkey feed to combat parasites. FDA tolerance residue is 2 ppm in uncooked fat of chickens; 3 ppm in uncooked muscle meat of chickens; 3 ppm in uncooked muscle meat and liver of turkeys; 6 ppm in uncooked liver and kidneys of chickens.

APPENDIX A
FOOD STORAGE GUIDELINES*

Supermarkets today have an amazing array of fresh, frozen, and prepared foods. Your store maintains rigid quality assurance and sanitation standards to make sure you always receive fresh, wholesome, and safe food products.

After selecting food items, though, it's up to you to take care of them properly. The following table provides valuable food safety and storage advice to help you maintain the freshness and quality of foods that you purchase.

*Reprinted by permission of the Food Marketing Institute.

Food	Refrigerator	Pantry	Freezer	Special
Apples	1 to 3 weeks			Do not wash. Store in crisper or moisture-resistant wrap. Wash individual apples before eating.
Asparagus	1 to 2 days		8 months	Keep in crisper.
Bacon (opened)	5 to 7 days		Not recommended	Keep wrapped. Store in coldest part of refrigerator or in meat keeper.
Bacon (unopened)	2 weeks		One month	Keep wrapped. Store in coldest part of the refrigerator or in meat keeper.
Bananas	Only when fully ripe			
Beans, dried		12 months		Keep in crisper or moisture-proof wrap.
Beans, green or wax	1 to 2 days		8 months	Keep in crisper or moisture-proof wrap.
Beans, lima (unshelled)	3 to 5 days		8 months	Keep in crisper or moisture-proof wrap.

Food	Refrigerator	Pantry	Freezer	Special
Beef casseroles			3 months	Freeze two weeks in original wrapper. Use suitable wrap for longer periods.
Beef chops	2 to 3 days		6 to 9 months	Freeze two weeks in original wrapper. Use suitable wrap for longer periods.
Beef, corned	5 to 7 days		Not recommended	Freeze two weeks in original wrapper. Use suitable wrap for longer periods.
Beef, dried	10 to 12 days			Freeze two weeks in original wrapper. Use suitable wrap for longer periods.
Beef, ground	1 to 2 days		2 to 3 months	Freeze two weeks in original wrapper. Use suitable wrap for longer periods.
Beef, roast	2 to 4 days		6 to 12 months	Freeze two weeks in original wrapper. Use suitable wrap for longer periods.
Beef sausage	2 to 3 days		1 to 2 months	Freeze two weeks in original wrapper. Use suitable wrap for longer periods.
Beef steaks	2 to 3 days		1 to 2 months	Freeze two weeks in original wrapper. Use suitable wrap for longer periods.
Beef stew meat	1 to 2 days		6 to 9 months	Freeze two weeks in original wrapper. Use suitable wrap for longer periods.
Beef TV dinners			6 months	Freeze two weeks in original wrapper. Use suitable wrap for longer periods.
Beef varieties (heart, liver, etc.)			1 to 2 months	Freeze two weeks in original wrapper. Use suitable wrap for longer periods.

Food	Refrigerator	Pantry	Freezer	Special
Beets	1 to 2 weeks			Remove leafy tops. Keep in crisper.
Berries	1 to 2 days		12 months	Store opened.
Biscuit mix		9 months		Keep cool and dry.
Bread, commercial			2 to 3 months	
Baked bread, quick			3 to 6 months	
Bread, yeast (baked)			1 month	
Bread, yeast (unbaked)	Check expiration date on label			
Broth (leftover)	2 days		1 month	
Brownie mix		9 months		Keep cool and dry.
Butter	1 to 2 weeks		6 to 9 months	
Buttermilk	10 to 30 days		No	
Cabbage	1 to 2 weeks		No	
Cakes, purchased		1 to 2 days		If butter cream, whipped cream, cream, or custard frosting/filling, refrigerate.
Cake, angel food			2 months	If butter cream, whipped cream, cream or custard frosting/filling, refrigerate.
Cake, chiffon sponge			2 months	If butter cream, whipped cream, cream or custard frosting/filling, refrigerate.
Cake, cheese			2 to 3 months	If butter cream, whipped cream, cream or custard frosting/filling, refrigerate.
Cake, chocolate			4 months	If butter cream, whipped cream, cream or custard frosting/filling, refrigerate.

Food	Refrigerator	Pantry	Freezer	Special
Cake, fruit			12 months	If butter cream, whipped cream, cream or custard frosting/filling, refrigerate.
Cake, yellow pound			6 months	If butter cream, whipped cream, cream or custard frosting/filling, refrigerate.
Cakes, frosted			8 to 12 months	If butter cream, whipped cream, cream or custard frosting/filling, refrigerate.
Cake, home-frozen			3 months	If butter cream, whipped cream, cream or custard frosting/filling, refrigerate.
Canned food all types (unopened)		Several years		
Canned food (opened)				Transfer all opened canned foods to plastic or glass containers before refrigerating.
Canned baby foods	2 to 3 days			Transfer all opened canned foods to plastic or glass containers before refrigerating.
Canned fish and shellfish	2 days			Transfer all opened canned foods to plastic or glass containers before refrigerating.
Canned fruit	1 week			Transfer all opened canned foods to plastic or glass containers before refrigerating.
Canned meats	2 days			Transfer all opened canned foods to plastic or glass containers before refrigerating.

Food	Refrigerator	Pantry	Freezer	Special
Canned pickles	1 to 2 months			Transfer all opened canned foods to plastic or glass containers before refrigerating.
Canned poultry	2 days			Transfer all opened canned foods to plastic or glass containers before refrigerating.
Canned sauce (tomato)	5 days			Transfer all opened canned foods to plastic or glass containers before refrigerating.
Canned vegetables	3 days			Transfer all opened canned foods to plastic or glass containers before refrigerating.
Carrots	1 to 2 weeks		8 months	
Catsup		12 months		Refrigeration recommended after opening.
Chili or cocktail sauce (unopened)		12 months		Refrigeration recommended after opening.
Celery	1 to 2 weeks		Does not freeze successfully	Keep in crisper or moisture-proof wrapper.
Cereals, ready-to-eat (unopened)		6 to 12 months		
Cereals, ready-to-eat (opened)		2 to 3 months		Refold package liner tightly.
Cereals, hot (require cooking)		6 months		
Cheese, cottage	10 to 30 days			Keep all cheese tightly packaged in moisture-proof wrap.
Cheese, cream (opened)	2 weeks			Keep all cheese tightly packaged in moisture-proof wrap.

Food	Refrigerator	Pantry	Freezer	Special
Cheese, Neufchatel (opened)	2 weeks			Keep all cheese tightly packaged in moisture-proof wrap.
Cheese, hard and wax-coated cheddar, Edam, Gouda, Swiss, brick, etc. (unopened)	3 to 6 months			Moisture-proof wrap. If outside gets somewhat moldy trim off $\frac{1}{2}$ inch. The cheese may become crumbly after freezing.
Cheese, hard and wax-coated cheddar, Edam, Gouda, Swiss, brick, etc. (opened)	3 to 4 weeks			Keep all cheese tightly packaged in moisture-proof wrap. If outside gets somewhat moldy trim off $\frac{1}{2}$ inch. The cheese may become crumbly after freezing.
Cheese, hard and wax-coated cheddar, Edam, Gouda, Swiss, brick, etc. (sliced)	2 weeks			Keep all cheese tightly packaged in moisture-proof wrap. If outside gets somewhat moldy trim off $\frac{1}{2}$ inch. The cheese may become crumbly after freezing.
Cheese, Parmesan, Romano (opened)		2 months		If it picks up moisture it will develop mold.
Cheese, Parmesan, Romano (unopened)	2 months	10 months		If it picks up moisture it will develop mold.
Cheese, ricotta	5 days		No	
Cheese, processed products	3 to 4 weeks		4 months	Refrigerate after opening. Keep tightly closed.

Food	Refrigerator	Pantry	Freezer	Special
Cherries	1 to 2 days		12 months	Do not wash. Store in crisper or moisture-proof wrap. Wash before eating.
Chicken	2 to 3 days		12 months	
Chicken livers	1 to 2 days		3 months	
Chicken TV dinners			6 months	
Chocolate, premelted		12 months		Keep cool.
Chocolate, semisweet		2 years		Keep cool.
Chocolate, unsweetened		18 months		Keep cool.
Chocolate syrup (unopened)		2 years		
Chocolate syrup (opened)		6 months		Cover tightly and refrigerate.
Corn	1 to 2 days in husks		8 months	
Clams, shucked	1 day		3 months	
Cocoa mixes		8 months		Cover tightly.
Coffee, cans (unopened)		2 years		Refrigerate after opening. Keep tightly closed. Use dry measuring spoon.
Coffee, cans (opened)	2 weeks			Refrigerate after opening. Keep tightly closed. Use dry measuring spoon.
Coffee lightener, dry (unopened)		6 months		Keep tightly closed.
Coffee lighteners, dry (opened)		6 months		Keep tightly closed.
Cookies, homemade		2 to 3 weeks	8 to 12 months	Put in airtight container.
Cookies, packaged		2 months	8 to 12 months	Keep box tightly closed.

Food	Refrigerator	Pantry	Freezer	Special
Cornmeal		12 months		Keep tightly closed (in refrigerator, especially in summer).
Cornstarch		18 months		Keep box tightly closed.
King crab			10 months	Keep in original wrap.
Crab, in shell	2 days			
Crackers (unopened)		8 months		Keep box tightly closed.
Cream, half & half	10 days		No	Cover tightly. To prevent bacteria from spreading to leftover cream, don't return unused cream to original container. Keep covered.
Cream, light/heavy	10 days		No	Cover tightly. To prevent bacteria from spreading to leftover cream, don't return unused cream to original container. Keep covered.
Cream, coffee lightener (liquid)	10 days		No	Cover tightly. To prevent bacteria from spreading to leftover cream, don't return unused cream to original container. Keep covered.
Cream, sour	2 to 4 weeks			Cover tightly. To prevent bacteria from spreading to leftover cream, don't return unused cream to original container. Keep covered.

Food	Refrigerator	Pantry	Freezer	Special
Cream, whipped, topping in aerosol can	3 month			Cover tightly. To prevent bacteria from spreading to leftover cream, don't return unused cream to original container. Keep covered.
Cream prepared from mix	3 days			Cover tightly. To prevent bacteria from spreading to leftover cream, don't return unused cream to original container. Keep covered.
Cream, dry		12 months		
Cream, frozen topping (after thawed)	2 weeks			Cover tightly. To prevent bacteria from spreading to leftover cream, don't return unused cream to original container. Keep covered.
Duck	2 days		6 months	
Eggs, in shell	4 to 5 weeks		No	
Egg whites	1 week		12 months	
Egg yolks	3 days		12 months	Yolks will thicken when frozen.
Eggs, hard-boiled	1 week			
Fish, lean (cod, flounder, haddock, sole)	1 to 2 days		6 months	Freeze in original wrap for up to 2 weeks. For longer periods wrap with suitable freezer wrap.
Fish, fatty (bluefish, perch, mackerel, salmon)	1 to 2 days		2 to 3 months	Freeze in original wrap for up to 2 weeks. For longer periods wrap with suitable freezer wrap.

Food	Refrigerator	Pantry	Freezer	Special
Fish, breaded			3 months	Keep purchased frozen fish in original wrap; thaw and follow cooking directions on package.
Flour, white		6 to 8 months		Keep in airtight container.
Flour, whole-wheat	6 to 8 months			Keep in airtight container.
Frosting, canned		3 months		Store leftover in refrigerator.
Frosting, mix			8 months	Store leftover in refrigerator.
Fruit, citrus	1 week			
Fruit, citrus (dried)			6 months	Keep cool in airtight container.
Fruit, citrus (sections)			6 months	
Gelatin (all types)		18 months		
Gravy (left over)	2 days		1 month	
Greens	1 to 2 days			
Ham, whole	1 week			Freezing cured meat not recommended.
Ham, canned (unopened)	6 months			Freezing cured meat not recommended.
Ham TV dinner			3 months	
Honey		12 months		If crystals form, heat in pan of water.
Hot roll mix		18 months		
Ice cream, ice milk			2 to 4 months	
Jellies (unopened)		12 months		Cover tightly. Storage-life lengthened if refrigerated after opening.

Food	Refrigerator	Pantry	Freezer	Special
Juices, canned		9 months		
Juices, citrus	6 days		6 months	
Juices, concentrated	6 days		12 months	
Lamb, ground	1 to 2 days		2 to 3 months	
Lamb steak and chops	2 to 3 days		3 to 4 months	
Lamb roasts	2 to 4 days		3 to 4 months	
Lamb stew meat	1 to 2 days		3 to 4 months	
Lamb meats, varieties	1 day		2 to 3 months	
Lettuce head (unwashed)	5 to 7 days			
Lettuce head (washed, thoroughly drained)	3 to 5 days			
Lettuce, Bibb	1 to 2 days			
Lobster tails	2 days in the shell		3 months	
Lunch meats	4 to 6 days	No	Freezing not recommended	
Margarine		2 to 3 months		Keep in airtight container.
Marshmallows		2 to 3 months		Keep in airtight container.
Marshmallow cream		3 to 4 months		Cover tightly. Refrigerate after opening to extend storage life. Use at room temperature.
Mayonnaise (opened)		2 to 3 months		Refrigerate after opening.
Meat substitutes, textured protein products (e.g., imitation bacon bits)		4 months		Keep tightly closed. For longer storage, refrigerate.

Food	Refrigerator	Pantry	Freezer	Special
Melon	1 week			
Metered-caloric products, instant breakfast		6 months		Keep in can, closed jars, or original packets.
Milk, condensed or evaporated (unopened)		9 months		Invert can every 2 months.
Milk, condensed or evaporated (opened)	4 to 5 days			
Milk, fresh	5 days		1 month	
Molasses (unopened)		12 months		
Molasses (opened)		6 months		Keep tightly closed. Refrigerate to extend storage life.
Nuts in shell (unopened)		4 months		Refrigerate after opening. Freeze for longer life. Unsalted and blanched nuts keep longer than salted.
Nutmeats, packaged in vacuum can (unopened)		1 year		Refrigerate after opening. Freeze for longer life. Unsalted and blanched nuts keep longer than salted.
Nutmeats, packaged in vacuum can (opened)		3 months		Refrigerate after opening. Freeze for longer life. Unsalted and blanched nuts keep longer than salted.
Nuts, salted			6 to 8 months	Package tightly in suitable freezer wrap.
Nuts, unsalted			9 to 12 months	Package tightly in suitable freezer wrap.

Food	Refrigerator	Pantry	Freezer	Special
Onions		3 to 4 weeks		Keep dry and away from sun.
Oysters	1 day		4 months	
Pancake mix		6 to 9 months		Once opened, store in airtight container.
Pasta (spaghetti, etc.)		2 years		
Peaches (ripe)		1 to 2 weeks	12 months	
Peanut butter (unopened)		6 to 9 months		
Peanut butter (opened)		2 to 3 months		Keeps longer if refrigerated.
Pears (ripe)		1 week	12 months	
Peas			8 months	
Peas, dried		12 months		Store in a cool, dry place in airtight container.
Peas, unshelled	3 to 5 days			Store in cool, dry place in airtight container.
Pectin, liquid (opened)			1 month	Recap and refrigerate.
Pies and pastries		2 to 3 days		Refrigerate whipped cream, custard, and chiffon fillings.
Pies and pastries, baked			1 to 2 months	Refrigerate whipped cream, custard, and chiffon fillings.
Pies and pastries, unbaked			8 months	Refrigerate whipped cream, custard, and chiffon fillings.
Pineapple	1 week		12 months	
Popcorn (unpopped)		2 years		Store in airtight container.
Pork chops	2 to 3 days		2 to 3 months	Original wrap up to 2 weeks. For longer period rewrap in suitable freezer wrap.

Food	Refrigerator	Pantry	Freezer	Special
Ground pork	1 to 2 days		1 to 2 months	Original wrap up to 2 weeks. For longer period rewrap in suitable freezer wrap.
Pork roast	2 to 4 days		3 to 6 months	Original wrap up to 2 weeks. For longer period rewrap in suitable freezer wrap.
Pork steaks	2 to 3 days		2 to 3 months	Original wrap up to 2 weeks. For longer period rewrap in suitable freezer wrap.
Pork TV dinners			3 months	Original wrap up to 2 weeks. For longer period rewrap in suitable freezer wrap.
Potatoes, fresh, white		2 to 3 months		Keep dry and away from sun. For longer storage keep at about 50 degrees F. Don't refrigerate potatoes.
Potatoes, sweet		2 to 3 weeks		Keep dry and away from sun. For longer storage keep at about 50 degrees F. Don't refrigerate potatoes.
Potatoes, instant		6 to 12 months		Keep in airtight package.
Pudding	1 to 2 days			
Pudding mixes		12 months		Keep cool and dry.
Radishes	1 to 2 weeks			
Rice, white		2 years		Keep tightly closed, cool, and dry.
Rice, flavored or herb		6 months		Keep tightly closed, cool, and dry.

Food	Refrigerator	Pantry	Freezer	Special
Rice mixes		6 months		Keep tightly closed, cool, and dry.
Rolls, yeast, baked			3 to 6 months	
Rolls, partially baked	Expiration date on label		2 to 3 months	Do not store in refrigerator door; temperature fluctuation and jarring lowers quality.
Salad dressings, bottled (unopened)		10 to 12 months		
Salad dressings, bottled (opened)		3 months		Refrigerate after opening or preparing.
Salad dressings made from mix		2 weeks		
Salad oils (unopened)		6 months		
Salad oils (opened)		1 to 3 months		
Sauces and gravy mixes		6 to 12 months		Keep cool and dry.
Scallops	1 day		3 months	
Sherbet			2 months	
Shortenings, solid		8 months		Refrigeration not needed.
Shrimp TV dinners			3 months	
Shrimp, frozen			12 months	
Shrimp, fresh (uncooked)	1 day			
Soup mixes		12 months		Keep cool and dry.
Spices, whole		1 to 2 years		Spices and herbs keep longer if refrigerated or frozen. Store in airtight containers in a dry place away from sunlight and heat.

Food	Refrigerator	Pantry	Freezer	Special
Spices, ground		6 months		Spices and herbs keep longer if refrigerated or frozen. Store in airtight containers in a dry place away from sunlight and heat.
Spices & Herbs		6 months		Spices and herbs keep longer if refrigerated or frozen. Store in airtight containers in a dry place away from sunlight and heat.
Spice/herb blends		6 months		Spices and herbs keep longer if refrigerated or frozen. Store in airtight containers in a dry place away from sunlight and heat.
Spice—paprika, red pepper		6 months		Best stored in refrigerator.
Spice—chili powder		6 months		
Spinach	3 to 5 days		8 months	
Sugar, brown		4 months		Put in airtight container.
Sugar, confectioners		18 months		Put in airtight container.
Sugar, granulated		2 years		Close tightly.
Sweetener, artificial		2 years		Close tightly.
Syrup		12 months		Keep tightly closed. Refrigerate to extend life.
Tea bags		18 months		Put in airtight container.
Tea, instant		3 years		Cover tightly.
Tea, loose		2 years		Put in airtight container.

Food	Refrigerator	Pantry	Freezer	Special
Toaster pastries		2 to 3 months		Keep in airtight packet.
Tomatoes	1 to 2 days		No	
Turkey	2 days		6 months	
Vanilla (unopened)		2 years		
Vanilla (opened)		12 months		Keep tightly closed; volatile oils escape.
Vanilla-type extracts (opened)		12 months		Keep tightly closed; volatile oils escape.
Veal, ground	1 to 2 days		2 to 3 months	Check for holes in trays and plastic wrap of fresh meat. If none, freeze in this wrap up to 2 weeks. For longer storage, wrap with suitable freezer wrap.
Veal steaks	2 to 3 days		3 to 4 months	Check for holes in trays and plastic wrap of fresh meat. If none, freeze in this wrap up to 2 weeks. For longer storage, wrap with suitable freezer wrap.
Veal chops	2 to 3 days		3 to 4 months	Check for holes in trays and plastic wrap of fresh meat. If none, freeze in this wrap up to 2 weeks. For longer storage, wrap with suitable freezer wrap.
Veal stew meat	1 to 2 days			Check for holes in trays and plastic wrap of fresh meat. If none, freeze in this wrap up to 2 weeks. For longer storage, wrap with suitable freezer wrap.

Food	Refrigerator	Pantry	Freezer	Special
Veal roasts	2 to 4 days			Check for holes in trays and plastic wrap of fresh meat. If none, freeze in this wrap up to 2 weeks. For longer storage, wrap with suitable freezer wrap.
Veal meat varieties	1 day			Check for holes in trays and plastic wrap of fresh meat. If none, freeze in this wrap up to 2 weeks. For longer storage, wrap with suitable freezer wrap.
Vegetables, home-frozen			10 months	
Vegetables, purchased frozen			8 months	
Vegetables, dehydrated flakes		6 months		
Vegetables, dried		1 year		If possible, refrigerate.
Venison and game birds			8 to 12 months	Check for holes in trays and plastic wrap of fresh meat. If none, freeze in this wrap up to 2 weeks. For longer storage, wrap with suitable freezer wrap.
Vinegar (unopened)		2 years		
Vinegar (opened)		12 months		Keep tightly closed. Slightly cloudy appearance doesn't affect quality. Distilled vinegar keeps longer.
Yeast, dry		Expiration date on package		Keep cool and dry.
Yogurt	7 to 10 days. Check date on package		No	

General Information

Proper food storage starts as soon as you select it at the store. Then the food must be handled carefully and safely at home. Check the product dating on the foods you purchase and use.

Filling Your Cart

- Shop for shelf-stable items such as canned and dry goods first.
- Buy refrigerated and frozen foods and hot deli items last—right before checkout.
- Don't choose meat, fish, poultry, or dairy products that feel warm to the touch or have a damaged or torn package.
- Place leaking packages in plastic bags.
- Choose only pasteurized dairy products.
- Choose only refrigerated eggs and make sure that they are not cracked or dirty.
- Check "sell-by" and "use by" dates on packages.
- Buy intact cans that are not bulging, leaking, or dented on the seam or rim.

Handling Food Safely at Home

Many cases of food poisoning occur each year due to improper handling of foods in the home. Once you purchase food, go directly home. If this is not possible, keep a cooler in the car to transport perishable items. Immediately put cold perishables in the refrigerator or freezer.

Hot perishable foods picked up from the deli department need to be kept warm and consumed within two hours. If you purchase hot deli foods to eat at a later time, place the food, in small portions, in shallow containers and refrigerate or freeze as soon as possible. Perishable foods should be kept at room temperature no longer than two hours.

Bacteria multiply rapidly at temperatures between 40°F and 140°F. Unfortunately, the harmful bacteria that cause most cases of food poisoning cannot be seen, smelled, or tasted. Therefore, it's important to:

Keep cold foods cold (40°F or below) and *hot foods hot* (above 140°F) and follow these other rules for handling food safely:

- Keep everything clean—hands, utensils, counters, cutting boards, and sinks.
- Always wash hands thoroughly in hot soapy water before preparing foods and after handling raw meat, poultry or seafood.
- Don't let raw juices from meat, poultry or seafood touch ready-to-eat foods either in the refrigerator or during preparation.

Food Product Dating

Dates are printed on many food products. After the date expires, must you discard that food? In most cases, no. A calendar date may be stamped on a product's package to help the store determine how long to display the product for sale. It is not a safety date. Product dating is not required by federal regulations, although dating of some foods is required by more than twenty states. Calendar dates are found primarily on perishable foods such as dairy products, eggs, meat, and poultry. Coded dates might appear on shelf-stable products such as cans and boxes of food.

There are several types of dates:

"Sell By"—tells the store how long to display the product for sale. You
  should buy the product before the date expires.

"Best If Used By (or Before)"—recommended for best flavor or quality. It is
  not a purchase or safety date.

"Use By"—the last date recommended for the use of product while at peak
  quality. The date has been determined by the manufacturer of the product.

Closed or coded dates—packing numbers for use by the manufacturer in
  tracking their products. This enables manufacturers to rotate their stock as
  well as locate their products in the event of a recall.

Baby Food

Do not buy or use infant formula and baby food past its "use-by" date. Federal regulations require a date on those products.

Expired Dates

As long as a product is wholesome, a retailer may legally sell fresh or processed meat and poultry products beyond the expiration date on the package.

Shelf-Stable Foods

Before opening, shelf-stable foods should be safe unless the can or packaging has been damaged. After opening, store products in tightly closed containers. The storage of many shelf-stable items at room temperature is a quality issue—unless the product is contaminated (bugs in flour, for example). Some foods must be refrigerated after opening, such as tuna or chili.

Foods Purchased Frozen

When shopping, place frozen foods in the cart last, immediately before checking out. Take the foods directly home and place in freezer.

Foods Purchased Refrigerated

Refrigerate foods to maintain quality as well as to keep them safe. Some bacteria grow and multiply—although very slowly—at refrigerator temperatures. There is a limit to the time various foods will stay fresh and safe in the refrigerator. Food kept continuously frozen at $0°F$ will always be safe, but the quality suffers with lengthy freezer storage.

NOTE: Storage times are from date of purchase unless specified on the chart. It is not important if a date expires after food is frozen.

Bakery Items

Bakery items containing custards, meat, or vegetables, and frostings made of cream cheese, whipped cream, or eggs must be kept refrigerated. Bread products not containing these ingredients are safe kept at room temperature, but eventually they will mold and become unsafe to eat.

Fresh Produce

Raw fruits are safe at room temperature, but after ripening, will mold and rot quickly. For best quality, store ripe fruit in the refrigerator or prepare and freeze. Some dense raw vegetables such as potatoes and onions can be stored at cool room temperatures. Refrigerate other raw vegetables for optimum quality and to prevent rotting. After cooking, all vegetables must be refrigerated or frozen within two hours.

Refrigerating Food

We keep food in the refrigerator to preserve its freshness and keep it safe. Cold temperatures keep food fresh and inhibit the growth of most bacteria. However, food spoilage microorganisms can still grow and multiply slowly over time, so there is a limit to the length of time various foods will stay fresh in the refrigerator. Eventually food will begin to look or smell bad and should be thrown out. Use the following temperature and storage tips to help keep perishable food safe.

TEMPERATURE

Set the refrigerator to maintain a temperature of $40°F$ or below. Keep a refrigerator thermometer in the unit or check the temperature periodically. The control may need to be adjusted seasonally. For example, a refrigerator set for 40°F in the summer may be too cold for the winter, resulting in frozen lettuce or milk. Don't overload the refrigerator. Air must circulate freely to cool all foods evenly.

STORAGE

Leave meat and poultry products in the store wrap before using, since repeated handling can introduce bacteria into the product or spread bacteria around the kitchen. Store opened food in foil, leakproof plastic bags, or airtight containers to keep food from drying out. Place meat, poultry, and fish in the coldest part of the refrigerator. Store eggs in their original carton on a shelf, not in the door.

Defrost frozen meats or marinate meats in the refrigerator where they will remain safe—never on the kitchen counter.

Clean the refrigerator regularly to remove spoiled foods so that bacteria can't be passed to other foods.

FREEZING FOOD

Foods frozen at peak quality will taste better than foods frozen near the end of their useful life, so quickly freeze items you don't plan to use in the next day or two.

PACKAGING

Proper packaging helps maintain quality and prevent "freezer burn." It is safe to freeze foods in their supermarket wrappings. Wrap foods with airtight heavy-duty foil, plastic wrap, or freezer paper, or place packages inside a plastic bag. Date packages and use the oldest items first.

FREEZER BURN

If frozen food gets "freezer burn," it is still safe to eat; it is merely dry in spots. Cut freezer-burned portions away either before or after cooking the food.

DEFROSTING

Freezing to 0°F inactivates but does not destroy microbes—bacteria, yeasts, and molds—present in food. Once thawed, however, these microbes can again become active, multiplying under the right conditions to levels that can lead to foodborne illness. Never defrost foods outdoors, in a cold room in the house such as the basement, or on the kitchen counter: these methods encourage growth of harmful bacteria that may be present.

There are three safe ways to defrost food: in the refrigerator, in cold running water, and in the microwave. Food thawed in the refrigerator is safe to refreeze without cooking. It is important to plan ahead because food takes longer to thaw in the refrigerator.

Pantry Storage

Shelf-stable foods such as canned goods, cereal, baking mixes, pasta, dry beans, mustard, and catsup can be kept safely at room temperature. To keep these foods at their best quality, store in clean, dry, cool (below 85°F) cabinets away from the stove or the refrigerator's exhaust.

Extremely hot (over 100°F) and cold temperatures are harmful to canned goods. Never use food from cans that are leaking, bulging, badly dented, or have a foul odor; cracked jars or jars with loose or bulging lids; or any container that spurts liquid when you open it. Never taste such foods. Throw out any food you suspect is spoiled. In general, most canned foods have a long "health life," and when properly stored, are safe to eat for several years:

- Low-acid canned goods—2 to 5 years (canned meat and poultry, stews, soups except tomato, pasta products, potatoes, corn, carrots, spinach, beans, beets, peas, and pumpkin)

- High-acid canned goods—12 to 18 months (tomato products, fruits, sauerkraut, and foods in vinegar-based sauces or dressings).

- Some canned hams are shelf-stable. But do not store ham or any foods labeled "keep refrigerated" in the pantry. Such foods must be stored in the refrigerator.

Reprinted with permission of:

Food Marketing Institute
800 Connecticut Ave.
Washington, D.C. 20006
202-452-8444
http//:www.fmi.org

APPENDIX B
SOURCES OF INFORMATION FOR FOOD ALLERGIES AND SENSITIVITIES

National Institute of Allergy and Infectious Diseases
31 Center Drive, MSC 2520
Building 31
Bethesda, MD 20892-2520
http://www.niaid.nih.gov

American College of Allergy, Asthma, and Immunology
85 W. Algonquin Road, Suite 550
Arlington Heights, IL 60005
(800) 842-7777
http://allergy.mcg.edu

American Academy of Allergy, Asthma, and Immunology
611 E. Wells St.
Milwaukee, WI 53202
(800) 822-2762
http://www.aaaai.org

Food Allergy Network
10400 Eaton Place, Suite 107
Fairfax, VA 22030
(703) 691-3179 or (800) 929-4040
http://www.foodallergy.org

Asthma and Allergy Foundation of America
1125 15th St. NW, Suite 502
Washington, D.C. 20036
(800) 7-ASTHMA
(202) 466-7643
http://www.aafa.org

Allergy and Asthma Network: Mothers of Asthmatics
2751 Prosperity Ave., Suite 150
Fairfax, VA 22031
(800) 878-4403
(703) 641-9595
http://www.aanma.org

Celiac Sprue Association
PO Box 31700
Omaha, NE 68131-0700
(402) 558-0660
http://www.csaceliacs.org

Feingold Association
127 E. Main St., Suite 106
Riverhead, NY 11901
(516) 369-9340
http://www.feingold.org

National Jewish Center for Immunology and Respiratory Medicine
Denver, CO
(800) 222-LUNG (RNs available to answer allergy questions).
http://njc.org

American Dietetic Association
(Recipes)
216 W. Jackson Blvd.
Chicago, IL 60606-6995
(312) 899-0040 or (800) 877-1600
http://eatright.org

APPENDIX C
THE HIDDEN THREAT
OF ANIMAL DRUGS

Medicated Meat

Why are animal drugs a problem? An estimated 80 percent of U.S. livestock and poultry, as pointed out, are treated with an animal drug during their lifetime. We are told that the availability of safe and effective drugs for use in food-producing animals has benefited us by increasing production at reduced cost, and improving the quality of these food items, while ensuring the safety of these foods. Bull?

The FDA's Dr. Friedman admits "the challenges faced by the FDA's Center for Veterinary Medicine [CVM] in the area of food safety have become more complex over the last several years as the technology of food production has advanced."

He noted before Congress:

> Animals are now grown in high-density production facilities which have increased the efficiency of food production, but which have also put additional stress on the animals and made control of diseases critical. Furthermore, recent changes in drug-manufacturing production technology have created new and more sophisticated types of animal drugs for the CVM to evaluate. Each of these advances presents a unique situation that must be evaluated before the drug can be approved. And because of the newness of the technology associated with some of these drugs, the CVM has also had to respond to concerns about the public's perceived threat from the use of these new technologies. Such as the case in recombinant bovine somatropin [see].

> Aside from the new safety issues in food production, technological advancement in recent years have also had a significant effect on the number of requests of drugs sponsors to CVM for review. During the last six fiscal years, CVM has experienced a 29 percent increase in the number of submissions for review. At the same time, the CVM's resources have decreased in terms of budget and manpower.

Dr. Friedman went on to tell Congress that the FDA has shifted the primary responsibility for validation of regulatory methods to the sponsor: "Instead of relying on government laboratories to schedule and complete a method trial, the sponsor may now contract with nongovernment labs to conduct method trials." We now have to hope that the manufacturers of potentially highly lucrative animal drugs will present a completely honest evaluation of their product to the FDA or else we will have "a fox in the hen house situation."

There are several serious problems with animals being laced with drugs. First of all, "high-density production facilities" are a cruel way to treat living creatures, and if animals were not raised this way, they would not need to be given so many drugs. Then there is the potential for human illness from medicated meats including allergic reactions, resistant bacterial infections, and cancer.

The Food and Drug Administration has been trying to rein in the use of antibiotics in animal feed since 1972, but cattle and poultry are still being fed antibiotic-laced feed to increase their growth. More and more antibiotic-resistant infections in humans are occurring, and scientists worldwide are blaming "animal husbandry practices" as an important cause.[1] The FDA, the USDA, and the Center for Disease Control and Prevention are cooperating in response to an American Society of Microbiology task force on antibiotic resistance, established in 1995. The program grew out of the concerns by the FDA and other scientific experts about how to best maintain antibiotic effectiveness, ensure safety, and increase the availability of new products to veterinarians and the food industry.

I first became interested in food safety many years ago when my daughter was small and had a case of intractable hives. The allergist finally determined that it was probably the penicillin in the milk. When asked what penicillin was doing in the milk, he said, "Farmers treat cows with mastitis [inflammation of the udder] with penicillin. They are supposed to throw away the milk from treated cows, but since milk is pooled, no one knows who put the penicillin in the pool."

Are antibiotic residues still a problem?

To catch dealers selling cattle contaminated with antibiotics, FDA investigators sent in "undercover cows" named Buttercup, Elsie, and a steer named Elmer. The animals were outfitted with internal transmitters. The FDA agents told the dealers the cattle had been treated with antibiotics and should not be sent to the slaughterhouse until the required waiting period had elapsed.

The sting operation worked. The FDA agents were able to follow the three bugged animals, and in each case, the animals were sold for human use before the waiting period was up.[2]

Hormone Enhancement

Could the great sale of the male potency pill, Viagra, be related in some way to hidden hormones men have been eating with their dinners?[3]

Consumers and scientists have been fighting for more than two decades to stop hormone use in cattle, swine, and poultry, but these powerful drugs are still widely

---

[1] Emilio Perez-Trallero, Mercedes Urbieta, Carmen Lopategul, Carmen Zigorraga, Isabel Ayestaran, "Antibiotics in Veterinary Medicine and Public Health," *Lancet* 342 (27 Nov. 1993), p. 1371.

[2] Laurie McGinley, "Where's the Beef?: Bugged Cows Help Send Shifty Dealers Packing," *Wall Street Journal,* 9 October 1996.

[3] Paul Foster, "Assessing the Effects of Chemicals on Male Reproduction: Lessons Learned from Di-*n*-Butyl Phthalate," *Chemical Industry Institute of Toxicology Activities* 17 (September 1997).

employed. Implantation of or injection of long-acting drugs with slow rates of absorption, such as anabolic steroids, are used to increase and speed the growth of cattle and poultry. For the same purpose, hormones are also put in animal feed. Three natural hormones are used—estradiol, progesterone, and testosterone—and two synthetic hormones, zeranol and trenbolone. The European Union (EU) has banned red meat from the United States because of the use of hormones as growth promoters since the 1980s. The USDA has been attempting to overcome this roadblock, which is costing U.S. beef producers $100 million annually.[4] As of this writing, the three natural hormones are approved for use in the EU itself, for therapeutic purposes, but not for growth promotion.

It is not just the hormones deliberately used in implantation and feed but other chemicals that act like hormones. As far back as 1993, the EPA reported evidence indicating that the insecticide, endosulfan, and other chemicals that imitate estrogen may be associated with instances of breast cancer.[5] Perhaps things will move more swiftly now that there are increasing reports that estrogen residues "in the environment" may also be responsible for the great drop in male sperm count.[6] Other chemicals that may find their way into our food supply and have hormone-like effects are bisphenol, the pesticide DDE and di-*n*-butyl phthalate, an insect repellent. The EPA has, in fact, formed the Endocrine Disrupter Screen and Testing Advisory Committee, to provide advice on what the nature of the screening and testing should be to deal with this problem.

The Food and Agriculture Organization of the United Nations (FAO) and the World Health Organization (WHO) Expert Committee on Food Additives agrees there is a problem with animal drug residues being ingested by humans, noting:[7]

> Of particular relevance to the Committee are residues of drugs used in animal medications or as aids to animal production, and the frequency with which the consumer might be exposed to them. A drug whose toxicity profile was unsatisfactory and that was used widely and for lengthy periods during food-animal production would cause the highest level of concern. Human exposure to such a drug in food could be expected to occur widely and repeatedly.

Also of concern to the Committee are drugs whose presence in food could result in a pharmacological effect in us despite the absence of conventional toxicological effects. Drugs still present in the animal at the time of slaughter and at a concentration compatible with a pharmacological effect pose the greatest risk in this respect.

The Committee said the sedative azaperone; the phenothiazine tranquilizers chlorpromazine and propiomazine; and the beta-blocker carazolol *(see all)* fall into this category. "In particular," the Committee said, "chlorpromazine is known to persist for very long periods in the human body (up to eighteen months), and it

[4]Foreign Agricultural Service, USDA Online, "Chronology of the European Union's Hormone Ban," April 1998.
[5]"EPA to Study an Insecticide for Links to Cancer," *New York Times*, 24 October 1993, p. 21.
[6]Cristophe Lambton, "Mamas Maketh Man," *Guardian*, 11 February 1993.
[7]World Health Organization, *Evaluation of Certain Veterinary Drug Residues*, Technical Report Series, 815 (1991): 1–64.

THE HIDDEN THREAT OF ANIMAL DRUGS 471

is therefore possible that repeated intake could result in accumulation of the drug, thereby increasing the pharmacological response."

The Committee said examples of types of use that may cause high levels of residues include:

- Administration of a drug before slaughter, as when pigs are given tranquilizer drugs by injection immediately before transport to slaughter (this indication requires the full pharmacological effect of the drug to be exerted right up to the moment of slaughter and renders a withdrawal period impossible). The potential of drug effect in the consumer is then of concern in addition to conventional toxicity.

- Veterinary drug treatment of animals slaughtered for human consumption before appropriate withdrawal times are observed.

- Implantation or injection of long-acting drugs with slow rates of absorption such as anabolics (hormones) in edible tissue.

"Such problems could be avoided" the Committee says, "by ensuring that the injection site is excised and discarded at slaughter. In practice, this is difficult to achieve because the site is not readily recognizable unless the drug is colored or implanted in an inedible tissue. The site, its dimensions, and the efficiency of its removal would be liable to considerable variation. To accommodate these variables, a relatively large amount of tissue would have to be discarded, and it is probable that this practice would be seen as uneconomic."

Elsie, Elmer, and Buttercup gave their lives to prove that antibiotic-laced meats are getting to the dinner table.

The Committee recommends that measures be taken to limit the need for drugs used immediately prior to slaughter and thus likely to leave significant levels of residues in food. With regard to pigs, such measures may include improved preslaughter handling, transport, and shelter, and the elimination of stress-susceptible pigs from production.

With respect to residues at sites of injected drugs, the Committee recommended that implants or injections of long-acting and slowly absorbed substances should preferably be located in tissues that are discarded at slaughter, such as in the ears of cattle.

Chemicals in animal feed are also a big problem. For example, consider this statement from the following dictionary entry:

CARBADOX • An antibacterial used in animal feed for swine. The FAO-WHO Expert Committee on Food Additives would not set an ADI or NOEL *(see both)* for this drug since it is a cancer-causing agent. FDA tolerance for carbadox residues in swine is zero.

You can't *see* carbadox in pork with the naked eye. It requires expensive chemical tests and trained personnel for detection. We must still today rely on the swine producer's honor to stop using the antibacterial so that the residue is zero, as the FDA tolerance is set.

APPENDIX D
THE HIDDEN THREAT
OF PESTICIDES

Pesticides and Potency

Pesticide residues in food have long been a worrisome problem to health professionals, environmentalists, and regulators. The U.S. Environmental Protection Agency (EPA) reviews the scientific data on pesticide products before they can be registered (or licensed) for use. If a product is intended for use on food crops, the EPA also establishes a tolerance. The Food and Drug Administration (FDA) is responsible for enforcing these tolerances on all foods except meat, poultry, and certain egg products, which are monitored by the U.S. Department of Agriculture (USDA). In this "alphabet soup" of regulators, the FDA works with the EPA to set "action levels"—enforcement guidelines for residues of pesticides that may remain in the environment after their use is discontinued. In the past fifty years, 8,500 separate residue tolerance licenses have been awarded for pesticides.[1]

The EPA in June 1993 acknowledged that federal safety guidelines for the use of pesticides on food crops should be made ten times more stringent. This move by the EPA to reduce the use of pesticides was in response to a $1.1 million, five-year study of children's health risks from pesticides commissioned by the National Academy of Sciences (NAS).[2] The residue amounts had been based on the effects on a 160-pound adult male. Nearly one billion pounds of pesticides are applied to crops each year.[3] When setting tolerances, the EPA now takes into account the special diets of twenty-two vulnerable subgroups, including infants, children, pregnant females, and nursing females.

The NAS report stated that infants and young children might be uniquely sensitive to pesticides on food. Early in life, youngsters consume more than sixty times the amount of fruits as adults for their body weight and so tend to get higher doses of the pesticides used on fruits. The report also stated that infants and children—as well as adults—routinely encounter residues from more than one pesticide on individual food items. Government risk-assessment procedures assume that we are exposed to only one pesticide at a time.

Prof. John Wargo of Yale, who spent five years with the NAS panel sifting through data on pesticide risks to infants and children and trying to make sense of

[1]John Wargo, Associate Professor of Natural Resource Policy, Yale School of Forestry and Environmental Studies, and chief policy analyst for the National Academy of Sciences, quoted in *Yale University Science News* 57, 30 September 1993.

[2]National Academy of Sciences, "Pesticides in the Diets of Infants and Children," report released 29 June 1993, Washington, D.C.

[3]Keith Schneider, "Pesticide Plan Could Uproot U.S. Farming," *New York Times,* 10 October 1993, p. 6.

the patchwork system of federal regulations, says: "Children are particularly vulnerable to having a neurological response called cholinesterase inhibition when exposed to toxic chemicals, which causes the pattern of electronic-signal transfer between nerves to be disrupted, and my research indicates that between one point two and five of two-year-old children consume pesticides at a level above that which the EPA has identified as safe."[4]

The findings to date are inconclusive. Several factors suggest that infants and children are more sensitive. Their vital organs are less developed and thus more susceptible to harm from toxic chemicals. In addition, their higher metabolic rate speeds the absorption of some chemicals. This characteristic, however, may provide some protection since it would speed the breakdown of some harmful chemicals.

NAS experts have recommended regulators to:

- Use more immature animals in their tests to determine how young organisms react to chemicals.

- Conduct annual food consumption surveys of children aged 0–5 years, 6–10, and 11–18.

- Consider nondietary sources of exposure to pesticides, such as the air, soil, lawns, and pets.

- Apply new statistical methods to estimate the risk to infants and children.

The Food Quality Protection Act of 1996 requires the government to upgrade its testing and risk-assessment methods to better protect children. As a result, the agencies that regulate pesticides are expected to adopt many of the NAS recommendations. In 1994 the FDA did increase its monitoring of foods eaten by infants and children. In its domestic monitoring, for example, the agency analyzed twice as many carrot samples and ten times as many fruit juice samples as in 1993. It also increased sampling of green beans, peaches, and oranges—both domestic and imported—as well as imported bananas.

The agency has denied tolerances for some pesticides over concern for the adverse effects on children. For example, it has barred the use of the pesticide pydrin over concern that children might drink milk with its residue since milk cows eat pyridin-treated alfalfa and sorghum.

Government bureaucracy moves slowly, however, and some environmental groups maintain a number of the established tolerance levels are still too high for safety. They believe that any pesticide residue on food is hazardous. The EPA's regulatory programs, they note, fail to consider:

- The effect of interaction among pesticides
- How health may suffer from consuming residues from many compounds over a lifetime
- The special vulnerability of infants and children

---

[4]Wargo, op. cit.

How Tolerant Is the Government of Cancer-Causing Pesticides?

Up until 1996, the EPA observed different safety standards for raw and processed foods. For the latter, it used the zero-risk standard established by the Delaney Amendment, a 1958 amendment to the Food, Drug, and Cosmetics Act. That standard, however, had proved to be impractical and even counterproductive, said pesticide-promoting lobbyists to government regulators. The promoters pointed out that the Delaney clause prohibited foods from carrying minute traces of carcinogenic compounds, while exempting many toxic chemicals that were registered before the clause was enacted. As a result, regulators were forced to allow the use of toxic chemicals while barring safer alternatives.

Congress substituted the "negligible risk standard" instead of the Delaney Amendment in the Food Quality Protection Act of 1996 to set pesticide tolerances for raw foods. This standard allows residues of potentially carcinogenic pesticides as long as there is a "reasonable certainty of no harm" to consumers. In practice, regulators will approve a pesticide application only if it will cause no more than one additional cancer case per million people who consume it over a lifetime. Of course, if you are that one in a million, you might be a little annoyed.

The EPA maintains its tolerances tend to err on the side of safety. They are set and enforced as residues appear on foods at the farm. Residue levels tend to decline during transport, storage, mixing with untreated crops, processing, and cooking.

The EPA also restricts the times pesticides may be applied during the growing season, along with the amounts and the crops on which they may be used. These measures are designed to control the residues. The EPA may revoke a pesticide's tolerance and cancel its registration for particular crops or all crops if new scientific data reveal health hazards.

The EPA has reduced pesticide risks through negotiated agreements with suppliers. In 1996 suppliers agreed to eliminate the use of the mite killer, propargite on ten fruit and vegetable crops. Cancer concerns and high residue levels led to this action. Cancer risks are also prompting the industry to restrict and phase out the use of cyanazine by 1999. It takes a long time to get a pesticide off the market. For years, the EPA wanted to remove DVVP (Dichlorvos), an organophosphate insecticide, but was unable to do so. Finally, the manufacturers themselves asked that their permission to use it on food products be rescinded. The EPA also allows manufacturers to use up current supplies of a pesticide it bans. And remember, some pesticides hang around the environment indefinitely, even after their use has ceased.

The Food Quality Protection Act requires the EPA to reevaluate more than nine thousand existing pesticide tolerances within the next ten years to ensure that all tolerances meet the more stringent standards set by the law. It also charges the EPA to establish a renewal program for reregistering pesticides on a fifteen-year cycle to ensure that tolerance levels and application controls are up to date with the most current scientific research.

What's wrong with the registration process? Many pesticides were registered long before the extensive research on cancer and other diseases in recent years. The EPA has been investigating the safety of all the older pesticides as part of a major reregistration effort expected to take many years. Advocacy groups charge that the EPA is taking too long—a position held by a number of food industry groups. In 1988 Congress accelerated the timetable in an amendment to the Federal Insecticide, Fungicide, and Rodenticide Act (FIFRA), which set a 1997 deadline for completing 614 reregistration cases. By the end of 1996, the EPA had completed action on just 380 cases. In well over half the situations, suppliers either suspended the reregistration review or voluntarily canceled the registration.

How Does the Government Monitor the Market for Unsafe Residues?

The FDA monitors food for pesticide residues as part of its responsibility to protect consumers. The USDA monitors the commodities in its domain: meat, poultry, and egg products. Many farm states, including California and Florida, complement federal efforts with their own monitoring.

Without sufficient funds and personnel to more than spot-check domestic and imported foods from one hundred nations, the FDA gives emphasis to sampling food commodities of major dietary importance. It also emphasizes foods most likely to contain residues at the time of consumption. Fresh produce is sampled before foods are processed. If illegal residues are detected or suspected in a region—foreign or domestic—the agency gives special attention to food products coming from that area.

Of the 9,394 samples tested in one year, only 0.8 percent were deemed "significant," meaning that the residue levels exceeded the legal limit, there was no tolerance level set for the pesticide on the commodity, or there was some other unusual finding. The data include both imported and domestic products.

The USDA's 1995 Pesticide Data Program also revealed few residue violations in 6,924 produce and grain samples from thirty-nine states and seventeen countries. Less than 4 percent of the samples (263) carried illegal residues. Imported products actually had a lower illegal residue rate—2 percent vs. 4 percent of the U.S. samples, according to the USDA.

The FDA also performs a Total Diet Study at the retail level. Inspectors visit supermarkets and other outlets and purchase about three hundred different items, including fresh, frozen, and packaged foods, fast foods, and wine. Four times a year, they make identical purchases in three cities in a particular region. The foods are prepared as they would be at home and analyzed by an FDA laboratory for pesticide residues. This program has found that the residue levels are consistently below the safe limits of exposure recommended by the World Health Organization (WHO), the United Nations agency that oversees food safety worldwide.

The FDA has been monitoring pesticides since 1965 and reports it has found that the residues in the foods that Americans eat fall well below the daily levels recommended by WHO. The fact is, however, that less than 2 percent of the food is sampled and the federal agencies have no tests to detect certain pesticides.

How Does the Government Enforce the Pesticide Laws?

State and federal agencies work with the food industry to remove from the market any food contaminated with illegal residues. Food that is deemed adulterated must be recalled. The FDA has the authority to seize adulterated foods, prevent further shipments, and initiate criminal actions against those responsible. The FDA is also authorized to refuse entry to imported foods that are adulterated. When the FDA identifies a contaminated product, the food industry responds to remove it from the market.

A producer that fails to follow the directions on the pesticide label is violating the pesticide laws and is subject to civil or criminal penalties. The label on a pesticide specifies exactly how it is to be used, when, the rate of application, and the interval between the last application and harvesting of the food product. When you factor in that pesticides are often applied by non-English-speaking persons who cannot read warning labels, this is not reassuring. For example, improper pesticide use led to recalls of milk contaminated with the pesticide heptachlor (from animal feed consumed by cows) and watermelons contaminated with aldicarb. The application of these two pesticides was illegal since they were not registered for use on animal feed or watermelons.

What If State and Federal Pesticide Regulations Disagree?

States are required by law to observe EPA tolerance levels and application restrictions. They may, however, adopt lower tolerance levels and stricter use restrictions. Food manufacturers object to this state authority because it promotes inconsistent regulations from state to state, which interferes with an orderly flow of commerce.

On the other side, environmentalists, consumer groups, and many governors want to strengthen states' rights. They argue that states should have the right to protect consumers and workers. They also would like states to have more staff and funds to regulate pesticides more extensively.

APPENDIX E
RECOMMENDED DIETARY
ALLOWANCES (RDA)

The Recommended Dietary Allowances (RDA) are a set of nutrient standards established by the National Academy of Sciences Committee on Dietary Allowances. Designed for the maintenance of good nutrition, the RDA are the average daily intakes of energy and nutrients considered adequate to meet the needs of most healthy people under usual environmental stresses. People are urged to base their diets on a variety of common foods in order to obtain other nutrients for which requirements have been less well defined.

Age (YR)	Weight (kg)	Weight (lb)	Height (cm)	Height (inches)	Energy (kcal)	Protein (g)	Vitamin A (µg RE)	Vitamin D (µg)	Vitamin E (mg α-TE)	Vitamin K (µg)	Vitamin C (mg)	Thiamin (mg)	Riboflavin (mg)	Niacin (mg NE)	Vitamin B6 (mg)	Folate (µg)	Vitamin B12 (µg)	Calcium (mg)	Phosphorus (mg)	Magnesium (mg)	Iron (mg)	Zinc (mg)	Iodine (µg)	Selenium (µg)
Infants																								
0.0–0.5	6	13	60	24	650	13	375	7.5	3	5	30	0.3	0.4	5	0.3	25	0.3	400	300	40	6	5	40	10
0.5–1.0	9	20	71	28	850	14	375	10	4	10	35	0.4	0.5	6	0.6	35	0.5	600	500	60	10	5	50	15
Children																								
1–3	13	29	90	35	1300	16	400	10	6	15	40	0.7	0.8	9	1.0	50	0.7	800	800	80	10	10	70	20
4–6	20	44	112	44	1800	24	500	10	7	20	45	0.9	1.1	12	1.1	75	1.0	800	800	120	10	10	90	20
7–10	28	62	132	52	2000	28	700	10	7	30	45	1.0	1.2	13	1.4	100	1.4	800	800	170	10	10	120	30
Males																								
11–14	45	99	157	62	2500	45	1000	10	10	45	50	1.3	1.5	17	1.7	150	2.0	1200	1200	270	12	15	150	40
15–18	66	145	176	69	3000	59	1000	10	10	65	60	1.5	1.8	20	2.0	200	2.0	1200	1200	400	12	15	150	50
19–24	72	160	177	70	2900	58	1000	10	10	70	60	1.5	1.7	19	2.0	200	2.0	1200	1200	350	10	15	150	70
25–50	79	174	176	70	2900	63	1000	5	10	80	60	1.5	1.7	19	2.0	200	2.0	800	800	350	10	15	150	70
51+	77	170	173	68	2300	63	1000	5	10	80	60	1.2	1.4	15	2.0	200	2.0	800	800	350	10	15	150	70
Females																								
11–14	46	101	157	62	2200	46	800	10	8	45	50	1.1	1.3	15	1.4	150	2.0	1200	1200	280	15	12	150	45
15–18	55	120	163	64	2200	44	800	10	8	55	60	1.1	1.3	15	1.5	180	2.0	1200	1200	300	15	12	150	50
19–24	58	128	164	65	2200	46	800	10	8	60	60	1.1	1.3	15	1.6	180	2.0	1200	1200	280	15	12	150	55
25–50	63	138	163	64	2200	50	800	5	8	65	60	1.1	1.3	15	1.6	180	2.0	800	800	280	15	12	150	55
51+	65	143	160	63	1900	50	800	5	8	65	60	1.0	1.2	13	1.6	180	2.0	800	800	280	10	12	150	55
Pregnant					+300	60	800	10	10	65	70	1.5	1.6	17	2.2	400	2.2	1200	1200	320	30	15	175	65
Lactating																								
1st 6 mo.					+500	65	1300	10	12	65	95	1.6	1.8	20	2.1	280	2.6	1200	1200	355	15	19	200	75
2nd 6 mo.					+500	62	1200	10	11	65	90	1.6	1.7	20	2.1	260	2.6	1200	1200	340	15	16	200	75

APPENDIX F
DAILY VALUES FOR FOOD LABELS

The Daily Values were developed by the FDA for use on food labels. In creating them the FDA first established two sets of reference values. The first set, the Reference Daily Intakes (RDI), are for protein, vitamins, and minerals and reflect average allowances based on the RDA (see Appendix E). The second set, the Daily Reference Values (DRV), are for nutrients and food components, such as fat and fiber.

*Reference Daily Intake**

Protein[a]	50 g
Vitamin A[b]	5000 IU
Thiamin	1.5 mg
Riboflavin	1.7 mg
Niacin	20 mg
Vitamin B$_6$	2 mg
Vitamin B$_{12}$	6 mcg
Vitamin C	60 mg
Vitamin D[b]	400 IU
Vitamin E[b]	30 IU
Biotin	0.3 mg
Copper	2 mg
Folate	0.4 mg
Calcium	1,000 mg
Iodine	150 mcg
Iron	18 mg
Magnesium	400 mg
Pantothenic acid	10 mg
Phosphorus	1000 mg
Zinc	15 mg

*Changed December 28, 1995.
[a]The RDI for protein varies for different groups of people: pregnant women, 60 g; nursing mothers, 65 g; infants under 1 year, 14 g; children 1 to 4 years, 16 g.
[b]The RDI for fat-soluble vitamins are expressed in International Units (IU), an old system of measurement. The current RDA and tables of food composition use a more accurate system of measurement. Equivalent values are as follows: for vitamin A, 875 μg RE: for vitamin D, 6.5 μg; for vitamin E, 9 mg alpha-TE.

Daily Reference Values

Food Component	DRV	Calculation
Fat	65 g	30% of kcalories
Saturated fat	20 g	10% of kcalories
Cholesterol	300 mg	Same regardless of kcalories
Carbohydrate (total)	300 g	60% of kcalories
Fiber	25 g	11.5 g per 1000 kcalories
Protein	50 g	10% of kcalories
Sodium	2400 mg	Same regardless of kcalories
Potassium	3500 mg	Same regardless of kcalories

The DRV were established for adults and children over 4 years old. The values for energy-yielding nutrients are based on 2000 kcalories a day.

BIBLIOGRAPHY

Adams, Catherine F. *Nutritive Value of American Foods in Common Units*. Washington, D.C.: Agriculture Handbook No. 456, U.S. Department of Agriculture, 1975.

Bowes, Helen N., and Charles F. Church. *Food Values of Portions Commonly Used,* 11th ed., rev. Philadelphia: J. B. Lippincott Co., 1970.

Chemicals Used in Food Processing. Washington, D.C.: National Academy of Sciences, Publication 1274, 1965.

Code of Federal Regulations: Food and Drugs, Parts 100 to 169, revised April 1, 1993.

Concise Encyclopedia of Foods & Nutrition. Edited by Audrey Ensminger, M. E. Ensminger, James Konlande, John R. K. Robson, CRC Press, Boca Raton, Fl., 1994.

The Condensed Chemical Dictionary, 11th ed. Revised by N. Irving Sax and Richard J. Lewis, Sr., New York: Van Nostrand Reinhold, 1987.

Done, Alan. "Toxic Reactions to Common Household Products." Paper read at the Symposium on Adverse Reactions sponsored by the Drug Service Center for Disease Control, December 1976, San Francisco.

Evaluation of Certain Food Additives and Contaminants. Forty-first report of the Joint FAO/WHO Expert Committee on Food Additives, WHO Technical Report Series 837, Geneva: 1993.

Fisher, Alexander A. *Contact Dermatitis,* 3d ed., Philadelphia: Lea & Febiger, 1986.

Food Additive Status List, Investigations Operations Manual, corrected to January 30, 1998. U.S. Food and Drug Administration.

Food Allergy: Adverse Reactions to Foods and Food Additives. Edited by Dean D. Metcalfe, M.D., Hugh Sampson, M.D., and Ronald A. Simon, M.D. Boston: Blackwell Scientific Publications, 1991.

Food Allergy and Intolerances. Bethesda, Md.: NIAD Publications, 1997.

Food Chemicals Codex, 1st ed. Washington D.C.: National Academy of Sciences, Publication 1406, 1966.

Food Labeling: Questions and Answers for Guidance to Facilitate the Process of Developing or Revision Labels for Foods Other than Dietary Supplements. Office of Food Labeling, Center for Food Safety and Applied Nutrition Food and Drug Administration, August 1993.

Gleason, Marion N., et al. *Clinical Toxicology of Commercial Products*. Baltimore: The Williams & Wilkins Co., 1969.

Gordon, Lesley. *A Country Herbal*. New York: Mayflower Books, 1980.

Handbook of Food Additives. Edited by Thomas E. Furia. Cleveland: Chemical Rubber Co., 1971.

Hawley's Condensed Chemical Dictionary, 11th ed., Revised by N. Irving Sax and Richard J. Lewis, Sr. New York: Van Nostrand Reinhold, 1987.

Lewis, Richard, Sr. *Food Additives Handbook.* New York: Van Nostrand Reinhold, 1991.

Martin, Eric W., et al. *Hazards of Medications.* Philadelphia: J. B. Lippincott Co., 1971.

The Merck Index. 8th, 9th, 10th, and 15th editions. Rahway, N.J.: Merck, Sharp and Dohme Research Laboratories, 1989.

The Merck Manual, 15th ed. Edited by Robert Berkow, M.D. Rahway, N.J.: Merck, Sharp and Dohme Research Laboratories, 1987.

Miall, L. Mackenzie, and D. W. A. Sharp. *A New Dictionary of Chemistry,* 4th ed. New York: John Wiley & Sons, Inc., 1968.

Physicians' Desk Reference. Oradell, N.J.: Medical Economics, 1993.

Present Knowledge in Nutrition, 5th ed. Washington, D.C.: The Nutrition Foundation, Inc., 1984.

Recommended Dietary Allowances, rev. ed. Washington, D.C.: National Academy of Sciences, 1980.

Smith, Jim. *Food Additives User's Handbook.* New York: Blackie and Sons Ltd., Van Nostrand Reinhold, 1991.

Sourcebook on Food and Nutrition, 3d ed. Edited by Joannis Scarpa, Ph.D., Helen Kiefer, Ph.D., and Rita Tatum. Chicago: Marquis Academic Media, 1982.

Steadman's Medical Dictionary, 25th ed. Baltimore: The Williams & Wilkins Co., 1989.

Suspected Carcinogens: A Subfile of the NIOSH Toxic Substance List. Rockville, Md.: Tracor Jitco, Inc., U.S. Department of Health, Education and Welfare, 1975.

Suspected Carcinogens: A Subfile of the Registry of Toxic Effects of Chemical Substances. Cincinnati: U.S. Department of Health, Education and Welfare, Public Health Services, Center for Disease Control, 1976.

Toxicants Occurring Naturally in Foods, 2d ed. Washington, D.C. National Academy of Sciences, 1973.

Toxicity Testing: Strategies to Determine Needs and Priorities. Washington, D.C.: National Research Council: National Academy Press, 1984.

Watt, Bernice, and Annabel Merrill et al. *Composition of Foods: Raw, Processed, Prepared.* Washington, D.C.: Agriculture Handbook No. 8, U.S. Department of Agriculture, 1963.

White, John Henry. *A Reference Book of Chemistry,* 3d ed. New York: Philosophical Library, 1965.

WHO. *Evaluation of Certain Veterinary Drug Residues in Food.* Technical Report Series, no. 800, 1991.

Winter, Ruth. *Cancer-Causing Agents: A Preventive Guide.* New York: Crown Publishers, 1979.

———. *Poisons in Your Food,* rev. ed. New York: Crown Publishers, 1991.

———. *A Consumer's Dictionary of Household, Yard and Office Chemicals.* New York: Crown Publishers, 1992.

————. *A Consumer's Guide to Medicines in Food: Nutraceuticals That Help Prevent and Treat Physical and Emotional Illnesses.* New York: Crown Publishers, 1995.

————. *A Consumer's Dictionary of Medicines: Prescription, Over-the-Counter, Homeopathic, and Herbal Plus Medical Definitions.* New York: Crown Publishers, 1996.